MODERN STEREOTACTIC NEUROSURGERY

MODERN STEREOTACTIC NEUROSURGERY

Edited by

L. Dade Lunsford, M.D.

Martinus Nijhoff Publishing
A member of the Kluwer Academic Publishers Group

BOSTON DORDRECHT LANCASTER

DISTRIBUTORS

for the United States and Canada:

Kluwer Academic Publishers, 101 Philip Drive, Assinippi Park, Norwell, MA, 02061, USA

for the UK and Ireland:

Kluwer Academic Publishers Group, Distribution Centre, P.O. Box 322, 3300 AH Dordrecht, The Netherlands

Library of Congress Cataloging-in-Publication Data

Modern stereotactic neurosurgery.

(Topics in neurological surgery; 1)
Includes index.
1. Nervous system—Surgery. 2. Stereoencephalotomy.
I. Lunsford, L. Dade. II. Series. [DNLM: 1. Neurosurgery—methods. 2. Stereotaxic Technics. WL 368 M689]
RD593.M63 1987 617'.48 87-14058
ISBN-13:978-1-4612-8418-5 e-ISBN-13:978-1-4613-1081-5
DOI: 10.1007/978-1-4613-1081-5

CONTENTS

CONTRIBUTING AUTHORS

Masamitsu Abe, M.D.
Clinical and Research Fellow in Neurosurgery
Massachusetts General Hospital
Boston, Massachusetts

John E. Adams, M.D.
Professor of Neurological Surgery
University of California, San Francisco
San Francisco, California

Michael L.J. Apuzzo, M.D.
Professor
Department of Neurological Surgery
University of Southern California
Director of Neurological Surgery
Kenneth R. Norris Cancer Hospital and Research Institute
Los Angeles, California

Jurgen Arndt, B.S.
Senior Staff
Hospital Physics
Karolinska Institute
Stockholm, Sweden

Erik-Olof Backlund, M.D., Ph.D
Professor and Chairman
Department of Neurosurgery
University of Bergen
School of Medicine
Bergen, Norway

Gordon E. Banks, M.D.
Associate Professor of Neurology
University of Pittsburgh School of Medicine
Pittsburgh, Pennsylvania

Nicholas M. Barbaro, M.D.
Assistant Professor of Neurological Surgery
University of California, San Francisco
San Francisco, California

Mats Bergström, Ph.D.
Associate Professor
Department of Neuroradiology
Karolinska Institute
Stockholm, Sweden

W. Birg
Department of Neurosurgery
Neurochirurgische Universitatsklinik
Abteilung Stereotaxie und Neuronklearmedizin
Freiburg, West Germany

Dennis E. Bullard, M.D.
3009 New Bern Avenue
P.O. Box 14027
Raleigh, North Carolina

John Clorius, M.D.
Department of Neurosurgery Tumor Center
Heidelberg-Mannheim Institute of Nuclear Medicine
German Cancer Research Center
University of Heidelberg
Heidelberg, West Germany

J. O. Dostrovsky, M.D.
Associate Professor of Physiology
University of Toronto
Toronto, Canada

Kaj Ericson, M.D., Ph.D.
Associate Professor of Neuroradiology
Karolinska Institute
Stockholm, Sweden

Craig A. Fredericks, M.D.
Department of Neurological Surgery
University of Southern California
Los Angeles, California

Andreas Gamroth, M.D.
Department of Neurosurgery Tumor Center
Heidelberg-Mannheim Institute of Nuclear Medicine
German Cancer Center
University of Heidelberg
Heidelberg, West Germany

Philip L. Gildenberg, M.D., Ph.D
Clinical Professor of Neurosurgery
University of Texas Medical School
Houston, Texas

Stephen J. Goerss, B.S.
Research Technician
Department of Neurological Surgery
Mayo Clinic
Rochester, Minnesota

Philip H. Gutin, M.D.
Associate Professor of Neurological Surgery
University of California, San Francisco
San Francisco, California

Walter Hall, M.D.
Department of Neurological Surgery
University of Pittsburgh School of Medicine
Pittsburgh, Pennsylvania

Tyrone L. Hardy, M.D.
Department of Neurosurgery
Lovelace Medical Center
Albuquerque, New Mexico

M. Peter Heilbrun, M.D.
Professor and Chairman
Division of Neurological Surgery
University of Utah School of Medicine
Salt Lake City, Utah

Alfred C. Higgins, M.D.
Neurosurgery
Hilton Head, South Carolina

Tomas Hindmarsh, M.D. Ph.D.
Associate Professor of Neuroradiology
Department of Neuroradiology
Karolinska Institute
Stockholm, Sweden

Anita Hirsch, M.D., Ph.D.
Senior Staff
Department of Audiology
Karolinska Institute
Stockholm, Sweden

Edward R. Hitchcock, M.D.
Professor and Head
Midland Center for Neurosurgery and Neurology
University of Birmingham
West Midlands
Birmingham, England

Skip Jacques, M.D.
Advanced Neurosurgical Laboratory
Huntington Medical Research Institutes
Pasadena, California

Bruce A. Kall, M.S.
Computer Scientist
Department of Information Processing and Systems
Department of Neurosurgery
Mayo Clinic
Rochester, Minnesota

Patrick J. Kelly, M.D.
Associate Professor
Department of Neurological Surgery
Mayo Medical School,
Mayo Graduate School of Medicine
Rochester, Minnesota

Raymond N. Kjellberg, M.D.
Associate Clinical Professor of Surgery
Harvard Medical School
Massachusetts General Hospital
Boston, Massachusetts

Stephan Kunze, M.D.
Department of Neurosurger Tumor Center
Heidelberg-Mannheim Institute of Nuclear Medicine
University of Heidelberg
German Cancer Research Center
Heidelberg, West Germany

Lauri V. Laitinen, M.D., Ph.D.
Associate Professor of Neurological Surgery and Chief of Stereotactic Surgery
Umeå Hospital
Umeå, Sweden

Sharon Lamb, R.N.
Department of Neurological Surgery
University of California, San Francisco
San Francisco, California

Richard E. Latchaw, M.D.
Professor of Radiology and Chief, Division of Neuroradiology
University of Pittsburgh School of Medicine
Pittsburgh, Pennsylvania

Steven A. Leibel, M.D.
Associate Professor of Radiation Oncology
University of California, San Francisco
San Francisco, California

Dan Leksell, M.D.
Department of Head and Neck Surgery
Karolinska Institute
Huddinge University Hospital
Huddinge, Sweden

F. Lenz, M.D.
Research Fellow
Division of Neurosurgery
Toronto General Hospital
Instructor of Medical Science
University of Toronto
Toronto, Canada

Allan B. Levin, M.D.
Associate Professor of Neurological Surgery
Division of Neurological Surgery
University of Wisconsin
Madison, Wisconsin

Robert Levy, M.D., Ph.D.
Assistant Professor
Division of Neurological Surgery
Northwestern University
Chicago, Illinois

Christer Lindquist, M.D.
Associate Professor of Neurological Surgery
Department of Neurosurgery
Karolinska Institute
Stockholm, Sweden

Walter J. Lorenz, Ph.D.
Department of Neurosurgery Turmor Center
Heidelberg-Mannheim Institute of Nuclear Medicine
University of Heidelberg
German Cancer Research Center
Heidelberg, West Germany

L. Dade Lunsford, M.D.
Associate Professor of Neurological Surgery and Radiology
University of Pittsburgh School of Medicine
Chief, Stereotactic and Functional Surgery
Presbyterian-University Hospital
Pittsburgh, Pennsylvania

Harold F. Lutes, O.D.
Advanced Neuorsurgical Laboratory
Huntington Medical Research Institutes
Pasadena, California

Yoshiaki Mayanagi, M.D., D.M.Sc.
Chief Neurosurgeon
Tokyo Metropolitan Police Hospital
Lecturer, University of Tokyo
Tokyo, Japan

Sean McLinden, M.D.
Department of Neurology
University of Pittsburgh School of Medicine
Pittsburgh, Pennsylvania

Björn A. Meyerson, M.D., Ph.D.
Associate Professor of Neurosurgery
Karolinska Institute
Stockholm, Sweden

Per Mindus, M.D.
Associate Professor of Psychiatry
Karolinska Institute
Stockholm, Sweden

Fritz Mundinger, M.D.
Professor and Director
Abteilung fur Stereotaxis und Neuronuklearmedizin and Director in charge of the Neurochirurgische Universitatsklinik,
Klinikum der Albert Ludwigs-Universitat
Freiburg, West Germany

Blaine S. Nashold, Jr., M.D.
Professor of Surgery (Neurological Surgery)
Duke University School of Medicine
Durham, North Carolina

Georg Norén, M.D.
Senior Staff
Department of Neurosurgery
Karolinska Institute
Stockholm, Sweden

Christoph B. Ostertag, M.D.
Professor and Direktor
Abteilung fur Stereotaktische Neurochirurgie
Neurochirugische Universitatsklinik
Homburg, West Germany

Chihiro Ohye, M.D.
Professor and Chairman
Department of Neurosurgery
Gunma University School of Medicine
Gunma-Ken, Japan

Arun-Angelo Patil, M.D.
Associate Professor
Division of Neurological Surgery,
University of Nebraska Medical Center
Omaha, Nebraska

G. L. Rea
Neurosurgical Department
University Hospital
Zurich, Switzerland

David W. Roberts, M.D.
Assistant Professor of Clinical Surgery (Neurosurgery)
Dartmouth-Hitchcock Medical Center
Hanover, New Hampshire

Keiji Sano, M.D., D.M.Sc.
Emeritus Professor
University of Tokyo
Director and Professor
Department of Neurosurgery
Teikyo University
Tokyo, Japan

C. Hunter Sheldon, M.D.
Director of Huntington Medical Research Institutes
Pasadena, California

Jean Siegfried, M.D.
Professor of Neurological Surgery
University Hospital
Zurich, Switzerland

Hansjörg Sinn, Ph.D.
Department of Neurosurgery Tumor Center
Heidelberg-Mannheim Institute of Nuclear Medicine
University of Heidelberg
Heidelberg, West Germany

Ladislau Steiner, M.D.
Professor of Neurosurgery
Karolinska Institute
Stockholm, Sweden

Ulrich Steude, M.D.
Department of Neurosurgery Tumor Center
Heidelberg-Mannheim Institute of Nuclear Medicine
University of Heidelberg
Heidelberg, West Germany

Volker Sturm, M.D.
Professor
Department of Neurological Surgery Tumor Center
Heidelberg-Mannheim Institute of Nuclear Medicine
German Cancer Research Center
University of Heidelberg
Heidelberg, West Germany

Ronald R. Tasker, M.D.
Head, Division of Neurosurgery
Toronto General Hospital
Professor of Surgery
University of Toronto
Toronto, Canada

Hans von Holst, M.D., Ph.D.
Associate Professor
Department of Neurological Surgery
Karolinska Institute
Stockholm, Sweden

John Vries, M.D.
Associate Professor of Neurological Surgery
Director, Epilepsy Center
University of Pittsburgh School of Medicine
Pittsbugh, Pennsylvania

K. Weigel
Neurochirurgische Universitatsklinik,
Klinikum der Albert-Ludwigs-Universitat
Freiburg, West Germany

Bernd Wowra, M.D.
Department of Neurosurgery Tumor Center
Heidelberg-Mannheim Institute of Nuclear Medicine
German Cancer Research Center
University of Heidelberg
Heidelberg, West Germany

K. Yamashiro, M.D.
Research Fellow
Division of Neurosurgery
Toronto General Hospital
Toronto, Canada

Ronald F. Young, M.D.
Professor and Chief
Division of Neurological Surgery
California College of Medicine
University of California, Irvine,
Orange, California

Dedication

Modern Stereotactic Neurosurgery is dedicated posthumously to Lars Leksell, one of the great innovators and investigators in modern neurological surgery. Professor Leksell died suddenly on January 12, 1986, at the age of 78, after completing a morning walk in the Swiss Alps. Characteristically, earlier that day he had telephoned his son and proposed another clinical study designed to further expand the usage of stereotactic surgery. He was buried in Rome next to his beloved wife, Ludmila, and is survived by five children and many grandchildren, all successful in their own right.

Lars Leksell was born in Fässberg, Sweden, on November 23, 1907. He completed his medical studies at the Karolinska Institute. In 1935, he began his neurosurgical training with Professor Herbert Olivecrona at the Serafimer lasarettet, a nesting place for many other neurosurgical pioneers. His 1945 Ph.D. dissertation, under the direction of 1967 Nobel Laureate Ragnar Granit, described the gamma motor system. Forty years later (1985), Professor Granit delivered the first "Lars Leksell Lecture" at the Karolinska Institute. Lars Leksell was Professor of Neurological Surgery at Lund between 1958 and 1960 and then Professor of Neurosurgery at the Karolinska Institute from 1960 until his "retirement" in 1974. For the next 12 years, Lars remained actively involved in the research and clinical activities of the Karolinska, continuing daily visits and monitoring all types of stereotactic surgery performed there.

His accomplishments include the combination of multiple imaging modalities with guided brain surgery: encephalography in 1949, echoencephalography in 1955, computed tomography in 1976, and magnetic resonance imaging in 1983. He was convinced that all forms of energy could be devoted to the ablation of tumors or the creation of therapeutic brain lesions.

Perhaps the most creative invention of this brilliant mind was the development of stereotactic radiosurgery (the gamma knife), a technique in which multiple cobalt sources are focused stereotactically in the brain to ablate brain tumors without the need for a surgical incision.

Honored internationally by many surgical and neurological societies and decorated by many governments, Lars Leksell remained a man always available to his peers, his patients, his family, and even to the unknown visitors who streamed to his side. He left a legacy of friends and trainees throughout the world.

Foremost a scientist, he was a linguist (Swedish, English, German, French, Italian), an adventurer (he often traveled to the Karolinska by motorcycle or boat), and a gregarious raconteur. In his later years, those who had the opportunity to spend many hours in conversation with him at the Diplomat Tea House can testify to his wide-ranging interests. He was a perfectionist: Each of his scientific

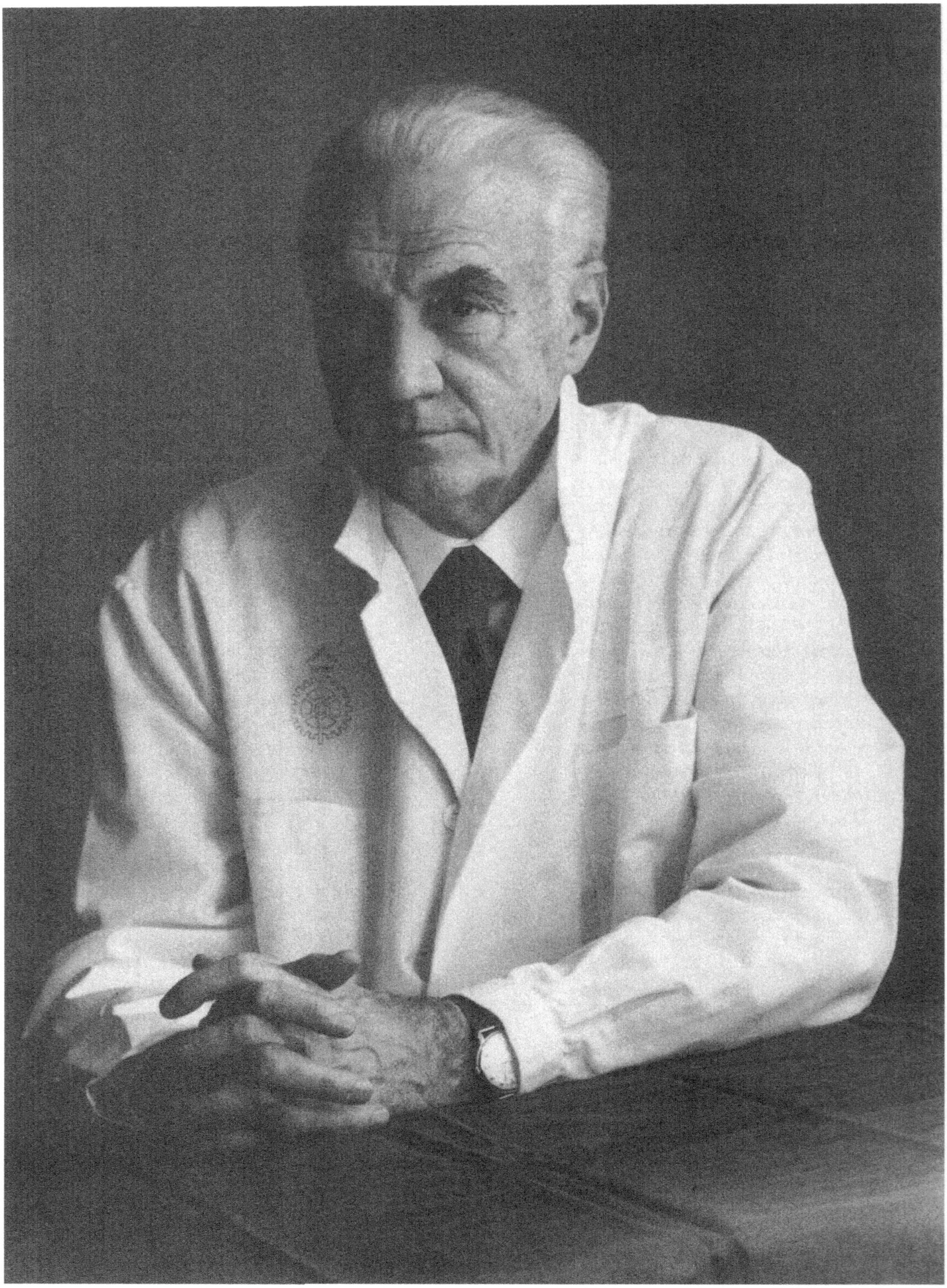

papers was remarkable for its succinct presentation, clarity, and literacy; regardless of the language in which he wrote, each punctuation mark was important. The stereotactic instrument over which he labored remained in evolution, as Lars continued to make even seemingly minor changes designed to perfect the device. He vociferously campaigned against the aggrandizement of bibliographies by the inclusion of inconsequential papers; his concern was quality, not quantity. His sparkling humor was manifest in his personal writings: Hjärnfragment *(a play on the Swedish double entendre* Hjärn *meaning both "brain" and "iron") is an autobiographical sketch ostensibly intended as a family memoir. He was a passionate humanist, intimately involved in the Swedish controversy over the definition of brain death, which culminated with his coauthorship (with Gerda Antti) of* Hjärn död?, *published in 1985.*

Lars Leksell trained in the infancy of neurological surgery, a time when families lined up outside the operating-room door to donate blood, lest exsanguination terminate the removal of a relative's brain tumor. He was convinced that all areas of the brain could be explored safely if only the proper tools were available. He lived to see one of his fondest dreams realized: the full integration of safe and effective stereotactic instrumentation into its rightful place in the field of neurological surgery.

L. Dade Lunsford

ACKNOWLEDGMENTS

"Words are but empty thanks."—Colley Cibber, *Woman's Wit*, Act 1, 1697

To the authors of this first edition of *Modern Stereotactic Nevro Surgery* I offer my gratitude and admiration. For some, it probably has proved difficult to transcribe into a few words what may be the result of much of a lifetime's efforts. For others, stereotactic technique represents only a small part of their contributions within the field of brain surgery.

Completion of this volume was impossible without the special help of three talented, patient, and tireless individuals. Helene Hochman reviewed, edited, and when necessary, revised each chapter. She brought great skill, humor, and expertise to the job of Editor, Department of Neurological Surgery, at the University of Pittsburgh. Phyllis Shoemaker and Mary Ann Vincenzini were the superb transcribers and organizers who laboriously prepared each manuscript for publication.

To my wife, Julie, and my children, Stephanie and Andrew, I convey my appreciation for support and time to complete the task.

The Department of Neurological Surgery, University of Pittsburgh, provided personnel and economic resources. Lastly, to Jeffrey Stier and the staff of Martinus Nijhoff Publishing, Boston, I give accolades for their efforts in presenting an attractive and, I hope, instructional survey of the contemporary field of human stereotactic surgery of the brain.

L. Dade Lunsford, M.D.
Pittsburgh, Pennsylvania

PREFACE

When I was first approached by the publisher of this volume, Martinus Nijhoff, Boston, I explored the possibility of writing a personal monograph on contemporary stereotactic surgery. After a review of available literature, several aspects became apparent. First, no current, readily accessible, multiauthored text designed to survey the field was available. Those books that were available tended to heavily emphasize theory, physiology, and anatomy. Second, stereotactic surgeons were considered abstruse and for too long were relegated to a status outside of the mainstream of neurosurgery. This attitude probably reflected the insufficient explanation of the practical uses and advantages of stereotactic technique. Third, in recent years, the field has expanded so rapidly that it has become a major component of any active neurosurgical teaching program. For example, at some centers, stereotactic technique may be used in 25%–30% of all neurosurgical procedures. My goal, therefore, changed to one of editing a general textbook designed to emphasize the practical role of stereotactic technique in the daily routine.

Modern Stereotactic Neurosurgery is divided into four sections. Section I, Basic Techniques, identifies and explains many, but certainly not all, of the currently commercially available stereotactic instruments. Section II, Morphological Surgery, discusses the use of these devices in the diagnosis and treatment of structural mass lesions of the brain. Section III, Functional Surgery, describes the role of stereotactic technique in the treatment of physiologic disorders of the brain. Section IV, Stereotactic Radiosurgery, introduces a quickly growing field that combines stereotactic precision with powerful radiotherapeutic treatment modalities.

As in any multiauthored textbook penned by writers of diverse backgrounds and interests, *Modern Stereotactic Neurosurgery* to some extent suffers from incompleteness. Future volumes no doubt will include many additions from other authors who also are important specialists in the field. Because not all authors write in the same style (or even language), we have attempted to achieve a more cohesive text in the editorial process. Each chapter has been subdivided into pertinent headings for easier reference. Because of my own background, some readers will note an Americanization (as opposed to anglicization) of the chapters. While many chapters comprise primarily summaries of the authors' work within the field, each author was encouraged to review the literature in that discipline if appropriate. In most chapters, the bibliography purposely was kept small so that interested readers might know precisely those references regarded as important by recognized authorities in the field.

The practice of stereotactic surgery progresses—new indications, new devices, and new techniques. Few specialities more successfully have combined the advantages of tremendously advanced imaging tools, computer technology, and therapeutic devices. In the process, the goal of reduced patient morbidity has been maintained in an era in which the preservation or improvement of neurological function after surgery has become a major achievement. Stereotactic surgery is firmly integrated within the neurosurgical armamentarium and, no doubt, future investigators will further expand its uses.

L. Dade Lunsford, M.D.
Pittsburgh, Pennsylvania

I. BASIC TECHNIQUES

1. GENERAL CONCEPTS OF STEREOTACTIC SURGERY

Philip L. Gildenberg

Stereotactic surgery is that field of neurosurgery in which an apparatus is employed to direct an electrode or probe to an intracerebral target with minimal damage to overlying structures. Stereotactic procedures are used to alter the function of deep structures within the brain, to treat various lesions, or to obtain tissue for study.

Before the advent of stereotactic surgery, it was necessary to incise the brain to visulize the target area in order to approach any target. If an anatomical structure were the target, it might not be identifiable by direct vision. If the lesion were deep and small, it might be difficult to locate, resulting in extensive damage to the surrounding brain. If the lesion underlay a functional area, it might not be possible to approach the target without causing an unacceptable neurological deficit. If a target lay near or beneath arteries, it might not be approachable without significant injury to blood supply. These considerations made most deep-seated targets off limits to the surgeon.

Even prior to the development of stereotactic surgery, neurophysiological information had been available to theorize how abnormal brain function might be alleviated by interrupting various pathways. Techniques that were devised to interrupt extrapyramidal fibers in the peduncle, for instance [28, 29], or infarct extrapyramidal structures by ligating an artery [6] had inconsistent results and unacceptable risk, so they did not become widely acepted and later became supplanted by stereotactic procedures. Stereotactic surgery made it possible to approach deep targets safely and accurately, leading to a new subspecialty of neurosurgery.

The principles of stereotactic surgery depend on a Cartesian coordinate system. Descartes observed that it is possible to define the location of an individual point in space by relating it to three planes intersecting at right angles to each other (figure 1–1) [9]. Therefore, to define a point, one must state three coordinates, each corresponding to the distance between the point and one of the planes. There is only one point that corresponds to each defini-

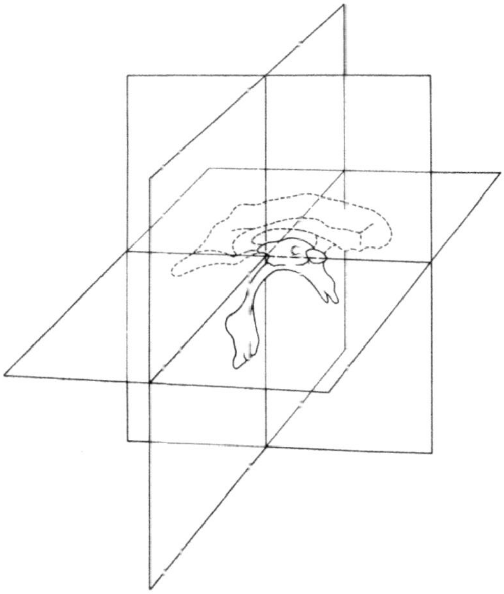

FIGURE 1–1. The Cartesian coordinate system on which stereoencephalotomy is based is related to landmarks about the third ventricle. Reprinted with permission from Gildenberg PL: Functional neurosurgery. In Schmidek H and Sweet H (eds): *Operative Neurosurgery* (2nd ed). New York: Grune & Stratton, 1987.

L.D. Lunsford (ed.) *MODERN STEREOTACTIC NEUROSURGERY*.

tion. For instance, only one point can be 4 mm to the right of the midsagittal plane, 6 mm above a horizontal plane at right angles to the first, and 8 mm anterior to a vertical plane at right angles to the other two. If the three planes are related to the brain, (e.g., if they intersect at the posterior commissure, with the sagittal plane in the midline and the horizontal plane passing through both commissures), the defined target point will lie at a specific location within the brain. If it is determined what anatomical structure ordinarily lies at a particular set of coordinates, it becomes possible to use those coordinates to define the location of the anatomical structure.

Let us proceed one step at a time. Three such reference planes were originally defined for experimental animals. One is the midsagittal plane (a logical choice). The horizontal or basal plane in animals is defined as a plane at right angles to the first, running through both external auditory meatus and the inferior orbital rims. This plane can be related approximately to the Frankfort plane used in anthropology for measurements of the skull, which is defined as a plane through both external auditory canals and one inferior orbital rim. Such reference avoids inconsistencies caused by asymmetry. By defining the planes in this manner, there is an additional advantage in that animal stereotactic apparatus are designed to secure the animal's head with earplugs and with tabs resting on the inferior orbital rim, automatically aligning the head with the basal and interaural planes. Because the basal plane, defined by the bony landmarks, ordinarily lies entirely below the brain, a parallel plane 10 mm higher is often taken for convenience as the stereotactic basal plane. By aligning the head in the center of the apparatus, the midsagittal plane is defined, as well.

Stereotactic Apparatus

The above original and revolutionary principle was described in 1908 by Horsley and Clarke in a classic paper, "The Structure and Functions of the Cerebellum Examined By a New Method" published in *Brain* [19]. Their amazing contribution, which should be read by any surgeon or neurophysiologist engaging in stereotactic surgery, is divided into five parts, although the title refers only to the physiologic study of the cerebellum presented in one part of the paper. To study the cerebellum, lesions were made at specific places, which required the development of a stereotactic apparatus. The general principles of the device are described in exquisite detail along with a description of the first stereotactic brain atlas. One part of the paper involves the production of electrolytic lesions with a direct current, a study that has not been improved upon in the 80 years since it appeared. The animal stereotactic device was so inventive and successful that it continues to be used to the present day with some mechanical modifications or revisions but no refinements in its basic principles.

Horsley and Clarke made these essential points:

1. Any irregular solid may be divided by three section planes in three dimensions into eight segments, in each of which the three internal surfaces are those of a cube.
2. In any solid body, a constant point (which can be measured from plane surfaces and represents the three dimensions of a cube) can be identified by three perpendiculars of correct length dependent from those surfaces, and it is the only point where those perpendiculars can meet.
3. A needle may be substituted for any of these perpendiculars, and in order for it to be directed mechanically to any required point in any of these rectilinear segments, an instrument is necessary that will introduce it in a direction perpendicular to one surface, and therefore parallel to the other two, to any required distance from the first surface, any required distance from the others, i.e., the needle must have a regulated movement in three dimensions [19].

Even as early as 1918, an adaptation of the Horsley and Clarke apparatus for humans was made by Mussen [31], but we do not know whether it was ever used.

Attempts to apply the experimental animal system to humans met with difficulty. Because there is great variability between landmarks on the skull and anatomical structures within the cerebrum of humans, the accuracy of the system did not approach that required for clinical use. Inaccuracies in electrode placement in experimental animals caused by anatomical variability were dealt with by using a number of animals, sectioning the brains at the conclusion of the experiment to examine the precise electrode placement, and using data from only those animals with satisfactory electrode placement. Obviously, this could not be done in humans, where every electrode placement had to be accurate.

In 1947, Spiegel and Wycis reported a technique to improve accuracy sufficiently to allow the adaptation of stereotactic surgery to humans [41]. They related the coordinate system not to landmarks about the skull but to internal cerebral landmarks as seen on anteroposterior (AP) and lateral roentgen films. Originally, they took as their basal plane a line (on lateral pneumoencephalography films) between the foramen of Monro and the pineal gland. The coronal plane passed through the pineal gland at right angles to the basal and midsagittal planes. They named their new technique *stereoencephalotomy*, a three-dimensional system based on encephalographic coordinates. The original Horsley and Clarke apparatus involved a translational system, that is, the electrode was moved longitudinally along a system of slides to move the vertically oriented electrode in the AP or lateral direction individually. Once the electrode was adjusted to lie immediately above, and pointing to, the target, it was lowered by a microdrive to the target. Later modification allowed angular adjustments so the electrode might be tilted to approach the target along a predetermined trajectory, but the major adjustments remained AP and lateral, performed by sliding the electrodes.

The original Spiegel-Wycis human apparatus, Model I, resembled the original Horsley and Clarke apparatus in that it contained only translational, and not angular, adjustments [41]. It was fixed not to the skull but to the scalp by a plaster cap manufactured for each individual patient, from which a base ring was suspended. The adjustable part of the apparatus was attached to the base ring. Later models of the Spiegel-Wycis apparatus incorporated angular adjustments and fixation to the skull but still depended primarily on translational movements for aiming the electrode (figure 1–2).

As the field has developed, most currently used stereotactic apparatus can be assigned to one of four categories, (a) the translational system; (b) burr-hole mounted; (c) the arc type; and (d) a system with interlocking arcs (figure 1–2).

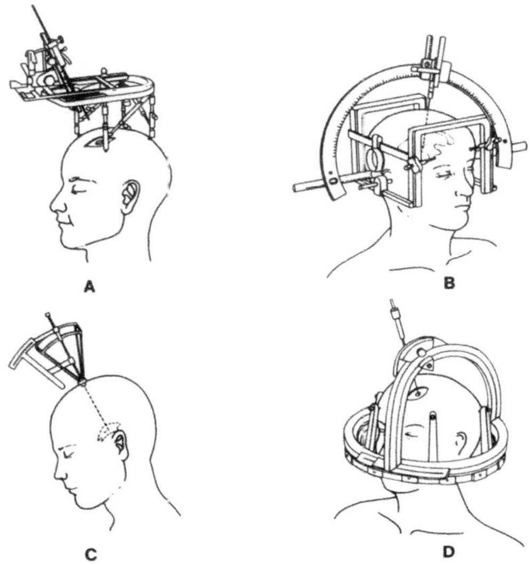

FIGURE 1–2. The four basic types of stereotactic apparatus are (a) the translational system, (b) burr-hole mounted, (c) the arc type, and (d) a system with interlocking arcs. Reprinted with permission from Gildenberg PL: Functional neurosurgery. In Schmidek H and Sweet H (eds): *Operative Neurosurgery* (2nd ed). New York: Grune & Stratton, 1987.

Some early systems were actually aiming devices that attached to a burr hole. The only adjustments possible were angular, in order to point the electrode at the target; possibly a microdrive was added to advance the electrode to a given depth. Lines were drawn on both the AP and the lateral roentgen ray films from the target through the fulcrum of the burr-hole-mounted apparatus. The AP and lateral angles of the apparatus were adjusted to correspond to the angles demonstrated on the films. It is very difficult to make angular adjustments accurately, because the error of even a fraction of a degree may produce an error of several millimeters at target depth, so there is an inherent inaccuracy in these devices. In addition, firm fixation to the burr hole is frequently suboptimal, and even the slightest movement can cause a great mechanical inaccuracy. More recent varieties of burr-hole-mounted stereotactic apparatus employ a base plate screwed to the skull for greater stability and use a phantom to adjust the angles with greater accuracy [4].

A major contribution to stereotactic surgery was the development of arc systems, such as the Leksell apparatus [25, 26]. These types of apparatus contain a semicircular arc on which an electrode carrier is mounted so that it always points to the center of the semicircle. In some systems, the arc is attached to a frame, which is attached to the patient's head in an adjustable measured manner so that the target lies in the center of the arc system. In other systems, the patient's head is moved within the arc system so that the target point lies at the center of the apparatus, as in the Todd-Wells system [49].

A modification of this apparatus relies on an arc system that is not centered on the target, such as that used in the Riechert device and its modifications [33]; instead, the arc is adjusted with a phantom. A head ring is applied to the patient and radiographs taken to define the target point in relation to the head ring. The arc system, or target bow, is applied to a similar head ring (a phantom) on which a device indicates the relative position of the target, and the arc is adjusted to advance the probe to the target. The arc system can then be transferred to the head ring on the patient's skull, and a probe can be advanced to the target without further adjustment.

The recently introduced Brown-Roberts-Wells apparatus uses a system of interlocking arcs to point the probe to the target [3, 17]. The target coordinates are determined in relation to a head ring. A computer is used to determine the four angular adjustments to direct the probe either from the location of a burr hole or along a specific angle and declination.

Other systems, such as the Talairach apparatus [45], use a grid system to introduce the electrode or multiple electrodes from a given angle to the target. Although such devices do not allow as much flexibility for the introduction of single electrodes, they allow the introduction of an array of electrodes, which is particularly useful for exploring an area for epileptiform activity or for the implantation of multiple radioisotope sources.

Atlases

In order to know at which coordinates a specific anatomical structure can be found, it is necessary to have a "road map," or atlas. To produce an atlas, a brain is fixed by a technique to minimize distortion and shrinkage. It is sectioned through planes parallel to, and a measured distance from, one of the three reference planes [38]. Most frequently, the sections are related to the coronal plane, but more recently, the horizontal plane has become more popular because of its relationship to images seen by computed tomography (CT) scanning. For instance, in an atlas involving coronal sections, it is indicated how far each plate lies anterior or posterior to the coronal plane, providing the AP coordinates. Along the top or bottom is a scale with the zero at the midsagittal plane, and along the side of the plate is a scale relating it to the basal plane, so that all three coordinates can be derived from measurement on the plate that bears the desired anatomical structure (figure 1–3).

After the original description of a human stereotactic apparatus in 1947, Spiegel and Wycis published the first human stereotactic atlas in 1952 [38]. It consisted of photographs of a sample brain along with coordinates relating it to the coordinate system then employed, based on a plane between the pineal gland and the foramen of Monro. The atlas contained several variability tables, derived from the measurements of a number of brains; the tables indicated the distribution of measurements between key structures in a limited sample population so that corrections might be estimated in very large or very small brains. Additional variability tables appeared in articles throughout the next 15 years, gradually adding to the statistical accuracy of the measurements.

Later atlases were also based on individual sample brains, but generally were related to the intercommissural plane, which passes through the center of the anterior and posterior commissures at right angles to the midsagittal plane. Often, these atlases included transparent overlays on which outlines of the nuclei and subnuclei were drawn [34]; finely detailed enlarged drawings of limited anatomical areas, such as the thalamus and brain stem [1, 50]; information about the location of major blood vessels [45]; and a host of physiological and anatomical data [48], concentrated on the cerebellum. All were based on the principle originated by Horsley and Clarke and elaborated on by Spiegel and Wycis.

As technology has advanced, however, we are entering a new generation of computer-

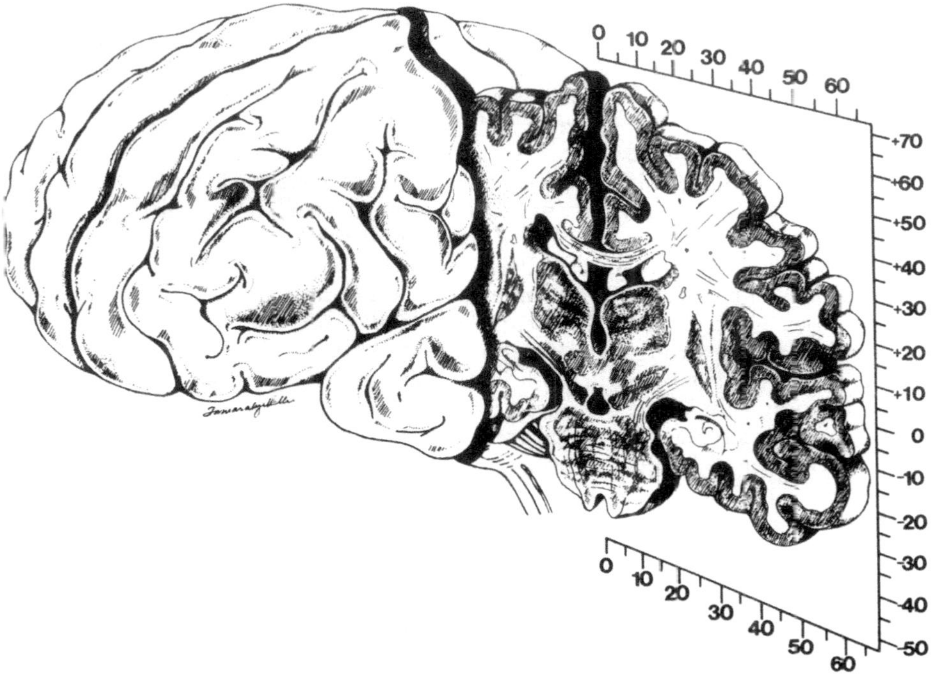

FIGURE 1–3. Each page in a stereotactic atlas provides all three coordinates of a visualized target. In coronal sections, the anteroposterior coordinate is obtained from the location of the image; the lateral and vertical coordinates are obtained from measurements made on the illustration.

based stereotactic atlases. They generally consist of graphic illustrations derived from a previously published atlas. These illustrations can be artifically distorted to fit the configuration of key structures of the individual patient's brain as demonstrated on radiographs or computed tomographic (CT) scans [22], or they can be magnified and manipulated in the operating room to provide information and views of value to the surgeon [15]. They provide a repository for anatomical and clinical information obtained in the operating room regarding the anatomical structures enabling correlation of physiological data and clinical results with specific foci [15, 47].

Radiography Requirements

Stereoencephalotomy requires the intraoperative roentgenographic visualization of anatomical landmarks upon which the coordinate system is based. Originally, the stereotactic surgeon required a pneumoencephalogram to visualize the foramen of Monro. Because it is difficult to demonstrate posterior structures with air, the pineal gland was taken as the posterior landmark. Later, ventriculography was employed, at first with air as the contrast medium. Better radiographic techniques made localization of the anterior commissure reliable, and its structure made it a more accurate landmark than the foramen of Monro. By instilling the air under controlled pressure, it was possible to demonstrate the posterior commissure, and that was adopted as the posterior landmark. This enabled the surgeon to have far more accuracy than using the pineal gland, which varies greatly in size and demonstrability.

The development of positive-contrast media improved demonstration of the landmarks even further. Pantopaque (iodophenylundecanoate) allowed excellent visualization when administered through a ventricular cannula, but since it is very hyperbaric, it could only be used with the patient in the sitting position, when the patient's head could be first flexed and then extended to enable visualization of both anterior and posterior commissures. Use of water-soluble contrast media made it possible to visulize the entire third ventricle along with both commissures accurately and reliably. This has become the technique of choice. Gains are being made, however, in using coordinates derived from landmarks visualized by CT or magnetic resonance imaging (MRI) scans, and that technique promises to be the future method of choice.

Consistent and precise placement of AP and lateral x-ray tubes is imperative to the accuracy demanded by stereotactic surgery. The central beam should reliably pass through the center of the apparatus and/or target point in both AP and lateral films to prevent image distortion by parallax; thus, each stereotactic system must have incorporated into it a method for alignment of roentgen x-ray sources [39].

Magnification must be controlled so that measurements taken on roentgenograms can be accurately related to actual distances. There are generally two basic techniques to compensate for roentgen x-ray magnification. The first involves using a standard tube-to-cassette distance to determine the magnification factor. Because magnification increases as one moves further from the central beam, the magnification factor will vary in different parts of the film. This problem can most easily be overcome by the use of a variable ruler, which can be either spiral-shaped [26] or linear [14]. The second way to control for magnification is to use very large tube-to-cassette distances, so-called teleradiography, so that magnification is negligible. This, however, may require building an extra-large dedicated operating room, possibly with a dome two stories high to house the AP x-ray tube.

CT Stereotaxis

Stereotactic surgery recently has entered a new era [10]. There is a natural affinity between stereotactic surgery and CT, because both are concerned with the accurate definition of internal cerebral structures in a three-dimensional array. The marriage was consummated with the development of devices and techniques that allow the insertion of a probe into any target that can be seen by CT or MRI scanning, whether a specific anatomical structure or mass lesion.

If one looks carefully at a CT image, one can see that the picture is made up of a grid of numerous squares organized in lines and rows, pixels arrayed as a natural coordinate system, as each has a specific position or address. The CT sections are piled upon each other to form a three-dimensional organized stack. When considered in three-dimensional volume, each address is referred to a voxel, and the organization of voxels in a scan represents a Cartesian coordinate system similar to that used with stereotactic coordinates.

One must be cautious in naming the coordinates because disparate routines have been adopted. It is common among stereotactic surgeons to refer to the AP coordinate as the "X" coordinate, the vertical coordinate as the "Y" coordinate, and the lateral coordinate as the "Z" coordinate. The radiologists, however, have adopted a different nomenclature, which may lead to considerable confusion.

The AP and lateral stereotactic coordinates can be demonstrated on an individual CT image, and various methods can be used to define a zero point from which measurements can be made. The difficulty lies, however, in defining the exact position of the image in relation to the head and/or the stereotactic apparatus, and several solutions have been employed.

One simple technique can be used with any CT scanner that demonstrates a translational image, such as the GE ScoutView® (General Electric Medical Systems, Milwaukee, WI) and with any stereotactic apparatus [13]. The AP and lateral coordinates are taken from the image bearing the target by measuring from the center of the head. The position of the target-bearing image is obtained by relating the target position in the images on the electronic sagittal radiograph (ScoutView®) to the target position on the lateral roentgenogram taken in the operating room. Those images that pass through identifiable landmarks at the base of the skull are drawn on the operating room roentgenogram, and the distance to the target image is measured taking magification into account.

Other techniques require the stereotactic apparatus or head ring to be attached to the scanner table; the distance the table moves between the scan of the head ring and the target represents the vertical coordinate.

Perhaps the most accurate system involves a localizer device, which is attached to the head ring and is included in the scan of each slice. The most common of these involves three N-shaped arrangements of three carbon rods each. As the CT slice cuts through a set of three rods, the relative distance between the center rod and the other two rods is proportionate to the height the slice lies above the base ring. Because the distance is determined at three separate points, it is possible to define the slice as a plane in space, even if the slice is not parallel to the base ring [17].

Simple aiming devices can be attached to a burr hole and the probe inserted under CT guidance, but this trial-and-error method leaves much to be desired.

Finally, the stereotactic apparatus can be built into the CT scanner and the position of the image and target indicated directly in stereotactic coordinates [23]. Such a system can be elegant and accurate, and the procedure can be monitored with the patient's head in the scanner, but it is elaborate and too costly for most stereotactic surgeons.

Indications

Indications for stereotactic surgery can be divided roughly into two groups, functional and CT-directed. In functional procedures, that is, procedures designed to change the function of the nervous system, specific anatomical sites or structures are the targets [11, 36, 39]. In CT-directed procedures the target is a lesion seen by CT or similar imaging techniques [10, 17]. Functional procedures may require the interruption of pathways by production of a lesion, stimulation of a region or anatomical structures (keeping in mind that electrical stimulation may actually cause a temporary inhibition or disruption of physiological activity), or pharmacological manipulation of an area. Often, electrical techniques are combined with recording of physiological activity. Ablative procedures generally employ a radiofrequency electrical current to heat a controlled volume of tissue to the point of denaturation [8], although controlled cutting with a leukotome and controlled freezing have been used [7].

The classic reason for ablative stereotactic operations has been the interruption of basal ganglion pathways for the alleviation of movement disorders, particularly tremor [11]. In the late 1950s and early 1960s, functional stereotaxy reached its peak in the treatment of Parkinson's disease, as many neurosurgeons ablated various targets, such as the ventral lateral nucleus of the thalamus [36], the globus pallidus [37], or the intervening pathways in the ansa lenticularis (ansotomy) or Forel's field H (campotomy) [39, 42]. Although there has been a sharp decline in this use since the introduction of L-dopa, there is still a role for surgery in those patients whose primary symptom is tremor [12] (see chapters 23 and 25). Other types of tremor such as intention or post-traumatic tremor may respond to similar lesions. An occasional patient with dystonia musculorum deformans may have a dramatic response to ventral lateral lesions, and half can be helped to some extent [5]. Whether spasmodic torticollis responds to stereotactic ablation is still under consideration [16], but the response may be partial or long delayed [24].

Ablative stereotactic procedures can be used for the treatment of pain, primarily cancer pain. The major targets are the lemniscal pathways in the midbrain [30, 43, 44, 46] or the extralemniscal pathways within the thalamus [11, 43, 44] or at the cervicomedullary junction [18, 35].

Although the original intention of Spiegel and Wycis was to develop stereotactic surgery as a refinement of psychosurgery (which then consisted of prefrontal lobotomy), that has become only a minor use for stereotactic techniques. Nevertheless, cingulotomy or dorsal median thalamotomy can be an invaluable treatment for patients with intractable depression or obsessive-compulsive behavior [2, 36].

There have been numerous attempts to employ ablative stereotactic surgery in the treatment of epilepsy, with targets in Forel's field or associated pathways [21, 36, 39, 40] or other basal ganglia areas. Theoretically, such procedures were designed to prevent propagation of abnormal cerebral activity, but they have not supplanted the more classic approaches to ablative epilepsy surgery. However, stereotactic insertion of recording electrodes has been an important part of the evaluation of epilepsy patients who may be considered for surgical resection of seizure foci. Indeed, depth recordings can be done whenever an electrode is stereotactically inserted for any reason, and information thus obtained has been the basis for our understanding of human neurophysiology [36, 39].

The development of implantable stimulating devices, such as those used for dorsal spinal cord stimulation, has further led to the development of implantable brain-stimulating electrodes that can be used with such stimulators. Stimulation of the somatosensory areas of the internal capsule is useful for denervation pain [20], and chronic stimulation of the periaqueductal or periventricular gray regions can inhibit chronic pain or cancer pain [32].

Today, neurosurgeons can insert a probe into any lesion seen by CT or other imaging techniques; stereotaxis thus can be used for the biospy of mass lesions, aspiration of abscesses or cysts, evacuation of intracerebral hematomas, insertion of radioisotopes, instillation of antibiotics or chemotherapeutic agents [10], and soon, for the insertion of tissue sources of neurotransmitters or embryonal tissue [27].

Stereotactic vs. Stereotaxic

There has been considerable disagreement about the proper usage of *stereotactic* versus *stereotaxic*. The latter term, used originally, involves the Greek root words for *three-dimensional* and *system*. However, at its 1973 meeting, the International Society for Research in Stereoencephalotomy voted to change the name of the organization to the World Society for Stereotactic and Functional Neurosurgery. The spelling was derived from the Greek work *stereo* for three-dimensional and the Latin word *tactus*, to touch. The feeling was that stereotactic surgery involved more than merely displaying the brain in three dimensions, but actually using a three-dimensional system to touch a structure deep within the brain.

References

1. Andrew J, Watkins ES: *Stereotactic Surgery: A Stereotactic Atlas of the Human Thalamus*. Baltimore: Williams Wilkins, 1969
2. Ballantine HT Jr, Levy BS, Dagi TF, et al: Cingulotomy for psychiatric illness: Report of 13 years' experience. In Sweet WH, Obrador S, Martin-Rodriquez JG (eds): *Neurosurgical Treatment in Psychiatry, Pain and Epilepsy*. Baltimore: University Park Press, 1977, pp 333–353
3. Brown RA, Roberts TS, Osborn AG: Stereotaxic frame and computer software for CT-directed neurosurgical localization. *Invest Radiol* 15: 308–312, 1980
4. Carol M: A true "advanced imaging assisted" skull-mounted stereotactic system. *Appl Neurophysiol* 48:69–72, 1985
5. Cooper IS: *Involuntary Movement Disorders*. New York: Hoeber, 1969
6. Cooper IS; Surgical occlusion of the anterior choroidal artery in parkinsonism. *Surg Gynecol Obstet* 99:207–219, 1954
7. Cooper IS, Lee AS: Cryostatic congelation. *J Nerv Ment Dis* 33:259–263, 1961
8. Cosman ER, Nashold BS Jr, Bedenbaugh P: Stereotactic radiofrequency lesion making. *Appl Neurophysiol* 46:160–166, 1983
9. Descartes R: *Discours de la Methode*. Leyen, 1637
10. Gildenberg PL: Computerized tomography and stereotactic surgery. In Spiegel EA (ed): *Guided Brain Operations*. Basel: Karger, 1982, pp 24–34
11. Gildenberg PL: Functional neurosurgery. In Schmidek HH, Sweet WH (eds): *Operative Neurosurgical Techniques*, Vol II. New York: Grune Stratton, 1982, pp 993–1043
12. Gildenbery PL: The present role of stereotactic surgery in the management of Parkinson's disease. In Hassler RG, Christ JF (eds): *Parkinson-Specific Motor and Mental Disorders*. New York: Raven, 1984, pp 447–452
13. Gildenberg PL, Kaufman HH, Murthy KSK: Calculation of stereotactic coordinates from the computed tomographic scan. *Neurosurgery* 10:580–586, 1982
14. Gildenberg PL, Murthy KSK: A simple technique for correcting for magnification in stereotactic surgery. *Appl Neurophysiol*, 1986 (In press)
15. Giorgi C, Cerchiari U, Broggi G, et al: Digital image processing to handle neuroanatomical information and neurophysiological data. *Appl Neurophysiol* 48:30–33, 1985
16. Hassler R, Dieckmann G: Stereotactic treatment of spasmodic torticollis. In Schaltenbrand G, Walker AE (eds): Stereotaxy of the Human Brain (2nd ed). Stuttgart, New York: Georg Thieme Verlag, 1982, pp 522–531
17. Heilbrun MP: Computed tomography-guided stereotactic systems. *Clin Neurosurg* 31:564–581, 1984
18. Hitchcock ER: Stereotactic cervical myelotomy. *J Neurol Neurosurg Psychiatry* 33:224–230, 1970
19. Horsley V, Clarke RH: The structure and functions of the cerebellum examined by a new method. *Brain* 31:45–124, 1908
20. Hosobuchi Y, Adams JE, Rutkins B: Chronic thalamic stimulation for the control of facial anesthesia dolorosa. *Arch Neurol* 29:158–161, 1973
21. Jinnai D, Nishimoto A: Stereotaxic destruction of Forel H for treatment of epilepsy. *Neurochirurgia* (Stuttg) 6:164–176, 1963
22. Kall BA, Kelly PJ, Goerss BS, et al: Methodology and clinical experience with computed

tomography and a computer-resident stereotactic atlas. *Neurosurgery* 17:400–407, 1985
23. Koslow M, Abele MG: A fully interfaced computerized tomographic-stereotactic surgical system. *Appl Neurophysiol* 43:174–175, 1980
24. Laitinen LV: Stereotaxic treatment of spasmodic torticollis. *Acta Neurol Scand* [Suppl 4] 39:231–236, 1963
25. Leksell L: The stereotaxic method and radiosurgery of the brain. *Acta Chir Scand* 102:316–319, 1951
26. Leksell L: *Stereotaxis and radiosurgery. An Operating System.* Springfield, IL: Thomas, 1971
27. Mark VH, Gildenberg PL, Franklin PO: Proceedings of the colloquium on the use of embryonic cell transplantation for correction of CNS disorders. *Appl Neurophysiol* 47:1–76, 1984
28. Meyers R: The modification of alternating tremors, rigidity and festination by surgery of the basal ganglia. *Res Publ Assoc Res Nerv Ment Dis* 21:602–665, 1942
29. Meyers R: Surgical experiments in the therapy of certain "extrapyramidal" diseases. *Acta Psychiat Neurol* [Suppl] 26:3–42, 1951
30. Nashold BS Jr: Extensive cephalic and oral pain relieved by midbrain tractotomy. *Conf Neurol* 34:382–388, 1972
31. Olivier A, Bertrand G, Picard C: Discovery of the first human stereotactic instrument. *Appl Neurophysiol* 46:84–91, 1983
32. Richardson DE, Akil H: Pain reduction by electrical brain stimulation in man. II. Chronic self-administration in the periventricular gray matter. *J Neurosurg* 47:184–194, 1977
33. Riechert T: *Stereotactic Brain Operations.* Bern, Stuttgart, Vienna: Hans Huber, 1980
34. Schaltenbrand G, Bailey P: *Introduction to Stereotaxis with an Atlas of the Human Brain.* Stuttgart: Thieme, 1959
35. Schvarcz JR: Spinal cord stereotactic techniques re trigeminal neucleotomy and extralemniscal myelotomy. *Appl Neurophysiol* 41:99–112, 1978
36. Spiegel EA: *Guided Brain Operations.* Basel: Karger, 1982
37. Spiegel EA, Wycis HT: Pallido-thalamotomy in chorea. *AMA Arch Neurol Psychiatr* 64:495–496, 1950
38. Spiegel EA, Wycis HT: *Stereoencephalotomy, Part 1.* New York: Grune & Stratton, 1952
39. Spiegel EA, Wycis HT: *Stereoencephalotomy, Part 2.* New York: Grune & Stratton, 1962
40. Spiegel EA, Wycis HT, Baird HW: Pallidotomy and pallidoansotomy in certain types of convulsive disorders. *AMA Arch Neurol Psychiatr* 80:714–728, 1958
41. Spiegel EA, Wycis HT, Marks M, et al: Stereotaxic apparatus for operations on the human brain. *Science* 106:349–350, 1947
42. Spiegel EA, Wycis HT, Szekely EG, et al: Campotomy in various extrapyramidal disorders. *J Neurosurg* 20:871–881, 1963
43. Spiegel EA, Wycis HT, Szekely EG, et al: Combined dorsomedial, intralaminar and basal thalamotomy for relief of so-called intractable pain. *J Int Coll Surg* 42:160–168, 1964
44. Spiegel EA, Wycis HT, Szekely EG, et al: Medial and basal thalamotomy in so-called intractable pain. In Knighton RS, Dumke PR, (eds): *Pain.* Boston: Little, Brown, 1966, pp 503–517
45. Talairach J, David M, Tournoux P, et al: *Atlas d'Anatomie Stereotaxique.* Paris: Masson, 1957
46. Tasker RR: Thalamic stereotaxic procedures In Schaltenbrand G, Walker AE (eds): *Stereotaxy of the Human Brain,* (2nd ed.). Stuttgart, New York: Thieme/Verlag, 1982, pp 484–497
47. Tasker RR, Hawrylshyn P, Row IH, et al: Computerized graphic display of results of subcortical stimulation during stereotactic surgery. *Acta Neurochir [Suppl]* (Wien) 24:85–98, 1977
48. Tasker RR, Organ LW, Hawrylshyn PA: *The Thalamus and Midbrain of Man. A Physiological Atlas Using Electrical Stimulation.* Springfield, IL: Thomas, 1982
49. Todd EM: *Todd-Wells Manual of Stereotactic Procedures.* Randolph, MA: Codman and Shurtleff, 1967
50. Van Buren JM, Borke RC: *Variations and Connections of the Human Thalamus.* Vol 2, *Variations of the Human Diencephalon.* New York: Springer, 1972

2. THE IMAGING-COMPATIBLE RIECHERT-MUNDINGER SYSTEM

Fritz Mundinger
Walter Birg

The Riechert-Mundinger stereotactic system [36, 37] as updated by Mundinger and Birg is compatible with computed tomography (CT) and magnetic resonance imaging (MRI) (figure 2–1) [1–4, 6]. Clinical experience with 9,000 operations in Freiburg, West Germany led to the development of this device, which offers some unique advantages. Any target within the brain can be reached from any site of the face or skull. After the base ring is attached to the patient's skull, it is completely unmovable, even by involuntary movement of the patient. The ring is attached to a holder that can be fixed anywhere, which allows the operation to be performed with the patient either sitting, prone, or supine. If necessary the device can be removed easily from the table holder, as when epileptic seizures occur. It can be fixed in a position that does not correspond exactly to the anterior commissure—posterior commissure line without affecting precision in reaching the target. A special version of the base ring is available for MRI. For CT and MRI stereotaxy, the ring can be fixed in position to the imaging devices by means of an especially adapted holder, making coordinate calculations unnecessary. The stereotactic coordinates are taken directly from the CT or MRI images [5, 7, 21].

The arc with the electrode holder can be attached to the patient's skull in 16 different positions, detailed later in this chapter. The electrode or probe position can be checked radiographically, because the brain and skull structures of interest are not covered by any parts of the device. Using conventional roentgen-ray techniques for target determinations, long distances between the roentgen-ray source and target are desirable but not mandatory, as an image converter can be used for radiography [30, 34]. No special operating room is needed for use of the apparatus; it can be used in any operating room or radiology suite (figure 2–2).

Various parts of the device are stored in a special box containing sterilizable insets, which enables the device to be used in a variety of clinical situations. The stereotactic base ring and target arc and some probes and electrodes are sufficient basic equipment. This equipment can be augmented modularly as warranted.

Theory

This stereotactic system works according to the polar coordinate principle (figure 2–3). Details of the mathematical deduction of the five setting parameters—alpha, beta, phi, psi, and NT—are described elsewhere [2, 3]. The final formulas for the determination of the parameters are as follows:

Alpha = arctan (W2/gx)

Beta = arctan (gz/gy)

Psi = arctan (W1/sqr [w2 * w2 − w1 * w1])

Phi = arctan (sqr [1 − w1 * w1/w2 * w2 − ex * ex]/ex) − alpha (if ex ⟨ ⟩ 0)

Phi = PI/2 − alpha (if ex = 0)

NT = 312.5 − L1

L.D. Lunsford (ed.) *MODERN STEREOTACTIC NEUROSURGERY*.

Martinus Nijhoff Publishing. Boston/Dordrecht/Lancaster.

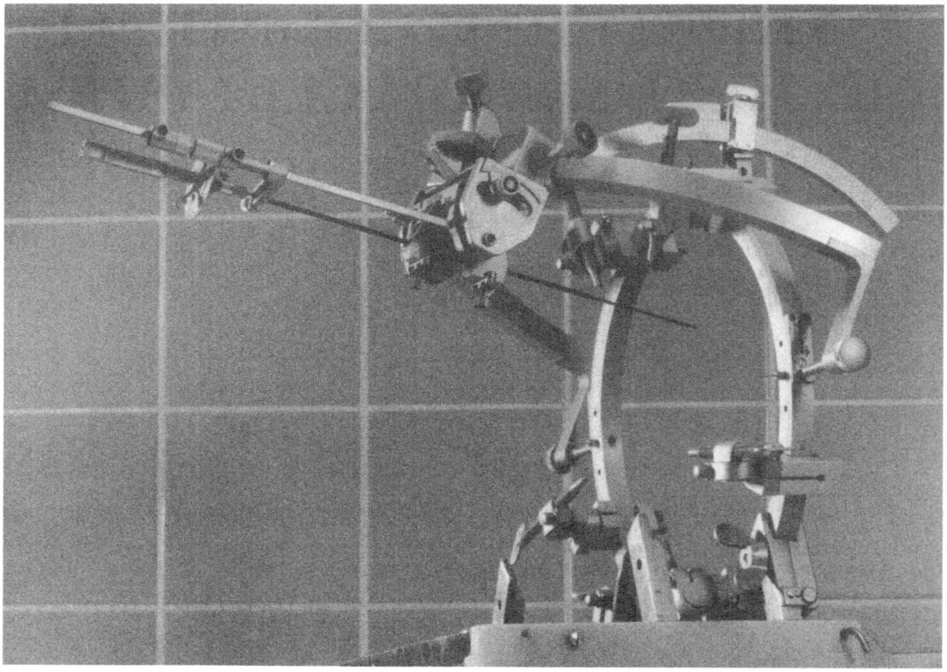

FIGURE 2–1. The Reichert-Mundinger stereotactic device in its computer-compatible version, designed by the authors. The target arc is fixed on the base ring by a segmental arc. For radiographic imaging, the ring is positioned on a fixation device on the operating table.

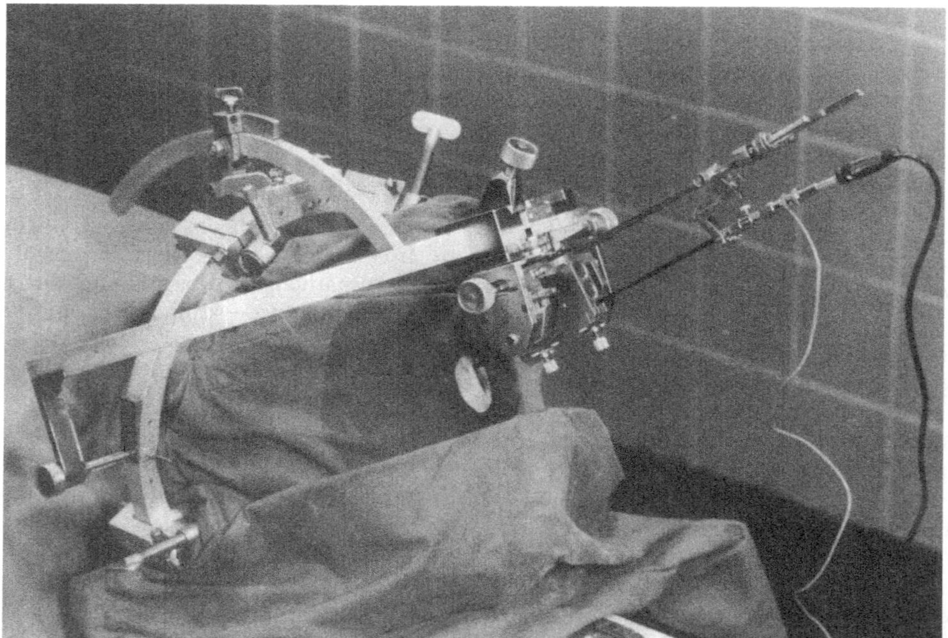

FIGURE 2–2. An operation in progress. The electrode path is calculated by a computer. The target arc and the electrode holder with vernier scales can be seen.

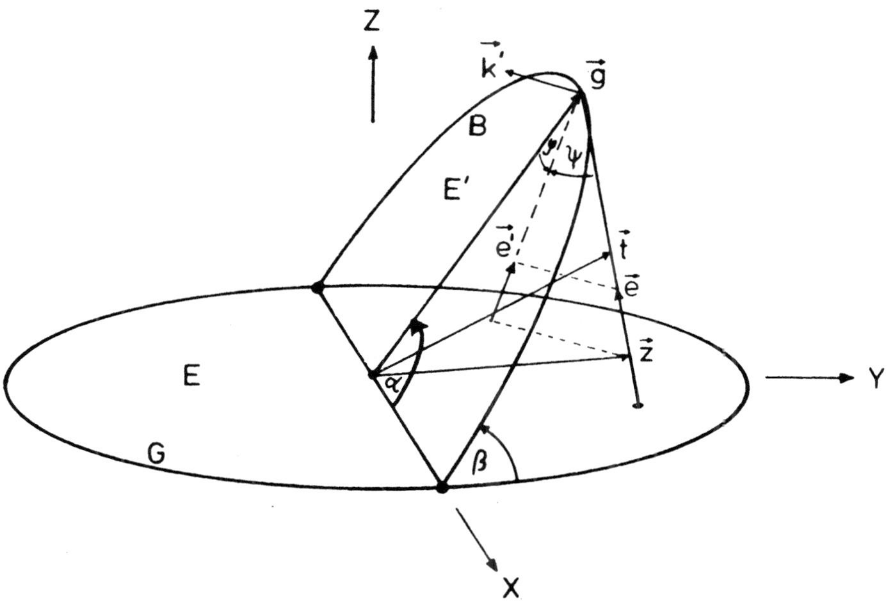

FIGURE 2–3. Mathematic principle of the stereotactic device. The four setting parameters are (α) alpha, (β) beta, (φ) phi, and (Ψ) psi. Plane E is the plane of the base ring; plane E′ is the (effective) plane of the target arc. T = the trephination point;
Z = the target. The position of the target arc is determined by the β angle, the position of the electrode holder by the α angle. The direction of the electrode is marked by the two polar coordinate angles, φ and Ψ. The needle depth corresponds to the distance GL − Z, denoted "NT."

The abbreviations are:

T = (tx, ty, tz) the trephination point

Z = (zx, zy, zz) the target point

r = Radius of the target arc

L1 = sqr [(t − z) * (t − z)]

ex = (tx − zx)/L1

ey = (ty − zy)/L1

ez = (tz − zz)/L1

L = −(z * e) + sqr ((z * e) * (z * e) − z * z + r * r)

gx = zx + L * ex

gy = zy + L * ey

gz = zz + L * ez

W1 = ey * gz − ez * gy

W2 = sqr (gy * gy + gz * gz)

The coordinates also can be determined without mathematically calculating the setting parameters by means of the phantom device. A ring marking the burr-hole point is set to the planned trephination point on the patient's head with a holder fixed to the base ring. In the same position, the holder is transferred to the base ring of the phantom device. The target marker of the phantom device then is set to the target point by means of a holder that can move in three axes. The target arc is adjusted empirically so that the introduced electrode hits precisely the predetermined target point. The angles and needle depths are documented, and the target arc with preset target parameters is transferred to the base ring on the patient's head.

Using mathematical calculations instead of the phantom, however, offers several advantages. Sterility problems resulting from the transfer procedure can be avoided. Also, this method is less time-consuming. Above all, the need for different or additional target points sometimes is not apparent until the operation is in progress; in such cases, it is much easier to determine the new setting with a computer than with the phantom. Cases in which exact predetermination of the trephination point is intended and procedures using CT and MRI also call for computer calculation.

Accuracy

The mechanical accuracy of the current Riechert-Mundinger device is very high (approximately ±0.1 mm) because of the limited setting precision. The effective accuracy, which takes into consideration slight electrode distortions, is approximately ±0.5 mm. Errors in target placement can result from intraoperative transfer of the radiography or CT coordinates. Errors that may result from roentgenogram transfer have been examined by Mundinger and Uhl [34], who studied the accuracy in transferring CT coordinates using a modified stereotactic phantom device secured directly to the CT scanner. In this study, the preset phantom coordinates were compared with the coordinates actually measured on the CT image. The accuracy was ±0.3 mm. For MRI, such results have not yet been established. However, the accuracy range probably will be approximately ±0.6 mm.

Modes of Fixation

As stated earlier, the stereotactic device can be fixed to the patient's head in any of 16 positions, which vary according to both the chosen height angle and the orientation of the target arc. The height angle (beta) can be set at approximately 45°, 135°, 225°, and 315°, and each angle has two possible target arc orientations. Additionally, the head fixation screws can be attached either above or below the base ring plane, making possible the 16 different placements. Thus, the optimal approach can be used, even in highly complicated surgical situations (e.g., an approach through the posterior cranial fossa or when patients are in the lateral position). The ability to fix the screws in two ways is a great advantage, because the base ring can be placed above or below the operation site.

Two of these 16 fixation modes are of special interest: target arc in a normal or rotated position. In both cases, the choice of coordinate axes is important. Usually, we direct the X axis toward the right ear, the Y axis toward the nose, and the Z axis toward the vertex. Use of these coordinates produces the correct setting parameters when the normal fixation modes are selected. With the target arc rotated, however, Y must be replaced with −Y in the computer calculations.

Range of Application

COMPUTED TOMOGRAPHY

Although the stereotactic device can be used independently, it frequently is combined with other diagnostic and therapeutic techniques, notably CT [5, 12, 13, 21–25] and MRI [7] as well as brachy Curietherapy or Curietherapy [18, 20].

To use our apparatus with CT (figures 2–4 through 2–6), we attach a holder to the CT-scanner bed. The base ring of the stereotactic device, attached to the skull in either a high cranial or low basal position, and thus can be adjusted precisely in the center of the CT gantry (see figures 2–4, 2–6). With the device fixed in this way, the same X and Y coordinates apply to both the stereotactic device [5, 21] and the CT image. Tumor implantation coordinates for Curietherapy can be determined on the CT images and calculated with the software of the CT scanner. The coordinates subsequently can be entered in the computer to calculate the final stereotactic coordinate settings.

It is also possible to choose the trephination point and the approach angle for the probe directly on the CT monitor. In this way, we have determined all parameters required for the operation immediately after the CT examination. For optimal documentation and for comparison with the intraoperative roentgenograms, the target and trephination points taken from the CT images also are transposed to the corresponding stereotactic roentgenograms (electronic radiographs).

MAGNETIC RESONANCE IMAGING

To adapt our stereotactic device for MRI (figure 2–7) [7], the base ring had to be modified. The metal alloy of the apparatus was replaced by a plastic material, because ferrous

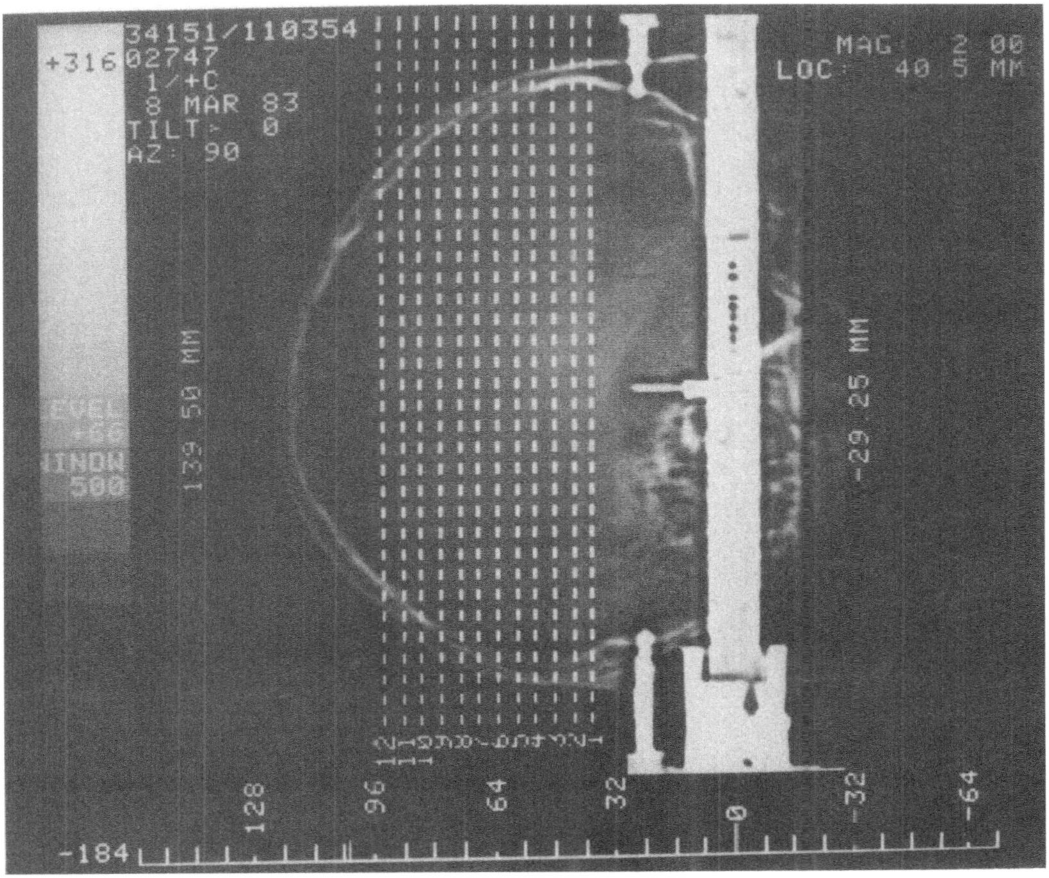

FIGURE 2–4. CT stereotactic surgery. By means of an electronic sagittal radiograph, the levels of the CT images are selected. The zero point of the ring coincides with the zero point of the CT system; the scan planes must be parallel to the ring plane.

metal parts in the examination area of the MRI scanner can produce artifacts. So it can be precisely located, the plastic base ring contains a concentrically arranged reservoir on the inside, filled with a paramagnetic liquid. This leads to projection of light "spots" on the sagittal and coronal images; these "spots" are used to define the coordinate axes. As with CT, coordinates corresponding to those of the stereotactic device can be obtained directly from the MRI image. The surgeon takes the required target and trephination coordinates directly from the MRI monitor and calculates the stereotactic coordinates as it has with the CT the stereotaxy (several thousand successful operations), this has proved to be a great advantage to us.

Clinical Indications

The stereotactic apparatus can be utilized without restriction for all current clinical indications [10, 19, 27, 29, 33, 35]. Because any point in the cranial cavity can be targeted precisely from any entry point of the face or skull, approaches ranging from frontal to occipital and parietal to temporal are possible. Approaches through the face are also possible, for example, transnasally for hypophysectomies, transbuccally for clival lesions, transorbitally for retroorbital lesions or for lesions in the facial region.

Using the transcerebellar approach, the cerebellum and cerebellopontine angles and the brain stem as far as the medulla area can be reached for both functional and nonfunctional

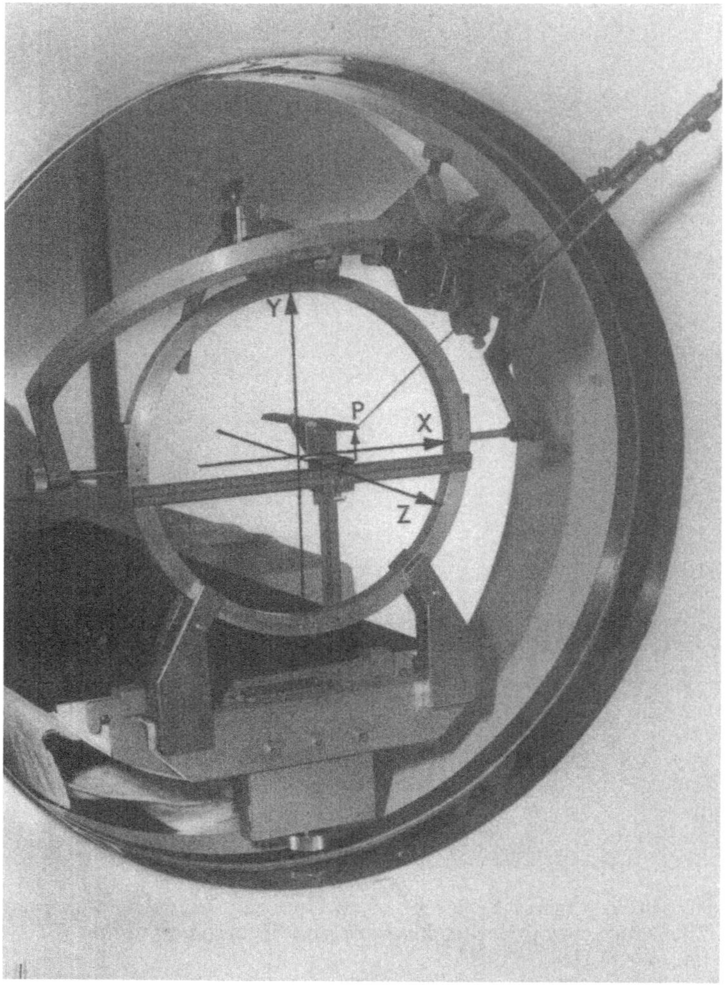

FIGURE 2–5. The stereotactic device inside the scanner gantry. If the zero point of the stereotactic device is in the origin of the CT scanner and the ring plane is parallel to the scan plane, the Cartesian target-point coordinates of the stereotactic device will be identical to the coordinate of the CT scanner.

stereotactic surgery. With ventral or dorsal and lateral-cervical approaches, lesions or structures in the region of the cervical vertebral column and the cervical region of the spinal cord can be reached. Clinical indications for functional and nonfunctional stereotactic surgery at our center are listed in tables 2–1 and 2–2.

Operative Technique

NONFUNCTIONAL NEUROSURGERY

As a rule, patients are given local anesthesia; general anesthesia is used only for children under six years of age or when the transcerebellar approach has been chosen. The operation is performed in an operating room adjacement to the CT scanner. In the operating room, the base ring is fixed to the patient's head in either a low or high position, and depending upon the location of the tumor, with screws either cranial or basal. After two roentgenograms are obtained, the patient is taken to the scanner room. With the aid of the laser-positioning system and by adjustment of the scanner table, the base ring is positioned so that its center corresponds to the center of the CT scanner and so that the scanning planes and base ring plane are parallel. The coordinates of the

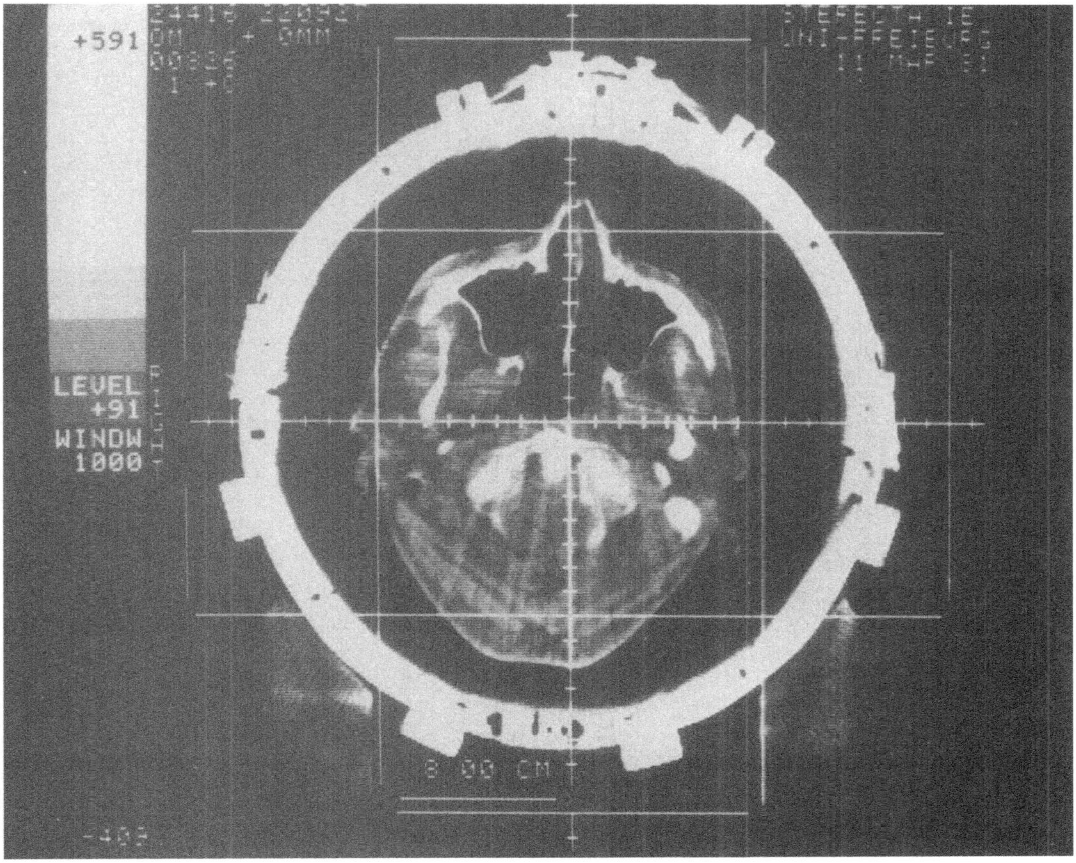

FIGURE 2-6. CT image on the zero level (Z = 0 mm). With the grid feature, coincidence of the coordinate systems of the scanner and the stereotactic device can be verified.

stereotactic system should coincide with those of the scanner; this is confirmed with the grid feature (see figure 2-6). After the necessary CT images are obtained, the area of the target structure is measured with the aid of the grid and circle features of the scanner software. For example, the tumor radius and the coordinates can be measured by means of the region-of-interest indicator. The tumor size parameters can be determined more precisely with the use of sagittal and coronal reformations; the direction of an approach is determined with a second (trephination) point (figures 2-8 and 2-9). The coordinates thus obtained are transferred to the original roentgenograms, and the coordinates for the stereotactic device are calculated. This calculation is performed using a separate personal computer, which also calculates the dosimetry.

The calculated parameters (four angles and the needle depth) are set and verified, and a 6-mm burr hole is made in preparation for the biopsy. After the dura is coagulated, the biopsy forceps are led slowly through the outer cannula. The first biopsies are taken before the tumor surface is reached; in cases where peritumoral edema or reactive gliosis is suspected, this is especially important for the demarcation of the tumor and for the dosimetry. Subsequent biopsies are performed every 1–2 mm until the target and, in many cases, until the other side of the tumor, is reached. Altogether, five to 20 tumor samples are taken for analysis (paraffin embedding and special staining) by the neuropathologist(s). Intraoperatively, a differential diagnosis of the tumor is carried out immediately, based on smear preparations and staining with methylene blue; thus, if necessary, radiotherapy of the tumor can follow immediately.

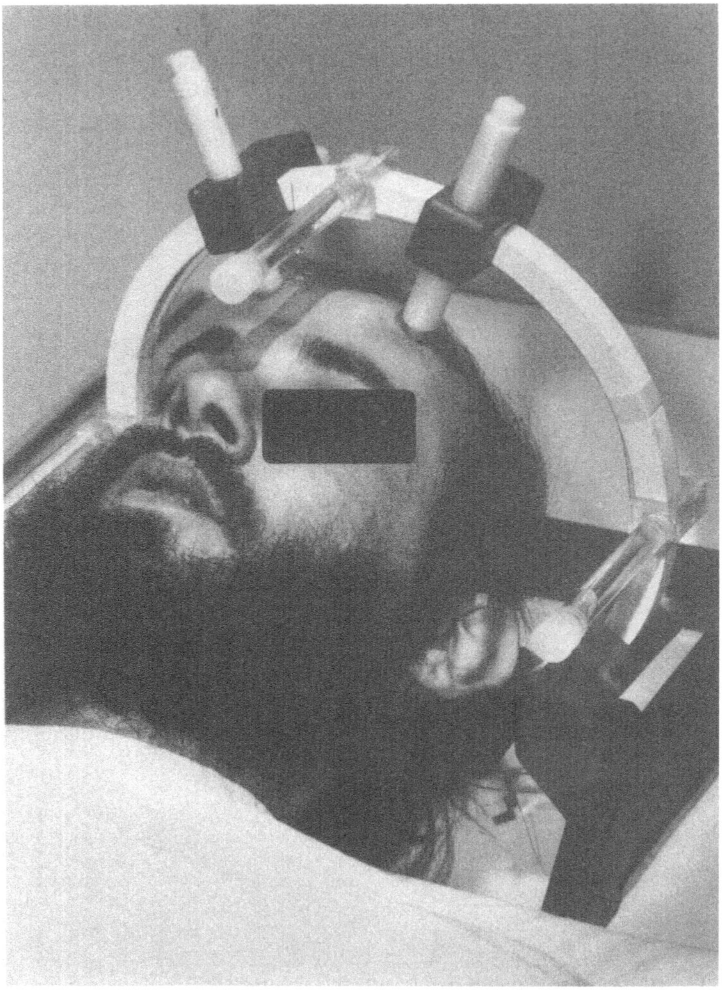

FIGURE 2-7. MRI stereotactic device developed by Mundinger and Birg et al. [7]. The stereotactic ring and the fixation screws are made from a special plastic material. Small steel pins which do not disturb the MRI process are attached to the tip of the screws.

TABLE 2-1. Clinical Indications for Stereotactic Radiotherapy at the University of Freiburg

Type of Therapy	Clinical Indications
Brachy Curietherapy + external irradiation (±chemotherapy)	Anaplastic glioma (grade III), astrocytoma, glioblastoma, malignant ependymoma, melanoma, medulloblastoma, sarcoma, metastatic tumors
Brachy Curietherapy alone	Small-volume malignant tumors that recur as malignant tumors after external irradiation
Curietherapy alone	Cyst; small-volume glioma; glial (grades I, II), nonglial, and extracerebral tumors; pituitary adenoma recurrences, ependymoma; dysontogenetic tumors; extracerebral benign or invasive tumors; malignant midline tumors
Curietherapy plus external irradiation	Anaplastic glioma (grades II, III); germinoma; pinealoblastoma and pinealtoma
External irradiation (including neuroaxis)	Inoperable large-volume anaplastic glioma; multiple metastases; medulloblastoma; germinoma; malignant extracerebral tumors; primitive neuroectodermal tumors

TABLE 2–2. Indications for CT-Stereotactic High-Dose-Rate Brachy Curietherapy (^{192}Ir or ^{125}I) of Intracranial Malignant Turmors[a]

Type of Therapy	Indications
Primary	Small volume hemispheric tumors
	Tumors in functionally important regions (central, temporal, parietal)
	Nonresectable deep-seated tumors
Secondary	Tumors recurring after operation and external beam irradiation[b]

[a] Temporary implantation technique after obligatory biopsy.
[b] Not indicated in lesions involving midline cerebral structures.

If radiotherapeutical measures are chosen, the following techniques may be used according to the type, grade, and location of the tumor; (1) permanent implantation of a radioisotope (iodine-125 [^{125}I] or iridium-192 [^{192}Ir] [8, 9, 14–17, 19, 26, 28, 31] or (2) irradiation of the tumor using the afterloading technique (^{125}I catheter or ^{192}Ir contact radiation device GammaMed®) [17]. Tables 2–1 and 2–2 show our criteria for using both methods. When permanent implantation of ^{125}I is planned, the radioactivity to be implanted and the configuration of the implanted sources first are calculated. Afterwards, the implanted cannula is placed at the predetermined parts of the tumor, and the seeds are implanted (figure 2–10).

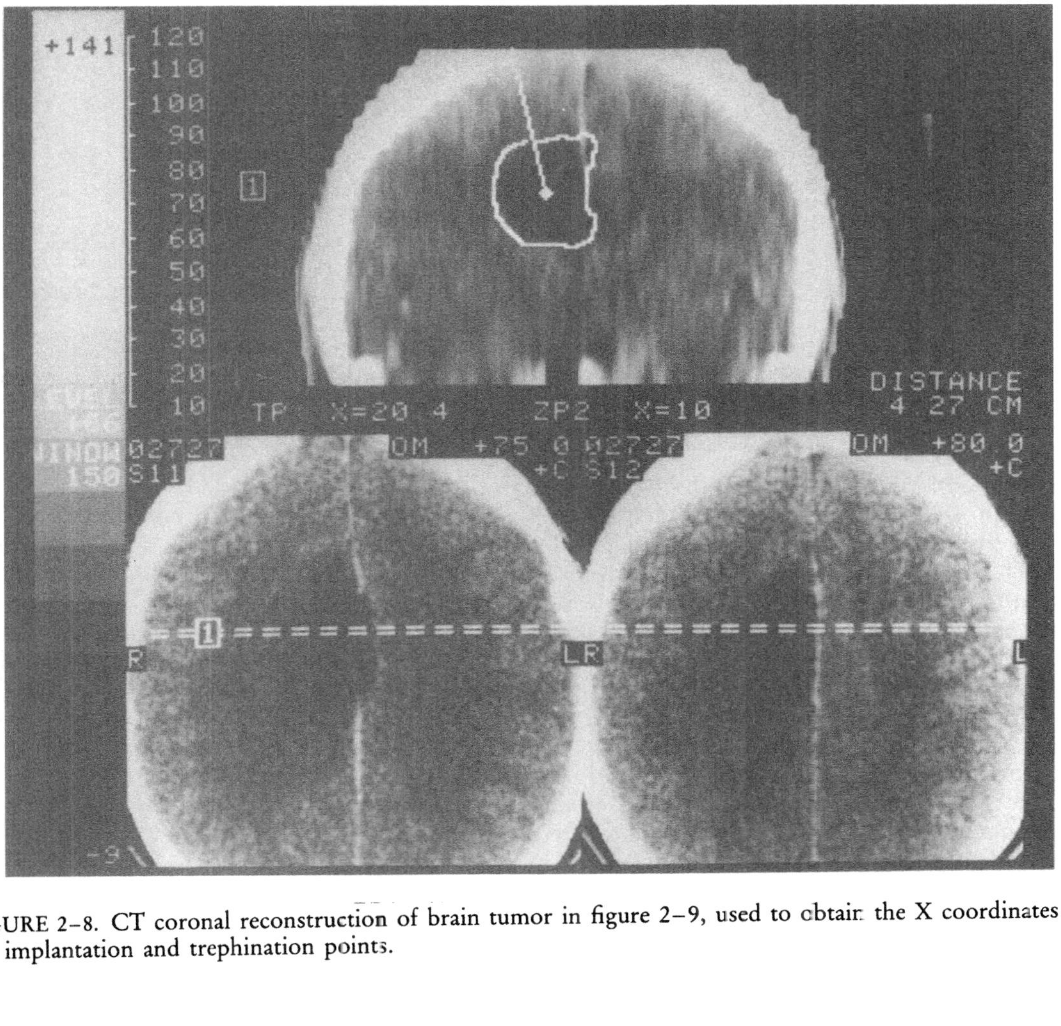

FIGURE 2–8. CT coronal reconstruction of brain tumor in figure 2–9, used to obtain the X coordinates of the implantation and trephination points.

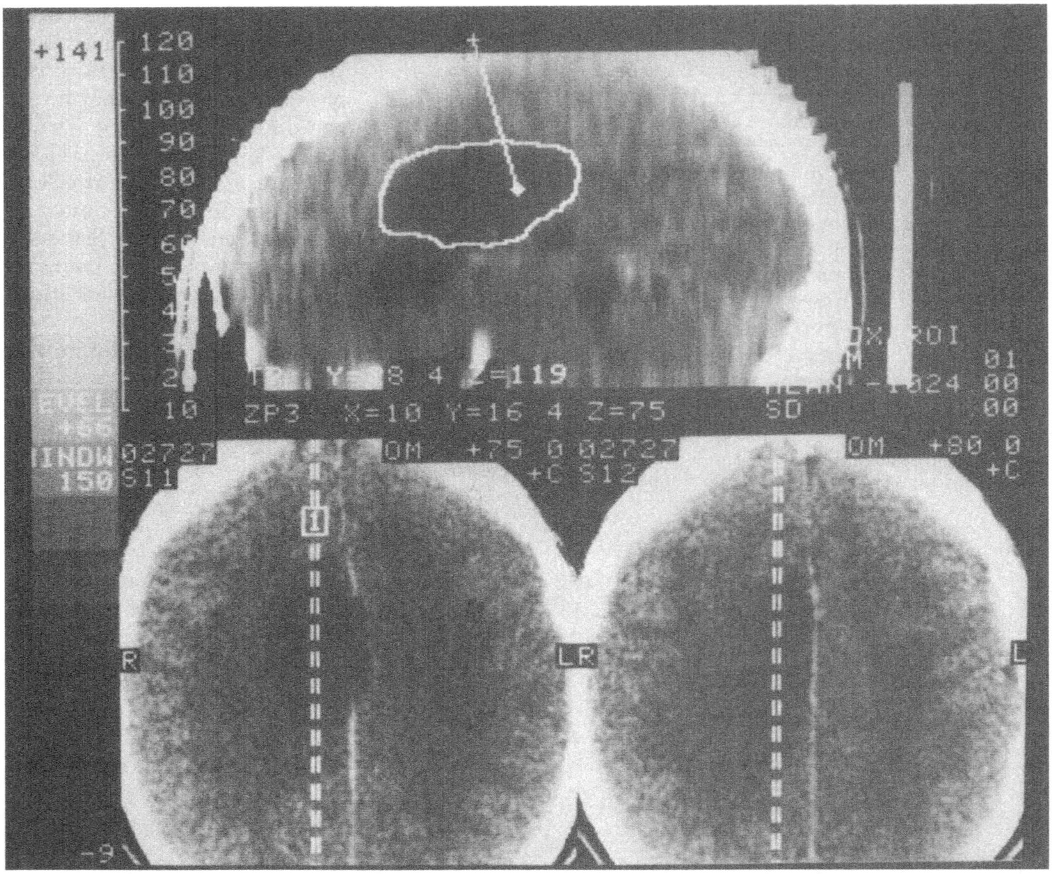

FIGURE 2–9. CT sagittal reconstruction of the brain tumor traced by the electronic trace feature of the CT scanner. The first implantation point and the trephination point are marked. Because the coordinate systems coincide, the coordinates measured by this procedure are the same as for the stereotactic device.

FUNCTIONAL NEUROSURGERY

Although we developed a method for determining the functional target points using CT [5, 21] or MRI, in most cases we still use contrast ventriculography. A regression technique is used to calculate the approximate coordinates for the foramen of Monro from the skull height and length on the sagittal and frontal films [11, 32]. Ventriculography then is performed. After calculating the foramen of Monro and posterior commissure locations and determining the target point from a stereotactic atlas, the target point coordinates are obtained through computer "streching" of the atlas topography [1, 4, 6, 36, 37].

A suitable trephination point 65° sagittal to the base line and 10° coronal to the midsagittal plane is determined. The coordinates of the trephination and target points are entered in the computer, which calculates the device parameters. After the stereotactic device is adjusted accordingly, the burr hole is drilled.

The coagulation electrode is introduced to the target point, and physiological stimulus checks are performed to confirm that the target has been reached. Using the appropriate coagulation parameters, temperature-regulated coagulation is performed with the side-exit electrode, which is adapted to the structure to be ablated.

Tables 2–3 and 2–4 list the indications for which we have performed stereotactic operations.

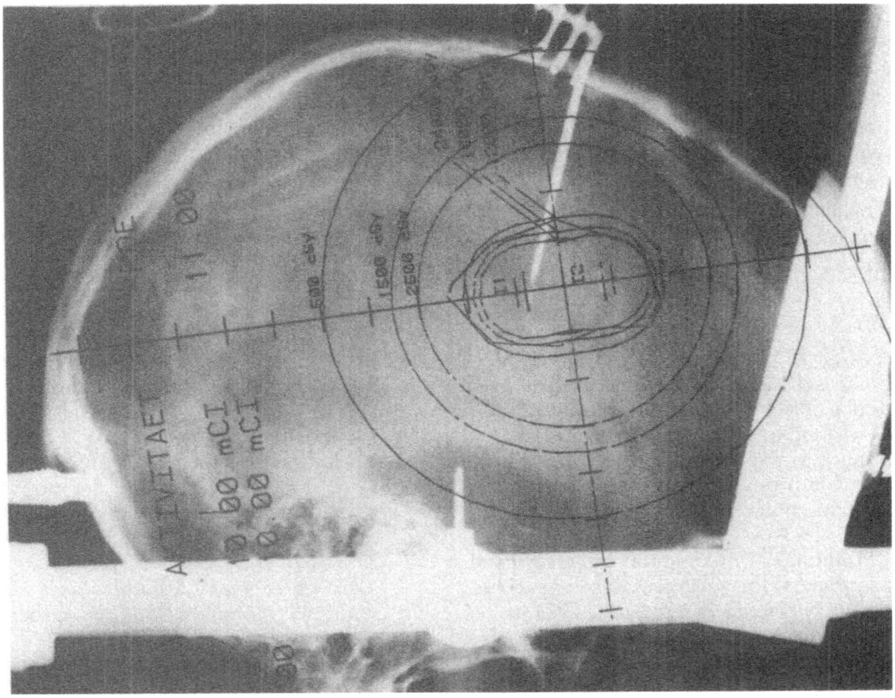

FIGURE 2-10. The computer-calculated isodose curves are transposed onto the roentgenogram.

TABLE 2-3. Stereotactic Operations Performed at University Hospital, Freiburg, West Germany[a]

Surgical Indication	No. of Operations
Parkinsonism	3,890
Hyperkinesia	1,331
Curietherapy	1,665
Biopsy only[b]	1,005
Intractable pain	415
Psychiatric surgery	174
Epilepsy	111
Angioma	17
Combined stereotactic/ open pituitary surgery	107
Other	473
Total	9,188

a. 1950–Dec. 31, 1985
b. After 1965

TABLE 2-4. Indications for Stereotactic Operations for Extrapyramidal Disorders Performed at University Hospital, Freiburg, West Germany, (1950–March 7, 1986)

Indication	No. of Operations
Parkinsonism	3,900
Choreoathetosis	215
Torsion dystonia	214
Spasmodic torticollis	231
Ballismus	26
Myoclonus	52
Gilles de la Tourette syndrome	18
Intention tremor (essential or hereditary) and action myoclonus (multiple sclerosis, trauma)	340
Mixed and spastic hyperkinesia	172
Total	5,168

Summary

The Riechert-Mundinger system has been used extensively at our center since 1950 (more than 9,000 stereotactic operations). Recent modifications have adapted this device to advances in computer and imaging capabilities. The versatility of this device has been shown in cases of both functional and morphological (tumor) neurosurgery of the brain.

References

1. Birg W, Klar M, Mundinger F: Programmierbare Taschenrechner bei stereotaktischen Hirnoperationen. *Med Klin* 72:135–136, 1977
2. Birg W, Mundinger F: Calculation of the position of a side-protruding electrode tip in stereotactic brain operations using a stereotactic apparatus with polar coordinates. *Acta Neurochir* (Wien) 32:83–87, 1975
3. Birg W, Mundinger F: Computer calculations of target parameters for a stereotactic apparatus. *Acta Neurochir* (Wien) 29:123–129, 1973
4. Birg W, Mundinger F: Computer programs for stereotactic neurosurgery. *Confin Neurol* 36: 326–333, 1974
5. Birg W, Mundinger F: Direct target point determination for stereotactic brain operations from CT data and the calculation of setting parameters for polar-coordinate stereotactic devices. *Appl Neurophysiol* 45:387–395, 1982
6. Birg W, Mundinger F, Klar M: Computer assistance for stereotactic brain operations. *Adv Neurosurg* 4:287–291, 1977
7. Birg W, Mundinger F, Mohadjer M, et al: X-ray and MR-stereotaxy for functional and nonfunctional neurosurgery. *Appl Neurophysiol* 48:22–29, 1985
8. Birg W, Schneider J, Bauer S, et al: An interactive program system for the stereotactic interstitial implantation of radionuclides in brain tumors. In Szikla G (ed): *Stereotactic Cerebral Irradiation* Inserm Symposium No. 12. New York: Elsvier/North-Holland Biomedical Press, 1979, pp 77–80
9. Dyck P: *Stereotactic Biopsy and Brachytherapy of Brain Tumors*. Baltimore: University Park Press, 1983
10. Hassler RF, Mundinger F, Riechert T: *Stereotaxis in Parkinson Syndrome*. Berlin, Heidelberg, New York: Springer, 1979
11. Hoefer T, Mundinger F, Birg W, et al: Computer calculation in localizing subcortical targets in plane x-rays for stereotactic neurosurgery. *Confin Neurol* 36:334–340, 1974
12. Mundinger F: CT-stereotactic biopsy for optimizing the therapy of intracranial processes. *Acta Neurochir* (Wien) 35:70–74, 1985
13. Mundinger F: CT-stereotactic biopsy of brain tumors. In Voth, D Gutjahr P, Langmaid C (eds): Tumors of the Central Nervous System in Infancy and Childhood. Berlin Heidelberg: Springer, 1982
14. Mundinger F: Implantation of radioisotopes. In Schaltenbrand G, Walker AE (eds): *Stereotaxy of the Human Brain*. Stuttgart: Thieme, 1982, pp 410–445
15. Mundinger F: Stereotactic biopsy and technique of implantation (instillation) of radionuclei. In Jellinger K (ed): *Therapy of Malignant Brain Tumors*. Wien, New York: Springer, 1987, pp 134–184
16. Mundinger F: Stereotactic interstitial therapy of nonresectable intracranial tumors with iridium-192 and iodine-125. In Karcher KH, et al (eds): *Progress in Radio-Oncology* (2nd ed). New York: Raven Press, 1982, pp 371–380
17. Mundinger F: Stereotaktische interstitielle Therapie nicht resezierbarer intracranieller Tumoren mit Ir-192 und Jod-125. In Wannenmacher M, Schreiber HW, Gauwerky F (eds): *Kombinierte Chirurgischeund Radiologische Behandlung. Maligner Tumoren*. Munich: Urban & Schwarzenberg, 1981, pp 90–112
18. Mundinger F: *Stereotaktische Operationen am Gehirn Grundlagen—Indikationen—Resultate*. Stuttgart: Hippokrates, 1975
19. Mundinger F: 30 Jahre stereotaktische Hirnoperationen beim Parkinsonismus (Ergebnisse im Vergleich pallido-thalamosubtahalamischer Ausschaltungen und Indikationen. In Gaenshirt H (ed): *Pathophysiologie, Klinik und Therapie des Parkinsonismus*. Editiones Roche, 1983, pp 331–357
20. Mundinger F: The treatment of brain tumors with interstitially applied radioactive isotopes. In Wang Y (ed): *Radionuclide Applications in Neurology and Neurosurgery*. Springfield, IL: Thomas, 1970, pp 199–265
21. Mundinger F, Birg W: CT-aided stereotaxy for functional neurosurgery and deep brain implants. *Acta Neurochir* (Wien) 56:245, 1981
22. Mundinger F, Birg W: CT-stereotaxy in the clinical routine. *Neurosurg Rev* 7:219–224, 1984
23. Mundinger F, Birg W: Stereotactic biopsy of intracranial processes. *Acta Neurochir* [Suppl] (Wien) 33:219–224, 1984
24. Mundinger F, Birg W: Stereotactic brain surgery with the aid of computed tomography (CT-stereotaxy). 32 Jahrestagung der Deutschen Gesellschaft fuer Neurochirurgie, Tubingen 4:22–25, 1981
25. Mundinger F, Birg W, Ostertag CB: Treatment of small cerebral gliomas with CT-aided stereotaxic curietherapy. *Neuroradiology* 16: 564–567, 1978
26. Mundinger F, Busam B, Birg W, et al: Results of interstitial iridium-192 brachy-Curietherapy

and iridium-192 protracted long-term irradiation, In Szikla G (ed): *Stereotactic Cerebral Irradiation*. Inserm Symposium No. 12. New York: Elsevier/North Holland Biomedical Press, 1979, pp 303–320

27. Mundinger F, Disselhoff J: Indications of stereotactic operations in torsion dystonia and choreoathetosis on the basis of long-term comparative studies. In *Progress in Pediatric Neurosurgery*, 1974, pp 237–240
28. Mundinger F, Metzel E: Interstitial radioisotope therapy of intractable diencephalic tumors by the stereotactic permanent implantation of iridium-192, including bioptic control. *Confin Neurol* 32:195–202, 1970
29. Mundinger F, Meyer-Tuwe W: Ergebnisse der stereotaktischen Behandlung des Parkinson-Rigors. In Fischer PA (ed): *Langzeitbehandlung des Parkinson-Syndroms*. Stuttgart, New York: Schattauer-Verlag, 1978, pp 179–188
30. Mundinger F, Mintert F, Gurkmann O, et al: Wie genau konnen vorausberechnete tiefliegende Hirnstrukturen mit dem stereotaktischen Zielverfahren mit einer Sonde erreicht werden? *Dtsch Med Wochenschr* 44:2224–2233, 1970
31. Mundinger F, Ostertag C, Birg W, et al: Stereotactic treatment of brain lesions, biopsy, interstitial radiotherapy (iridium-192 and iodine-125) and drainage procedures. *Appl Neurophysiol* 43:198–204, 1980
32. Mundinger F, Reinke MA, Hoefer T, et al: Determination of intracerebral structures using osseous reference points for computer-aided stereotactic operations. *Appl Neurophysiol* 38:3–22, 1975
33. Mundinger F, Riechert T: Indikationen und Langzeitergebnisse von 1400 uni-und bilateralen stereotaktischen Eingriffen beim Parkinson syndrom. *Wien Z Nervenheilk* 23:147–177, 1966
34. Mundinger F, Uhl H: Uber die Genauigkeit der roentgenologischen Zielpunktbestimmung bei stereotaktischen Hirnoperationen. *Fortschr Roentgenstr* 103:419–431, 1965
35. Mundinger F, Wunsch W: 7-Jahres-Langzeitergebnisse der stereotaktischen Tremorbehandlung beim Parkinson syndrom. In Fischer PA (ed): *Parkinson-Syndrom: Kombinations- und Begleit-Therapien*. Stuttgart, New York: Schattauer, 1980, pp 199–210
36. Riechert T, Mundinger F: Beschreibung und Anwendung eines Zielgerates fur stereotaktische Hirnoperationen (II-Modell). *Acta Neurochir* (Wien) 3:308–337, 1956
37. Riechert T, Mundinger F: Stereotaktische Geraete. In *Einfuhrung in die stereotaktischen Operationen mit einem Atlas des menschlichen Gehirns*. Stuttgart: Thieme, 1959

3. THE LEKSELL SYSTEM

L. Dade Lunsford
Dan Leksell

Impressed by the work of Spiegel and Wycis in Philadelphia in 1947 [13], Lars Leksell returned to Stockholm with the goal of developing a stereotactic apparatus that was "easy to handle and practical in routine clinical work" [5]. The first Leksell instrument was reported in 1949 [5], and all succeeding versions of this device have remained constant to the goals of practicality, accuracy, and versatility (figure 3–1). Leksell was one of the first to recognize the role of stereotactic surgery in both functional and morphological neurosurgery and was also one of the first to apply stereotactic technique to the diagnosis and treatment of brain lesions. In 1951, he introduced what has since been called stereotactic radiosurgery, the production of intracerebral lesions by means of stereotactically guided ionizing radiation. Intracavitary treatment of cystic craniopharyngiomas with radioactive phosphorus-32 was reported in the same year [9]. At about the same time, Leksell suggested that stereotactic surgery be used to retrieve bullet fragments from the brains of soldiers injured in combat.

The principle of the Leksell stereotactic instrument is simple (figure 3–2):

> Essentially, it consists of a semicircular arc with a movable electrode (probe) carrier. The arc is fixed to the patient's head in such a manner that its center corresponds to the selected cerebral target. The electrodes are always directed towards the center and hence to the target. Rotation of the arc around the axis rods in association with lateral adjustment of the electrode carrier enables any convenient point of entrance of the electrodes to be chosen, independent of the site of the target [6].

For the operation, the arc is attached to a coordinate frame fixed to the patient's head. The frame is used to define the target by various radiological techniques. Frame modifications over the past 37 years have been concomitant with advances in neuro-imaging, beginning with pneumoencephalography and proceeding to angiography, computed tomography (CT), and magnetic resonance imaging (MRI). Paralleling the leaps in imaging technology, each generation of the instrument has expanded the role and the advantages of stereotactic surgery. The Leksell stereotactic system is used at more than 350 neurosurgical centers in 60 countries world-wide.

General Description of the Device

The modern Leksell stereotactic instrument (all-imaging-technique-compatible Model D) is fully compatible with all currently available imaging techniques. The device consists of a cubical rectilinear coordinate frame, 180 mm in each dimension, and a semicircular arc, which is attached to the frame at the chosen coordinates after target selection is completed. The arc has a sliding instrument carrier to hold the probes necessary for the planned surgical intervention. The Y (anterior-posterior) and Z (superior-inferior) coordinates are set on the frame by means of two side bars. The X (right-left) coordinate is set on one of the axes of the arc frame (figure 3–3).

The X, Y, and Z axes of the coordinate system conform with the X, Y, and Z nomenclature used in CT and MRI scanning. The frame origin (X, Y, Z = 0) is outside the upper posterior corner on the right side of the frame (figure 3–4).

Depending upon the imaging tool selected, one of three pairs of indicator plates is attached to the left and right sides of the frame (figure 3–5). When conventional radiography is used, the coordinates of the targets are selected in

L.D. Lunsford (ed.) *MODERN STEREOTACTIC NEUROSURGERY*.

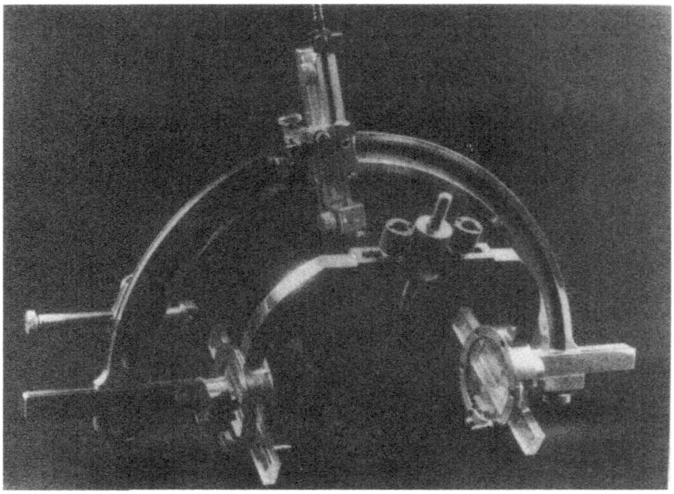

A

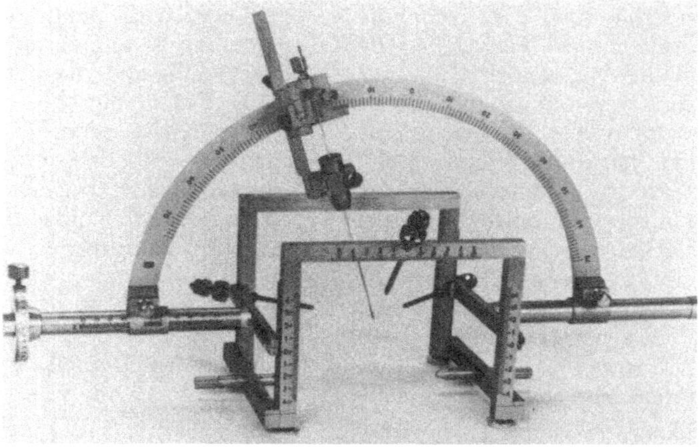

B

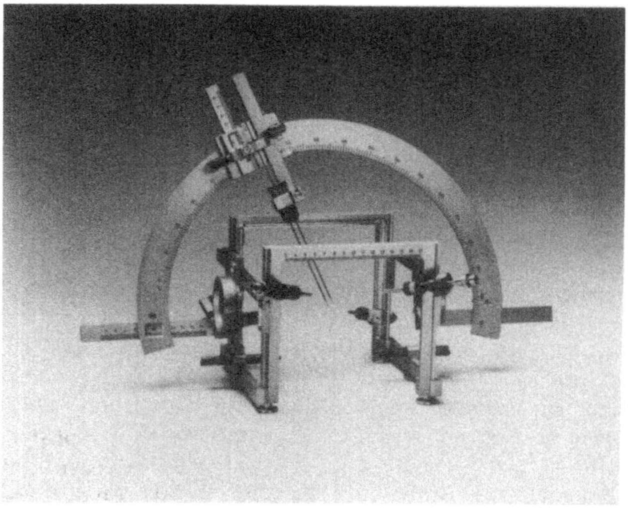

C

FIGURE 3-1. First Leksell stereotactic instrument, 1949, (A); Mark I, 1951 (B); Model D (all-imaging-technique-compatible) instrument (C).

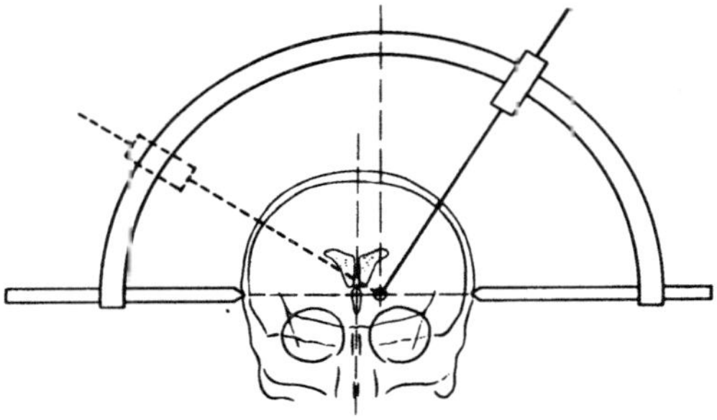

FIGURE 3–2. The arc principle of the instrument.

reference to the coordinate scales of the frame. In CT or MRI scanning, they are derived from fiducials generated by the coordinate indicators. To reach the target, the arc is attached to the frame at the chosen coordinates, an anatomically and functionally safe trajectory is selected, and the probe is advanced through the brain to a depth corresponding to the radius of the arc (190 mm). When the probe stop on the instrument carrier of the arc is set at zero, the tip of the probe hits the target with an accuracy of ±0.25 mm. The instrument is made of aluminum and weighs 1.8 kg.

Application of the Coordinate Frame

The coordinate frame is attached to the patient's head by means of four stainless steel drill bits. In most cases, application is performed with the patient in a sitting position. The skin at the proposed drill site is infiltrated with a local anesthetic.

Premedication with an anticholinergic and an

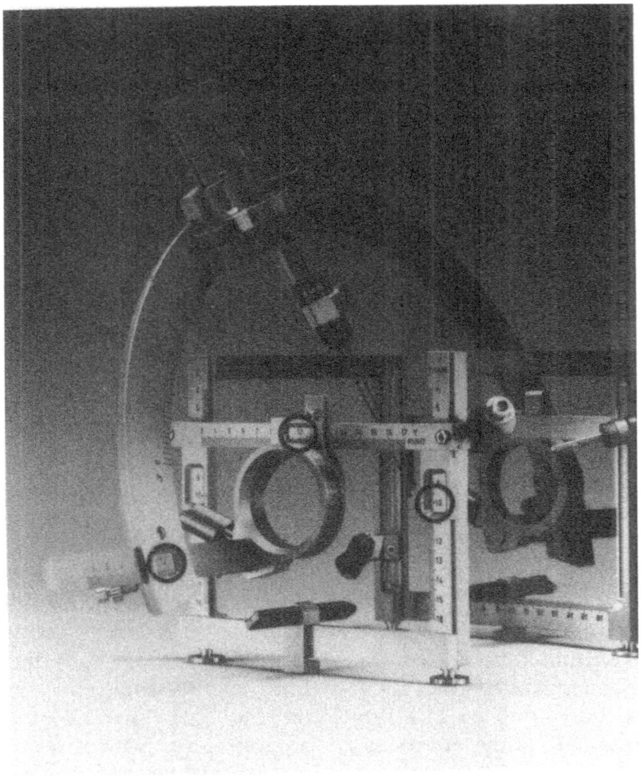

FIGURE 3–3. Setting the X, Y, and Z coordinates with the side bars and arc.

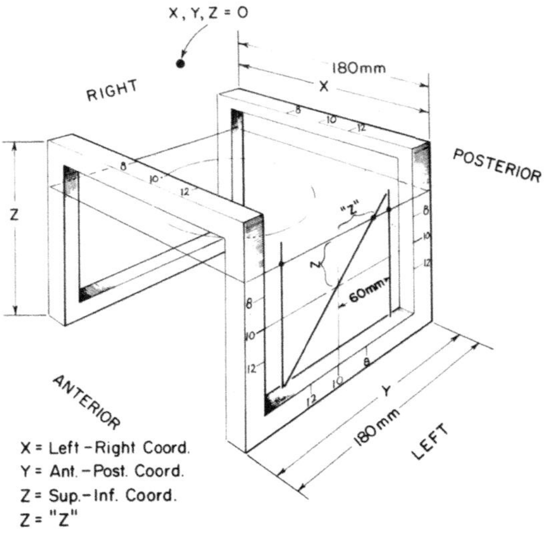

FIGURE 3-4. Origin of the coordinate system and the rectilinear X, Y, and Z coordinate system.

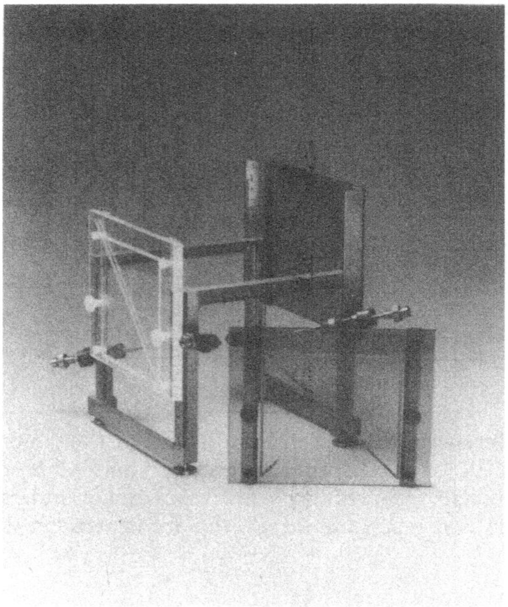

FIGURE 3-5. The three different coordinate indicator plates for radiography, CT and MRI.

anxiolyticdrug, occasionally supplemented by a narcotic, provides sufficient sedation in patients with mild to moderate anxiety. When necessary, the frame can be applied easily with the patient under general anesthesia and supine, the head supported by a suitable headrest [10]. Routine prepping of the entire head with alcohol prior to frame application ensures sterility and does not risk the image degradation seen when iodine preparation solutions are used with CT localization.

The position of the frame on the head is adjustable by means of ear plugs placed in the unanesthestized external auditory canals. Generally, the midline of the head should correspond to the midline of the frame. A steel sleeve containing the drill bit is used to punch through the scalp, after which bits 3.2 mm in diameter are drilled 3.5 mm into the outer table of the skull. The drills should be inserted diagonally to ensure proper tension of the frame against the skull. Standard drill bits are 110 mm in length, but longer bits (130 mm) are available for pediatric patients. Only those patients with the most severe macrocephaly are not able to fit satisfactorily within the frame. If CT is the imaging tool, the steel bits are replaced by carbon-fiber pins (materials of low atomic number are superior for CT imaging). Short fiberglass pins are used for MRI localization. The tips of these pins fit snugly into the previously made holes in the skull. Prior to imaging, the pins are checked serially to ensure proper tension and location within the drill holes. Secure attachment of the frame is tested by lifting the frame from above to verify that head and frame move together. Because the frame is light in weight, delays between frame application and imaging portions of the procedure are tolerated well by the patient.

Conventional Roentgenographic Target Localization

The x-ray–indicator side plates contain radiographically visible coordinate scales (tungsten); with the appropriate set attached to the frame, target coordinates can be obtained with plain film roentgenography, in cases with visible targets, or by means of encephalography and angiography. Both anterior-posterior and lateral films are necessary. The films are kept parallel to the coordinate frame by a coupling arm connecting the x-ray tube head to the frame (figure 3-6). A short-distance radiography unit, which maintains the frame in a constant

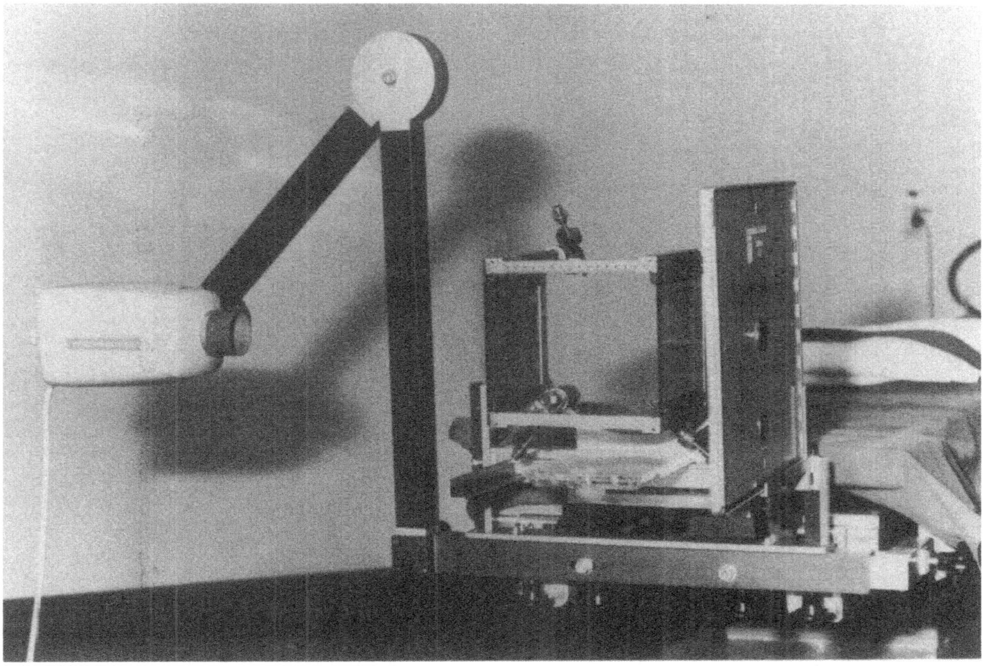

FIGURE 3–6. The table-mounted, short-distance radiography unit.

relationship to both tube head and cassette, considerably simplifies the target localization. It also ensures the repeatability of roentgenogram exposures, which can be exactly superimposed on each other. Leksell's ingenious construction of a geometric spiral diagram permits target-coordinate determination without the need for magnification, because of the short-distance roentgenogram exposures. His text eloquently discusses the usage of the spiral diagram [6]. Other localization methods include a graphic scale technique [12] and a desk-top stereotactic computer program. Both provide accurate coordinate determination, and neither requires anything more than the ability to visualize the target on the same film as the proximal and distal frame. With these methods, magnification becomes irrelevant, and any distance between tube head and film can be chosen. These methods for coordinate determination are particularly useful in combination with angiography.

CT Target Localization

The Leksell instrument is compatible with any advanced-generation CT scanner. Various frame adapters are available; their design depends on the CT manufacturer (figure 3–7). These adapters anchor to the scanner bed and keep the coordinate frame perpendicular to the gantry, which is not angled during imaging. The frame is attached to the magnetic adapter by iron footplates, which allow both rapid detachment and secure fixation.

Head fixation is maintained by the carbon-fiber pins, and then the CT-coordinate indicator plates are attached to the frame. Embedded in the indicator plates are three metallic bars, two vertical and one diagonal. These bars generate the necessary fiducial markers for target determination from axial CT images. The diagonal indicator descends from posterior-superior to anterior-inferior and determines the height of the CT scan within the frame, which is the Z coordinate of the target (figure 3–8) [7].

CT imaging is performed with a technique that is appropriate for the size of the target and the type of surgery. Most brain lesions undergoing stereotactic biopsy can be visualized well with 5-mm images incremented by 5-mm table movement. Three-millimeter images (5-mm thick, 3-mm table movement) increase detail as

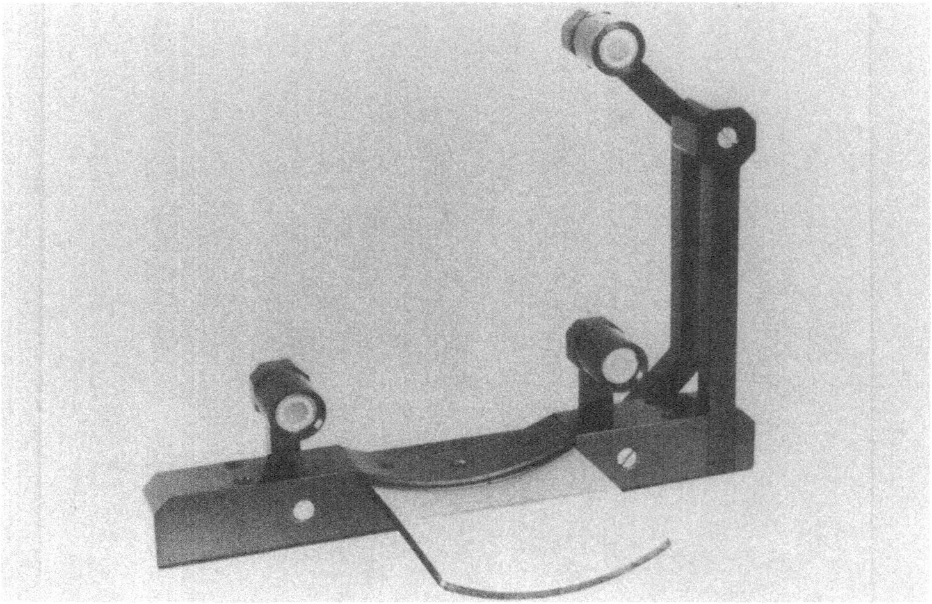

FIGURE 3–7. The CT adapter for anchoring the frame to the CT table.

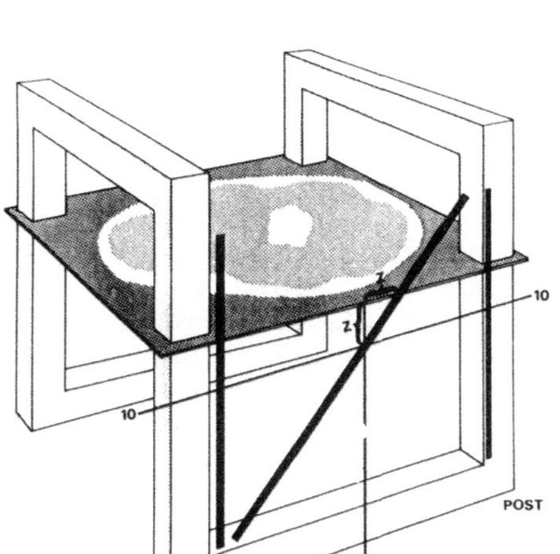

FIGURE 3–8. The diagonal indicator defines the Z coordinate.

well as quality of subsequent reformatted multiplanar images but are more time-consuming. Thicknesses of either 3 mm or 1.5 mm are used for functional procedures. Intravenous contrast infusion is performed in all patients except those with extreme contrast allergies. Both indicator plates have an additional short diagonal bar in the inferior-posterior corner that can be seen on the inferior CT images. These are used to confirm that the frame is perpendicular to the scanner gantry and that the two plates are correctly positioned on the frame. An axial CT image is obtained of sufficient reconstruction size (24 cm) to include both the head and the frame. Target coordinate determination can be performed on any axial CT image using one of the three possible techniques outlined below.

MANUAL GRID TECHNIQUE

A semitransparent scale placed on a viewing light box is used for manual coordinate determination. The scale, which is printed on a plastic disk, is magnified to correspond to the CT-film size preferred by the surgeon. As a rule, a large image is better than a small one. The fiducials on the CT film are aligned with the scale, whereupon the X, Y, and Z coordinates of the target are read directly (figure 3–9). This manual localization procedure is fast and accurate. It allows the target to be localized or modified in the operating room, and it safeguards the surgical procedure against computer malfunctions.

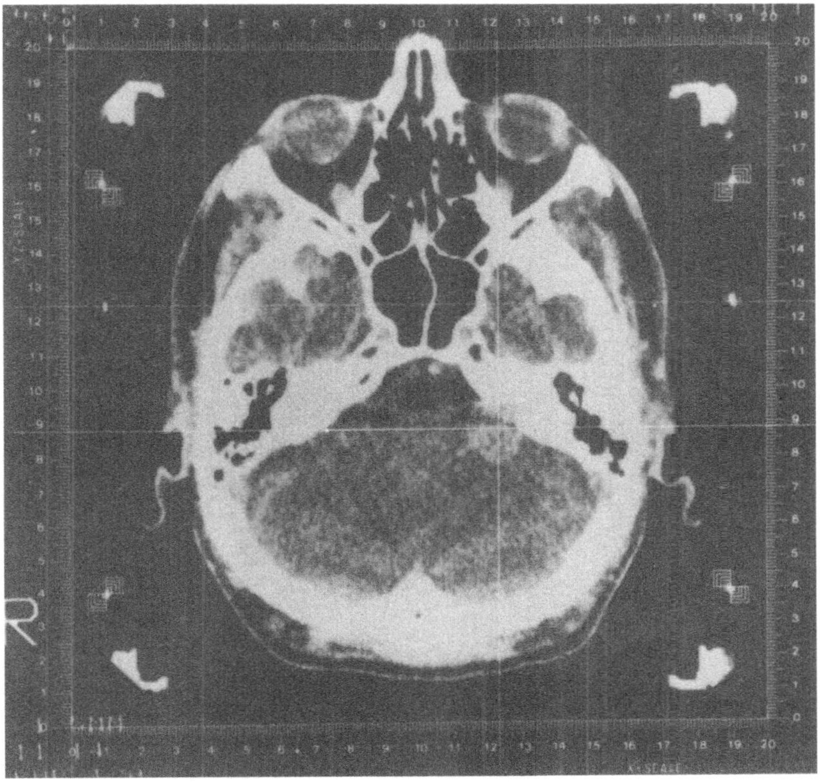

FIGURE 3–9. Manual target-coordinate determination is performed with a scale over a CT image placed on an roentgenogram viewbox. The dotted line intersecting the middle fiducials reveals the Z coordinate to be 125 mm. The X coordinate (123 mm) and Y coordinate (88 mm) are also read directly from the scale.

STANDARD CT-SCANNER SOFTWARD TECHNIQUE

Virtually all commercially available advanced-generation CT scanners include standard software with optional functions such as "deposit cursor" and "measure distance." These functions are used to determine the X, Y, Z coordinates of the selected target on the CT image. The cursor is deposited on each of the four vertical (e.g., corner) fiducials in a diagonal fashion, and lines are generated along the cursor's diagonal path (measure distance); the intersecting point of these two lines defines the center of the frame (figure 3–10A). The cursor is repositioned onto the frame center; the diagonal lines are erased by "erase graph," and the deposit cursor is depressed again. This procedure is repeated with the cursor placed on the target. When the measure-distance key is depressed, the computer software (GE 8800 or 9800) will display the X and Y coordinates of the target and the frame center (figure 3–10B). The actual stereotactic coordinates represent the sum of, or differences, between these values. When the signs of the two values are the same, the actual coordinate is represented by the difference of these two values (regardless of the sign); whereas, if the sign of the X coordinate of the target and that of the frame center are different, the actual stereotactic coordinate is represented by the sum of these two coordinates, whatever their signs. The reason for this is quite simple: The GE CT-scanner coordinate system is assigned numerical signs in four quadrants: upper right is positive/positive, lower right is positive/negative, lower left is negative/negative, and upper left is negative/positive. This technique mathematically defines the distance, right-left or anterior-posterior, between the target and

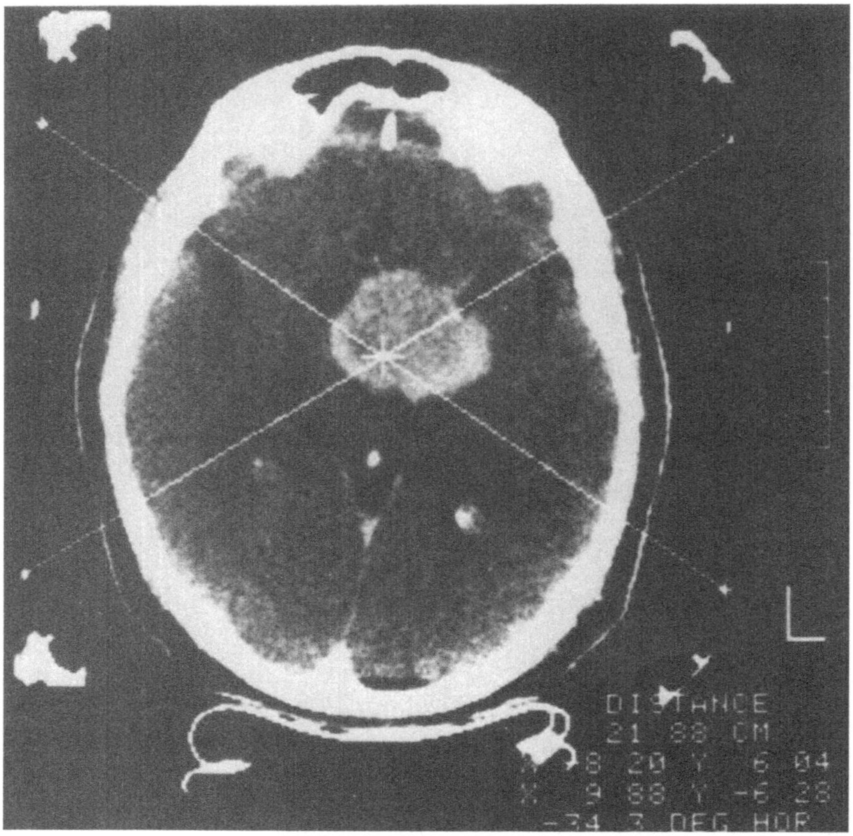

A

FIGURE 3–10. The frame center is defined with a CT computer cursor used to connect the vertical fiducial markers seen on the axial CT image (A). The CT X and Y coordinates of the frame center and the target are displayed on a GE scanner console; the actual stereotactic coordinates are the difference between these two values (B). The CT Z coordinate is determined by measuring the distance between the posterior vertical fiducial and the descending diagonal fiducial (C).

the frame center. Other scanners can provide the same information using measure-distance functions alone.

The Z coordinate (scan plane) is determined by measuring the distance between the posterior vertical fiducial and the center of the diagonal, which is the middle fiducial (figure 3–10C). If the distance measured is less than 60 mm, it is subtracted from 60, in which case the target is positioned in a CT plane superior to the frame center (Z = 10). The result represents the number of millimeters above the frame center at which the scan lies, and this is also the actual stereotactic Z coordinate. If the target plane is inferior to the Z = 10, the measured distance will be greater than 60, and 60 should be subtracted from it. This figure indicates the number of millimeters inferior to the Z = 10 and again represents the actual stereotactic Z coordinate. Other standard software features include multiplanar reformatted images based on the axial scans used for target selection. The target position can be displayed on the reformatted images, and different trajectories to the target also can be displayed (figure 3–11).

STEREOTACTIC SCANNER SOFTWARD PROGRAMS

Special stereotactic software options have been developed for the GE 8800 CT scanner [12] as well as the Siemen's CT and MRI scanners [8].

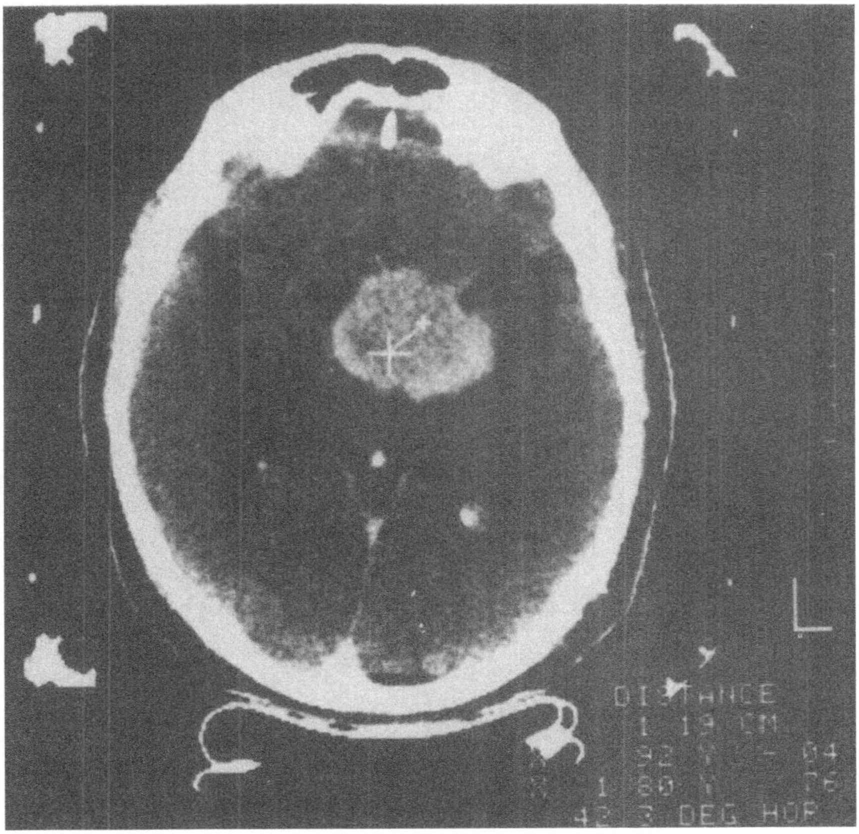

B

FIGURE 3-10. (cont.)

When the cursor is placed upon the target, these programs automatically display its X, Y, and Z coordinates (figure 3-12). They also permit the preoperative display of phantom probe trajectories on the axial CT images (figure 3-13) and determine the arc angles necessary to set such trajectories. The target and the pathway of the probe are equally well displayed both on the sagittal or the coronal electronic radiograms (figure 3-14) and on sagittal or coronal MRI scans (figure 3-15). In addition, the stereotactic programs can be used to display a millimeter grid on each potential target image such that the coordinates can be manually determined or the targets modified at any time, even when access to the computer is no longer available (figure 3-16). Ideally, a computer terminal dedicated to surgery is installed in the operating room (figure 3-17); this is particularly beneficial in centers where the radiological department lies at some distance from the operating room or where access to the scanners is limited.

MRI Localization

In contrast to CT, target selection with MRI can be performed from direct axial, coronal, or sagittal scans (figure 3-18). The Leksell coordinate frame has been modified to eliminate artifacts caused by eddy currents. Plastic feet replace the standard iron feet used for CT and for fixation of the frame; pins of fiberglass are used instead of carbon-fiber pins. The square coordinate frame fits within the diameter of most standard MRI radiofrequency coils. Special adapters have been designed to keep the frame in position during imaging. To localize a target from MRI scans, the coordinate indicator plates contain channels filled with a liquid having suitable magnetic properties. A vertex plate is used to permit coordinate determina-

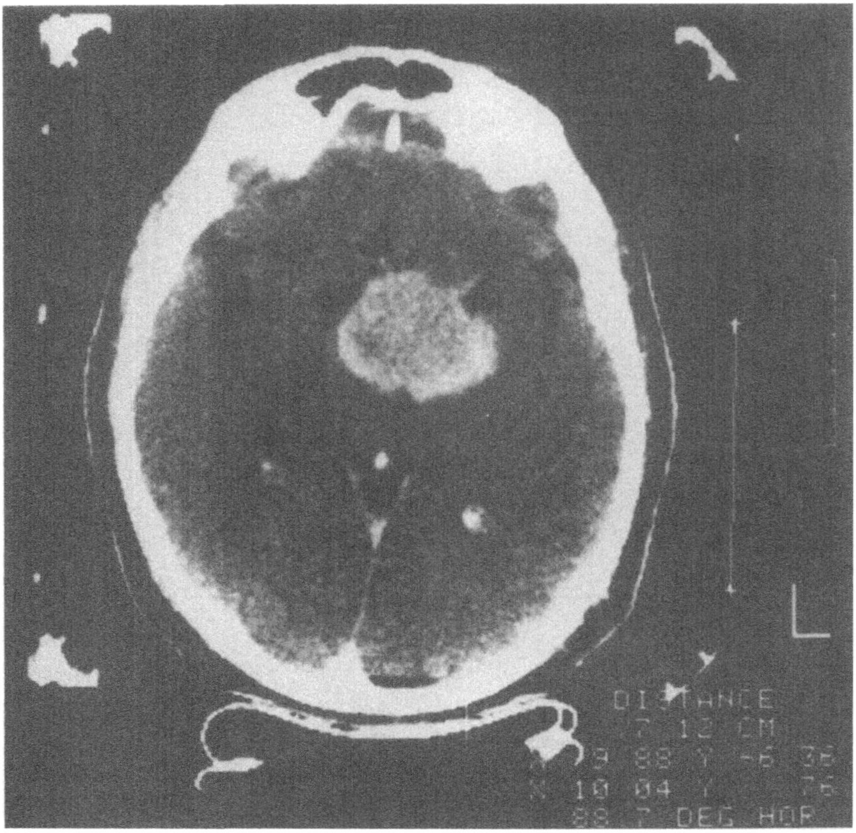

C

FIGURE 3–10. (cont.)

tion from sagittal images [8]. The fiducials can be seen on both T_1- and T_2-weighted images.

MRI-guided stereotactic surgery has several advantages, including significant reduction in image artifacts (the frame gives no nuclear magnetic resonance signal) and improved contrast resolution. Lesion definition can be accentuated by variation in the emphasis of T_1 and T_2 relaxation times (figure 3–19). Although this will probably change in the future, current acquisition times are considerably longer with MRI than with CT. Therefore it is particularly important that the frame be prevented from moving in the axial direction during imaging. This is ensured by the MRI adapter design. Increased distortion of the image during selection of targets peripheral to the frame center (i.e., RF coil center) has not been noted in the GE 1.5 tesla unit (General Electric Sigma, Milwaukee, WI) at the University of Pittsburgh. White matter tracts and deep-brain nuclei for functional intervention are visualized well with MRI (figure 3–20).

Target coordinates are determined from axial, coronal, and sagittal MRI images in the same manner as previously described for CT. Techniques for both the computer-based (standard and special stereotactic software) and manual localization (with a transparent plastic scale) are available also for MRI.

General Information

APPROACHES USED

The versatility of the Leksell stereotactic instrument is demonstrated by the remarkable freedom that the surgeon has to select various approaches or trajectories to the target. It is necessary only that the target be enclosed within the coordinate frame and that the fiducials be visible for the coordinate derivation. Trans-

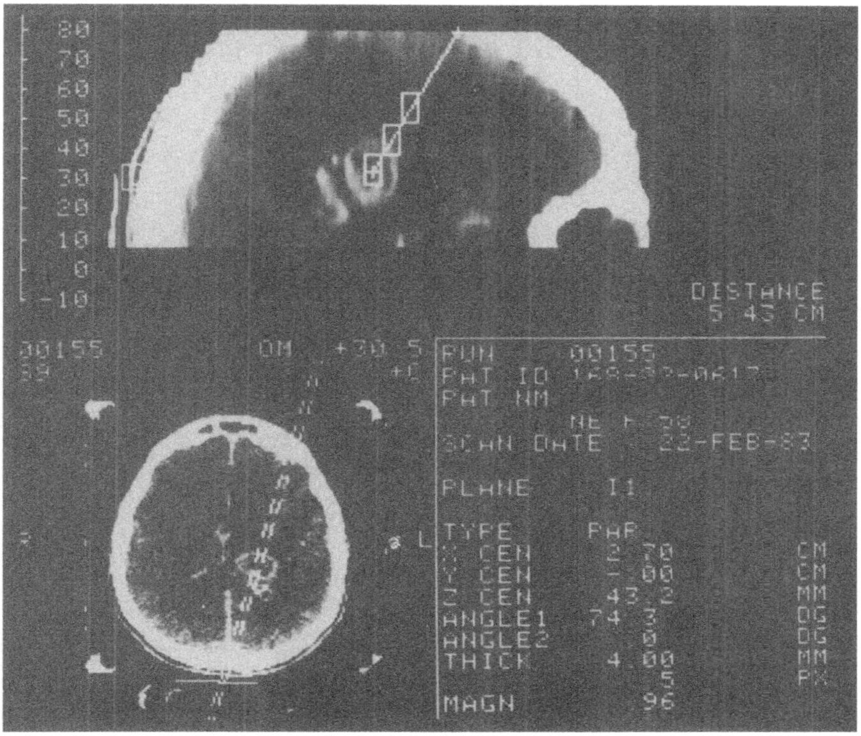

FIGURE 3–11. Paraxial reformatted CT images demonstrate the plane of the probe and biopsy sites (glioblastoma multiforme).

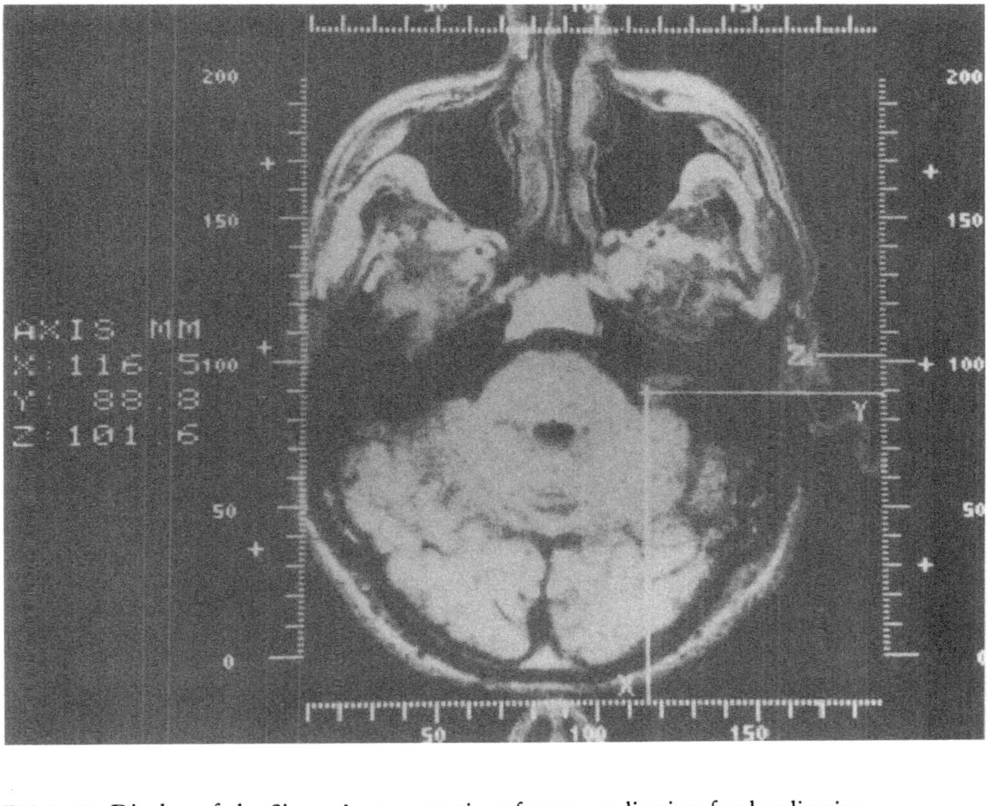

FIGURE 3–12. Display of the Siemen's stereotactic software application for localization.

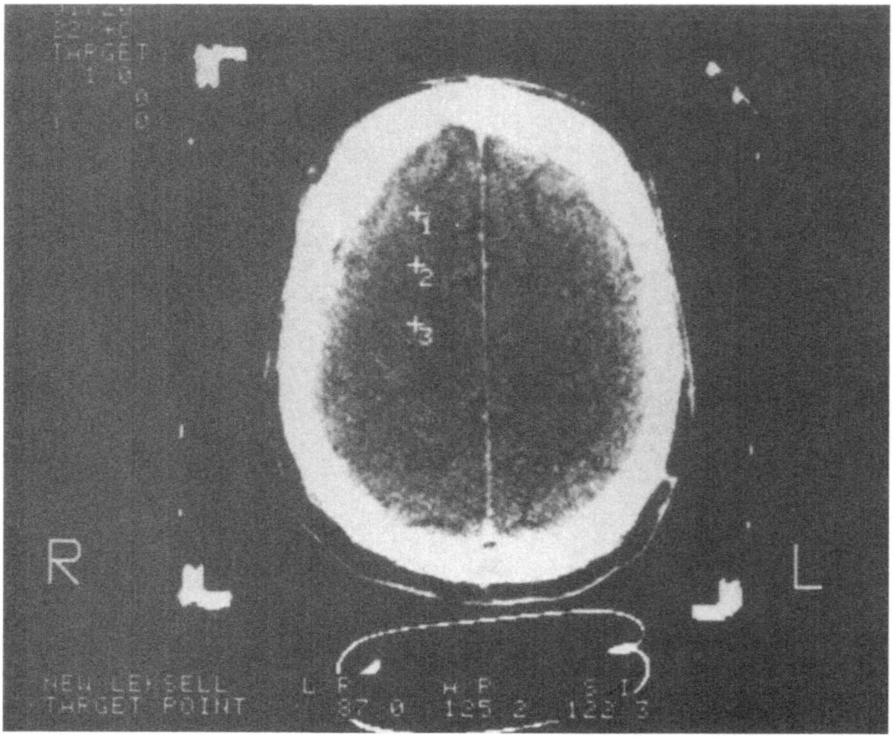

A

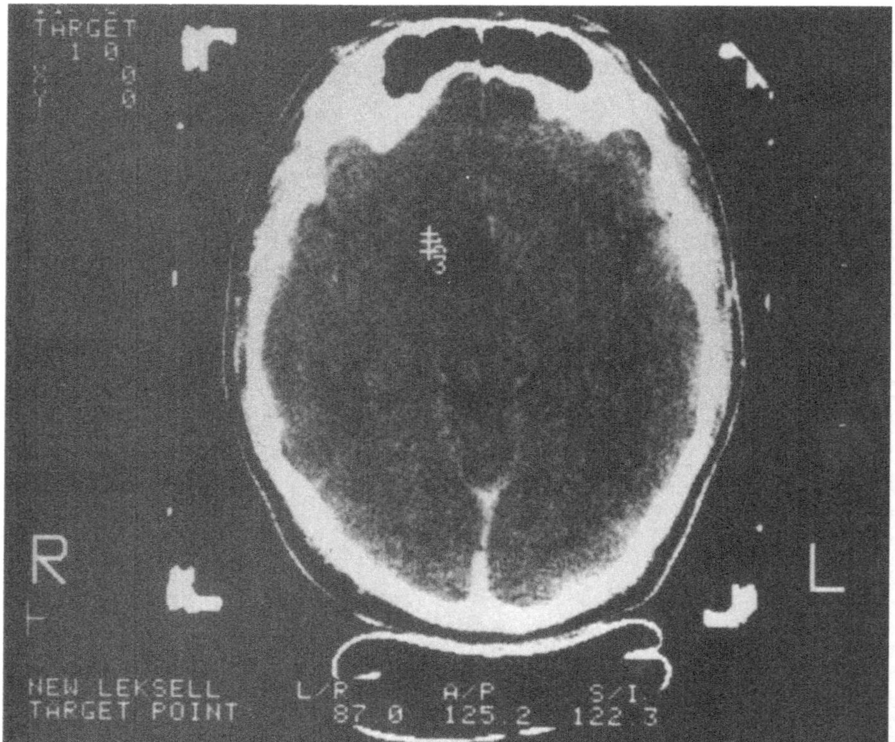

B

FIGURE 3–13. Three potential converging probe pathways are displayed at the cortical entry site, (A), level of the lateral ventricles, (B), just superior to the target, (C), and at the target, (D). The actual stereotactic frame coordinates are displayed on the CT image (cf. [12]).

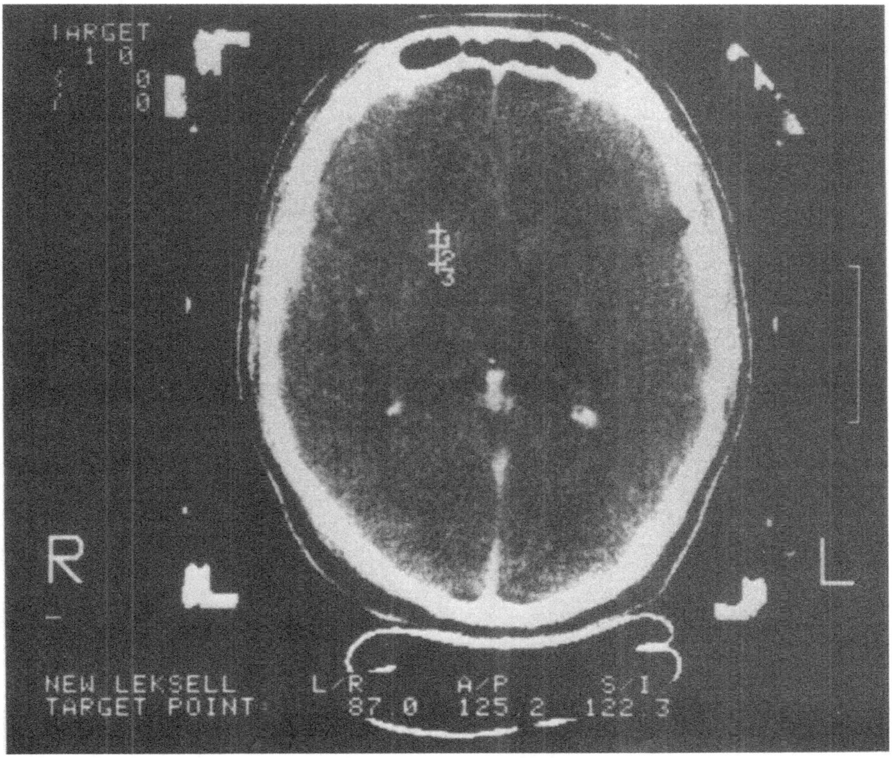
TARGET
1 0
R
L
NEW LEKSELL L/R A/P S/I
TARGET POINT 87 0 125 2 122 3

C

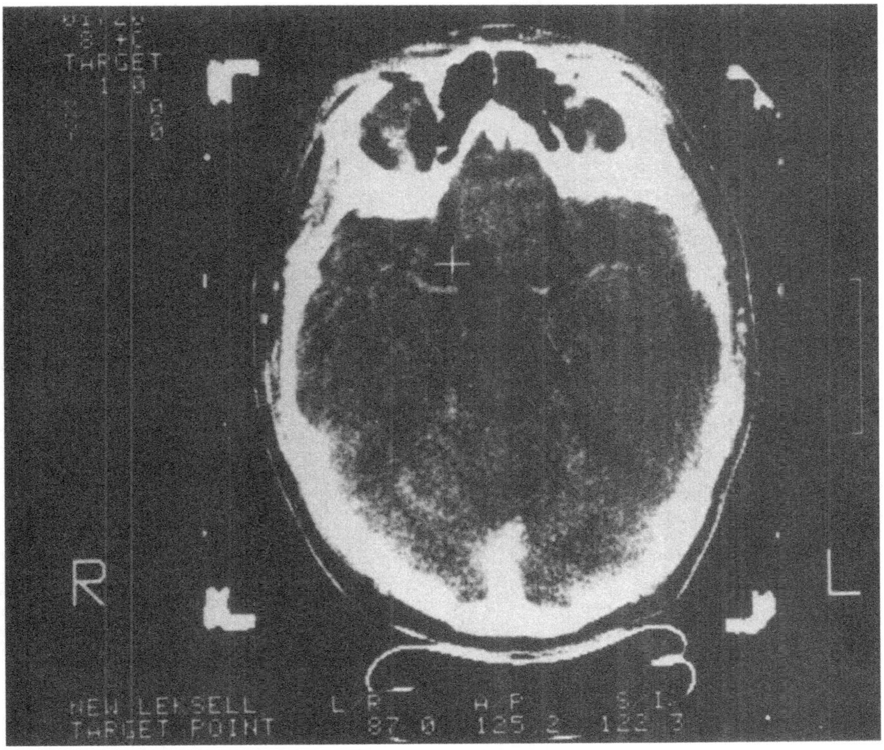
TARGET
1 0
R
L
NEW LEKSELL L/R A/P S/I
TARGET POINT 87 0 125 2 122 3

D

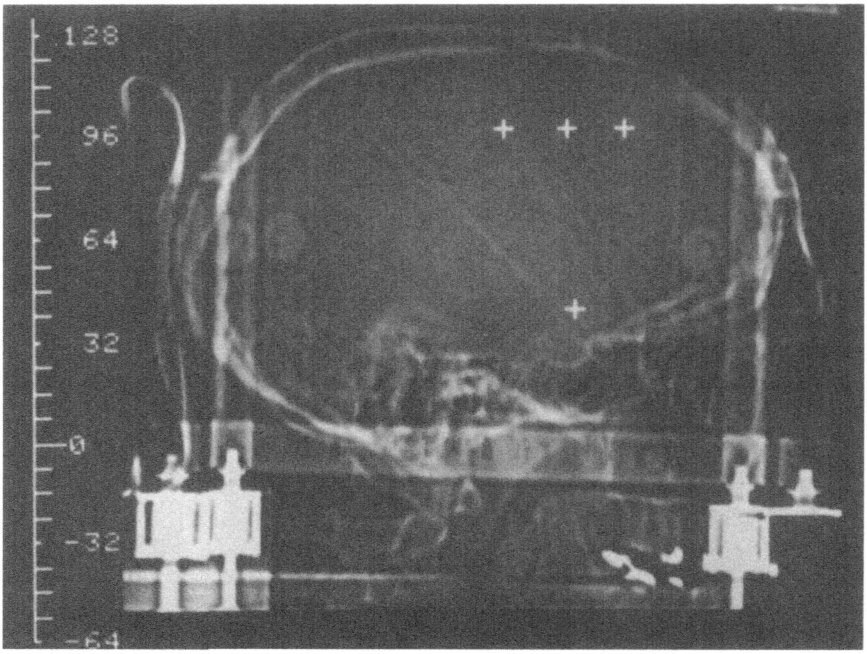

A

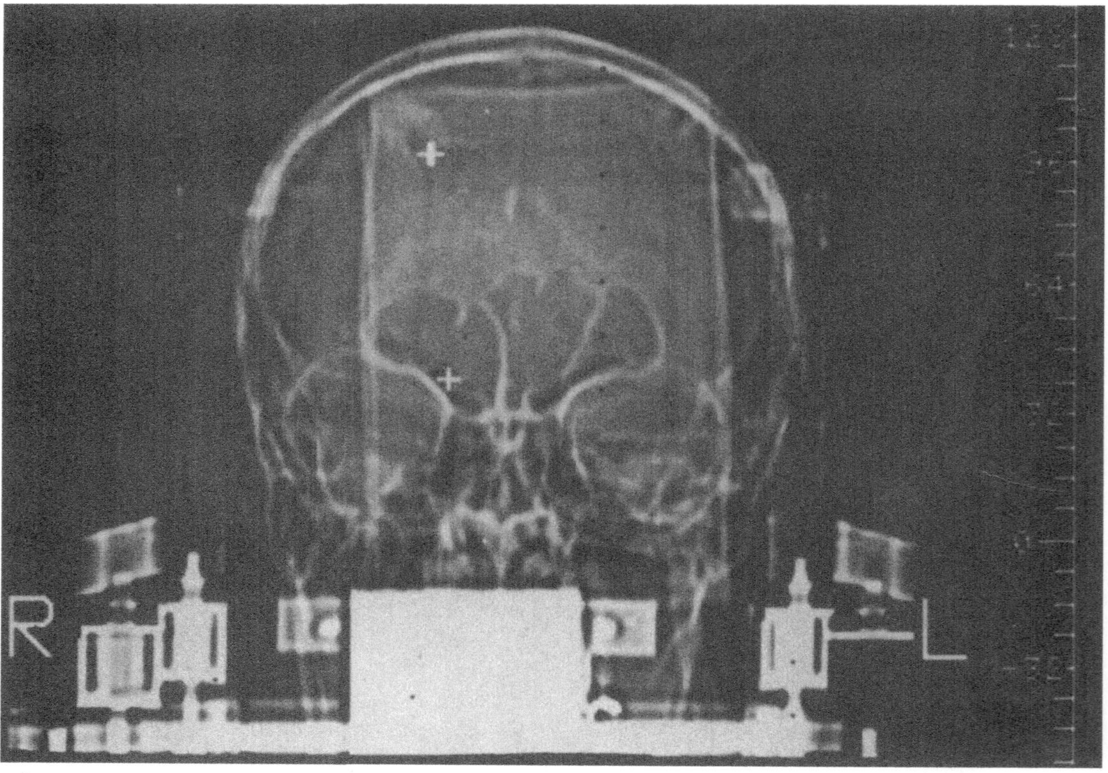

B

FIGURE 3–14. Saggital electronic radiograph (Scoutview®, General Electric Medical Systems) demonstrating the probe entry sites shown in figure 3–13 (A), and the target. Coronal electronic radiogram demonstrating the entry site for a probe and the target (B).

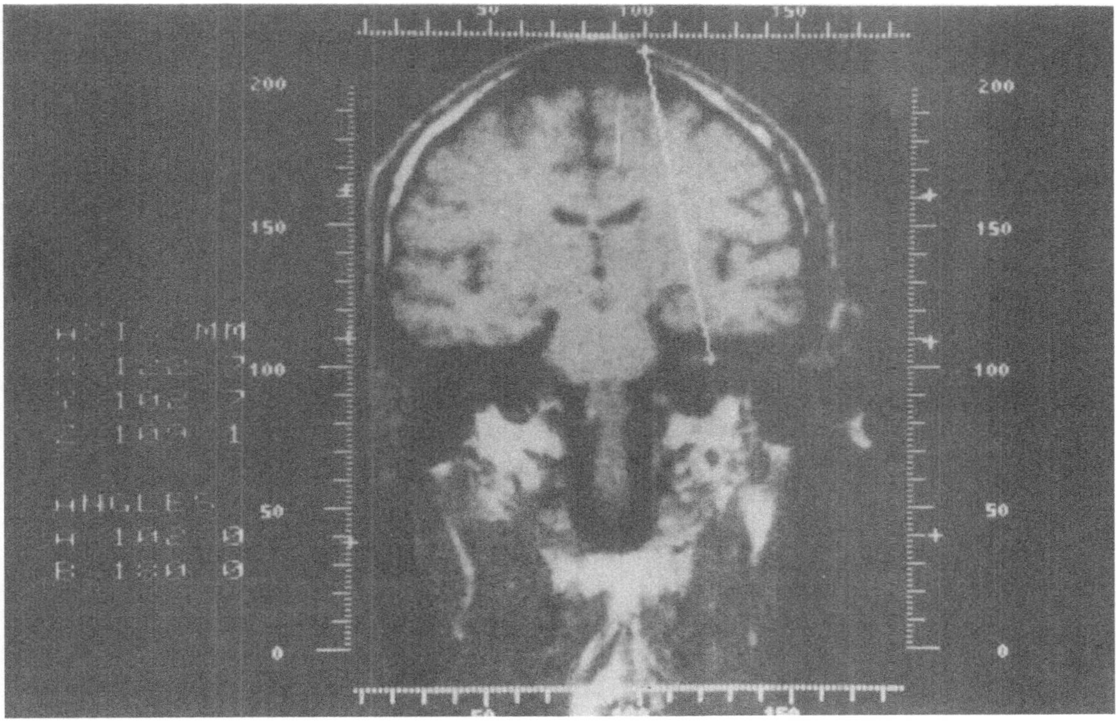

FIGURE 3–15. A coronal MRI (T_1-weighted) scan demonstrating a small acoustic tumor.

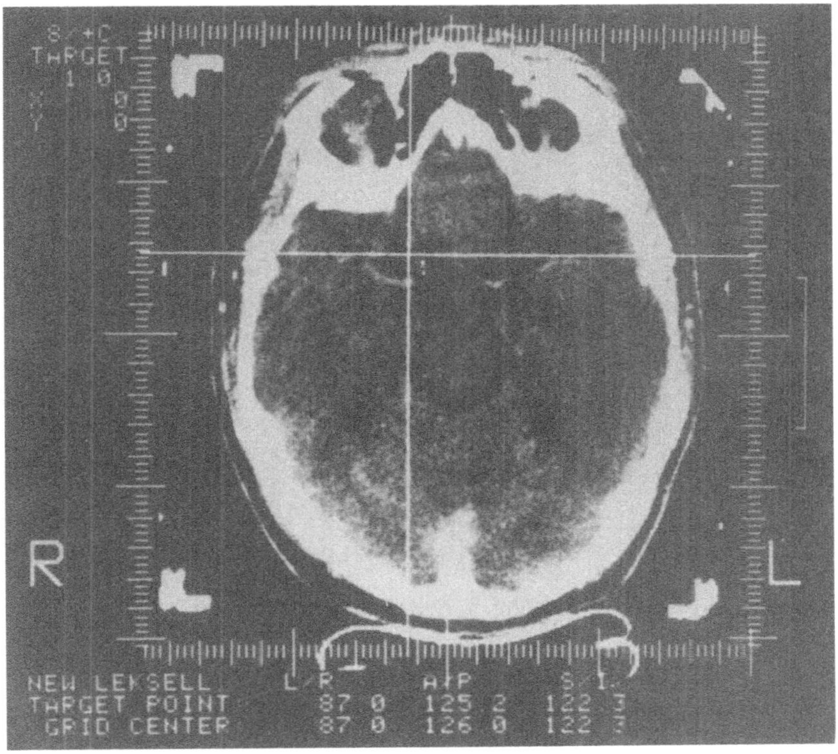

FIGURE 3–16. A grid can be displayed over the CT image containing the target by means of a special software package. The coordinates can be read directly.

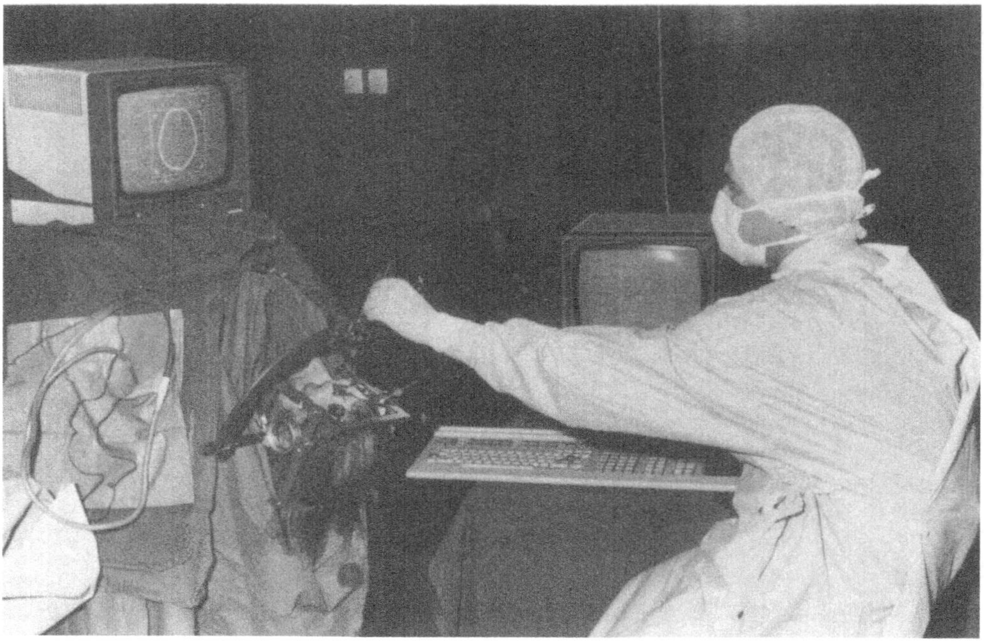

FIGURE 3-17. The integration of the imaging and the localization with the operation increases surgical flexibility.

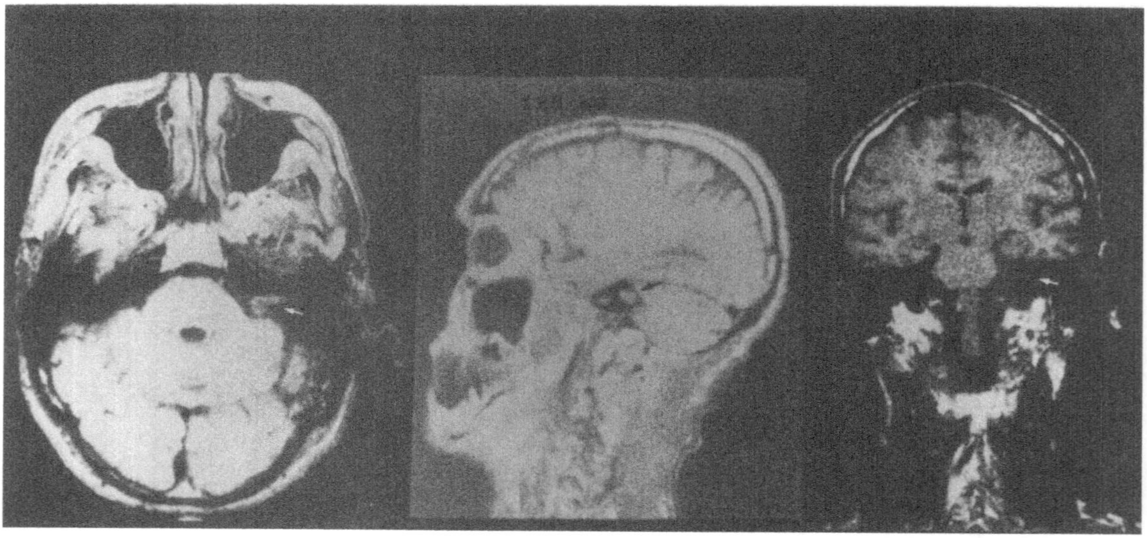

FIGURE 3-18. Small left-sided acoustic tumor visualized in three orthogonal planes with stereotactic MRI.

sphenoidal, suboccipital, and direct lateral approaches through the rings of the sidebars are possible. Patients undergoing posterior fossa procedures, such as transcerebellar biopsies, can be operated upon in either the sitting or prone positions. By reversing the semicircular arc on the coordinate frame, supraorbital approaches are readily performed. Transsphenoidal approaches are made equally easy by swinging the arc anteriorly over the face.

ACCESSORIES

A variety of instruments for both morphological and functional neurosurgery are avail-

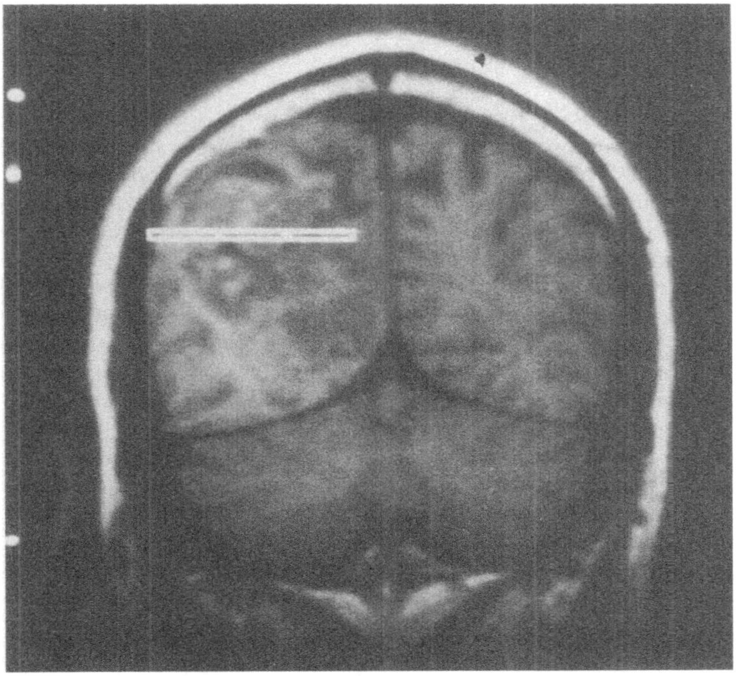

A

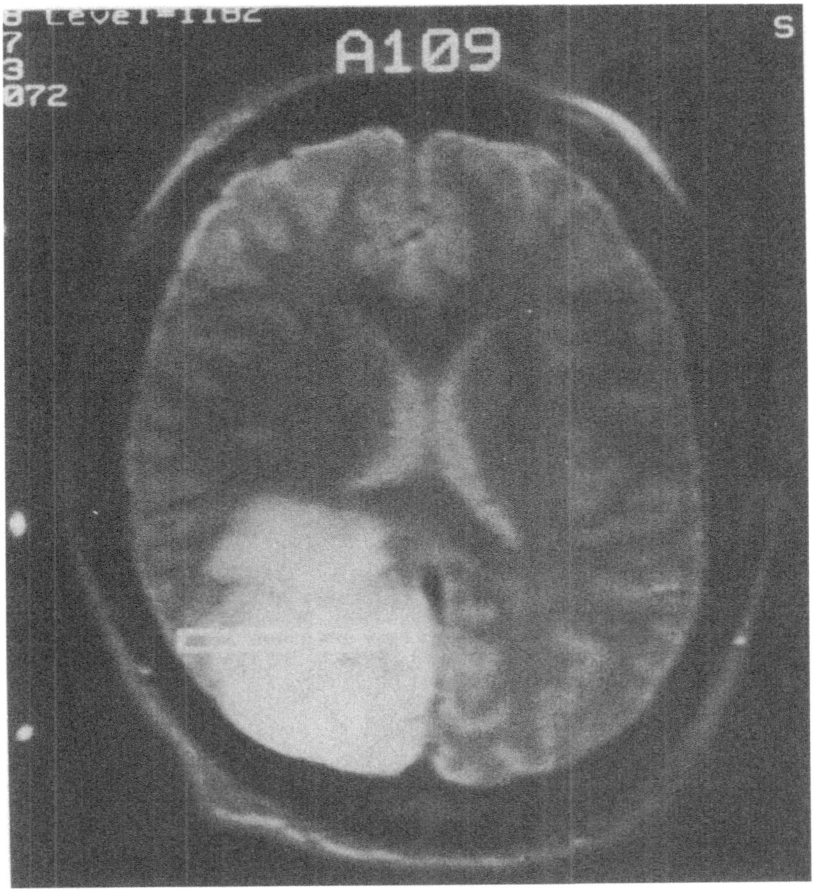

B

FIGURE 3–19. Stereotactic T_1-weighted coronal MRI of a mixed glioma (A). T_2-weighted image shows the tumor to advantage (B). (Biopsy site displayed).

able for the Leksell instrument (table 3–1). The Backlund biopsy kit [2] includes needles for corkscrew spiral and aspiration biopsies. Transcranial access for the probe is obtained either by the conventional burr-hole technique or by the use of a percutaneous drill set. Leksell performed the first operation designed to stereotactically reconstruct the occluded aqueduct of Sylvius. Backlund subsequently designed an instrument for this procedure.

Other available instruments in this stereotactic system include a hematoma evacuator [3] and a guide holder that permits intraoperative CT imaging with the arc removed (figure 3–21) [11]. A lesion generator with monopolar or bipolar thermocouple electrodes is also available. The design of the instrument makes it easily adaptable to other technologies, such as fiberoptics and lasers. Accessories for interstitial irradiation, including special dose-planning software, are under development.

CARE OF THE INSTRUMENT

After gentle washing with a soap solution, sterilization with steam autoclaving is recommended for all aluminum parts of the unit. Blood and debris should be removed from all instruments to ensure that they function smoothly and do not stick. All carbon-fiber or fiberglass pins should be gas-autoclaved. These pins wear out after approximately ten to 20 uses and must be replaced periodically. Stereotactic biopsy for suspected slow virus infections is not recommended, because the neces-

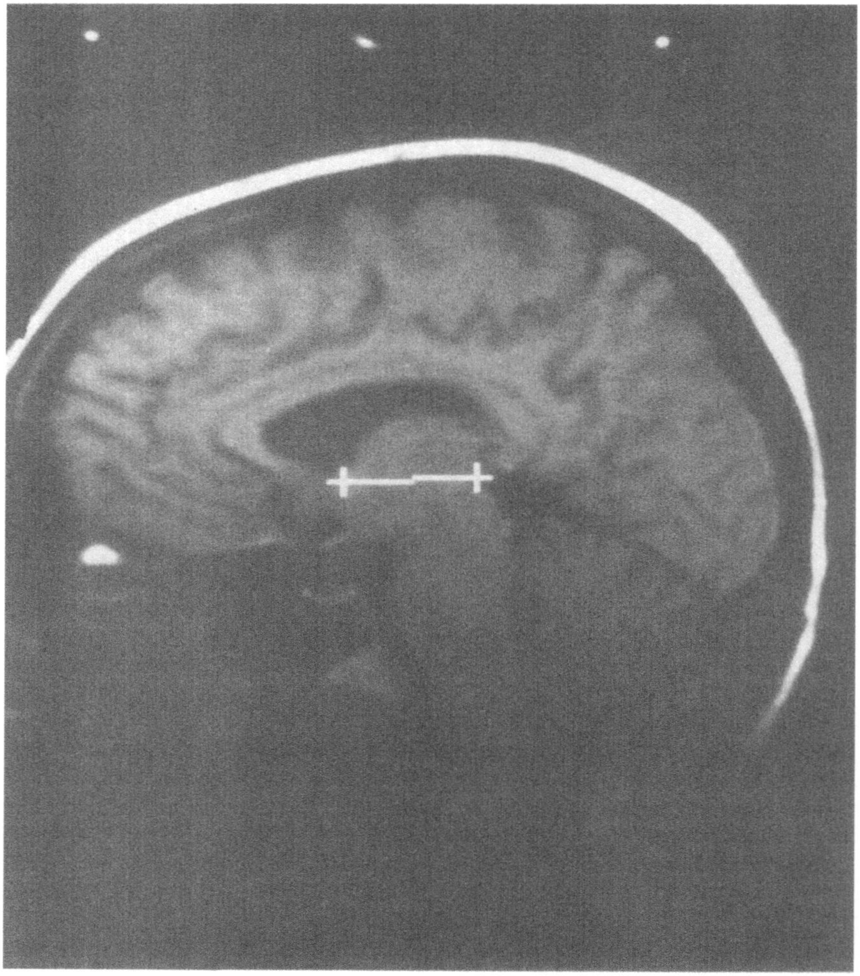

FIGURE 3–20. Sagittal stereotactic MRI anatomic (T_1-weighted) image, demonstrating the intercommissural line prior to thalamotomy.

TABLE 3–1. Accessories for the Leksell Stereotactic System

Functional Surgery
1. Short distance radiography units
   a. Ceiling-mounted
   b. Table-mounted
2. Leksell radiofrequency brain-lesion generator
3. Thermocouples and electrode system
   a. Monopolar
   b. Bipolar
4. Desktop Hewlett Packard calculator and printer with stereotactic software for radiographic localization

Morphological Surgery
1. Backlund biopsy kit
2. Salcman/Leksell percutaneous drill kit
3. Leksell/Bunge biopsy needle
4. Backlund hematoma evacuator kit
5. Lunsford intraoperative CT guide holder
6. Special stereotactic CT and MRI scanner software (or "computer programs")

Other
1. Universal CT and MRI adapters
2. Mayfield headrest adapter and adjustable headrests
3. Stereotactic operating chair

sary sterilization process requires the use of hypochlorite solutions, which react unfavorably with the anodized aluminum parts.

Conclusions

For more than 37 years, the Leksell stereotactic system has proved to be practical, understandable, and accurate. The term system is used to stress the idea of a complete range of interchangeable and compatible components, which together form a self-contained independent unit for all kinds of stereotactic procedures, regardless of the imaging technique used. Minor modifications have made the instrument compatible with all modern imaging modalities including CT and MRI. Continued clinical research has accompanied the progressive development of this stereotactic system. Practical surgical aspects are given great attention in the design of its various components. When evaluating a stereotactic device, users might well ask the following questions to ensure that the system selected meets their goals and needs:

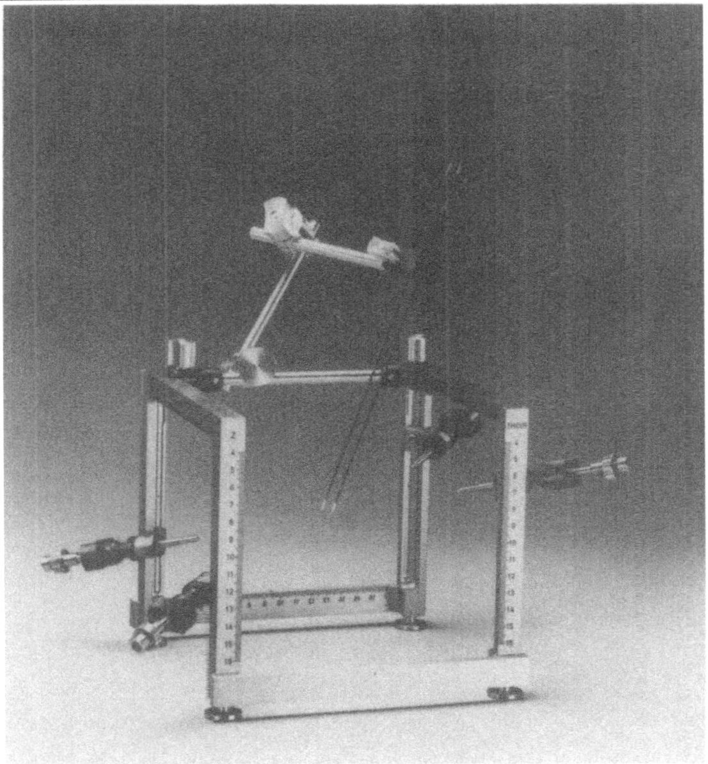

FIGURE 3–21. CT guide holder that replaces the semicircular arc for surgery performed under CT control.

1. Is it a complete system?
2. Is it simple?
3. Is it dependable?
4. Is it versatile?
5. Is it accurate?
6. Is it compatible with multiple-imaging modalities?
7. Is it both computer-compatible and independent?
8. Is its development keeping pace with developments in other related technologies?

Experience with the Leksell stereotactic system indicates affirmative answers to all these questions. Although many stereotactic devices are now available, few have proved as versatile or as simple to understand and operate as the Leksell stereotactic instrument.

References

1. Alberts WW: Simple graphic stereotaxic localization. *J Neurosurg* 18:561–562, 1961
2. Backlund EO: A new stereotaxic instrument for stereotaxic brain tumor biopsy. *Acta Chir Scand* 137:825–827, 1971
3. Backlund EO, Von Holst H: Controlled subtotal evacuation of intracerebral hematomas by stereotactic technique. *Surg Neurol* 9:99–101, 1978
4. Bergstrom M, Greitz T, Steiner L: An approach to stereotaxic radiography. *Acta Neurochir* (Wien) 54:155–165, 1980
5. Leksell L: A stereotaxic apparatus for intracerebral surgery. *Acta Chir Scand* 99:229–233, 1949
6. Leksell L: *Stereotaxis and Radiosurgery: An Operative System*. Springfield IL: Thomas, 1971
7. Leksell L, Jernberg B: Stereotaxis and tomography: A technical note. *Acta Neurochir* (Wien) 52:1–7, 1980
8. Leksell L, Leksell D, Schwebel J: Stereotaxis and nuclear magnetic resonance. *J Neurol Neurosurg Psychiatry* 48:14–18, 1985
9. Leksell L, Liden K: A therapeutic trial with radioactive isotopes in cystic brain tumors. In *Radioisotope Techniques*. Vol 1, *Medical and Physiological Applications*. London: HRI Stationery Office, 1951
10. Lunsford LD: Stereotaxy and the role of CT in morphological and functional surgery of the human brain. In Latchaw, RE (ed): *Computed Tomography of the Head, Neck and Spine*. Chicago: Yearbook, 1985, pp 743–764
11. Lunsford LD, Leksell L, Jernberg B: Probe holder for stereotactic surgery in the CT scanner: A technical note. *Acta Neurochir* (Wien) 69:297–304, 1983
12. Lunsford LD, Listerud JE, Rowberg A, et al: Stereotactic software for the GE 8800 CT scanner. *Neurol Research* (in press), 1986
13. Spiegel EA, Wycis HT, Freed H, et al: Stereoencephalotomy. *Proc Soc Exp Biol Med* 69:175–177, 1948

4. THE HITCHCOCK SYSTEM

Edward Hitchcock

The Hitchcock System developed from the need for an accurate, versatile stereotactic instrument for use in spinal procedures [1, 2]. The instrument also can be used for a wide variety of posterior fossa and intracranial procedures. Ideally, a stereotactic instrument should be extremely accurate and practical for a variety of patient postures yet simple, to reduce operator error. Many systems require expensive additional equipment for fixed-beam radiography or image intensification. Although the Hitchcock apparatus can accommodate their use, they are not essential for the system, which uses a standard portable roentgen machine or computed tomography (CT) scan.

When conventional radiography is used, simplicity is achieved by teleradiography, which greatly reduces magnification (0.96 magnification factor at 3 m); a radioopaque ruler adjusted to the target plane makes exact centration unnecessary. The principle is that with parallel rays, parallax equally affects all objects in the same plane; radiological distortion is therefore eliminated if the reference measurements can be made in the same plane as the target. Thus, the apparatus need not be set exactly 90° in relation to the x-ray source, and any obliquity or magnification in the target plane is mirrored exactly in the ruler. With the elimination of time-consuming centration and magnification correction, target coordinates are obtained directly by projection of lines onto the radio-opaque ruler. For teleradiography, the distances between the x-ray source and film should be 4.0 m (magnification factor: 0.98); short-distance radiography also can be used, in which case the magnification factor is determined from the radiopaque ruler. (In practice, teleradiography at 3 m has proven satisfactory.) If the target is localized by a proportional system, (e.g., two-thirds down the anterior commissure–posterior commissure line) or directly visualized (foreign body), no correction is necessary. An arc is then attached to the rectilinear system so that the target point is at the center of the spherical system and can be approached by any route.

The square base is rigid, strong, and simple, which enables it to be interfaced easily with any imaging system: conventional radiography, including angiography, as well as CT and nuclear magnetic resonance (NMR). In conventional radiography, target coordinates are obtained by direct reading from the radiopaque ruler; in stereotactic CT or NMR scanning, the coordinates are directly read from the video display unit without further calculation. The simple skull-fixation device facilitates "open" stereotactic procedures, including craniotomy and posterior fossa exposures; self-retaining retractors and instrument racks can be anchored to points on the square. A full range of ancillary equipment, such as radiofrequency electrodes, deep-brain stimulating or recording electrodes, can be used together with biopsy aspiration needles, forceps, or endoscopes. Laser-beam variable-focus systems can be attached directly to the arc or to a primary laser arc.

We believe that the design and construction of this device make it one of the most accurate, adaptable, and simple modern stereotactic instruments.

I am grateful to W. Mitchell (Senior Technician) for help in development and to the Photography Department, (A. Rose), especially for photographs. My particular thanks to Veronica Turner for typing and checking the manuscript.

Components

CARRYING CASE

All components are secured in an aluminum alloy case with adjustable vents for gas or auto-

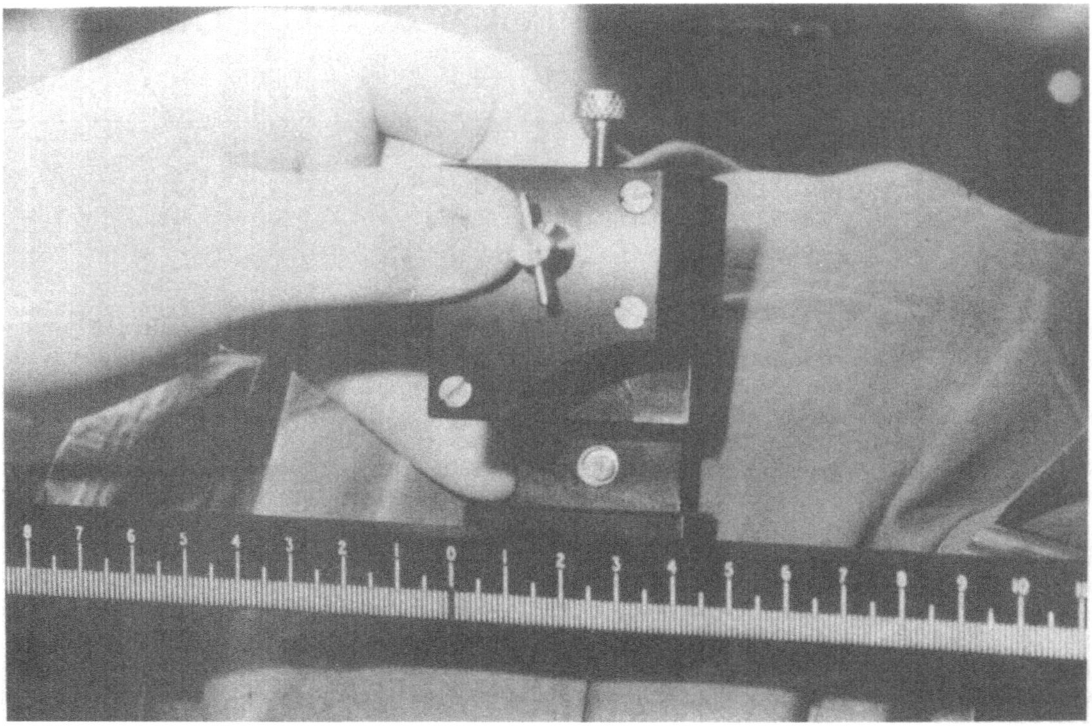

FIGURE 4–1. Grid/block holder is shown being applied to frame.

clave sterilization. Gas sterilization is recommended, but the instruments have been sterilized by heat autoclaving many times without damage. After sterilization, the vents are closed, and the instrument is ready for use.

SQUARE

The hollow "square" (26 square cm) of 15-square-mm cross-section is constructed without joints from a single plate of anodized aluminum alloy. The outer surface of each side of the square is engraved at 1-, 5-, and 10-mm intervals from the midpoint of the square, which is the center of the horizontal plane (figure 4–1). Either the top or bottom edge of the square or any point between can be used for the vertical plane zero; usually, the bottom edge is selected. Each corner and the center of one side holds "fixation pins" of interchangeable steel or CT-compatible aluminum. Extension pieces of CT-compatible aluminum can be fitted to the corners. The fixation pins are screwed to the skull by removable "bolts" with 2-mm scales; the depth of fixation can be noted for subsequent reproduction. After skull fixation, the patient's head and the square can be placed on the operating table without external fixation, but it is more convenient (especially if the sitting or semisitting position is used) to secure the square to the operating table by "fixation bars." The patient then can be placed in either the sitting or supine, or (the less comfortable) prone position.

CASSETTE HOLDER

The cassette holder (figure 4–2) can be attached to any side of the square and is adjustable to various heights. It is arranged so that, with conventional lateral radiography, the horizontal and vertical portions of the L-grid appear on the radiograph.

L-GRID

The L-grid is an L-shaped bar (2-cm-square cross-section) constructed from a single aluminum plate without joints (figure 4–3). Horizontal and vertical radiopaque markings are at 1-, 5-, and 10-mm intervals from the horizontal and vertical plane zero (see figure 4–3). The

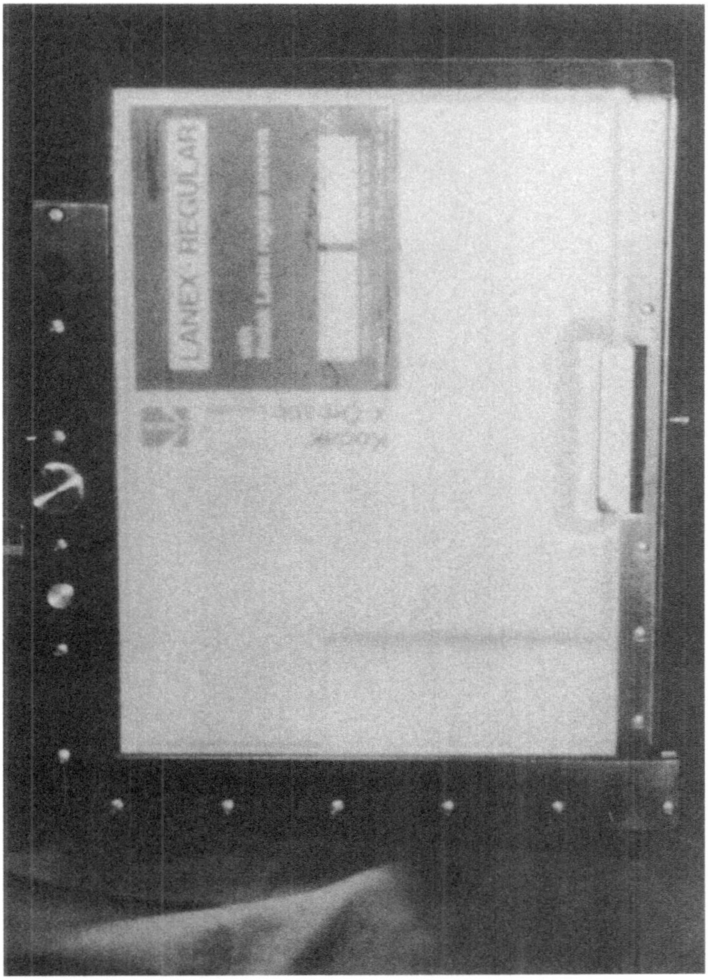

FIGURE 4–2. Cassette holder; holes permit adjustment of height.

grid is usually fixed on the right or left side at zero for the anteroposterior (AP) picture of the third ventricle. This assumes that the third ventricle lies in the lateral zero plane. If a lateral radiograph reveals that it does not, the grid is placed at the anterior or posterior distance from the zero that corresponds to the structures, and another AP view is taken. In practice, this is rarely necessary; for targets very far anterior or posterior, such as the pituitary fossa or fourth ventricle, a careful estimate of target position in respect to the frame enables accurate positioning of the L-grid. A line projected at right angles from the AP target to the horizontal ruler gives the lateral offset of the image (Z_S). The grid is then fixed at this lateral offset and at the zero setting on the vertical arm of the grid. Lines projected at right angles to the horizontal and vertical rulers of the grid indicate the anterior/posterior (X_S) and superior/inferior (Y_S) coordinates. (NB: To avoid confusion of stereotactic and CT coordinates, it is advisable to use an identifying subscript thus: $X_{stereo} = Y_{image}$; $Y_{stereo} = Z_{image}$ and $Z_{stereo} = X_{image}$).

GRID/BLOCK HOLDER

This device can be attached to any side of the square. It is used to hold the vertical limb of the L-grid or the cylinder block of the arc assembly at the chosen horizontal or vertical plane as shown in figure 4–1.

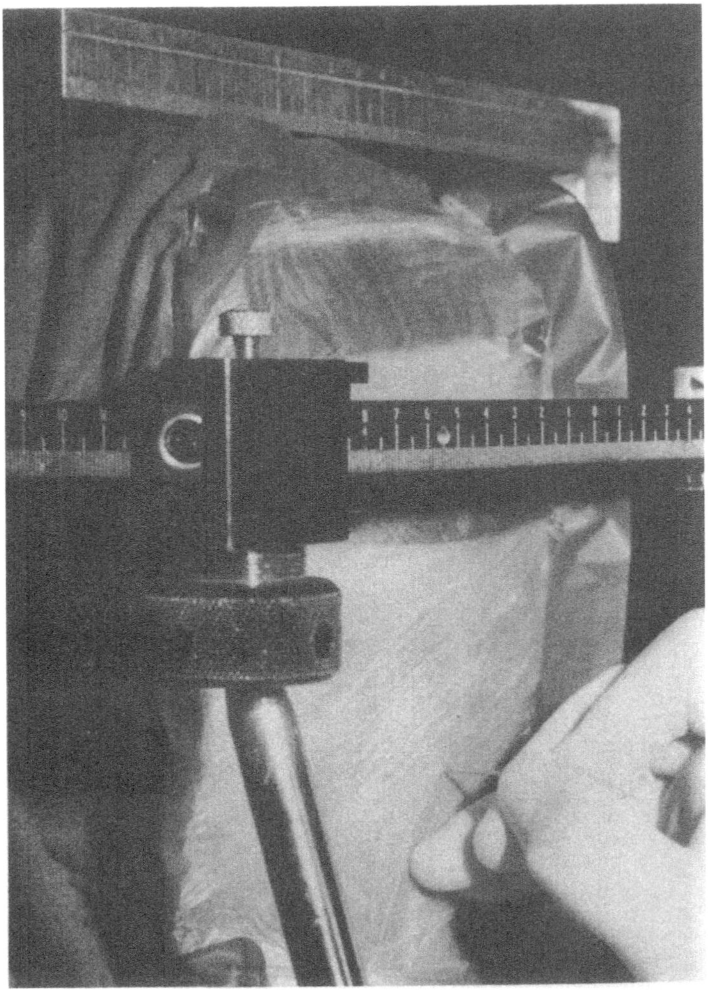

FIGURE 4–3. L-grid in place for AP view during a cisternal puncture for stereotactic cordotomy.

ARC ASSEMBLY

The "cylinder block" is anchored by the grid/block holder to any side of the square (figure 4–4). It is engraved at vertical intervals of 1, 5, and 10 mm and at 5° intervals on the cylinder hole. The grid/block holder secures the cylinder block at the desired X_S and Y_S (horizontal and vertical planes) or Z_S and Y_S (lateral and vertical planes) coordinates. The "arc cylinder" fits into the block and can be rotated 360°. Along its length, it is engraved at 1-, 5-, and 10-mm intervals with numerals indicating the distance of the target from the square's central zero. If the cylinder is arranged on the right or left side of the square, its length is the lateral offset of the Z_S coordinate. If (less commonly) it is applied to the anterior or posterior side, its length is the anterior/posterior plane. A transparent "glass sighting rod" with a central hole fits into the cylinder. The length of the electrode or other ancillary instrument is confirmed or adjusted by advancing the instrument until the tip appears at the sight hole. The "quadrant arc" is marked in degrees and can be fixed to the cylinder at the selected Z_S or X_S coordinate. Its eccentric construction ensures correct attachment of the slide assembly. As the cylinder revolves, the quadrant describes a hemisphere at the center of which is the target point. The "slide assembly" slides along the quadrant so that an instrument can be introduced through it at any desired trajectory. Un-

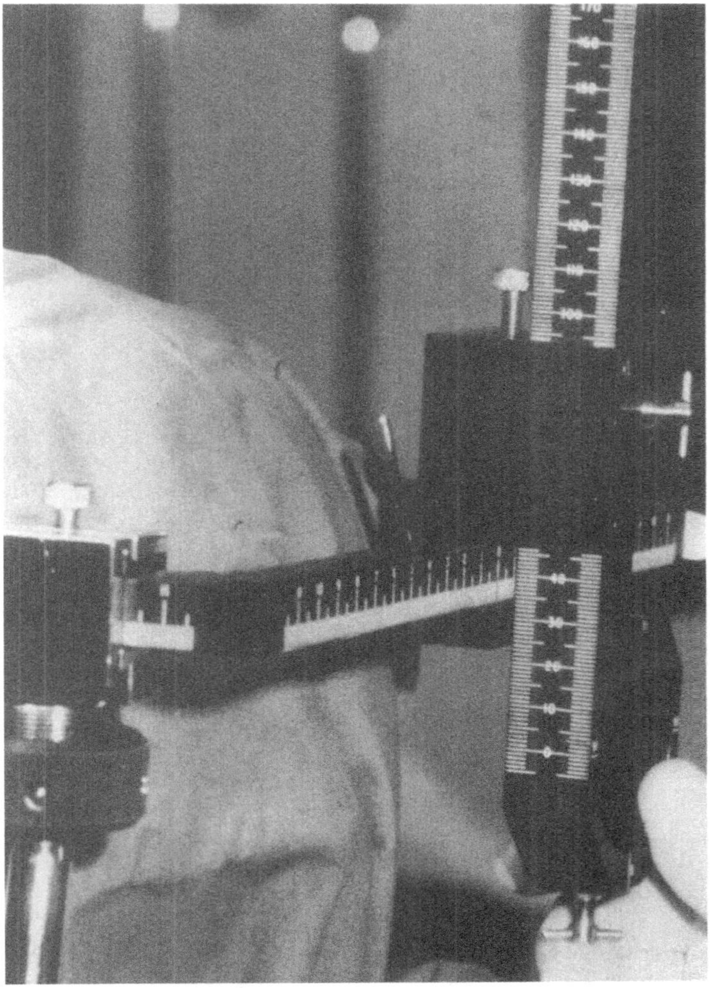

FIGURE 4–4. Cylinder block secured to grid/block holder.

approachable areas are limited to the thickness of the square (15 mm) and can be avoided by fixing the square well above or below the presumed target. The assembly has a graduated "electrode holder" (with a 0.1-mm vernier scale), that is advanced by a wheel that drives a rack and pinion. The electrode holder is designed to accept a variety of electrodes (figure 4–5). Very fine electrodes are stabilized by cannulas or by "stops" held in the "extension arm."

ALIGNMENT PLATES

Made of aluminum alloy with a thin steel fiducial marker, the "alignment plates" fasten to the side of the square at selected heights. CT alignment is verified by squaring the pillars as they appear in axial CT images. For large targets, such as tumors, fixation to the CT gantry is unnecessary after the head and square are placed securely on the table by means of a bean-bag support and the alignment beam is centered. X_I, Y_I, and Z_I coordinates then can be obtained by simple calculation.

For more precise measurement, the square is fixed to the CT gantry by a "gantry attachment" (figure 4–6). The laser alignment beam of the scanner is zeroed to the chosen vertical plane (usually the inferior edge of the square) and the horizontal coronal plane of zero. The superior laser alignment light then will be adjusted to the midline zero. Thereafter, all coor-

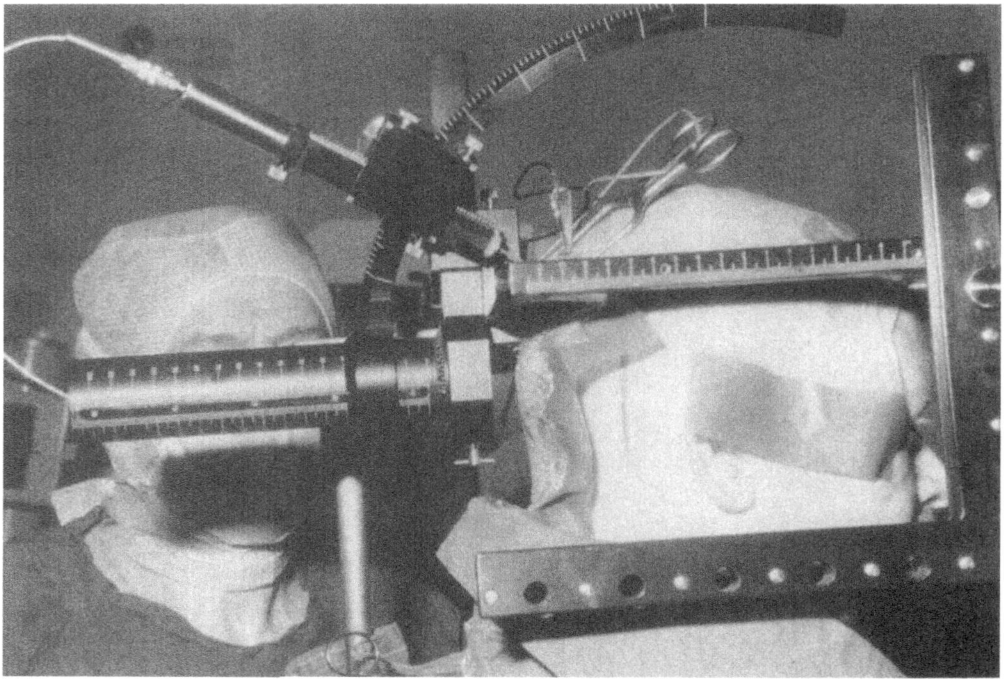

FIGURE 4–5. Arc assembly fixed to cylinder with electrode in slide assembly.

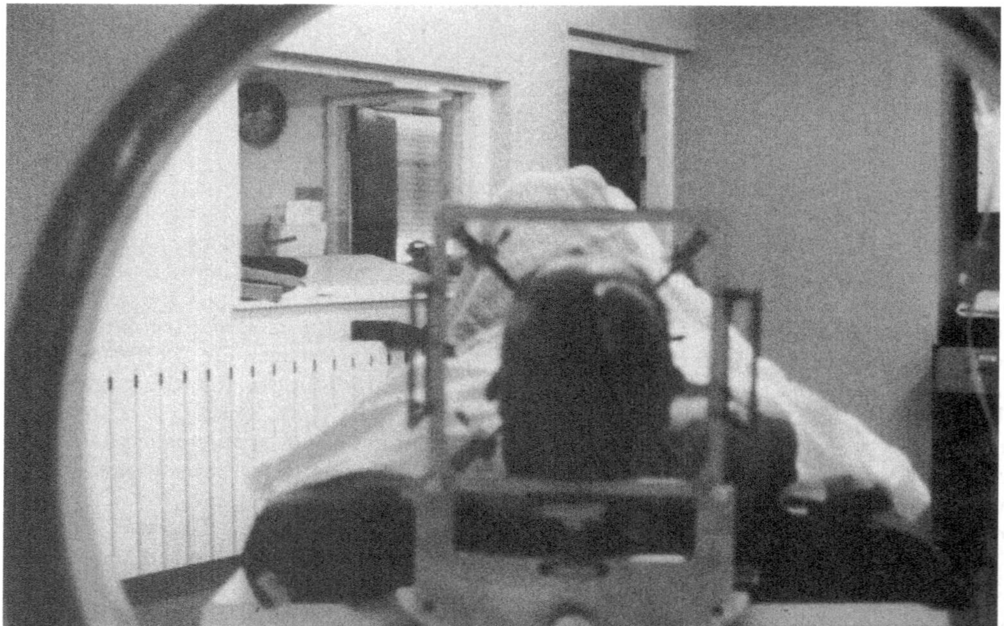

FIGURE 4–6. Gantry attachment; alignment plates fixed to square.

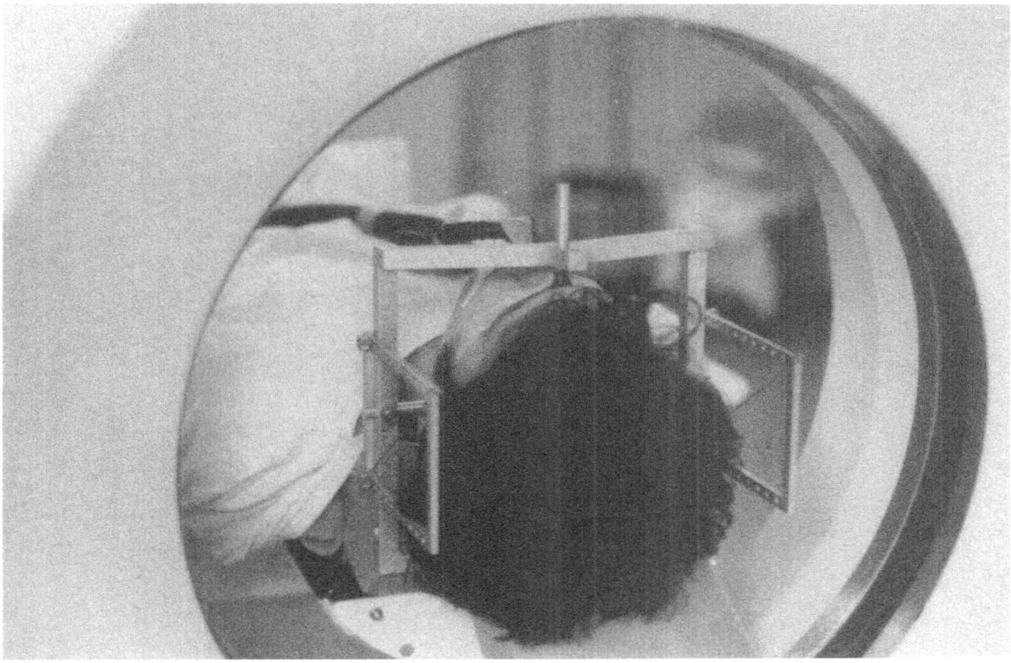

FIGURE 4-7. SCID with alignment plates and gantry fixation.

dinates are directly related to the stereotactic square at the X, Y, and Z coordinates, which are found in the usual way with the scanner computer.

STEREOTACTIC CT SCAN INTERFACE DEVICE (SCID)
The SCID can be fixed temporarily to the head by nasion rests and meatal plugs; skull fixation is also possible. The meatal and nasion measurements are noted and the device fixed to the gantry attachment (figure 4-7). After the scanner is zeroed to the SCID zeros, all coordinates are directly related to the SCID, and the X, Y, and Z coordinates can be displayed by the scanner computer. The SCID may be reattached at a later date and fixed to the stereotactic square (figure 4-8). The SCID is removed; the coordinates are transferred to the stereotactic instrument and the height is adjusted. The device permits outpatient and repeat scanning and eliminates the need for fixation of the stereotactic instrument by pins.

ADDITIONAL ATTACHMENTS
A sighting mirror can be attached to the base to enable exact centering of laser alignment beams. The glass sighting rod may be replaced with a multiple-electrode holder, which facilitates direct perpendicular insertion of a recording electrode for epilepsy. A nasion rest and meatal plugs can also be attached to the base; they are not needed for fixation generally, but are useful for CT-guided stereotaxy that employs the SCID. A series of self-retaining retractors, instrument trays, etc., are available for use with stereotactic open surgery and craniotomy. A fixation and cassette-holding platform that attaches to the floor is available for operating rooms with two-plane fixed-beam radiography or for use with primary laser arc surgery.

Method

CONVENTIONAL RADIOGRAPHY USAGE
The patient is placed in the semisitting position, appropriate fixation points are chosen, and local anesthesia is injected. The anterior fixation pins are pressed into the frontal bone midline while the square is held parallel to the interpupillary line; the fixation pins are tightened. The fixation bars are attached to the square and fixed to the table (figure 4-9).

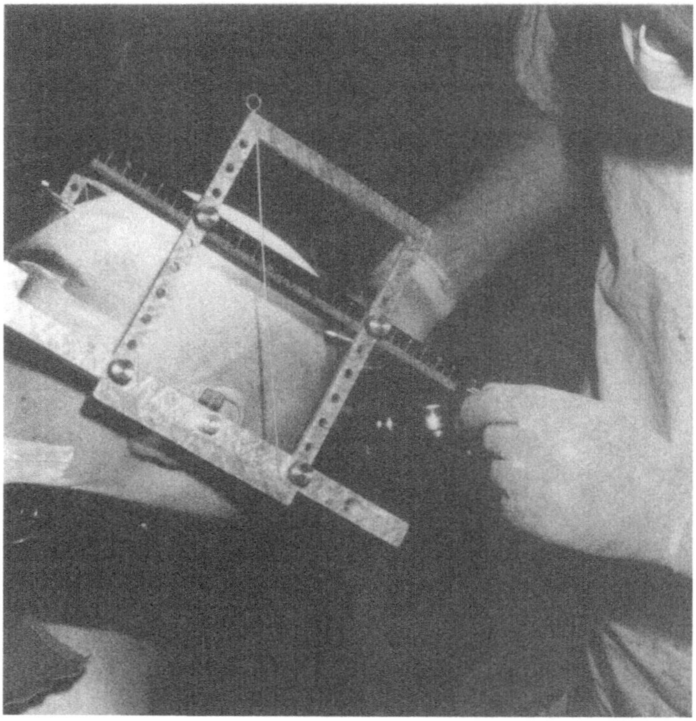

FIGURE 4–8. Square attached to SCID at appropriate height.

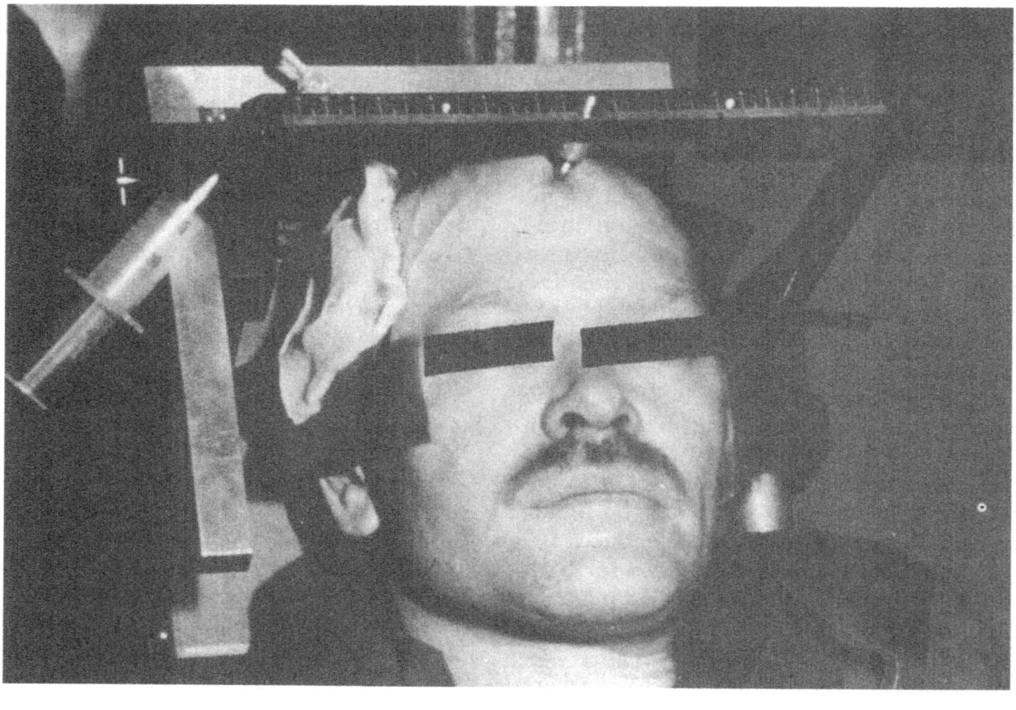

FIGURE 4–9. Patient is in a sitting position with the L-grid placed for the AP view and the square fixed to the table.

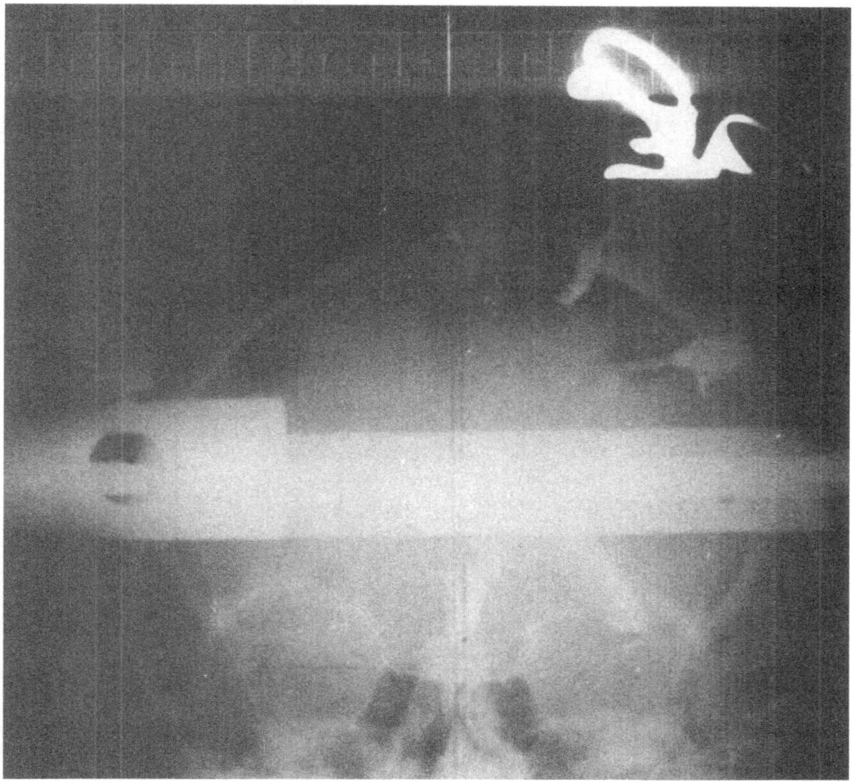

FIGURE 4-10. AP ventriculogram; the 90° projection from the middle of the third ventricle indicates laterality.

Next, the L-grid is secured in the grid block holder on the patient's right side in the reference plane (zero is chosen for the third ventricle). The cassette holder is attached to the posterior side and the cassette is inserted. The light beam or laser beam of the x-ray source is directed 3 m to zero of the square. (A light-beam box or laser-alignment mirror aids in centralization.) The light beams and the square should be parallel to the floor. A contrast agent is introduced and an AP image is obtained (figure 4-10). The line should be projected at right angles from the reference point (third ventricle) to the horizontal ruler. The lateral offset of the Z_S coordinate (right or left) is noted.

The L-grid is fixed posteriorly at Z_S coordinate and the zero vertical marks at the inferior edge of the square. The cassette holder is moved to the side square so that a lateral image can be obtained. The lines are projected at right angles from the selected target to the horizontal and vertical rulers (figure 4-11). The X and Y coordinates are noted. (If the reference point is more that 10 mm from the estimated plane, the L-grid is placed at the correct plane for the second AP image. Theoretically, this procedure could be repeated ad infinitum, providing progressive improvement of accuracy. In practice, one AP and one lateral ventriculogram are sufficient.)

The lateral coordinate of the target is selected from an atlas plus or minus the Z_S already determined. The cylinder block is fixed at the X and Y coordinates, and the arc cylinder, arc quadrant, and sighting rod are assembled. The arc is moved to the calculated Z_S. The electrode is advanced toward zero until its tip appears at the sight hole; the electrode then is fixed at zero on the vernier scale, and the electrode holder and electrode are removed. Next, the arc assembly is secured to the cylinder block (figure 4-12). The trajectory is adjusted by the rotating cylinder and moving the

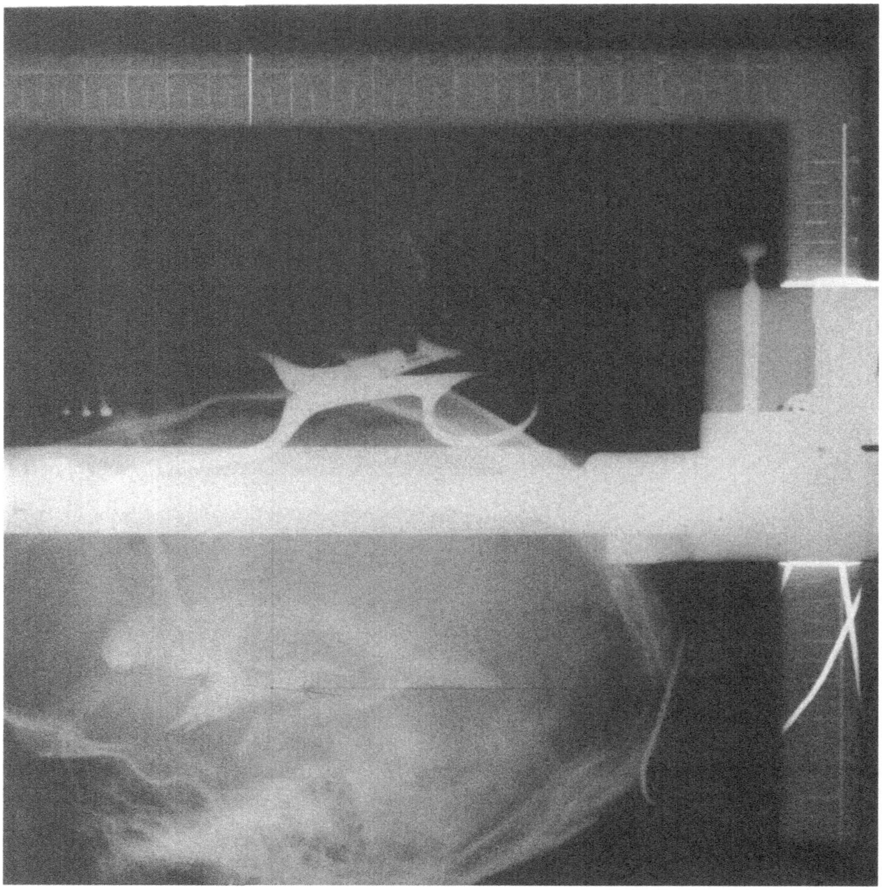

FIGURE 4–11. Lateral ventriculogram with 90° projections to horizontal and vertical arms of L-grid.

slide assembly along the quadrant until the electrodes can pass through the burr hole. Alternately, the cylinder rotation and arc degrees can be set in advance, and the burr hole placed at the trajectory point on the skull. The electrode now is advanced to the target, and its position is confirmed radiographically (figure 4–13).

STEREO CT SCANNING

The square is attached to the skull with either CT-compatible pins for three-point fixation or with extension pieces for four-point fixation. After the alignment plates are connected to the side of the square, the square is secured to the *gantry attachment*. The laser alignment light is used to align the zeros for the vertical and horizontal planes (the zero mark on the square and its inferior edge, respectively). The superior laser alignment should be zero. All coordinates are now in reference to the reference points of the square. Selected CT images are performed and the square is removed from the scanner.

Next, the cursor is moved to diagonally opposite pillars of the alignment plate and a line is drawn from one to the other. This step is repeated for the opposite diagonal. The cursor is moved to the point at which the diagonal lines cross (center of square) and the X, Y, and Z coordinates are obtained. The cursor is moved next to the target and the X, Y, and Z coordinates are determined conventionally. Selected reformatted images can be displayed with the target coordinates (figure 4–14). Alternatively, a selected section of a large film can be used, and the X_I and Y_I coordinates obtained by direct measurement from the superimposed grid (figure 4–15). If the square or SCID is fixed to the scanner gantry, the height is calcu-

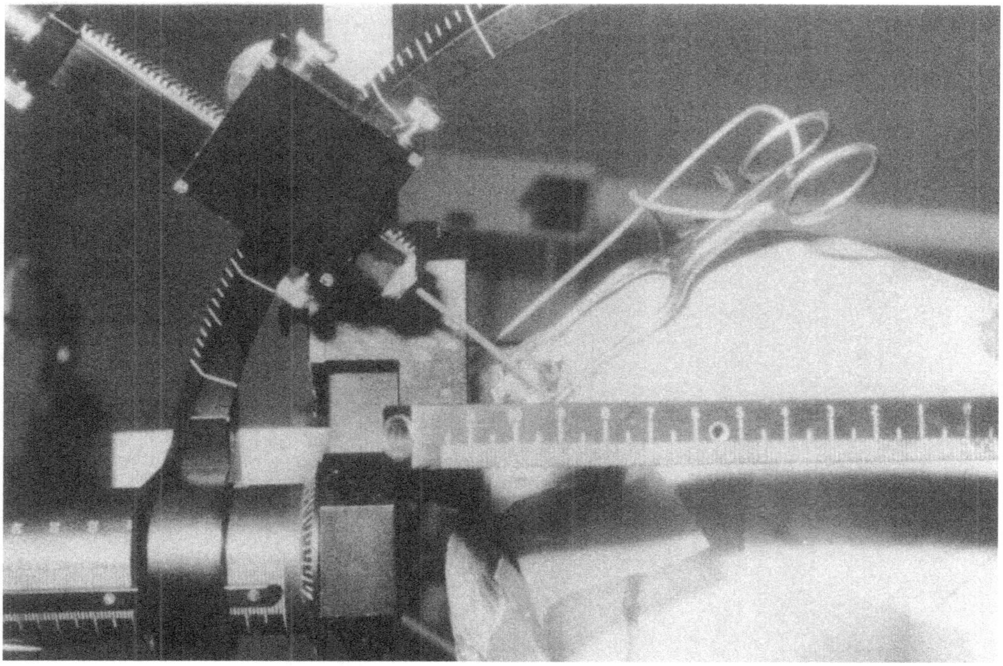

FIGURE 4–12. Close-up view of block and arc assembly.

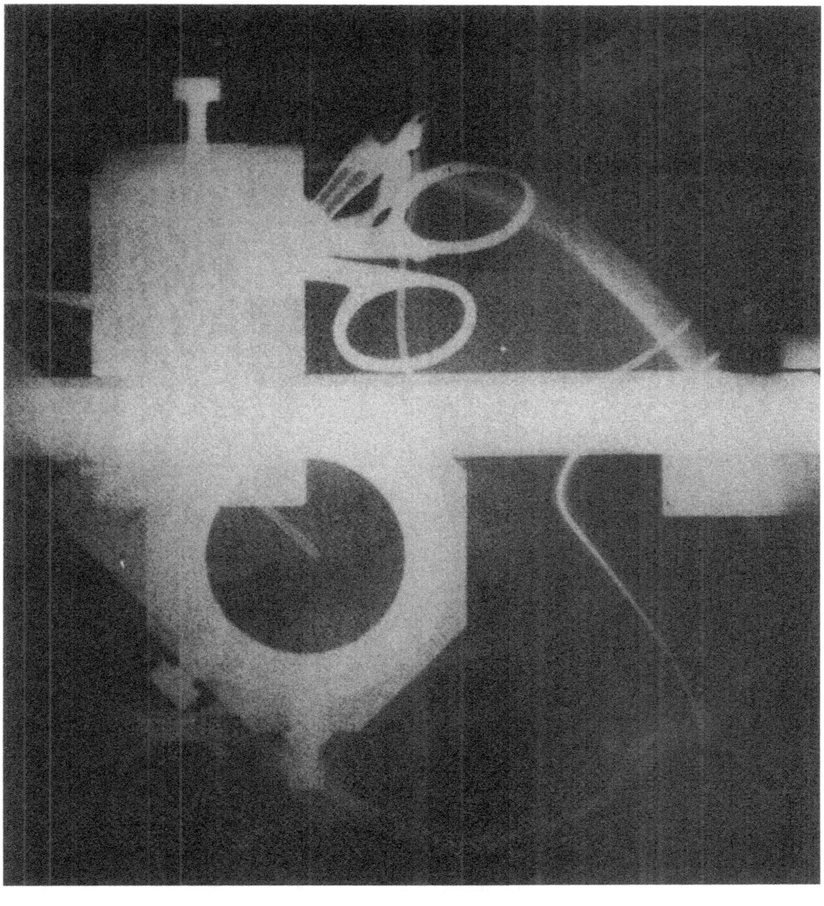

FIGURE 4–13. Roentgenogram shows position of target electrode.

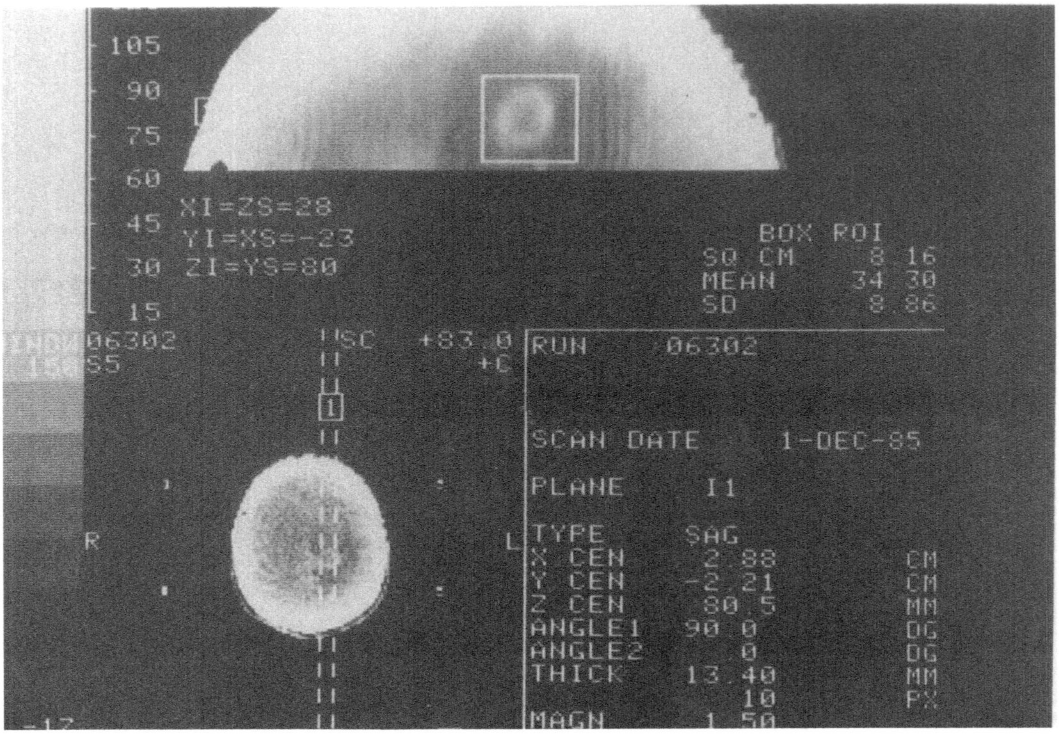

FIGURE 4–14. Reformatted image of the target and display of target coordinates.

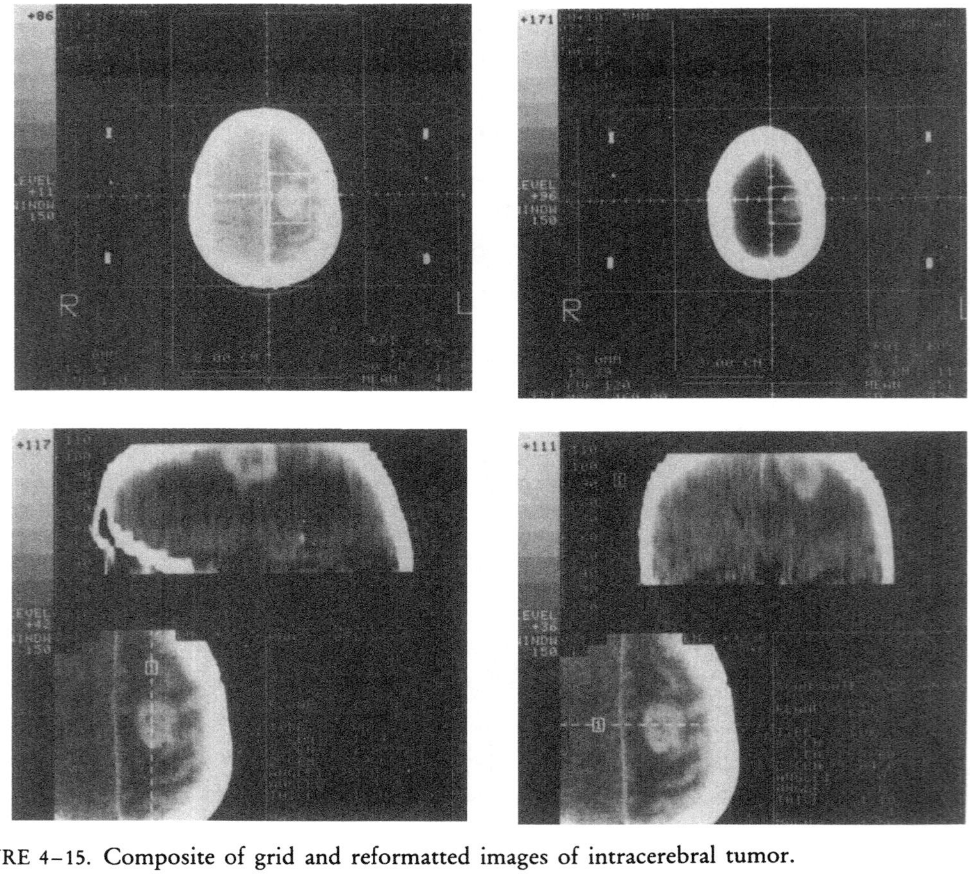

FIGURE 4–15. Composite of grid and reformatted images of intracerebral tumor.

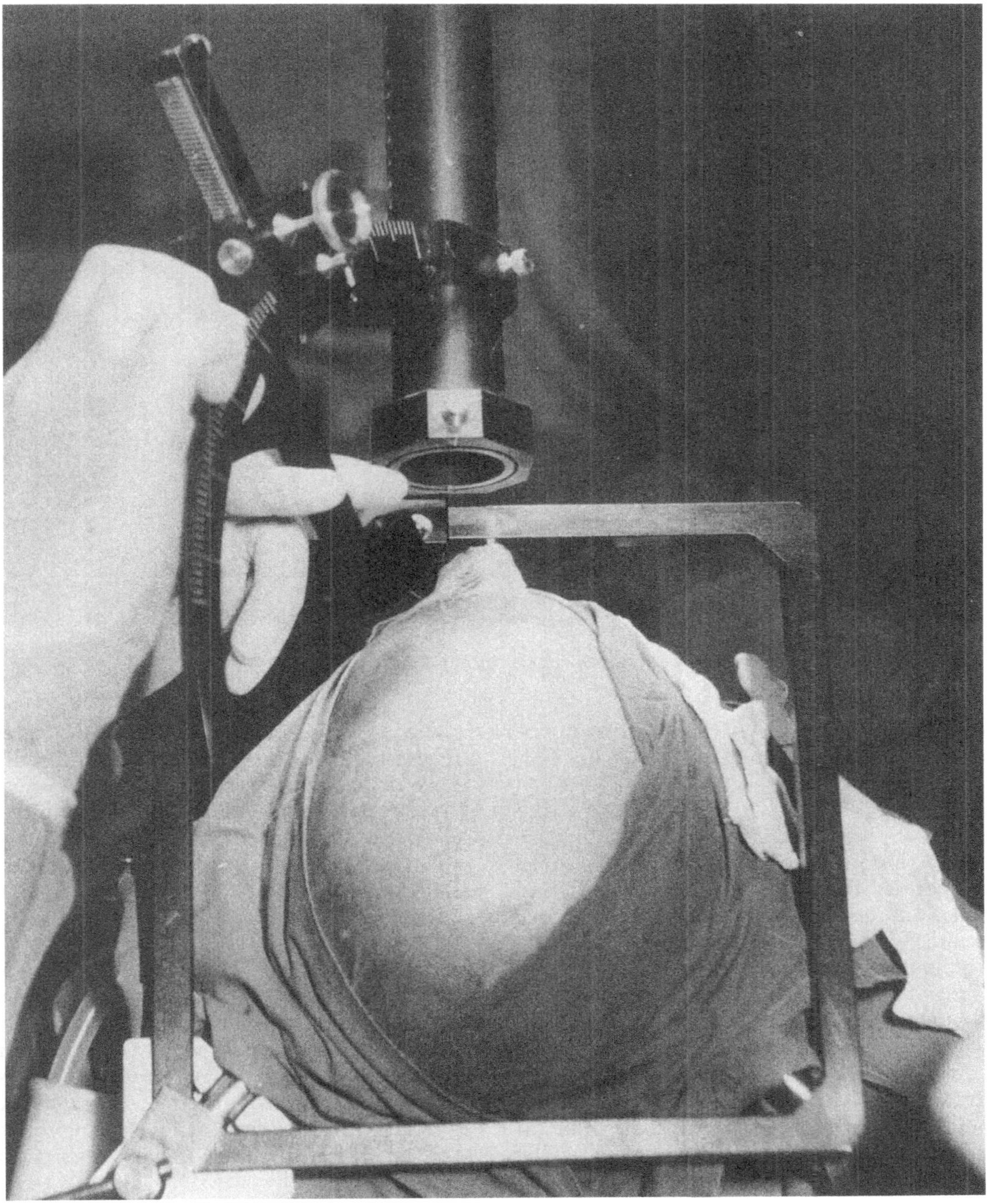

FIGURE 4–16. Open stereotactic surgery. The flat plane of the stereotactic square permits wide exposure for craniotomy.

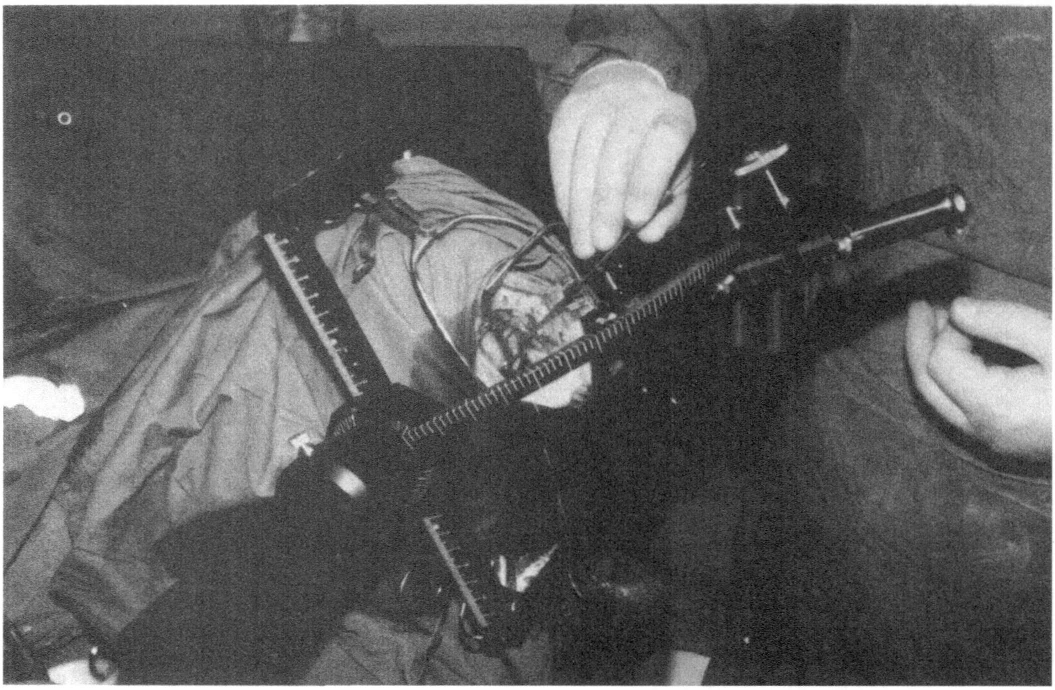

FIGURE 4–17. Open craniotomy for lesion localized by stereotactic CT scan.

lated by the computer (Z_S); otherwise, it can be read from the fiducial points.

SCID USAGE

The meatal plugs are inserted with comfortable pressure to equal depths in the external auditory meatus. The plugs are then secured, and the nasion rest is adjusted to a comfortable pressure. When complete, the nasion and meatal readings are recorded.

Next, the SCID is secured to the gantry attachment. The laser alignment light is used to align zeros for the vertical and horizontal planes (center of meatal plug and inferior edge, respectively). The superior laser alignment should be zero. All coordinates are now in reference to the SCID reference points. The selected section is scanned, and both the SCID and the patient are removed from the scanner.

The square is attached to the SCID by the aligned plates at the selected distance "D" above the SCID zero. The nasion rest and meatal bars, at previous readings are used to apply the SCID to the skull. The fixation pins then are inserted in the skull and both the SCID and the alignment plates are removed.

The AP (Y_S), and lateral (X_S) SCID targets are also those for the square. The target will be above or below the vertical zero of the square. The target height "T" can be determined as follows: if T is greater than D, then true height is T minus D *above* the square. If T is less than D, the true height is D minus T *below* the square.

OPEN STEREOTACTIC SURGERY

If a large craniotomy is required, the square should be fixed as low on the skull as possible, with the extension pieces, if necessary. Whenever possible, the simple three-pin fixation should be used (figure 4–16) to take advantage of the small single plane of the square, which presents fewer obstructions (figure 4–17).

Conclusions

Improvement in imaging has encouraged surgeons, including the author, to use only the coordinates obtained from CT scans in performing functional stereotactic procedures. SCID scanning is convenient because the coordinates can be obtained before the frame is applied, and it interferes less with scanning an operating room schedules. Although less precise than stereotactic CT scanning, SCID scanning is perfectly adequate for tumors.

The whole system has been in use for several years and has been employed in a large variety of procedures. Some of the recent developments described have improved the fundamental use of this instrument, which requires no more calculations than addition or subtraction.

References

1. Hitchcock E: An apparatus for stereotactic spinal surgery. *Lancet* 705–706, 1969
2. Hitchcock E: Stereotaxic spinal surgery: A preliminary report. *J Neurosurg* 31:386–392, 1969

5. THE BROWN-ROBERTS-WELLS SYSTEM

Micheal L.J. Apuzzo
Craig A. Fredericks

The Brown-Roberts-Wells (BRW) stereotactic system is the result of collaborative efforts between the Division of Neurosurgery at the University of Utah and the biomedical engineering developer, Trent Wells, in South Gate, CA. This system materialized from conceptual goals defined and elaborated by mathematician and medical student Russel Brown and neurosurgical director Theodore Roberts. These objective included [5–9]:

1. Location of a three-dimensional (X, Y, Z) point in space by using two dimensions (X, Y) defined by imaging studies and adding of a vertical coordinate (Z).
2. Provision of an infinite number of positions from which a three-dimensionally defined point in space could be reached directly with a probe.
3. Development of a methodology for verifying those established points and positions before surgery.

To transform two dimensions to three dimensions, a system was devised in which a reference plane is fixed with two vertical rods and a connecting diagonal rod (forming an N-shaped localizing system). The height above the reference plane is a function of the ratio of the constant distance between the two vertical rods to the variable distance between them and the diagonal rod. The final system is composed of three sets of N's around or within the reference plane, which fix the position and allow determination of X, Y, and Z coordinates for any point in that plane.

This configuration permits flexibility in patient positioning within the computed tomographic (CT) scanner gantry. It also makes remote computation and derivation of target coordinates possible, independent of the scanner computer. Because the localizing system is fixed to the patient only, the BRW apparatus can be used with a variety of CT scanners, and the surgeon has the freedom to complete the procedure in a separate operating room.

A previously designed general stereotactic arc system defined basal midline structures with the target at the center of the arc. This required moving the arc until the target was at the center and necessitated either a very large arc or remote placement in reference to the skull unless the target was midline. That design limited the approach to lesions not in the basal midline. The ultimate design of the BRW arc guidance system allows selection of any skull entry site for any intracranial target. Infinite probe tract versatility was accomplished by two movement parameters, which were incorporated into an arc system and allowed both vertical and horizontal rotation and pivot. Two vertical parameters (called alpha and beta) define 360° of rotation about the base ring and 40° of pivot,respectively. This feature allows the vertical matching of any entry point with its corresponding target. The horizontal counterpart is defined by gamma and delta movements. Gamma indicates 200° of rotation of the radial slide along the arc; delta is 110° of pivot about the radial slide itself.

A phantom base simulator was developed as a method for verifying the accuracy of the target computation and the frame setting. The user can establish the precision of all coordinates in relation to a phantom point that is identical to the real anatomical target.

L.D. Lunsford (ed.) *MODERN STEREOTACTIC NEUROSURGERY*.

Components of the BRW System

In its final form, the BRW stereotactic guidance system (Radionics, Inc., Burlington, MA) consists of a head ring, a localizer unit, an arc guidance system, and a phantom base simulator [9–11].

The head ring is composed of nickel-plated aluminum and is fixed to the cranium at four points by graphite epoxy posts with nylon and steel pins. It provides the base for the N-localizer which is used during imaging studies, and the arc guidance system which is applied during the invasive part of the procedure.

The localizing unit contains two rings connected by nine graphite rods arranged in the three N-shaped configuration's described earlier. It is applied to the head-ring platform during imaging for calculation of the X and Y coordinates. The relative positions of the vertical and diagonal rods seen on different CT images are mathematically correlated to the intracranial target point.

The arc guidance system consists of a base ring that attaches to a rotatable ring and to a perpendicular arc with a radial slide. This assembly can be affixed firmly to the patient's head ring or to the phantom base by three mounting balls. The rotatable ring defines the alpha and beta movements in the vertical arc. The radial slide (gamma) on the perpendicular arc has a pivotable sleeve (delta). This sleeve accepts various bushings that act as carriers and direct the trajectory of the surgical instruments to the target point.

The combination of the four angle settings (alpha, beta, gamma, delta) are computed in a programmable calculator, allowing the user to choose entry points to reach intracranial target points anywhere within the sphere of the guidance arc.

The phantom base includes a base ring (equivalent to the head ring) and a movable pointed tip, designated a "phantom target." This tip can be set to any precalculated (with the arc system) X, Y, and Z coordinates for either target or entry points. The scan coordinates and entry point data derived from the phantom are entered in the portable computer which then calculates the arc frame settings and the distance to the target. The target coordinates are set in the phantom. Trajectory coordinates are designated on the arc and confirmed on the phantom target. The arc system on the phantom ring bears the same relationship to the phantom target as it will to the intracranial target when it is affixed to the patient base ring. This provides an extracranial check of the target settings, arc coordinates, and distances for the intracranial instrument placement.

The software for the system utilizes data from the X and Y coordinates of the central CT or magnetic resonance imaging (MRI) pixel of each of the nine localizer rods and the target. The program transforms the two-dimensional (X and Y) coordinates to three-dimensional coordinates (X, Y, and Z) and relates the position of the localizer rods and the targets to the image plane, which indicates the vertical height from the base ring. With the X, Y, and Z coordinates of the target thus derived, the arc system allows the user to plot a course and distance between any two points in space, the entry point (scalp or dura) and the target. The software permits selection of multiple targets, entry points, and parallel transits in each scan plane.

Steps in Target Point Access

The time required to complete all steps from initiation of base ring application to target point access is 60 minutes (table 5–1).

APPLICATION OF BASE RING

(Figures 5–1 through 5–5)

The scalp is prepared and with the patient in the sitting position, and appropriate post and pin positions are selected. This step is achieved

TABLE 5–1. Average Time to Accomplish Steps Toward Target Point Access Using the BRW System

Step	Average Time (minutes)
1. Base ring assembly and application	10
2. Target scanning	10[a]
3. Data collection and processing	15
4. Entry point selection	5
5. Arc setting	5
6. Phantom base target confirmation	5
7. Instrumentation (infiltration, incision, drill, cannula introduction)	10
Total (point access)	60[b]

[a] Exact time depends on number of images obtained.
[b] Does not include time required to transport patient to and from CT scanner.

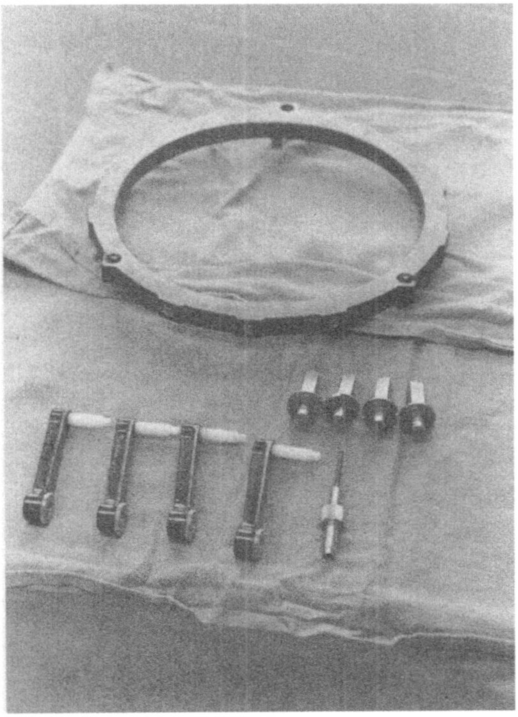

FIGURE 5-1. A disassembled base ring unit with carbon-fiber posts; an adjusting tool is at the lower right.

easily if the patient is on an operating room table in an anesthesia preparation room [1, 2, 4]. In many cases (i.e., lesions in the third ventricular region), the base ring is positioned in a plane defined by the tip of the nose and the inion. The ring is secured during placement fixation by a Velcro strap. Observers at the foot of the operating table and at the patient's side monitor ring position during placement. The assistant on the side of the patient assesses ring position and manually maintains the sagittal suture parallel to the floor. The neurosurgeon is free to direct and to infiltrate the scalp at the four fixation points with 1% lidocaine with epinephrine. The nylon drive pins are advanced to the scalp, the tracks adjusted, and the four carbon-fiber posts are advanced to secure the pins to the pericranium. Generally, intravenous contrast medium is infused during the early stages of this procedure. The patient is transported to the scanner, accompanied by the anesthesiologist.

SCAN TARGET (Figures 5-6 through 5-9)
With the patient in the CT scanner, the localizer unit is applied to the base ring. Because detailed imaging studies have been performed previously, an abbreviated study defining

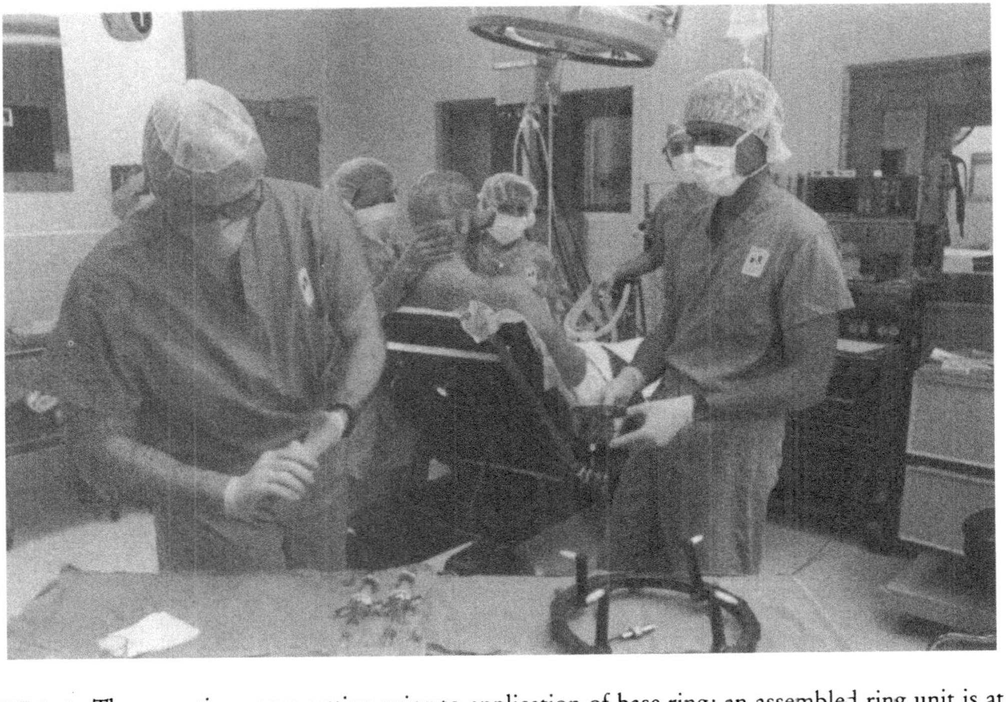

FIGURE 5-2. The operating room setting prior to application of base ring; an assembled ring unit is at lower right.

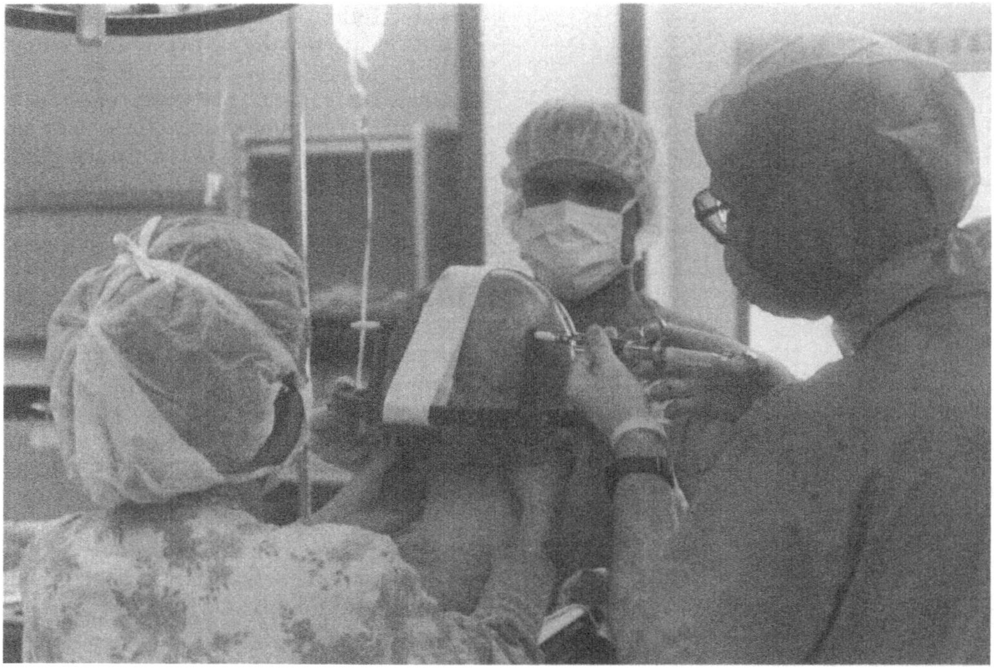

FIGURE 5–3. Local anesthetic is infiltrated for application of base ring unit while the patient's head and ring unit are stabilized by two assistants and the aid of a Velcro strap.

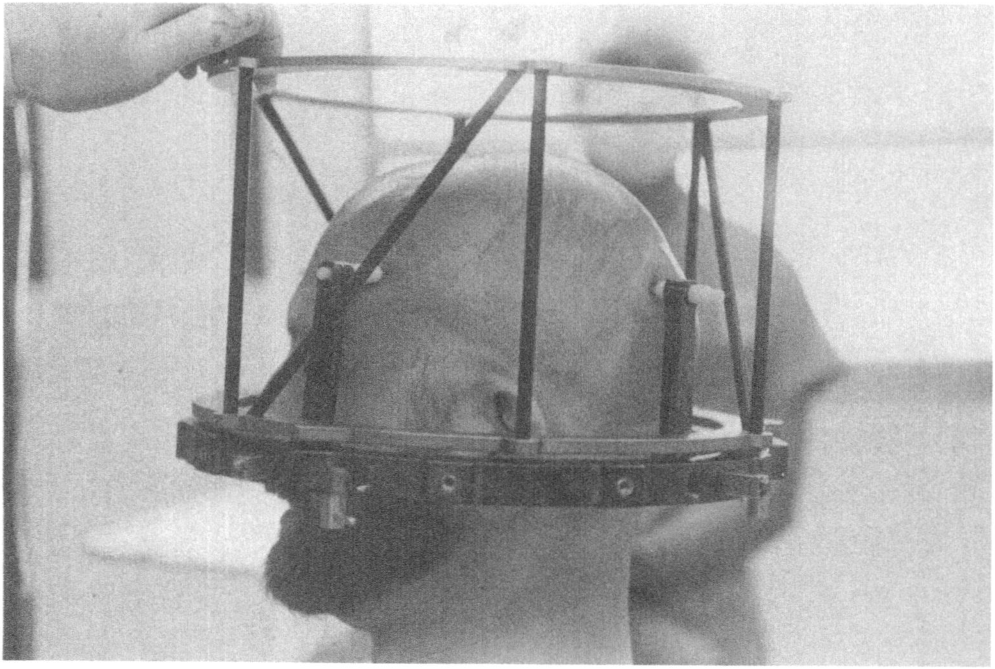

FIGURE 5–4. Final placement of ring with localizing unit attached. Note ring position in relation to the nose and mouth.

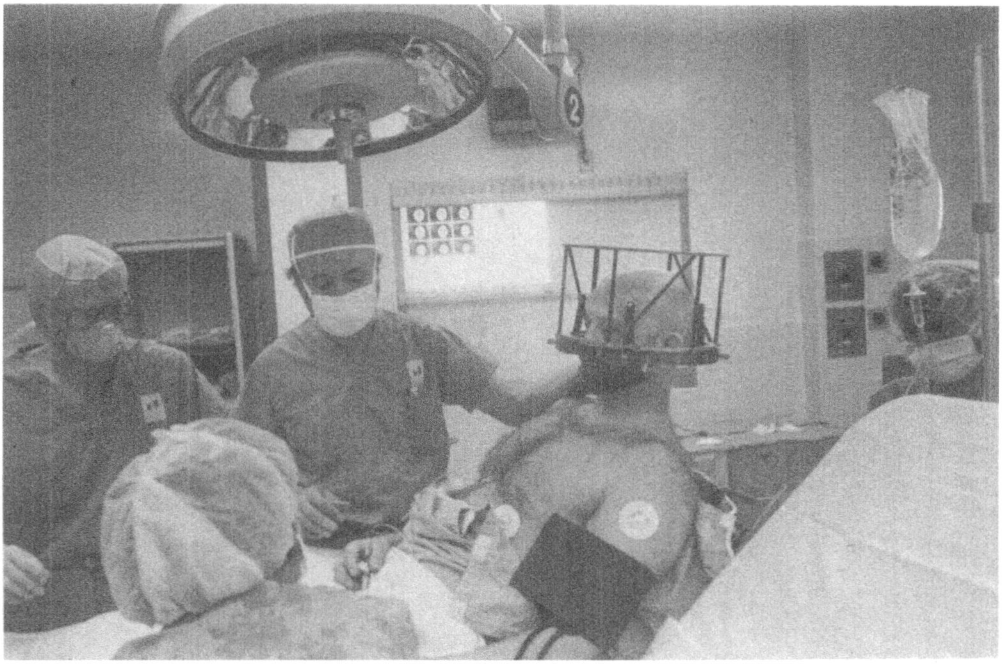

FIGURE 5–5. The anesthesiologist initiates the patient is transfer to CT suite.

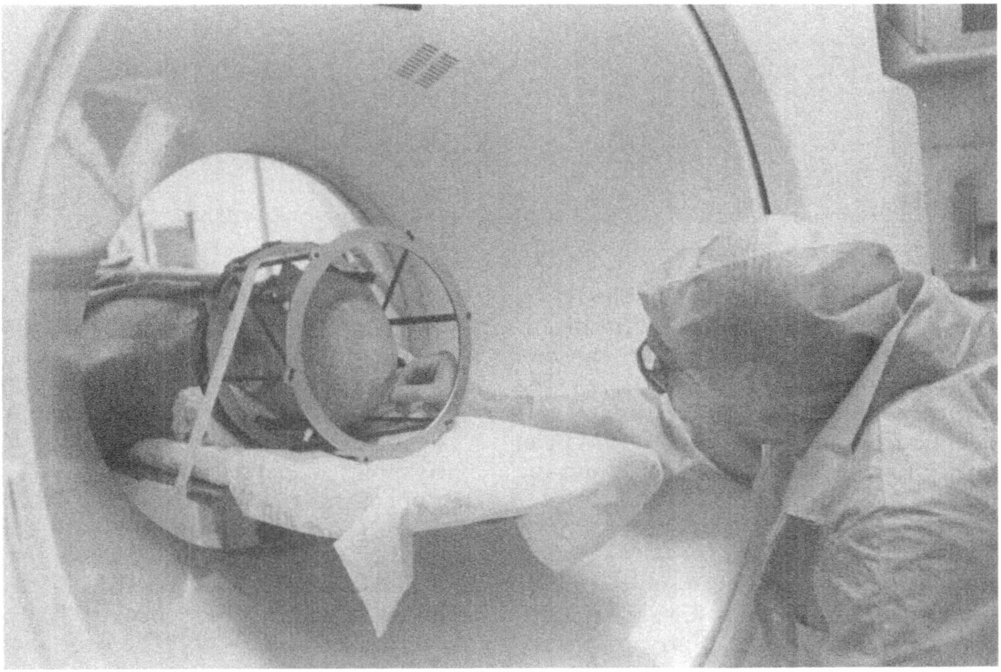

FIGURE 5–6. With the patient in the scanner gantry, the surgeon marks the proposed entry site for reference during imaging.

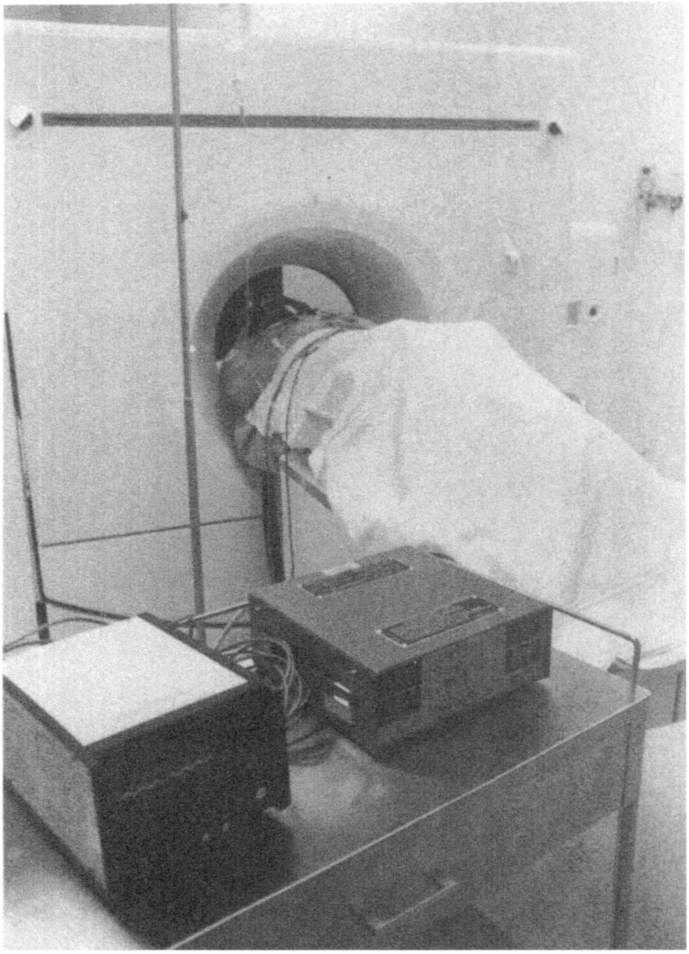

FIGURE 5–7. Cardiovascular and neurological status are monitored during scanning.

desired aspects of the target region should be adequate. Afterwards, the patient is returned to the operating room and prepared for the formal surgical aspect of the procedure. The surgeons then study the CT images, select one for use in targeting, and derive and record pixel coordinates for the nine localizer rods and the targets.

ENTRY POINT SELECTION

Entry points and trajectories are not standardized; they are selected individually with regard to the certain variables. Entry points are selected according to the target position. A well-chosen entry point is critical to establish a safe trajectory. Considerations in choosing an entry point are: the location, size, and suspected composition of the lesion; the intervening neural and vascular structures; the target point; and the objective of the procedure.

Once a point on the scalp is selected, the arc system is attached to the base ring, and the entry point is marked by a probe directed to the point and rigidly fixed in the arc system. The arc is detached from the head ring and applied to the phantom base, where the X, Y, and Z coordinates are derived from the three appropriate scales (anteroposterior [AP], lateral, vertical, figure 5–10). The coordinates are recorded.

Optimal entry point selection may be attained within the scanning unit. Given the

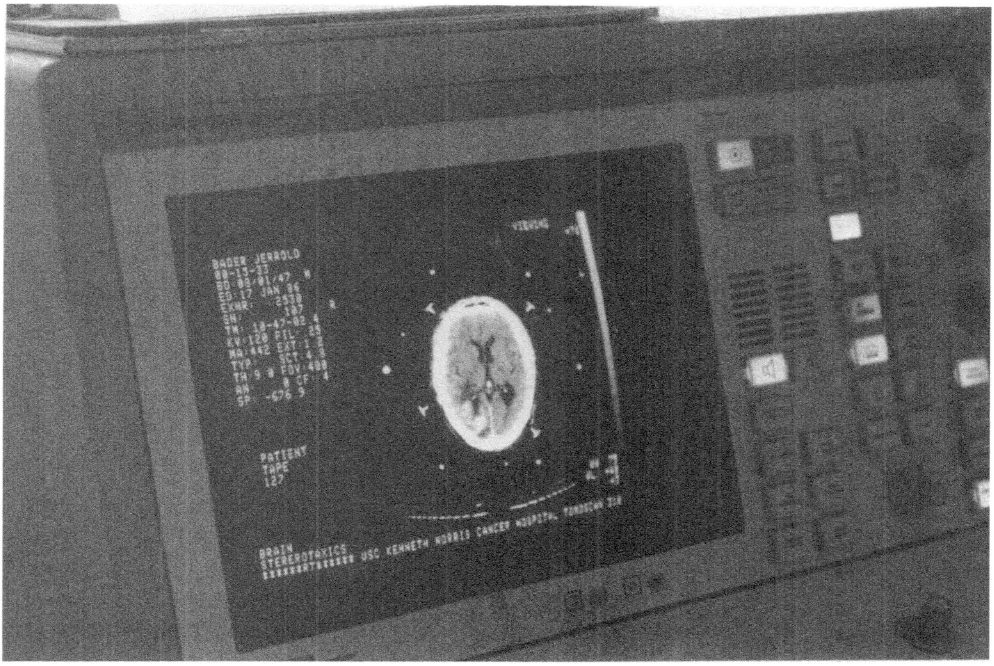

FIGURE 5–8. The nine rods of the localizer unit appear as dots around the target image, serving as external reference fiducials.

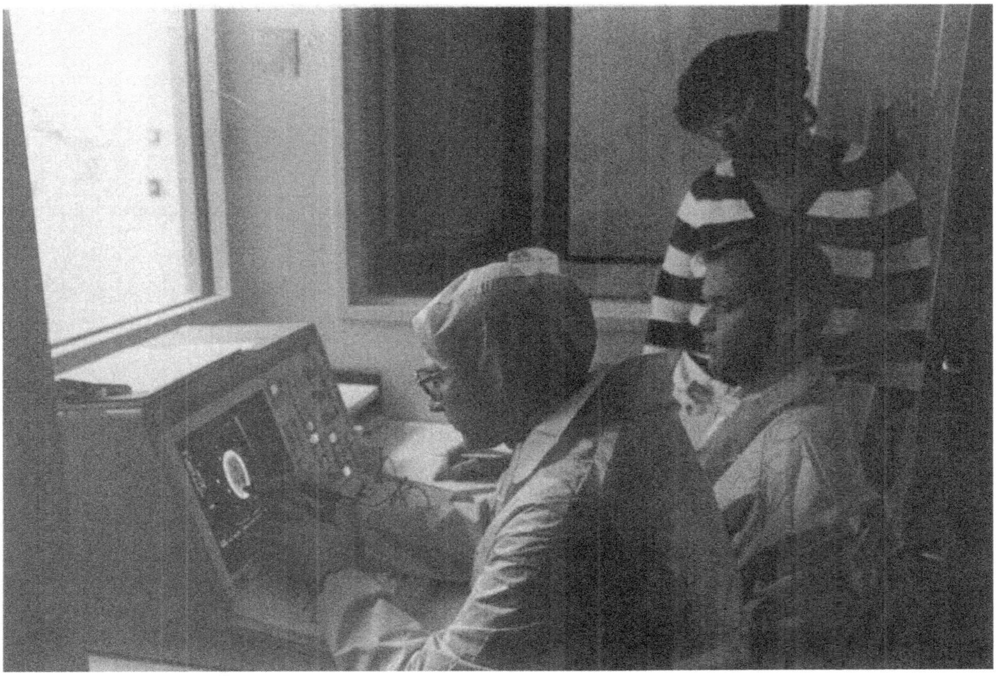

FIGURE 5–9. The surgeon selects the target and derives coordinates for the fiducials and target.

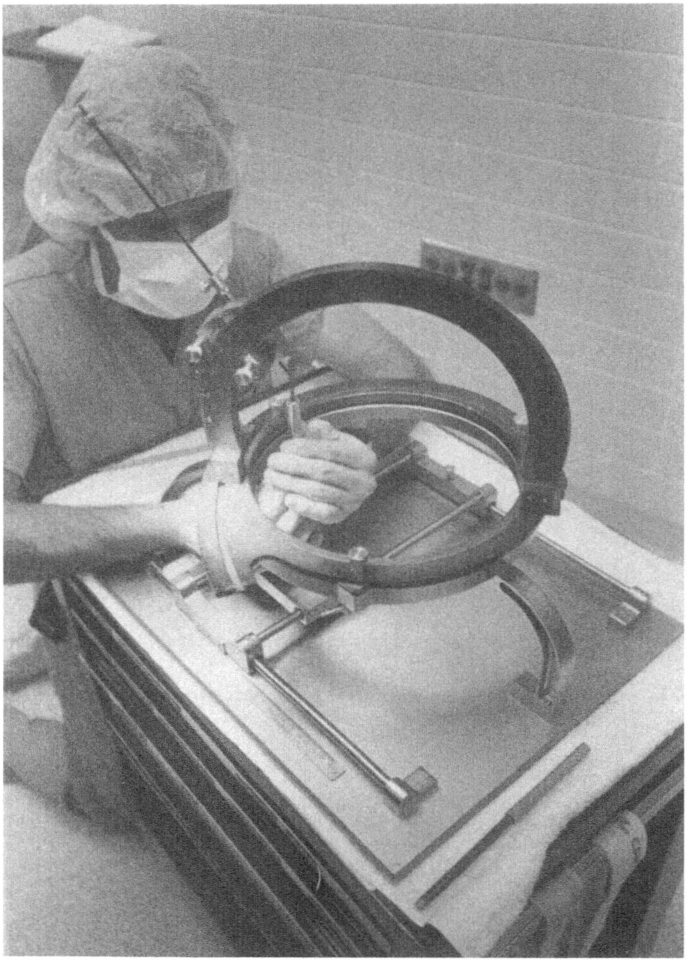

FIGURE 5–10. The phantom base is used to determine X, Y, and Z coordinates for the entry point (selected by the surgeon).

appropriate scanner software, an entry site can be marked during imaging, and planes of transit can be reconstructed to the target point. This technique, used concurrently with rapid bolus contrast infusion to define vascular structures, will increase the safety and control of the entry.

DATA PROCESSING

All X, Y imaging coordinates obtained from the nine localizer rods, the target(s), and the entry point(s) are entered in the programmable computer, which determines appropriate alpha, beta, gamma, and delta settings for the arc system. Data describing the depth of the target from the arc slide bushing also are indicated. Finally, coordinates for localization of the phantom are calculated (figures 5–11, 5–12).

ARC SETTINGS AND PHANTOM

The settings for the arc are entered and initially verified on the phantom base, using the X, Y, and Z coordinates for the phantom entry point. The target coordinates in the vertical, lateral, and AP planes (X, Y, Z) are placed on the phantom, thereby defining the phantom target. The probe is used to confirm the arc coordinates and the distance to the phantom target point, thus providing the preoperative (extracranial) assessment of the arc settings, trajectories, and target depth. Additionally, instruments to be introduced to the true target

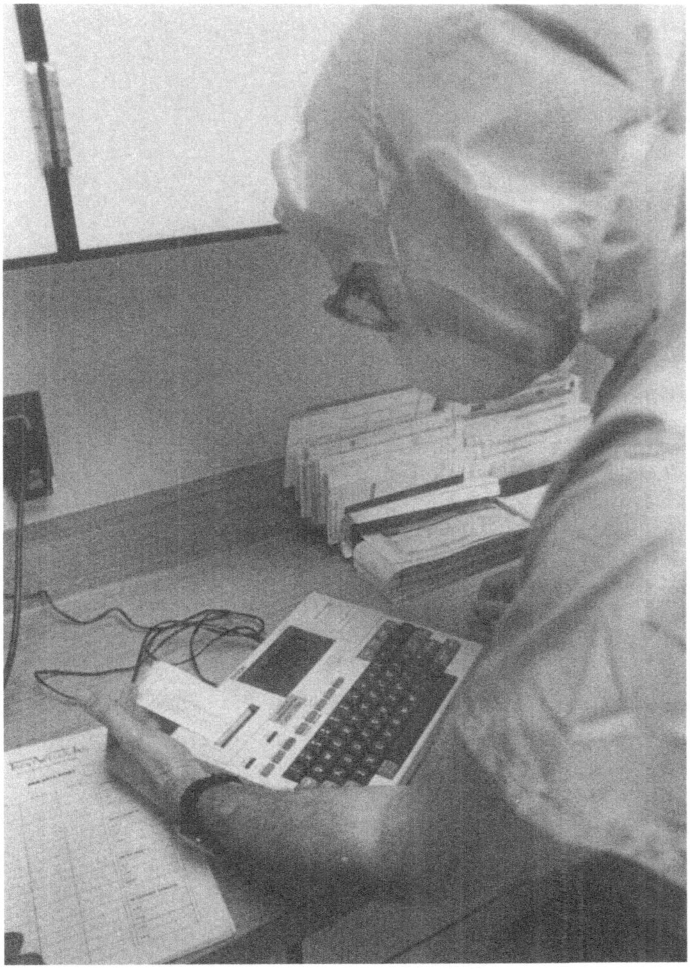

FIGURE 5–11. Fiducial, target, and entry coordinates are entered into the microcomputer system.

point can be calibrated precisely to the phantom target (figures 5–13, 5–14).

FINAL ACCESS TO INSTRUMENTATION AT TARGET POINT

At this point, various surgical procedures can be performed. For a biopsy, 13-gauge cannula with a blunt stylet and flexible bronchoscopy-cup biopsy forceps are used. In preparation for introducing this instrument to the target point, the biopsy forceps are advanced through the cannula, and the distance to the emergence of the cups is carefully marked with sterile tape.

Next, the arc system is attached to the patient's head ring. The scalp entry point is infiltrated with 1% lidocaine with epinephrine and a 7- to 10-mm incision is made. A guide tube suitable for stabilizing a long 4.5-mm twist drill is advanced and secured within the arc slide bushing (figure 5–15). The skull is penetrated with the twist drill. The patient feels minimal discomfort as the dura is entered. A 2.7-mm guide tube replaces the drill guide tube in the slide bushing, and a sharp probe is inserted to penetrate the dura. The blunt 13-gauge cannula then is advanced to the target site through the rigid fixation of the arc guidance system (figure 5–16). The inner stylet is removed, and the biopsy forceps are advanced to the tape marker; the forceps are opened to obtain specimens at various rotations of the cup and, if appropriate, at various depths. An assistant opens and closes the cups while the

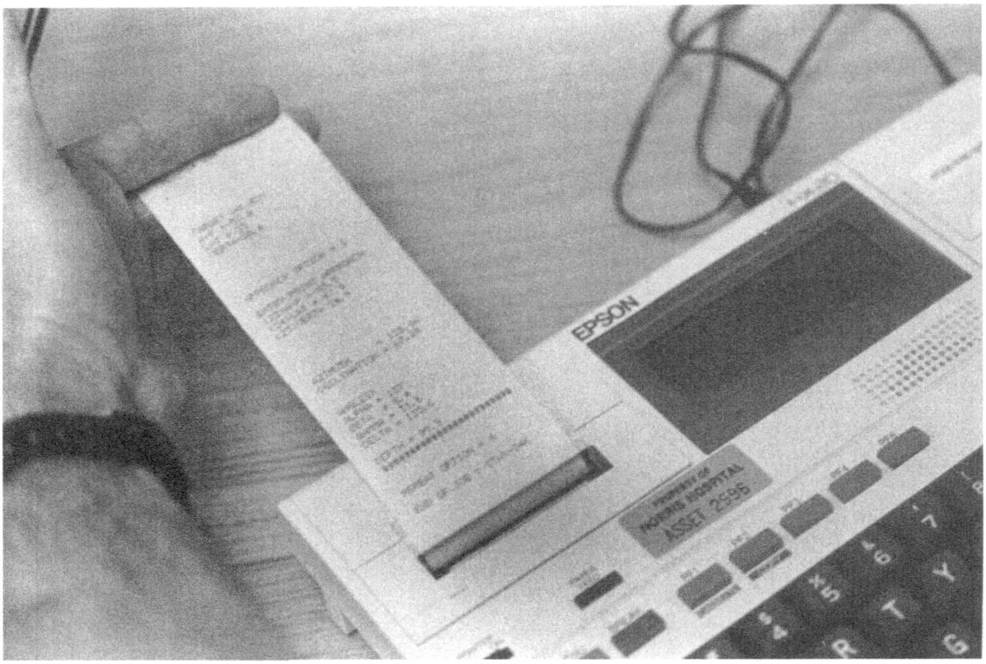

FIGURE 5–12. Target coordinates, arc settings, and depth of target in relation to arc bushing are calculated by a portable computer.

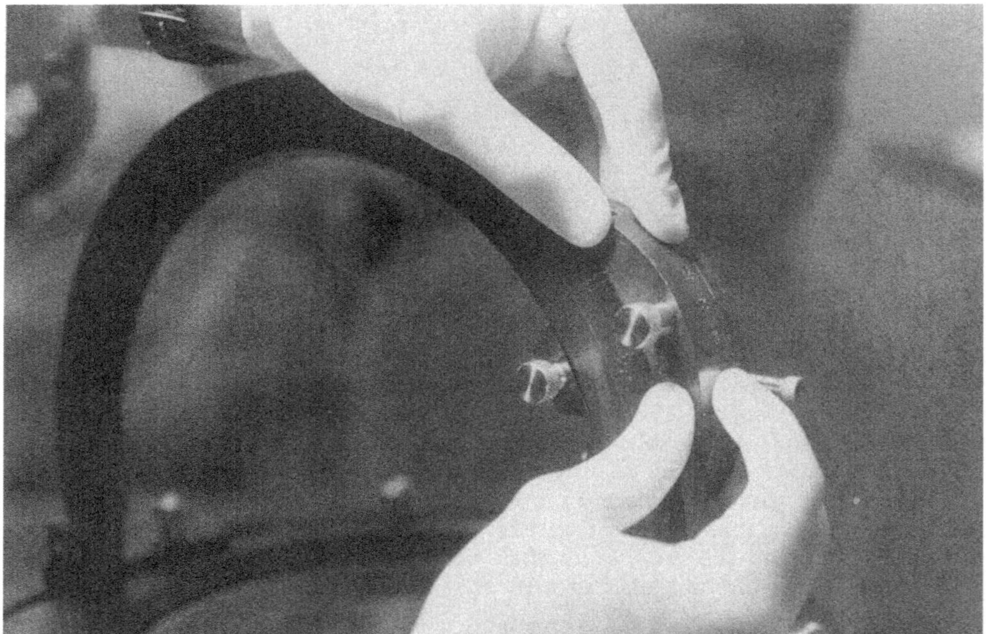

FIGURE 5–13. Arc settings are entered on the phantom base.

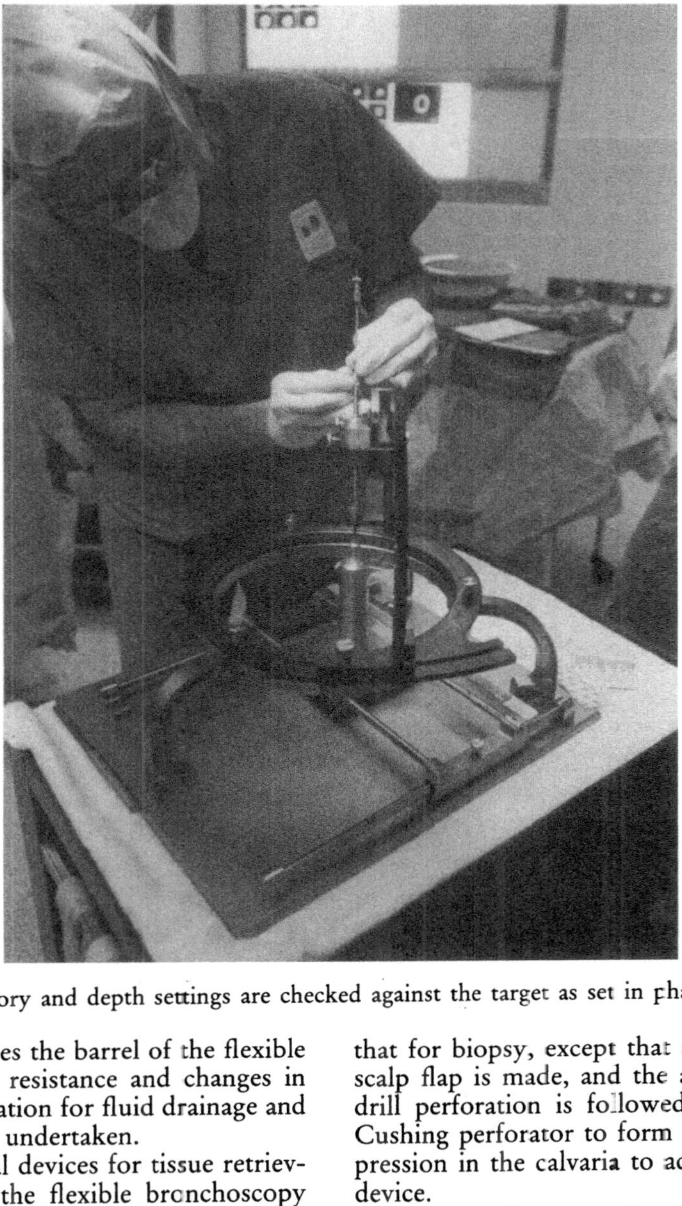

FIGURE 5-14. Trajectory and depth settings are checked against the target as set in phantom.

neurosurgeon palpates the barrel of the flexible forceps, monitoring resistance and changes in tissue texture. Aspiration for fluid drainage and analysis also can be undertaken.

After using several devices for tissue retrieval, we have found the flexible bronchoscopy biopsy forceps to be the best universal instrument. These forceps have afforded satisfactory tissue samples with very low morbidity, whereas the slotted and coiled instruments depend on minimal tissue resistance for removal of satisfactory samples.

For insertion of a permanent drainage conduit, we have used a 22-cm (working length) catheter (2.5 mm in diameter) with a rigid stylet. The catheter is connected to a large Rickham reservoir. The technique is similar to that for biopsy, except that a 3-cm curvilinear scalp flap is made, and the arc-directed twist-drill perforation is followed by the use of a Cushing perforator to form a cone-shaped depression in the calvaria to accept the Rickham device.

Catheter placement for interstitial brachytherapy is expedient with this method [3, 4]. The available software facilitates the implantation of parallel arrays of brachytherapy catheters at CT-derived target points. The basic method is the same as that for biopsy and conduit placement, except that multiple planar targets are used. Each target and trajectory is planned separately and verified on the phantom. Although a "shortcut" grid method is available, we prefer individual targeting and

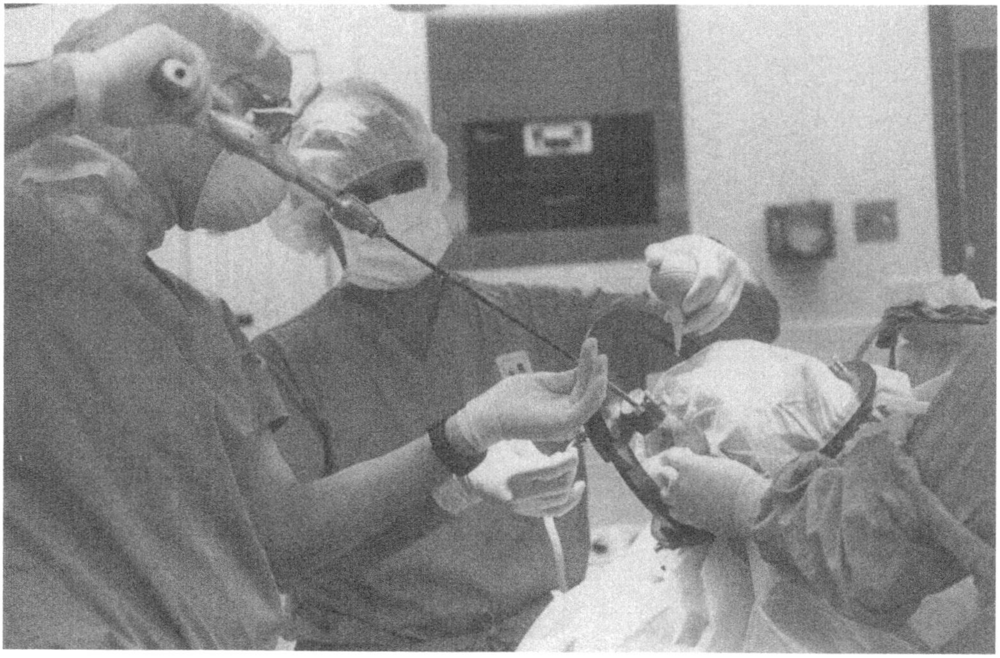

FIGURE 5–15. Following local anesthetic infiltration and scalp incision, the calvaria is perforated with a one-fourth-inch twist drill set in a guide tube with a trajectory to the target. A drill stop prevents dural dissection from the inner table.

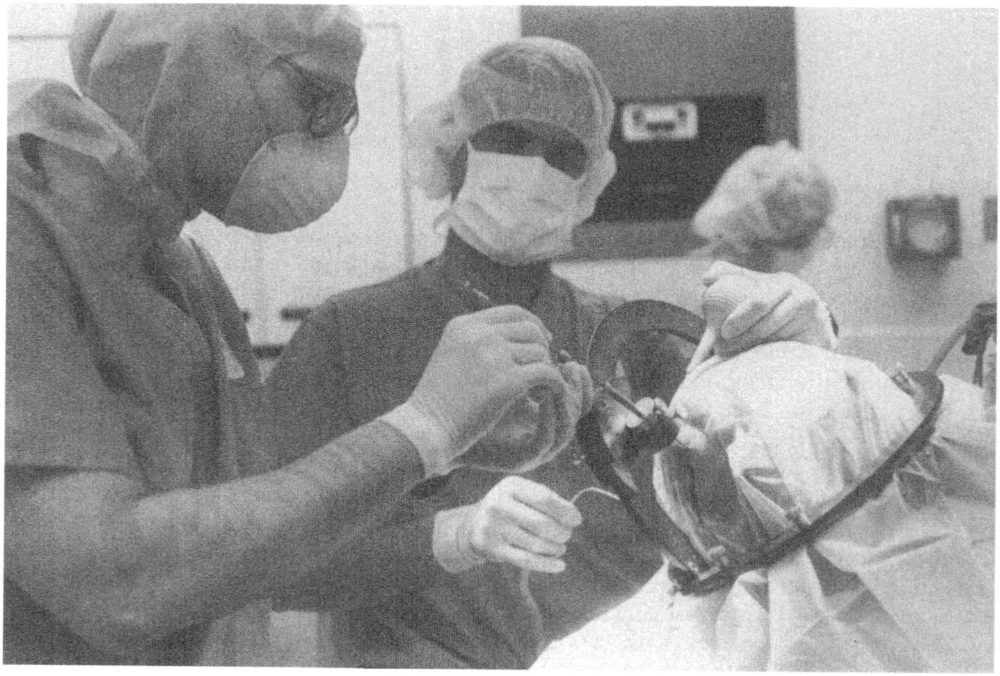

FIGURE 5–16. A 13-gauge cannula is introduced to the target.

target-point checks. Four to six catheters can be placed precisely in parallel array in less than two hours from the time of base ring application.

Endoscopy also is possible with the BRW system. We have used a 6.2-mmdiameter endoscope (Karl Storz Endoscopy, Tuttlingen, West Germany) with a 20-cm barrel both within the brain and the ventricles.

Experience and Critique

Because of the potential capabilities and value of the BRW instrument, it was readily assimilated into the neurosurgical armamentarium at the University of Southern California Medical Center Hospitals in 1981.

Since that date, the BRW system has been used in more than 600 procedures. Thus far, the system has been used almost exclusively to evaluate and manage mass lesions. Indications for our use of the device have included:

1. A deep, intrinsic cerebral lesion that could be approached by open surgery only with high risk of adverse functional sequelae (i.e., lesions of the basal ganglia and deep cerebral centrum).
2. An intracranial lesion that was poorly defined in imaging studies and for which either surgical or nonsurgical management was considered (i.e., deep midline and certain pineal region masses).
3. An intracranial lesion for which the value of open surgery was considered debatable (i.e., invasive intrinsic neoplasms without mass effect or lesions of possible infectious etiology).
4. An intrinsic cerebral lesion in a patient whose general medical condition made craniotomy an inordinately high risk (i.e., elderly patients or those with fragile cardiovascular or pulmonary status).
5. Patients for whom imaging stereotactic guidance techniques offered potentially lower-risk alternatives to craniotomy (i.e., colloid cysts, lateral ventricular cysts, suprasellar and primary or recurrent parasellar cystic craniopharyngiomas).
6. Patients for whom imaging/stereotactic methods offered the only feasible mode of surgical management (i.e., cerebral lesions less than 1 cm in diameter, deep intra-axial cerebral or pontomesencephalic masses, potential candidates for brachytherapy by contemporary methods).

Target regions of our first 400 cases are shown in figures 5–17 to 5–19. No false targeting was noted and no instrument failure was encountered.

The system has proven to be elegantly simple, mechanically rapid, and safe. Although concentration and attention to detail are required to ensure fluid utilization of the system, complications (0.8%) have not been related in any way to the system or its inherent metho-

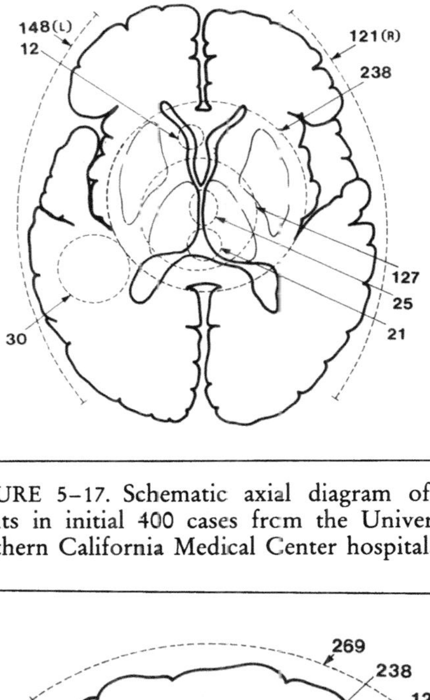

FIGURE 5–17. Schematic axial diagram of target points in initial 400 cases from the University of Southern California Medical Center hospitals.

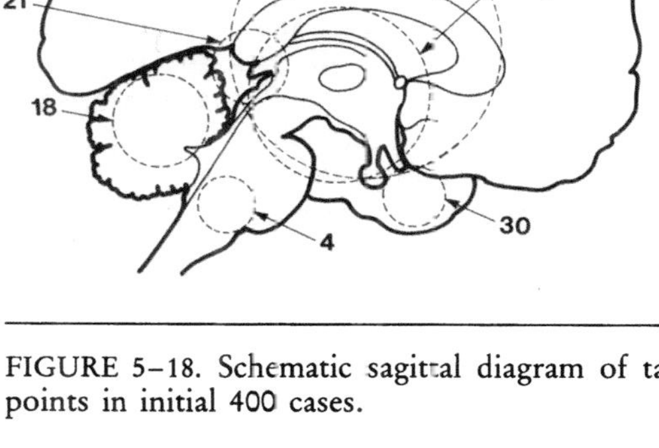

FIGURE 5–18. Schematic sagittal diagram of target points in initial 400 cases.

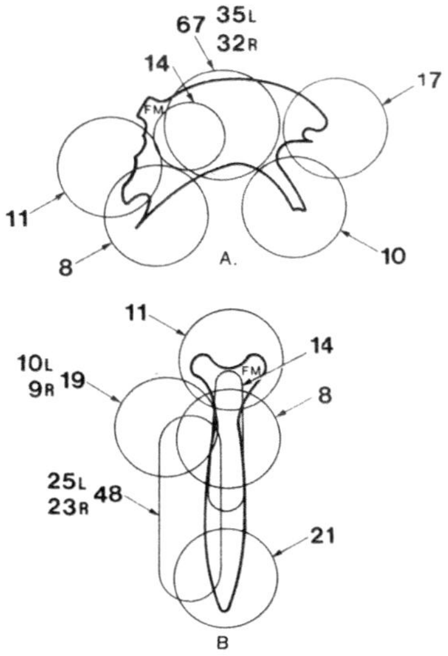

FIGURE 5–19. Lateral (A) and frontal (B) views of third ventricular outline. FM = foramen of Monro; circles = target site; numbers = frequency in 127 cases harboring lesions near or within the third ventricle.

dology. The phantom unit adds a vital element of protection against operator or mechanical error. The system is sturdy and generally has withstood the rigors of sterilization and handling throughout a 600-case series. The carbon-fiber posts do require frequent inspection and occasionally have fractured at the base; also, threading the nylon fixation pins is sometimes troublesome. The instrument has been easy to use in all supratentorial targets, including those with transtemporal and occipital entry points. We have not used a transcerebellar approach, favoring transtentorial trajectories to the cerebellum and transaxial or transincisural trajectories to central posterior fossa targets. During craniotomy or craniectomy, target points have been localized with the base ring used as a head-holder; subsequent precision localization of vascular elements was performed in functionally treacherous regions.

Of great practical importance has been the capability for rapid and accurate transmission of imaging data to the neurosurgical operating suite where the setting, material resources, and personnel are appropriate for a neurosurgical procedure. Scanning sessions usually last 15 minutes or less, placing little demand on busy imaging-facility schedules.

The Epson HX-20 (Epson-American, Inc., Torrance, CA) is a reliable, compact data-processing unit with software that provides target data for both single and multiple trajectories. However, the program does not allow computations when a target is at the base-ring level, a limitation that must be considered during initial base-ring fixation. In addition, software for rapid multiplanar trajectory definition and volume determination of target masses in brachytherapy is not adaptable to all imaging facilities. This is an important gap in an otherwise cohesive system.

Investigators at the University of Utah recently developed an improved methodology for data processing that is applicable to the BRW system in concert with the General Electric and Siemens imaging devices (M.P. Heilbrun, personal communication, April 1986). The system takes advantage of microcomputer development to enhance the capabilities of the BRW CT stereotactic guidance system. A Digital Equipment Corporation (DEC) Microvax II performs all standard BRW computations for localizing the target and determining frame settings. The stereotactic computations then are translated into a computer graphics display with multiple capabilities. Development and expansion of such an economically feasible and technically flexible methodology will provide the major effort for improvement in this system.

References

1. Apuzzo MLJ: Applications of stereotaxis. In Apuzzo MLJ (ed): *Surgery of the Third Ventricle*. New York: Williams Wilkins (In press)
2. Apuzzo MLJ, Chandrasoma T, Zelman V, et al: Computerized tomographic guidance stereotaxis in the management of lesions of the third ventricular region. *Neurosurgery* 15:502–508, 1984
3. Apuzzo MLJ, Jepson JH, Luxton G, et al: Ionizing and nonionizing radiation treatment of malignant cerebral gliomas: specialized approaches. *Clin Neurosurg* 31:470–496, 1984
4. Apuzzo MLJ, Sabshin JK: Computed tomographic guidance stereotaxis in the management of intracranial mass lesions. *Neurosurgery* 12:277–285, 1983
5. Brown RA: A computerized tomography-computer graphics approach to stereotaxic localization. *J Neurosurg* 50:715:720, 1979

6. Brown RA: A stereotactic head frame for use with CT body scanners. *Invest Radiol*, 14:300–304, 1979
7. Brown RA, Roberts TS, Osborn AG: Simplified CT-guided stereotaxic biopsy. *AJNR* 2:181–184, 1981
8. Brown RA, Roberts TS, Osborn AG: Stereotaxic frame and computer software for CT-directed neurosurgical localization. *Invest Radiol* 15:308–312, 1980
9. Heilbrun MP: Computed tomography-guided stereotactic systems. *Clin Neurosurg* 31:564–581, 1983
10. Heilbrun MP, Roberts TS, Apuzzo MLJ, et al: Preliminary experience with Brown-Roberts-Wells (BRW) computerized tomography stereotaxic guidance system. *J Neurosurg* 59:217–222, 1983
11. Heilbrun MP, Roberts TS, Wells TH Jr, et al: *Technical Manual: Brown-Roberts-Wells (BRW) CT stereotaxic Guidance System.* Burlington, MA: Radionics, Inc., 1982

6. MODIFICATION OF TODD-WELLS SYSTEM FOR IMAGING DATA ACQUISITION

Patrick J. Kelly
Stephen J. Goerss
Bruce A. Kall

The incorporation of computed tomography (CT) into stereotactic surgery brought about a renaissance in methodology. CT scanning provides a precise three-dimensional database, which can easily be incorporated into a stereotactic coordinate system. As a result, many neurosurgeons began rethinking their approaches to traditional surgery. New diagnostic and therapeutic stereotactic procedures have been developed that were not practical before CT.

Two approaches to CT-directed stereotactic procedures have been described. Some advocate performing surgery in the CT scanning unit, where CT images identify targets directly and confirm probe placement [9, 18, 23]. Others recommended the transfer of the CT database into the coordinate system of a stereotactic instrument located in the operating room [1–8].

Our group has favored the latter approach for several reasons. First, CT scanning suites lack a sterile environment and are ill-equipped to manage a complication, should it occur. Secondly, performing surgery in the CT scanner precludes use of other databases, such as magnetic resonance imaging (MRI), arteriography, standard teleradiography, neurophysiological information, and ultrasonography, all of which can increase the accuracy with which stereotactic procedures are performed. Third, except in unusual circumstances, CT scanners are controlled by radiologists who must consider their busy diagnostic work loads. As a result, surgery performed in a diagnostic CT scanning unit will be hurried and limited to the expedient positioning of probes intracranially. Few significant advances in technique can occur in this environment. However, the operating room is the surgeon's domain; new stereotactic procedures can be developed and refined there.

Various methods for transposing CT data into stereotactic space have been reported. Reconstructed CT data can be transposed onto anteroposterior (AP) and lateral roentgenograms relative to respective coronal and midline cranial landmarks. Alternatively, stereotactic coordinates can be determined from the scout view and inherent software packages available on most newer-generation CT scanners [6].

However, several systems for the convenient and accurate utilization of CT data in stereotactic procedures have been developed. Some were designed exclusively for CT scanning [5, 9, 18, 20, 22]. Others represent modifications of stereotactic frames developed in the pre-CT era that render them CT-compatible [2, 3, 7, 19]. Although it is probably unimportant which system a surgeon selects, there is a philosophical advantage to modified pre-CT-era systems: the surgeon is reminded that CT scanning is just another database. Stereotactic accuracy and progress will depend on the incorporation of other databases into the coordinate system of the instrument being used. Further-more, devices such as the Leksell, Talairach, Mundinger-Riechert, and Todd-Wells were developed, modified, and refined to

L.D. Lunsford (ed.) *MODERN STEREOTACTIC NEUROSURGERY*.

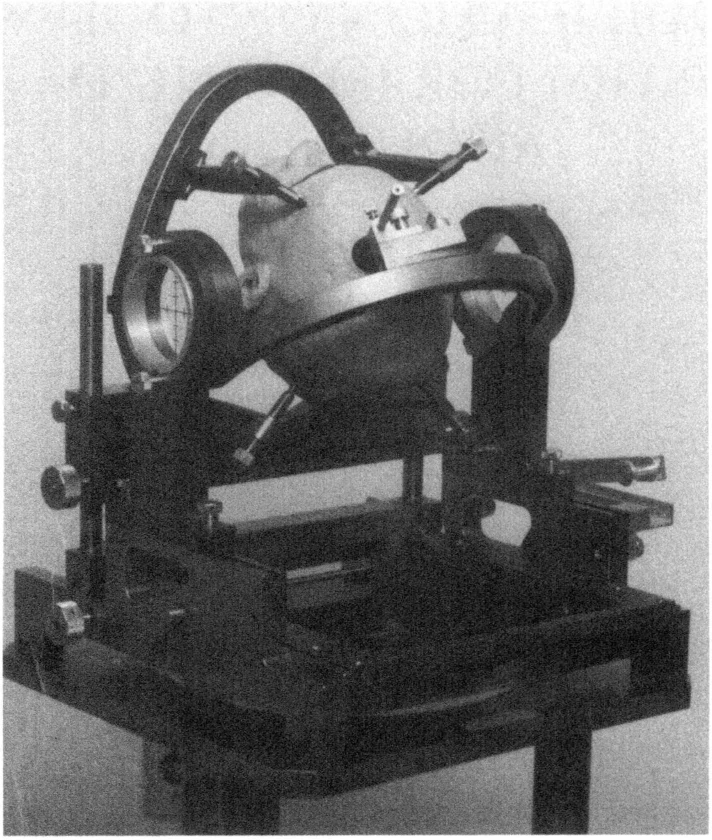

FIGURE 6-1. Todd-Wells stereotactic frame. Guide tube held in slide on arc is directed perpendicular to the tangent of sphere described by arc and collar.

perform specialized tasks. All can be modified to incorporate CT data as well as new imaging databases that become available.

We began using CT data with the Todd-Wells device in 1978 [17]. First, AP and lateral x-ray scatter films obtained during CT scanning, and demonstrating the level and inclination of each CT image, were superimposed on stereotactic radiographs. Then, sagittal and coronal reconstructions were used, as CT scanning units provided this capability [12]. Finally, the Todd-Wells head frame was modified for CT compatibility, and a localization system was developed for rapid and convenient calculation of target points and reconstructed volumes in stereotactic space by an operating room computer system [7, 10, 13-16]. This chapter describes our modifications of the Todd-Wells stereotactic frame for the incorporation of CT and other databases as well as subsequent developments in the surgical instrumentation.

The Todd-Wells Stereotactic System

The Todd-Wells system is rugged, versatile, and accurate and is the most popular stereotactic instrument in the United States. It employs the arc-quadrant principle: the patient's head in a rigid head holder is moved with three orthogonal degrees of freedom to position an intracranial target point at the focal point of a fixed sphere that is defined by the arc quadrant (figure 6-1). All approaches to the target point are described by two angles: collar (the angle from the horizontal plane) and arc (the angle from the vertical plane). The arc quadrant has a fixed radius (135 mm). One need only measure this distance on a probe (plus the length of the guide tube extending outside of the arc), and

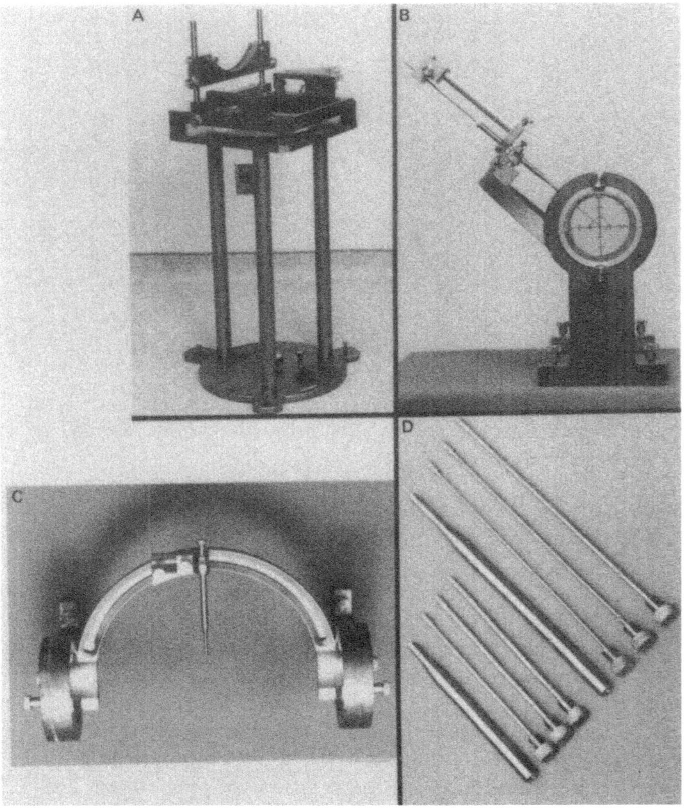

FIGURE 6–2. Components of the Todd-Wells system. (A) Base unit. (B) Horizontal arc quadrant. The micrometer advance fits onto the guide tube. (C) Top view of horizontal arc quadrant. (D) Guide and reducing tubes.

the probe will always arrive at the desired intracranial target point, which has been moved into the focal point. Thus, there are six simple mechanical adjustments: three axes (X, Y, and Z), two angles (collar and arc), and a probe depth.

Instrument Components

BASE UNIT AND XYZ STAGE

The base unit secures to the operating-room floor by a vacuum attachment. In another version, the base unit can attach to the operating table. The head holder attaches to a receiving yoke on the base unit. A reference mark on the head holder base ring must align with a reference mark on the receiving yoke. The receiving yoke is moved with three degrees of freedom by racks and pinions (superior-inferior and anterior-posterior) and slide (right-left) on the base unit (figure 6–2). Vernier scales for each axis display the position of each. Arc quadrants index into tracks on the base unit. Cassette holders attach to the base unit for performing lateral radiographs. Anterior posterior x-ray cassettes slide into a slot beneath the AP zero-reference reticle.

ARC QUADRANTS

Reference marks on the arc quadrants must be aligned with reference marks, which are inscribed on the tracks of the base unit. A slide on the arc of the arc quadrant directs guide tubes perpendicular to the tangent of the arc quadrant. Right and left reticles fit onto the arc quadrant for radiographic collimation. The center of the cross on the reticle indicates the focal point of the frame. A lateral-approach

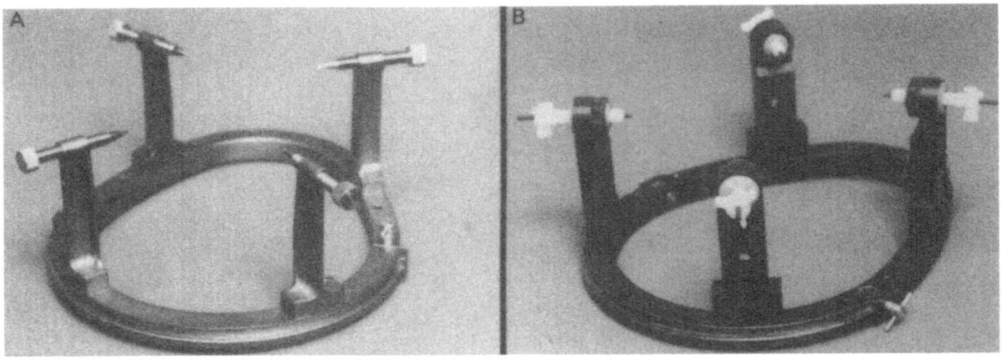

FIGURE 6–3. (A) Original head holder with metal vertical supports and skull fixation pins. (B) CT-compatible vertical supports with fixation sleeves and carbon-fiber pins secured by caps.

micropositioner is used for lateral targets when an orthogonal approach is desired.

GUIDE TUBES
The guide tubes insert into a slide on the arc and are used to direct stereotactic instruments to the focal point of the instrument. Several reducing tubes insert into the lumen of the guide tube to dilate it to the approximate diameter of the stereotactic probe in use. A micrometer also fits onto the guide tube for controlled advancement of instruments to the focal point of the arc quadrant (figure 6–2).

HEAD HOLDER
The head holder consists of a metal base ring and four metal vertical supports. Four metal fixation screws extend from each vertical support to the outer table of the patient's skull (figure 6–3).

MODIFICATIONS FOR CT COMPATIBILITY
Only two changes must be made in the Todd-Wells head frame to render it CT-compatible. First, the metal vertical supports and fixation screws on the head holder must be replaced with CT-compatible materials. Secondly, a CT localization system that creates reference marks on CT images is used to facilitate accurate calculation of stereotactic coordinates.

If the standard head holder is placed low enough on the patient's skull, the metal fixation screws and vertical supports may be below the CT image of interest, and no artifacts will be noted. However, images obtained below these metal components will be completely distorted by artifact. To have an efficient and versatile stereotactic system, the metal vertical supports and fixation pins should be replaced.

We used molybdenum disulfide to construct CT-compatible vertical supports which have the same dimensions as the original metal supports and attach to the base ring of the head holder (see figure 6–3). This material is structurally strong and results in no discernible CT artifact (figure 6–4). A collet in each vertical support holds the skull fixation system, which consists of a sleeve and a fixation pin.

The sleeves are hollow nylon cylinders, which extend through and are secured by the collet on the vertical supports. They maintain a fixed distance between the depressed scalp and each vertical support. A carbon-fiber fixation pin will be inserted through these hollow cylinders and held in place by a cap, which screws onto and crimps the end of the fixation screw.

The fixation pins are 3 mm in diameter and are constructed of molded carbon fiber. Four millimeters from the tip, the diameter narrows to 2.5 mm (figure 6–5). This creates a flange that will rest on the outer table of the patient's skull.

Miscellaneous Head Holder Modifications

AIRWAY WINDOW
The carbon-fiber fixation system relieves the base ring from the distracting forces produced when the metal fixation screws of the original device were tightened against the patient's scalp. With the new fixation system, it is possi-

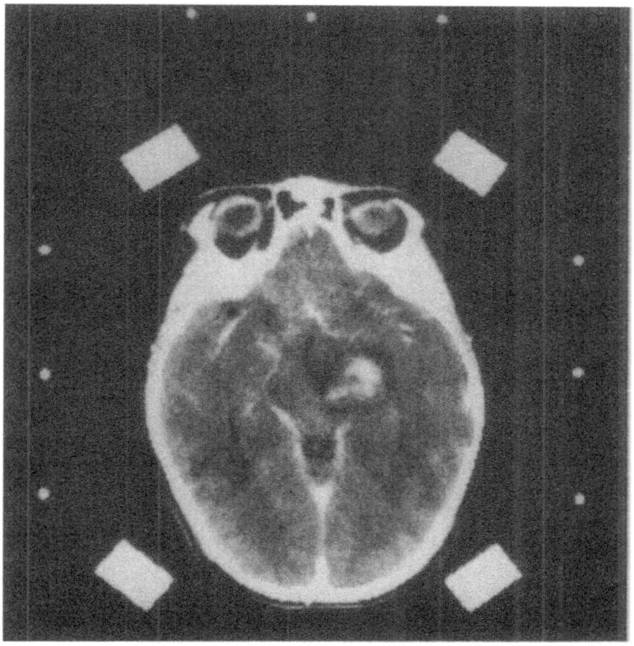

FIGURE 6–4. Stereotactic CT image demonstrating an absence of artifact when molybdenum disulfide vertical supports are used.

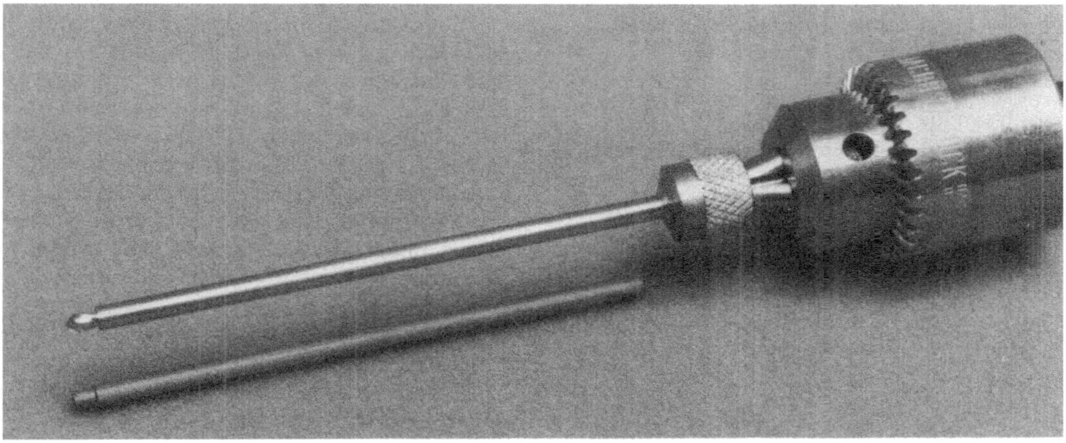

FIGURE 6–5. Carbon-fiber fixation pin. A skin punch over a drill is advanced to the proper depth for pin placement.

ble to incorporate a removable segment in the anterior part of the base ring to provide the anesthesiologist with convenient access to the patient's airway (figure 6–6).

ROUND HEAD FRAME

The original oval head frame is adequate for procedures performed with the patient in the supine position. However, it is cumbersome for procedures in which patients are in the prone or lateral positions. A round base ring was therefore developed to allow a 360° rotation of the patient's head for any desired surgical approach. With the round base ring, the patient may undergo CT scanning or other studies in the most comfortable position (i.e.,

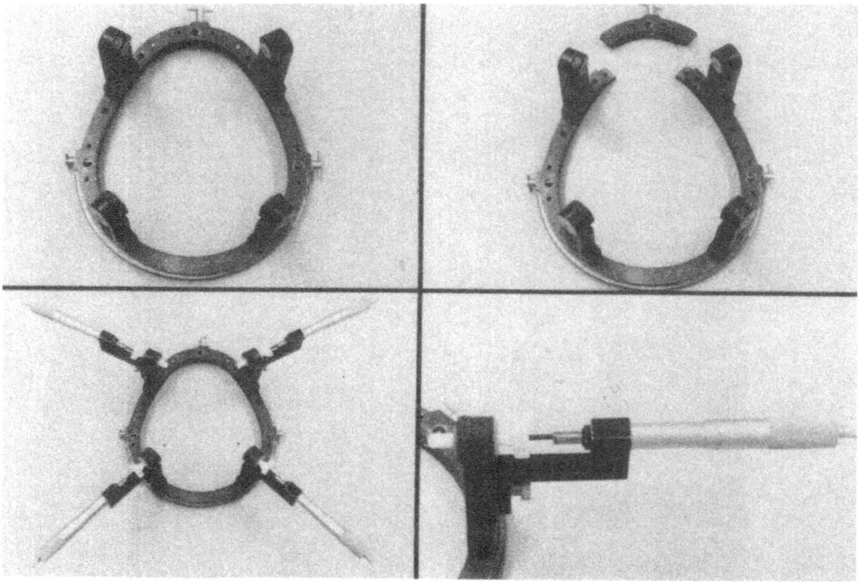

FIGURE 6–6. Removable segment for airway access (*top*). Micrometer attachments to vertical supports for reproducible frame replacement (*bottom*).

supine). Computer software will allow rotation of target points and volumes and recalculation of stereotactic frame settings that take into account rotation of the patient.

MICROMETER ATTACHMENTS

These connect conveniently with the vertical supports and allow precise measurement of the distance between the carbon-fiber pins and the vertical supports (figure 6–6, figure 6–7). This system provides a mechanism for accurate replacement of the frame if the data acquisition and surgery are not performed on the same day or if further stereotactic procedures are contemplated.

CT LOCALIZATION SYSTEM

A localization system attaches to the base ring of the stereotactic head holder during stereotactic CT scanning and MRI. This creates reference marks on each CT/MRI image from which the stereotactic coordinates of points on the image can be calculated. In principle, the known positions of the reference elements in the localization system establish a coordinate system in reference to the base ring of the stereotactic head holder. Our localization system consists of nine carbon-fiber rods in three sets of three rods each, arranged in the shape of the letter **N** (figure 6–8A, 6–8B). This attaches to the base ring of the stereotactic headholder such that a set of three **N**-shaped rods is located on either side of the head and anteriorly. The localization system produces nine reference marks on each CT image from which three vertical heights above the base ring are calculated, three points in space derived thereby, and the position and inclination of the CT image plane above the base ring established. The zero point of the coordinate arcs (defined by the localization system) is related to mechanical adjustments of the stereotactic instrument by bias factors.

The zero point of the localization system is defined on the point at which all three of the rods on each N set are equidistant. To derive the biases, the head holder, with localization system attached, is positioned in the Todd-Wells frame such that the oblique bars intersect in the reticles upon visual inspection (figure 6–8C) and by radiographic confirmation (figure 6–8D). The X, Y, and Z frame settings are recorded and included as parameter constants within the computer program, which calculates future stereotactic coordinates by the use of equations 1–14 in the appendix to this chapter.

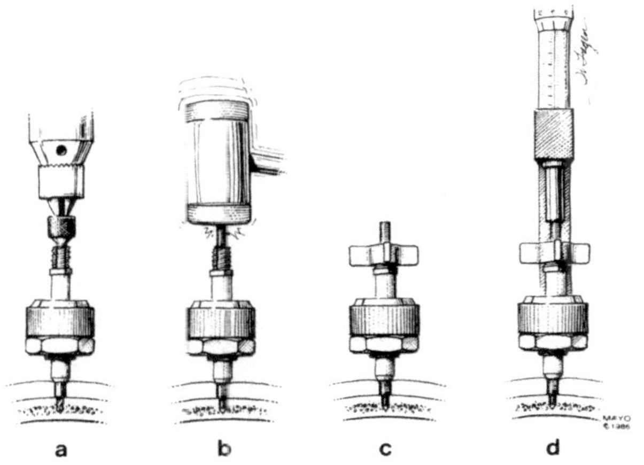

FIGURE 6-7. Setting the carbon-fiber pin. (A) The drill is advanced to the hub of the skin punch. (B) The carbon-fiber pin is tapped into place. (C) The pin is secured to the sleeve by the cap. (D) The micrometer records the distance from the end of the carbon-fiber pin to vertical support.

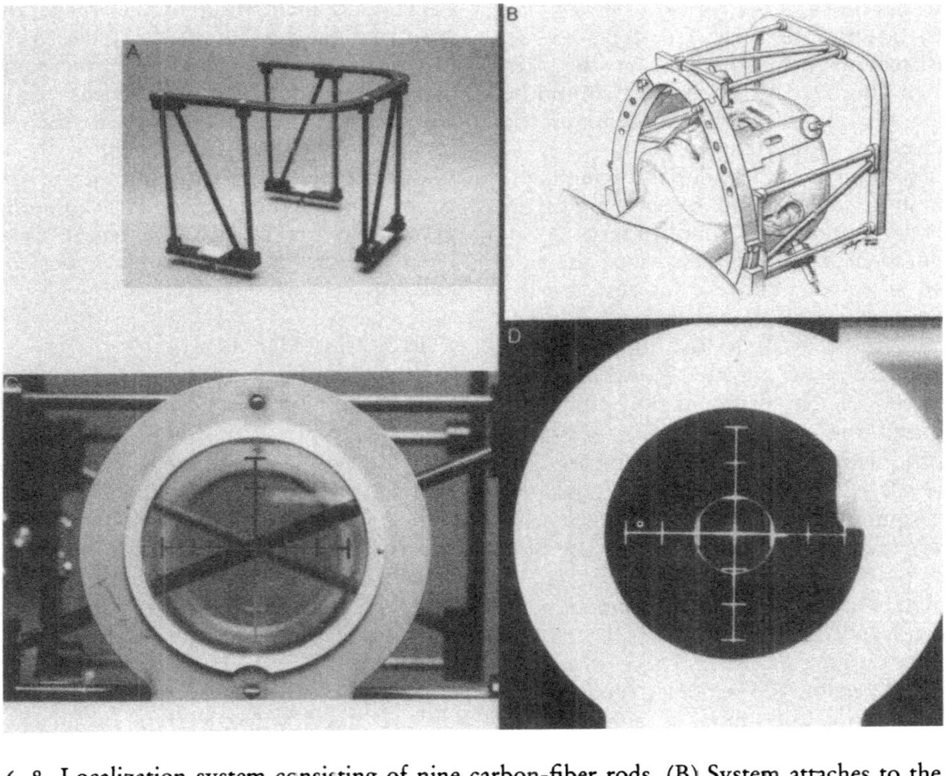

FIGURE 6-8. Localization system consisting of nine carbon-fiber rods. (B) System attaches to the CT head holder. The zero point of the localization system is identified visually (C) and by radiograph (D). X, Y, and Z frame settings are read from vernier scales on the stereotactic frame and retained in the computer as bias factors.

Procedural Aspects

APPLICATION OF THE HEAD FRAME

Patients are sedated with neuroleptic analgesia. The patient's head is rested on a support unit, and the CT-compatible head holder is placed over the patient's head. A nose support is adjusted to obtain the desired frame height anteriorly and posteriorly. Lateral ear bars, which fit into the external auditory canals, are adjusted to position the frame to the right or left. The inclination of the base ring with respect to the cantho-meatal line is adjusted by a slide on the nose support. The fixation sleeves are then advanced to depress the scalp at four points and are secured by tightening the collet on the vertical support. The scalp then is infiltrated at these four points with a 1% lidocaine–bupivacaine hydro-chloride mixture.

A power drill with a 7/64-inch bit is used as follows: The length of the bit is set so as to penetrate the skull the precise distance of the flanged end of the carbon-fiber pin. A skin punch that fits through the fixation sleeves may be used to facilitate this step (see figure 6–5). The measurement from the end of the skin punch to the shoulder of the drill bit should be identical to the distance from the end of the carbon-fiber pin to its flange.

The skin punch is advanced through the hollow fixation screw to the outer table of the skull, thereby removing a small plug of scalp. The measured drill bit is inserted into the skin punch and advanced until the bit rests on the outer table of the skull. A hole is drilled in the outer table of the skull to the diploe as the chuck of the drill is advanced to the skin punch (see figure 6–7A). The drill and skin punch are removed, and the carbon-fiber pin is gently tapped into place with a nylon hammer (see figure 6–7B). After placing all four pins, the collets are tightened with a special wrench, and the fixation caps are applied to secure the pins (see figure 6–7C).

Micrometers are attached to the vertical supports and advanced to the end of the carbon-fiber pin (see figure 6–7D). These measurements are entered on the patient's record.

Reapplication of the frame is simple: The surgeon taps the four fixation pins into the previously drilled holes, slides the sleeves over them, and secures the sleeves with the collets and caps after reproducing the micrometer measurements.

Frame Application for Posterior Fossa Procedures. Posterior fossa procedures are performed with the patient in the prone position and with the round stereotactic head holder applied in the inverted position (figure 6–9). This makes unobstructed access to the posterior fossa possible.

STEREOTACTIC CT SCANNING

A CT-scan table adaptation plate attaches to the table of the GE 8800 or 9800 scanning unit (figure 6–10). This device is similar to the receiving yoke on the Todd-Wells base unit and has a slot in which the base ring of the stereotactic head holder is fixed. Reference marks on the head frame are aligned on the adaptation plate as they are to the receiving yoke of the stereotactic base unit during the surgical procedure.

The localization system described previously is attached to the base ring of the head holder. This creates nine reference marks (A-I, figure 6–11) on each CT image from which the height and inclination of the image above the base ring can be measured [7, 11, 15]. Following CT scanning, the stereotactic calculations can be determined by a program on the CT computer (which is identical to the computer located in the operating suite), or the archived CT data tape can be entered into the operating-room computer system. The computer programs are for stereotactic target calculations based on the equations in the appendix of this chapter.

STEREOTACTIC MRI

Stereotactic MRI examinations are performed on a Picker .15 tesla Resistive unit or a General Electric Signa 2.0 tesla superconducting system. An MRI-compatible base ring, constructed of molybdenum disulfide, utilizes the same vertical support and fixation system described previously (figure 6–12A). The transverse localization system resembles that designed for CT (figure 6–12B). It consists of nine capillary tubes filled with copper sulfate ($CuSO_4$) solution. These create nine reference marks on each image (figure 6–12D). A multiplanar localization system calculates stereotactic coordinates from coronal, sagittal, and transverse images (figure 6–12C). Following the MRI scan, the archived data tape is also loaded into the operating-room computer system for stereotactic target calculations.

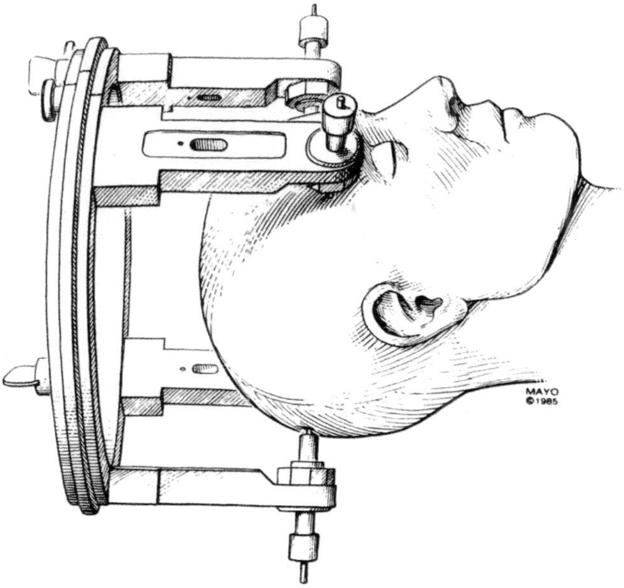

FIGURE 6-9. Frame placement for posterior fossa procedures.

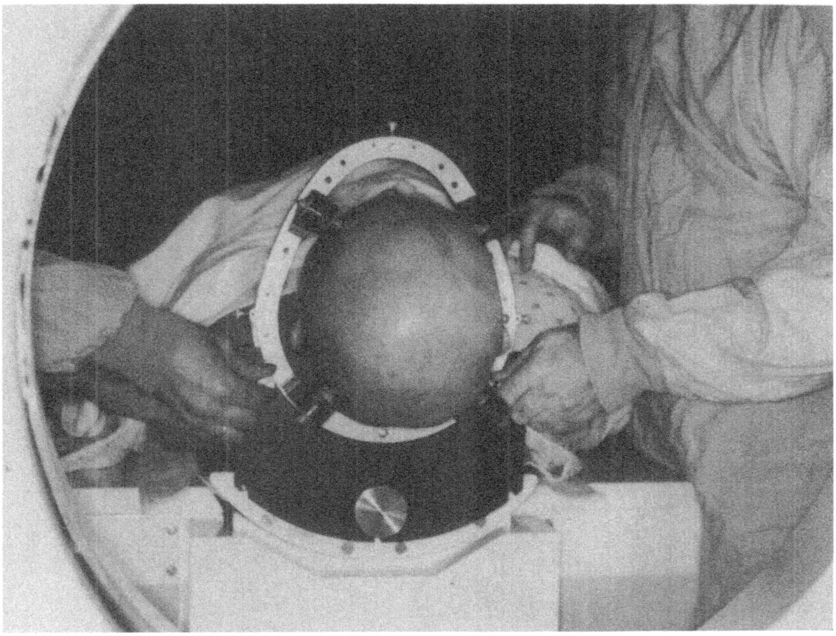

FIGURE 6-10. CT scan table adaptation plate receives stereotactic headholder.

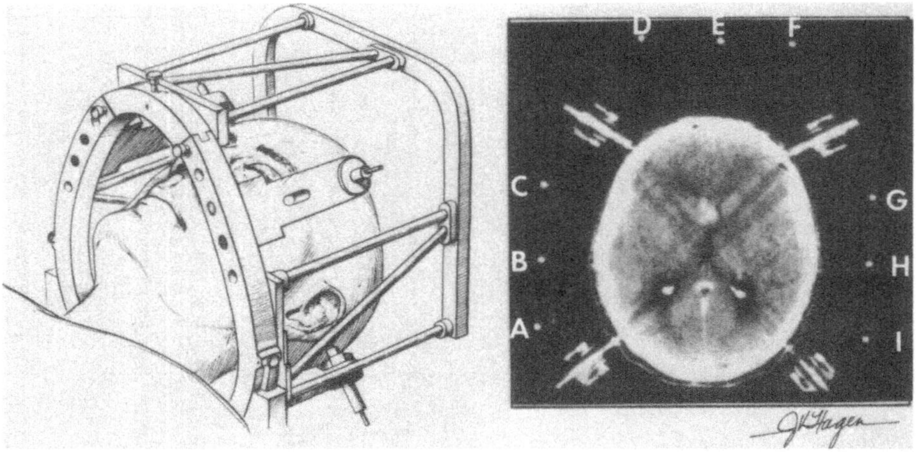

FIGURE 6–11. CT localization system (*left*) creates nine reference marks (A–I) on each CT image (*right*).

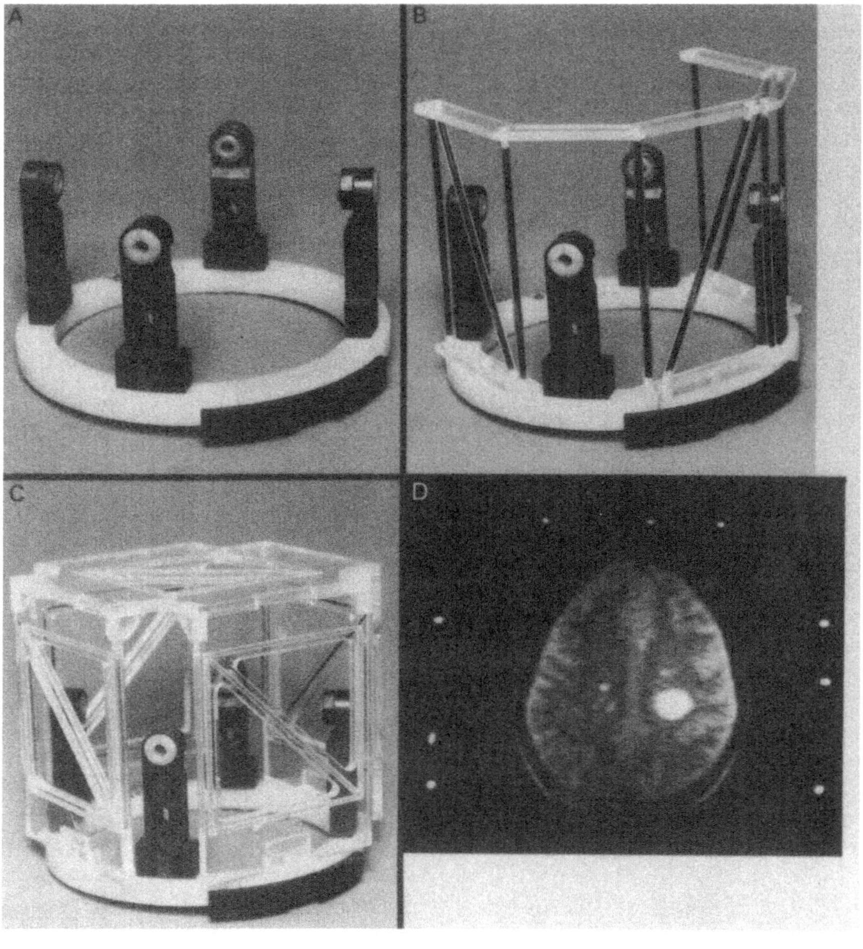

FIGURE 6–12. (A) MRI compatible head holder. (B) Transverse MRI localization system. (C) Multiplanar localization system. (D) (Stereotactic) MRI demonstrating nine reference marks.

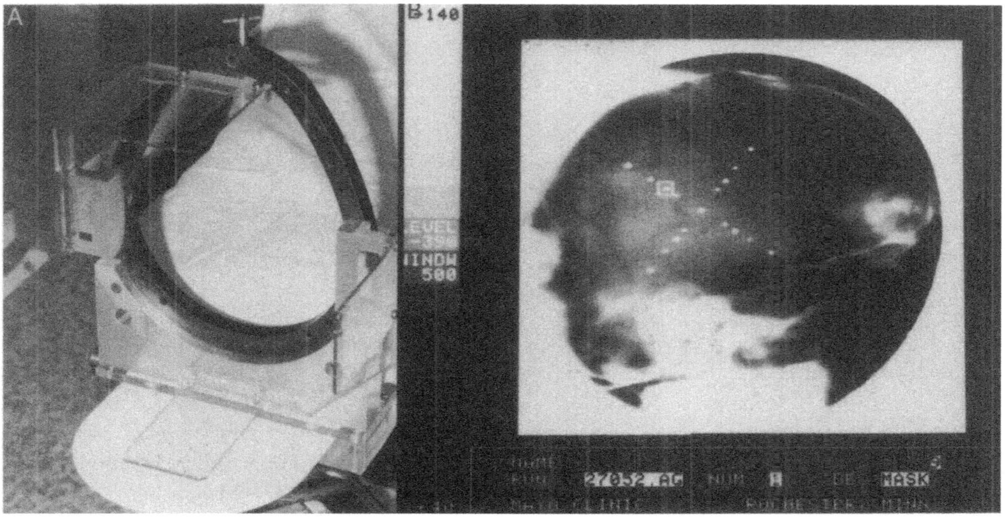

FIGURE 6-13. (A) Head frame secured on DA table by adaptation device. Fiducial reference plates for ARS. (B) DA lateral mask image demonstrating 18 reference marks created by ARS.

STEREOTACTIC DIGITAL ANGIOGRAPHY (DA)

Patients undergo DA examination with their heads fixed in the CT/MRI-compatible stereotactic head holder as previously described. A DA table adaptation system for the General Electric DF 3000 or 5000 units receives the head holder. An arteriographic reference system (ARS) fits onto the head holder (figure 6-13A). The ARS contains arrays of nine points suspended in radiolucent reference plates, which attach to each side of the base ring of the head holder. The reference plates are positioned bilaterally, anteriorly, and posteriorly. These create 18 reference marks on each DA image (figure 6-13B). The reference marks define coordinate axes of the ARS and provide grids for computer calculation of x-ray magnification at any three-dimensionally defined point in space. A computer program transforms X, Y, and Z points in space (from stereotactic CT and MRI calculations) as a function of distances from the central x-ray beam and ARS reference plates and interpolates the magnification factor for the correct annotation of that point on the DA images.

THE STEREOTACTIC OPERATING ROOM

Two adjoining operating rooms are equipped for stereotactic surgery (figure 6-14). A computer system (Data General Eclipse S-140 with 192 megabytes disk storage and Ramtek raster display console) is located directly above the operating rooms. Display consoles are located in the treatment-planning computer room and in an induction room between the operating rooms. Computer display monitors are suspended in both stereotactic operating rooms for display of stereotactic CT, MRI, and DA images; biopsy trajectories; angiograms; scaled stereotactic atlas sections; tumor volumes; and reformatted images. X-ray tubes for 4-m teleradiography are suspended on wormgear, servomotor-controlled slide systems for collimation with the stereotactic frame. HE-NE laser beams coaxial with the central x-ray beam AP and lateral tubes facilitate collimation.

DATA INPUT

The archived data tapes from the CT, MRI, and DA examinations are transferred to the operating-room computer system. Decoding programs for CT, MRI, and DA images formats make possible the display of each on the central Ramtek console, affording convenient calculation of stereotactic coordinates and treatment planning. The surgeon communicates with the operating-room computer by means of an alphanumeric keyboard, a trackball that manipulates a cursor on the display screen, and a deposit key. User-friendly programs allow rapid calculations of stereotactic targets and

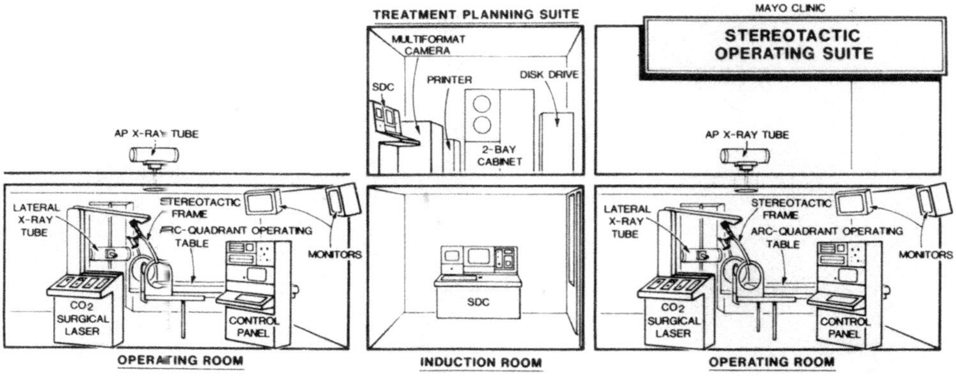

FIGURE 6-14. Stereotactic operating suite with computer treatment planning facility on upper level and the display console in the induction room between two stereotactic operating rooms.

cross-correlation of target points among CT, MRI, DA and a computer-resident stereotactic atlas. Probe simulations, radionuclide-source isodose configurations, and tumor-volume displays and reconstructions can be viewed with respect to the MRI, CT, and DA databases.

The surgeon selects target points from CT or MRI, utilizing the cursor and trackball subsystems (figure 6–15). A computer program determines screen coordinates for the target point (Xs/Ys) and converts these to stereotactic mechanical adjustments on the frame (X_{AQ}, Y_{AQ}, Z_{AQ}) (see chapter appendix).

NOMENCLATURE

Tridimensional coordinates in stereotactic surgery have varied from one surgical system to another. Since the incorporation of CT scanning and MRI into stereotactic surgery, most centers have adopted the coordinate system defined by these imaging modalities.

X = right (+), left (−)

Y = anterior (+), posterior (−)

Z = superior (+), inferior (−)

The frame adjustments are calculated instantaneously, displayed on the computer screen or a line printer, and then duplicated on the stereotactic instrument, bringing the target points selected on CT or MRI into the focal point of the stereotactic arc quadrant. The measured accuracy of this system for CT is ±500 microns in the X and Y planes and within one-half the image thickness in the Z planes. The treated accuracy of the MRI localization system is 1.1 mm in X and Y and within one-half the image thickness in Z.

The DA images are displayed on the screen. The surgeon digitizes all of the 18 reference marks, using the cursor and trackball subsystem. This establishes reference points within a three-dimensional computer-image matrix, which can be related to the coordinates established for CT and MRI.

POINT IN SPACE

The surgeon selects the target from displayed CT or MRI images, using the cursor and the deposit key. The mathematical manipulations for the simple translation of a point selected on a CT image to mechanical adjustments in a stereotactic frame can be accomplished with a hand-held calculator or an inexpensive microprocessor-based computer. However, many more useful options exist when a more capacious microcomputer or minicomputer is available. The surgeon can simulate probe trajectories on arterial and venous phases of the arteriogram (figure 6–16). After the optimal trajectory has been selected, the computer calculates arc and collar settings that represent these approach angles on the stereotactic instrument. Probe trajectories through contiguous CT and MRI images, given the calculated target coordinates and trajectory angles, can also be displayed (figure 6–17).

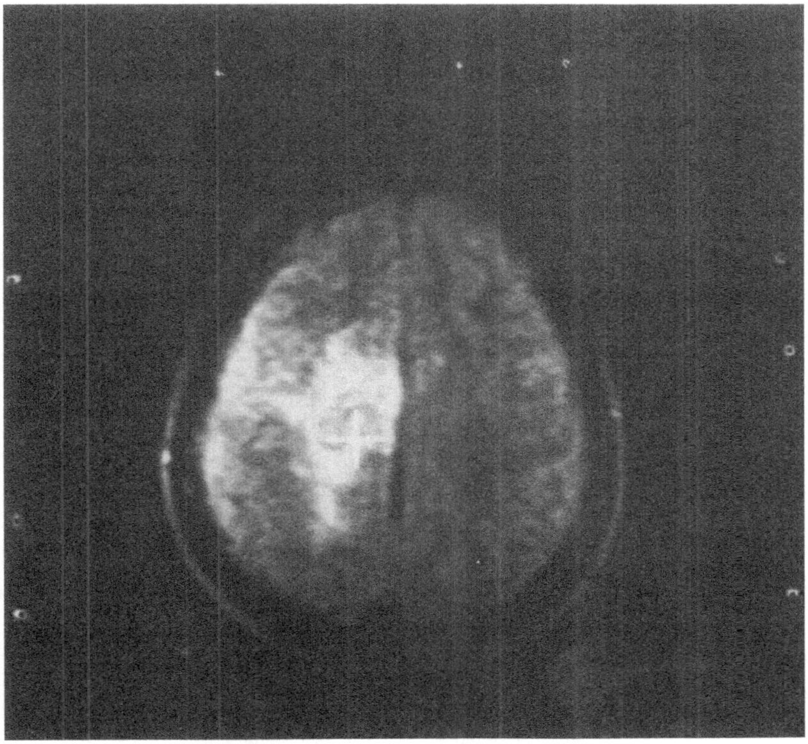

FIGURE 6–15. Digitizing target point on stereotactic MRI in patient with grade III astrocytoma in right medial central area.

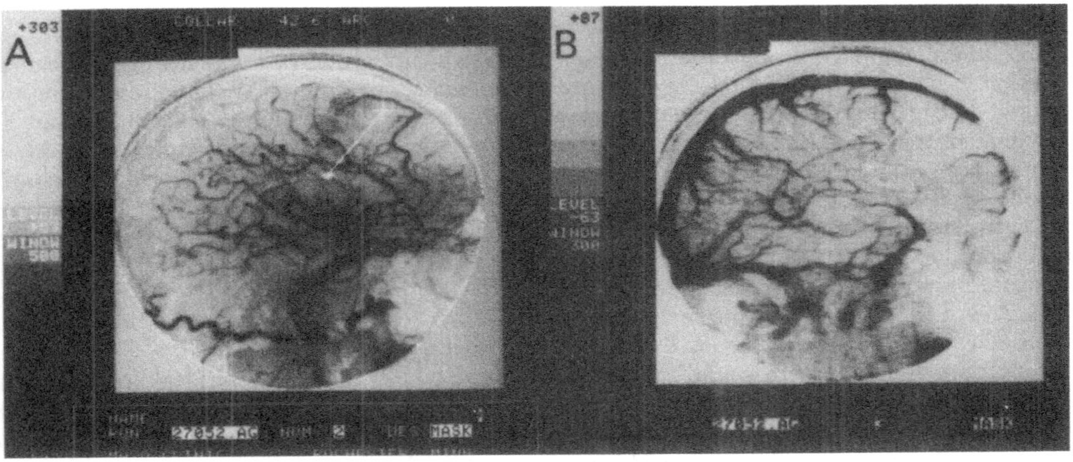

FIGURE 6–16. Selection and computer simulation of probe trajectories during stereotactic biopsy procedures. Cross cursors show position of target point digitized from CT or MRI. The surgeon manipulates cursor to select an entry point on the skull. The computer calculates and displays approach angles (collar and arc).

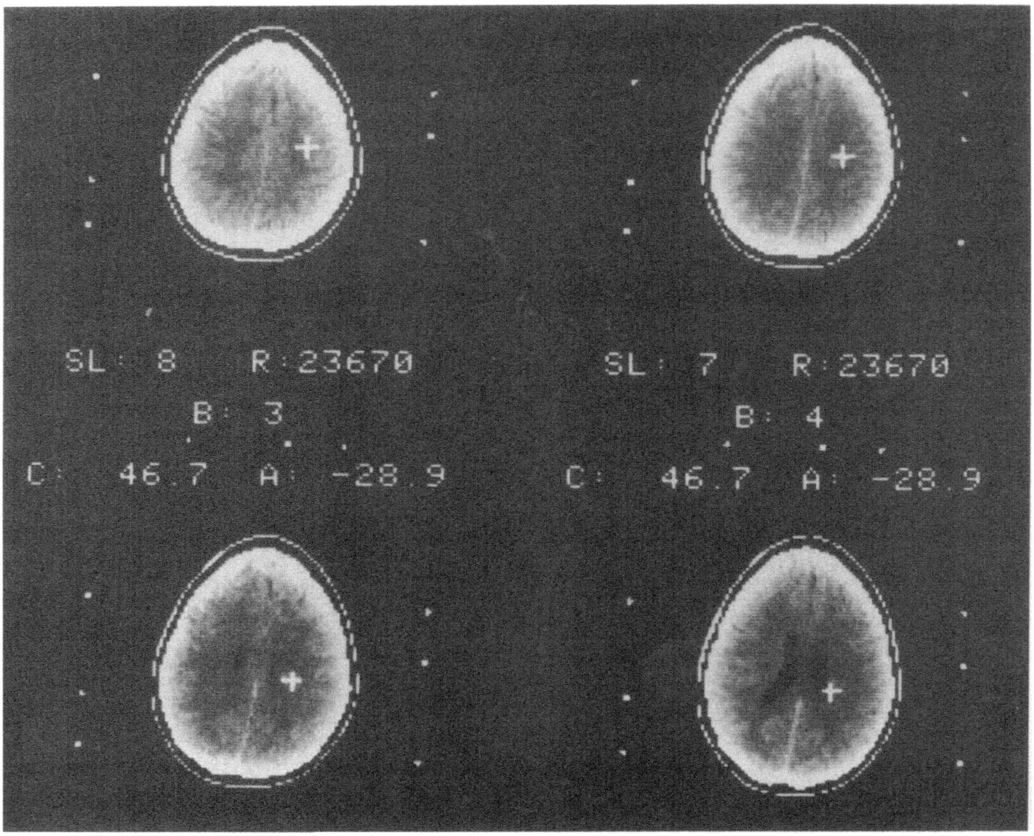

FIGURE 6–17. The computer demonstrates a probe tract on the contiguous CT images of a patient with a low-grade astrocytoma in the left frontoparietal region.

VOLUME IN SPACE

Multiple points digitized around the boundary of a lesion visualized on CT images or MRI are deposited into a three-dimensional computer-image matrix in precise relationship to their stereotactic coordinates, according to the calculations described in the appendix. The computer connects the points, forming a series of closed contours, and then interpolates intermediate contours at 1-mm intervals (figure 6–18). A volume within the image matrix is created when each of the digitized and interpolated contours are filled with 1-mm^3 voxels.

The volume is seen as a shaded surface display, a stereo pair, or a series of two-dimensional images scanned orthogonal to a viewline specified by arc and collar angles on the stereotactic frame. Stereotactic reconstruction of image volumes is useful for simulating isodose contours against tumor margins in patients who have intracranial neoplasms that will be treated by interstitial radiation. Computer reconstruction of volumes is also necessary for computer-assisted stereotactic resection of deep-seated intra-axial lesions and for selective stereotactic resection of the amygdala and hippocampus in patients with medically intractable partial-complex seizures.

Subsequent Modifications

The Todd-Wells frame is ideal for functional procedures, stereotactic biopsies, and posterior fossa approaches. However, as the number and variety of our cases increased, certain limitations became apparent. First, all adjustments on the frame were manual and cumbersome during procedures requiring more than one

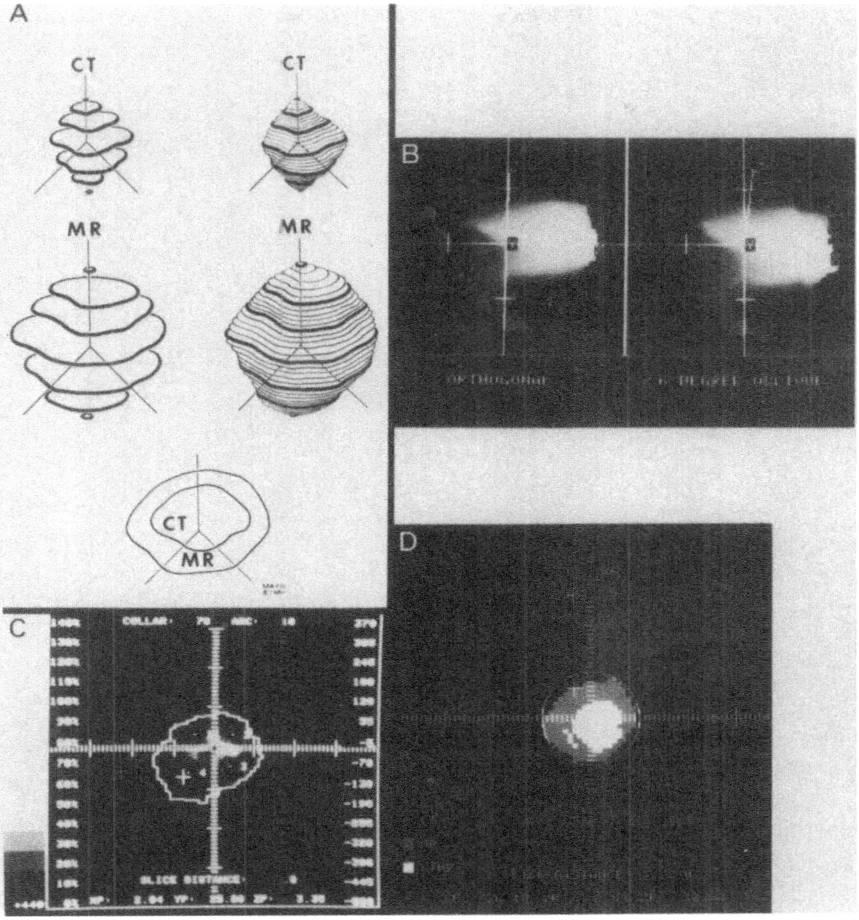

FIGURE 6–18. (A) The computer suspends CT and MRI images in a three-dimensional image matrix, then interpolates these at 1-mm intervals and creates volume for CT and MRI. (B) Display of volumetric information is shown as shaded graphics or as stereo pairs (stereotactic coordinate axes shown). (C) Images orthogonal to the viewline are specified by arc and collar angles for simulation of radionuclide source placements. (D) Position of laser (*cursor*) and stereotactic retractor (*circle*) are shown in relationship to the image of the tumor defined by stereotactic CT and MRI data in computer-assisted stereotactic resection.

target point. For example, in the implantation of multiple afterloading catheters for interstitial irradiation or in computer-assisted stereotactic laser resections of larger tumor volumes, multiple adjustments on the frame were needed to access different target points or different regions within a tumor volume. Second, the vernier scales for the X, Y, and Z mechanical adjustments on the frame were difficult to read, especially if the patient were draped during an operation; indeed, stereotactic frame settings were confirmed by a surgeon wielding a flashlight under the drapes. Third, convenient access to lateral targets was limited, due to the relatively small radius of the arc quadrant. Finally, the arc quadrant and base assembly were obstacles during the opening of a stereotactic craniotomy. For these reasons, we developed a new frame that utilizes the arc quadrant principle and many of the accessories of the old Todd-Wells instruments.

The basic system consists of a three-dimensional servomotor-controlled slide system attached to a large base plate, which is secured the a special operating table (figure 6–19). A receiving yoke (to which the stereo-

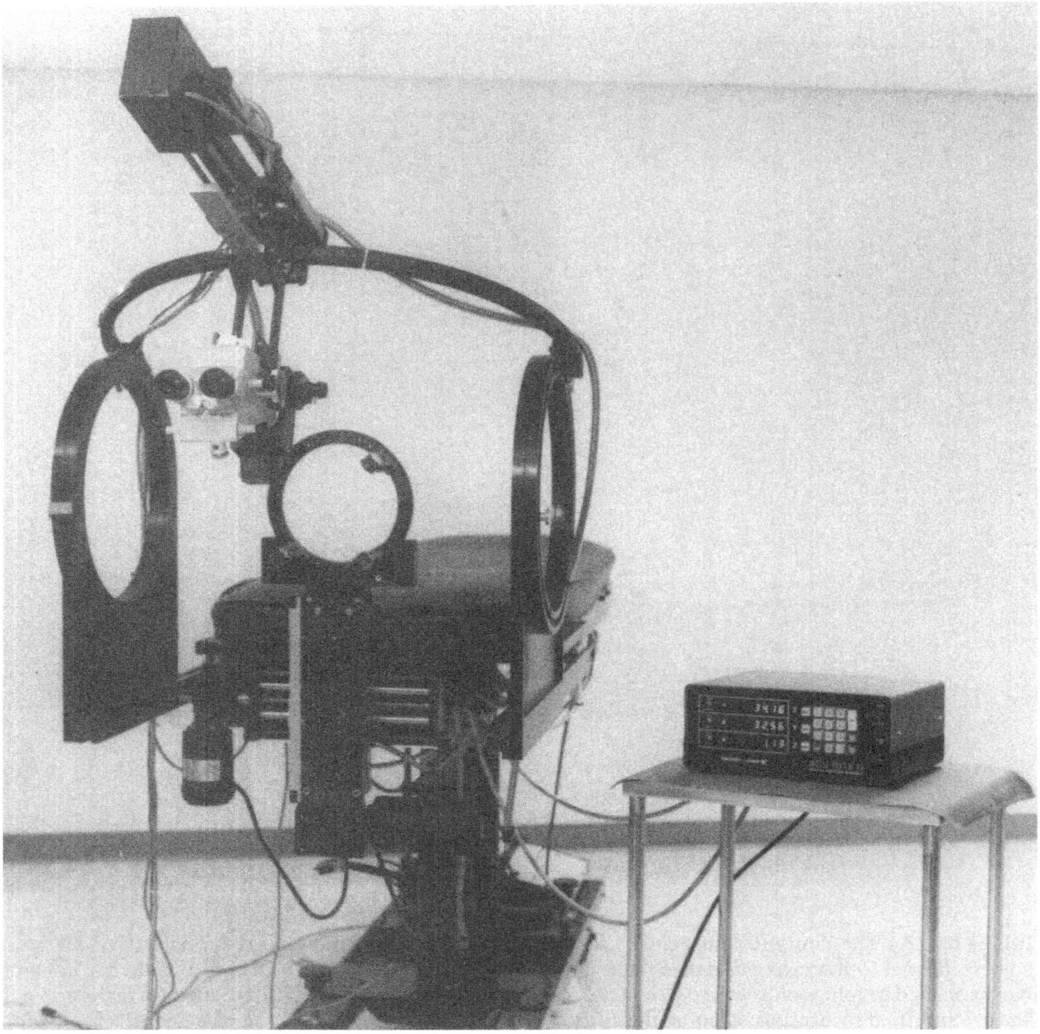

FIGURE 6–19. Stereotactic servomotor-controlled three-dimensional slide system demonstrating inner and 400-mm arc quadrants. Control panel for stereotactic frame with computer monitors, keyboards, and digital readout of (stereotactic) frame positions (right side of photograph).

tactic head holder attaches) is fixed to the three-dimensional slide. Fork assemblies containing tracks and index marks for 135-mm and 160-mm radius arc quadrants secure to the base plate. The fork assemblies can be attached or removed at any time during the surgical procedure. The stereotactic positions of the three-dimensional slides are detected by three-axis optical encoder systems (Bausch and Lomb, Accu-Rite II) and relayed to a digital display on a control panel. Finally, a 400-mm arc quadrant, which holds an operating microscope and laser manipulator apparatus, slides and locks into place on a track assembly, which is also attached to the base plate. The 400-mm arc quadrant is used during stereotactic tumor resections.

System Utilization

The system described has been employed in more than 600 stereotactic operations (table 6–1). It has proven to be versatile and accurate in performing a wide variety of stereotactic procedures. In addition, multiple databases can be used in treatment planning and in the sur-

TABLE 6–1. Stereotactic Procedures Performed with Custom Arc Quadrant Stereotactic System

Procedure	No. of Patients
Stereotactic biopsy	352
Stereotactic craniotomy	146
Third ventriculosotomy	31
Ventrolateral thalamotomy	40
Stereotactic resection of hippocampus and amygdala	9
Cyst aspirations	9
Interstitial irradiation	11
Ommaya reservoir placements	5
^{32}P instillation	2
Total	605

gical procedures. Furthermore, this system can be used conveniently and efficiently in a busy stereotactic neurosurgical practice.

In our practice, we frequently perform four to five stereotactic procedures per day and occasionally as many as 12. To accommodate the work load, we fabricated 12 stereotactic base rings, to which the vertical supports are attached for each use. A series of head frames are applied to patients requiring database acquisition the same day. Frames are reapplied to other patients for whom a database has been required, treatment planning completed, and stereotactic coordinates calculated, and who are to have surgery that day.

The ability to attach the stereotactic head frame for data acquisition and to remove and replace it for surgery becomes more necessary as the demand for the stereotactic operating room increases. With this system, the database acquisition and surgery can be done on separate days, and an operating room does not have to be held vacant until a patient returns from CT scanning, MRI, and angiography.

Treatment planning can take place at the surgeon's leisure on a nonoperating day in the room in which CT, MRI, and DA images are viewed; target points selected; probe trajectories simulated; and volumes reconstructed. Thus the surgical approach can be carefully considered without the pressure of attending to a patient already on the operating table. A computer-resident stereotactic atlas can be superimposed on reformatted CT slices to aid in treatment planning and target selections for functional procedures [11].

During the surgical procedure, the computer system is used interactively to display actual and reformatted images relative to the stereotactic frame settings. New target selections can be displayed rapidly on the preoperative database. For instance, points selected on CT or MRI can be displayed on arteriograms, and new entry points and probe trajectories will be selected quickly. In addition, the computer can display the position of surgical instruments relative to lesional volumes digitized from stereotactic CT and MRI to guide aggressive resection.

The future development of stereotactic surgery to its true potential will depend on the capacity, availability, and versatility of computer systems and software. The computer is a stereotactic surgical instrument as indispensable to the stereotactic surgeon as the microscope is to the aneurysm surgeon. In summary, the critical factor in our setup is not a particular stereotactic instrument but the computer, which has become essential to all phases of our procedures: data acquisition from a number of sources, treatment planning, and interactive surgery.

Appendix

METHOD OF COORDINATE TRANSFORMATION

A series of screen coordinates (X–Y pixels converted to millimeters) are entered for each of the CT/MRI localization system reference marks (A–I) as Xa, Ya, Xb, Yb . . . Xi, Yi. The target point is selected, and its two-dimensional screen coordinates (Xs, Ys) are determined. The computer then instantaneously transforms this screen point into the three-dimensional coordinate system of the arc quadrant device (X_{AQ}, Y_{AQ}, Z_{AQ}).

1. The zero points (origin) of the localization (X_0, Y_0, Z image) are calculated:

$$X_0 = \frac{Xa + Xg + Xc + Xi}{4} \tag{6.1}$$

$$Y_0 = \frac{Ya + Yg + Yc + Yi}{4} \tag{6.2}$$

$$Z\ image = \frac{Z_1 + Z_2 + Z_3}{3} \tag{6.3}$$

where Z_1, Z_2, and Z_3 are vertical heights above the base ring for each N-locator set of fiducials, and A is the angle between the vertical and oblique reference bars.

$$Z_1 = \frac{(Xc - Xb)^2 + (Yc - Yb)^2}{\tan(A)}$$

$$Z_2 = \frac{(Xe - Xd)^2 + (Ye - Yd)^2}{\tan(A)}$$

$$Z_3 = \frac{(Xh - Xi)^2 + (Yh - Yi)^2}{\tan(A)}$$

2. The angular tilts (alpha = right-left) (beta = anteroposterior) in reference to the stereotactic frame axis and the rotation of the image on the screen (gamma) are then determined.

$$\text{Alpha} = \tan^{-1}[(Z_1 - Z_3)/2X0] \quad (6.4)$$

$$\text{Beta} = \tan^{-1}[(2Z_2) - Z_1 - Z_3/2Y0] \quad (6.5)$$

$$\text{Gamma} = \tan^{-1}[(Ya - Yi)/Xa - Xi)] \quad (6.6)$$

3. The screen coordinate is translated in relation to the screen origin, adjusted by the screen rotation (equations 6.7–6.8) and adjusted for lateral and anteroposterior tilts (equations 6.9–6.11) to place the point in three-dimensional space (X_{3D}, Y_{3D}, Z_{3D}).

$$\text{Xrel} = (Xs - X0) * \cos(\text{gamma}) + (Ys - Y0) * \sin(\text{gamma}) \quad (6.7)$$

$$\text{Yrel} = (Ys - Y0) * \cos(\text{gamma}) - (Xs - X0) * \sin(\text{gamma}) \quad (6.8)$$

$$\text{X3d} = \text{Xrel} * \cos(\text{alpha}) \quad (6.9)$$

$$\text{Y3d} = \text{Yrel} * \cos(\text{beta}) \quad (6.10)$$

$$\text{Z3d} = \text{Z slice} + \text{Yrel} * \sin(\text{beta}) + \text{Xrel} * \sin(\text{alpha}) \quad (6.11)$$

4. These three-dimensional points are then placed in the coordinate system of the arc quadrant device (X_{AQ}, Y_{AQ}, Z_{AQ}):

$$X_{AQ} = \text{X3d} + Bx \quad (6.12)$$

$$Y_{AQ} = \text{Y3d} + By \quad (6.13)$$

$$Z_{AQ} = \text{Z3d} + Bz \quad (6.14)$$

where Bx, By, Bz are the bias factors relating the focal point of the stereotactic arc quadrant to the zero point of the localization system.

Reference

1. Apuzzo MLJ, Sabshin JK: Computed tomographic guidance stereotaxis in the management of intracranial mass lesions. *Neurosurgery* 12:277–285, 1983
2. Bergstrom M, Greitz T: Stereotaxic computed tomography. *AJR* 127:167–170, 1976
3. Birg W, Mundinger F: The direct target point determination for stereotactic brain operations from CT data and the calculation of setting parameters for polar-coordinate stereotactic devices. Presented at the Eighth Meeting of the World Society for Stereotactic and Functional Neurosurgery; Zurich, Switzerland, July 11, 1981
4. Boethius J, Bergstrom M, Greitz T: Stereotaxic computerized tomography with a GE 8800 scanner. *J Neurosurg* 52:794–800, 1980
5. Brown RA: A computerized tomography-computer graphics approach to stereotactic localization. *J Neurosurg* 50:715–720, 1979
6. Gildenberg PL, Kaufman HH, Murthy KSK: Calculation of stereotactic coordinates from the computed tomographic scan. *Neurosurgery* 10:580–586, 1982
7. Goerss SJ, Kelly PJ, Kall BA, et al: A computed tomographic stereotactic adaptation system. *Neurosurgery* 10:375–379, 1982
8. Heibrun MP, Roberts TS, Apuzzo MLJ, et al: Preliminary experience with Brown-Roberts-Wells (BRW) computerized tomography stereotaxic guidance system. *J Neurosurg* 59:217–222, 1983
9. Huk W, Baer U: A new targeting device for stereotaxic procedures within the CT scanner. *Neuroradiology* 19:13–17, 1980
10. Kall BA, Kelly PJ, Goerss SJ: Interactive stereotactic surgical system for the removal of intracranial tumors utilizing the CO_2 laser and CT-derived database. *IEEE Trans Biomed Eng* 32:112–116, 1985
11. Kall BA, Kelly PJ, Goerss SJ, et al: Methodology and clinical experience with computed tomography and a computer-resident stereotactic atlas. *Neurosurgery* 17:400–407, 1985
12. Kelly PJ, Alker GJ Jr: A stereotactic approach to deep-seated central nervous system neoplasms using the carbon dioxide laser. *Surg Neurol* 15:331–334, 1981
13. Kelly PJ, Alker GJ Jr, Goerss SJ: Computer-assisted stereotactic laser microsurgery for the treatment of intracranial neoplasms. *Neurosurgery* 10:324–331, 1982
14. Kelly PJ, Alker GJ Jr, Kall BA, et al: Method of computed tomography–based stereotactic biopsy with arteriographic control. *Neurosurgery* 14:172–177, 1984
15. Kelly PJ, Kall BA, Goerss SJ: Transposition of volumetric information derived from computed

tomography scanning into stereotactic space. *Surg Neurol* 21:465–471, 1984
16. Kelly PJ, Kall BA, Goerss SJ, et al: Precision resection of intra-axial CNS lesions by CT-based stereotactic craniotomy and computer monitored CO_2 laser. *Acta Neurochir* (Wien) 68:1–9, 1983
17. Kelly PJ, Olson MH, Wright AE: Stereotactic implantation of Iridium[192] into CNS neoplasms. *Surg Neurol* 10:349–354, 1978
18. Koslow M, Abele MG, Griffith RC, et al: Stereotactic surgical system controlled by computed tomography. *Neurosurgery* 8:72–82, 1981
19. Leksell L, Jernberg B: Stereotaxis and tomography: A technical note. *Acta Neurochir* (Wien) 52:1–7, 1980
20. Patil AA: Computed tomography–oriented stereotactic system. *Neurosurgery* 10:(3) 370–374, 1982
21. Penn RD, Whisler WW, Smith CA, et al: Stereotactic surgery with image processing of computerized tomographic scans. *Neurosurgery* 3:157–163, 1978
22. Perry JH, Rosenbaum AE, Lunsford LD, et al: Computed tomography-guided stereotactic surgery: Conception and development of a new stereotactic methodology. *Neurosurgery* 7:376–381, 1980
23. Rhodes ML, Glenn WV, Azzawi YM, et al: Stereotactic neurosurgery using 3-D image data from computed tomography. *J Med Syst* 6:105–119, 1982

7. THE LAITINEN SYSTEM

Lauri V. Laitinen

The Laitinen stereotactic system consists of the Stereoguide and the computed tomography (CT)/magnetic resonance imaging (MRI) adapter. This chapter provides a detailed description of the system and its use with all currently available imaging modalities.

The Stereoguide

The Laitinen Stereoguide [4] consists of an oval base ring with four screwholders for bony fixation, two symmetrical cylinder components, and a semicircular arc with an electrode carrier (figure 7–1). Four holes lie parallel to, and in the midplane of, the base ring: one anterior, one posterior, and two lateral holes at right angles. The anterior and the posterior holes form the sagittal midplane of the base ring, to which the lateral coordinate (X) of the target is related. The lateral holes form the origin of the anteroposterior (Y) and superior-inferior (Z) coordinates.

The cylinder components are positioned at the lateral aspects of the base ring according to the Y and Z coordinates of the target, which will lie at the common axis of the cylinders. Cogwheel mechanisms permit positioning of the cylinder components. A vernier ensures an accuracy of ±0.25 mm. The semicircular arc is positioned on the cylinders according to the X coordinate (figure 7–2). The brain target is located now at the midpoint of the spherical system of the Stereoguide and can be reached from any suitable direction.

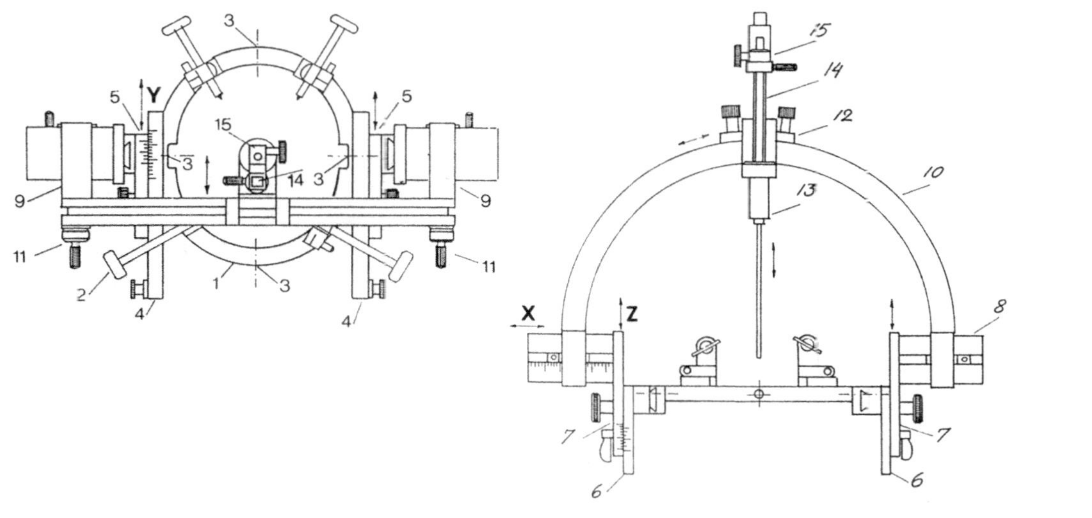

FIGURE 7–1. Laitinen Stereoguide. The left panel shows the view from above; the right panel, the anteroposterior view. The parts shown are: the base ring (1), the cylinder components (6, 7, 8), the semicircular arc (10), and the four origin holes (3).

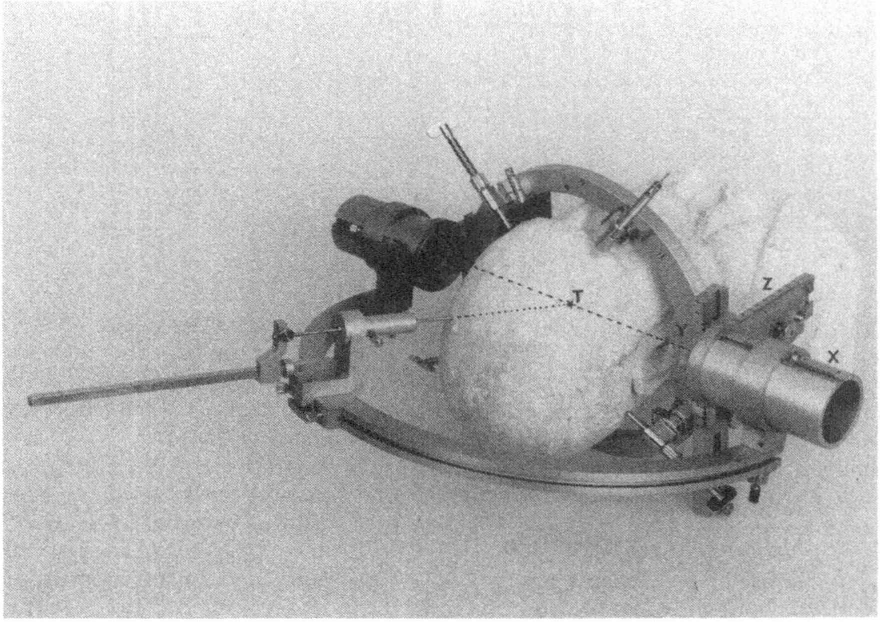

FIGURE 7–2. The target (T) lies at the midpoint of the spherical system of the Stereoguide and can be reached from any practicable direction.

The Stereoguide can be used for transnasal hypophysectomy (figure 7–3), and, when turned upside down, can be used for stereotactic surgery in the posterior fossa and upper cervical spinal canal (figure 7–4). The depth of a probe is determined using the semicircular arc with the probe carrier fixed to an arc stand (figure 7–5). The probe is advanced as far as the cone tip of the stand. The position of a stop screw is locked and read. The cone tip corresponds to the midpoint of the spherical system of the instrument.

Determination of a Brain Target Using Contrast Ventriculography

Previously, when brain targets were determined by contrast-enhanced ventriculography, a special floor stand and a teleradiographic system were needed in the operating room. Although CT or MRI study now is believed to permit more accurate localization of brain targets than does ventriculography [4], the latter will be described.

The floor stand is mounted firmly to the floor of the operating room but can be detached and remounted easily. An x-ray tube is fixed to the ceiling and another to the wall of the operating room in a position so that a central x-ray beam passes through the anterior, posterior, and lateral holes, respectively, of the base ring locked on the stand (figure 7–6). These holes form the origin of the Cartesian rectilinear coordinate system; the brain target, defined in relation to ventricular landmarks, can be coordinated with the holes (figure 7–7). The target is projected onto the X and Y axes, respectively, and the three coordinates X, Y, and Z are read directly. The distance between the floor stand and the two x-ray tubes is chosen so that the x-ray magnification coefficient is the same for both the anteroposterior (AP) and lateral radiographs. A special ruler with a corrected millimeter scale directly indicates real coordinate values.

Recent evidence demonstrated that CT determination of brain targets is more accurate than ventriculographic technique [6]. These advances promise to save considerable time and money and to increase the accuracy of surgery while reducing its risks.

The CT/MRI Adapter

The CT/MRI adapter (U.S. patent 4, 617, 925) permits all stereotactic surgery to be performed

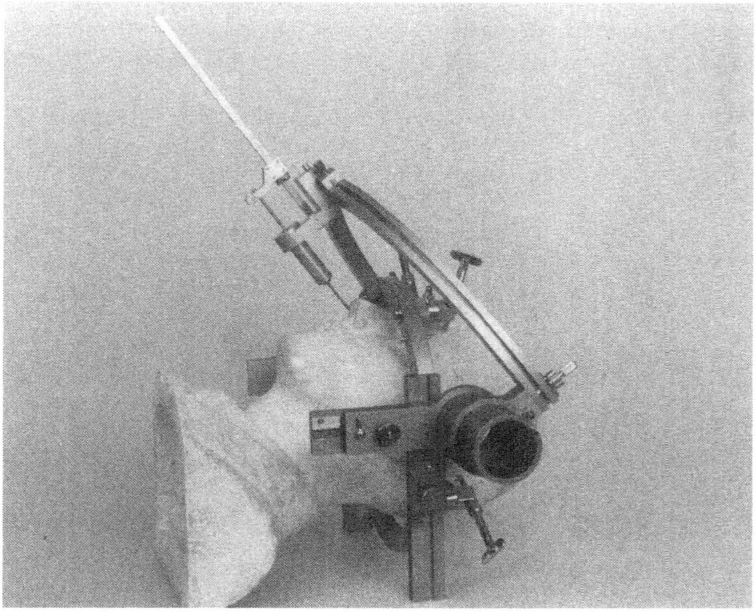

FIGURE 7–3. Transnasal approach.

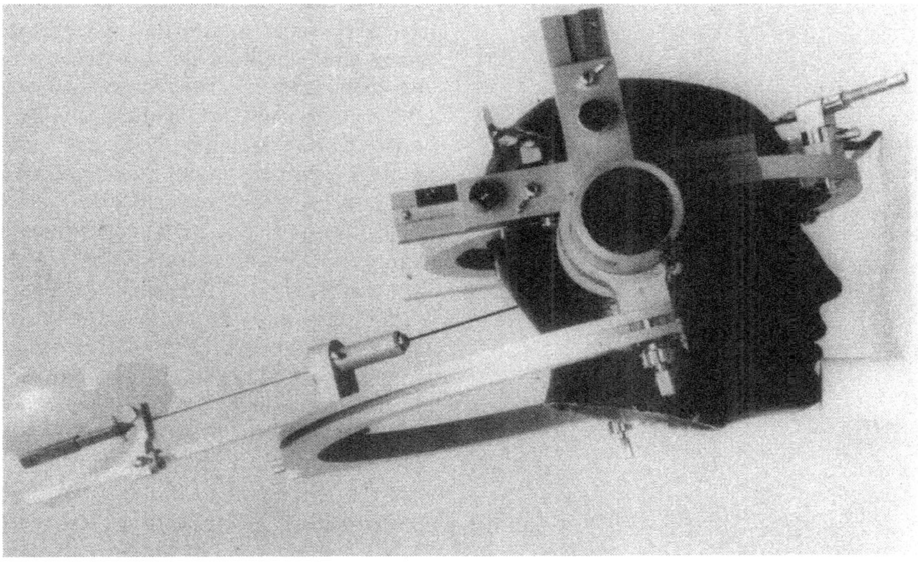

FIGURE 7–4. Posterior fossa approach.

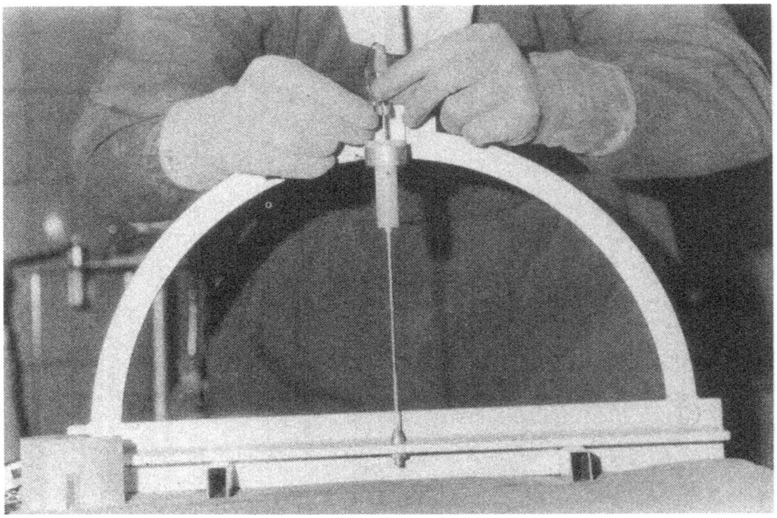

FIGURE 7–5. Determining the depth of the electrode.

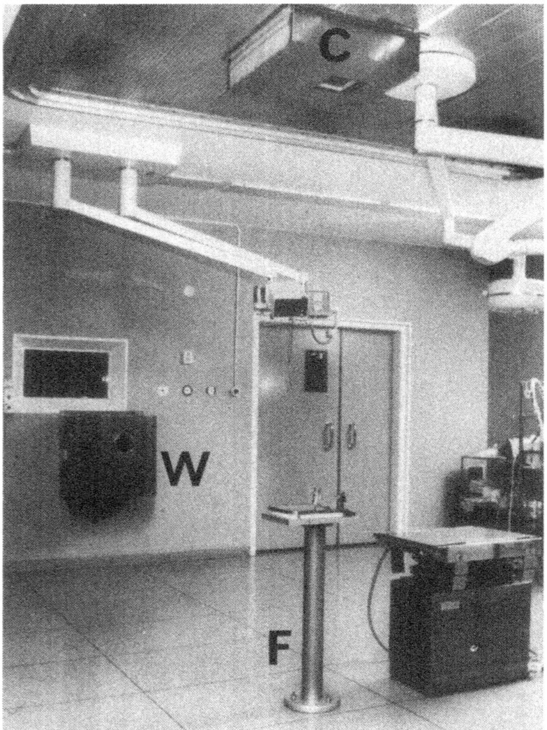

FIGURE 7–6. The detachable floor stand (F) and the rigidly fixed x-ray tubes at the ceiling (C) and on the wall (W) of the operating room.

without contrast-enhanced ventriculography and without x-ray apparatus in the operating room. The adapter can also be used in stereotactic angiography, stereotactic irradiation of brain targets with a linear accelerator, and in stereotactic location of subcortical brain tumors scheduled for open surgery.

The adapter consists of an aluminum and plastic frame (figure 7–8). It is mounted to the patient's head in a noninvasive way by means of two ear plugs and a nasion support. A threaded lever at the nasion support serves to press the ear plugs steadily against the external auditory canals. Two cogwheel screws press the nasion support against the bridge of the nose. Both posterior "laterality" indicators are fixed by hooks at the posterior ear arms and strapped against the scalp with an elastic band. An aluminum pin between the nasion support and a connector plate at the vertex functions as the frontal "laterality" indicator. These "laterality" indicators form the midplane of the adapter, to which the "laterality" coordinate (X) is related. The anterior margins of the posterior ear arms form the reference plane for the AP (Y) coordinate. Four transverse arms perpendicular to the posterior ear arms form the reference plane for the superior-inferior (Z) coordinate. The uppermost transverse arms lie at the average level of the anterior cingulum; the second pair at the level of the intercommissural

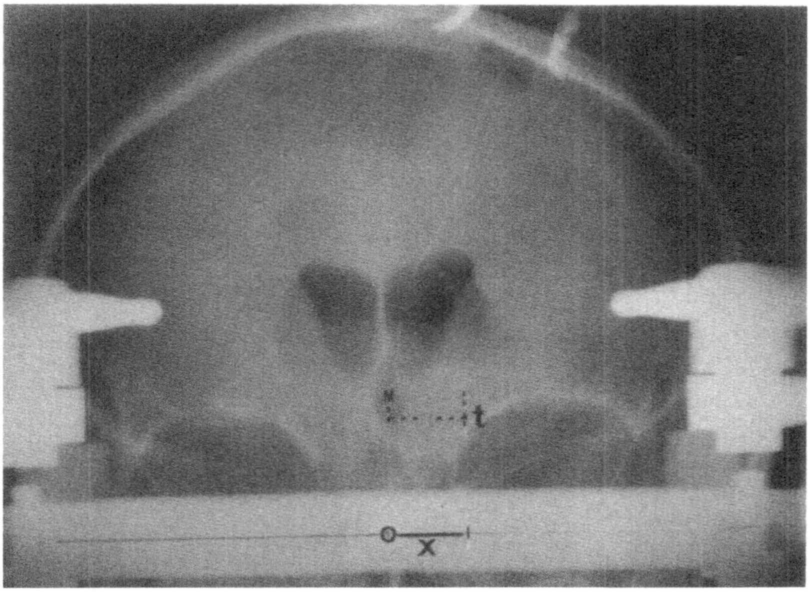

A

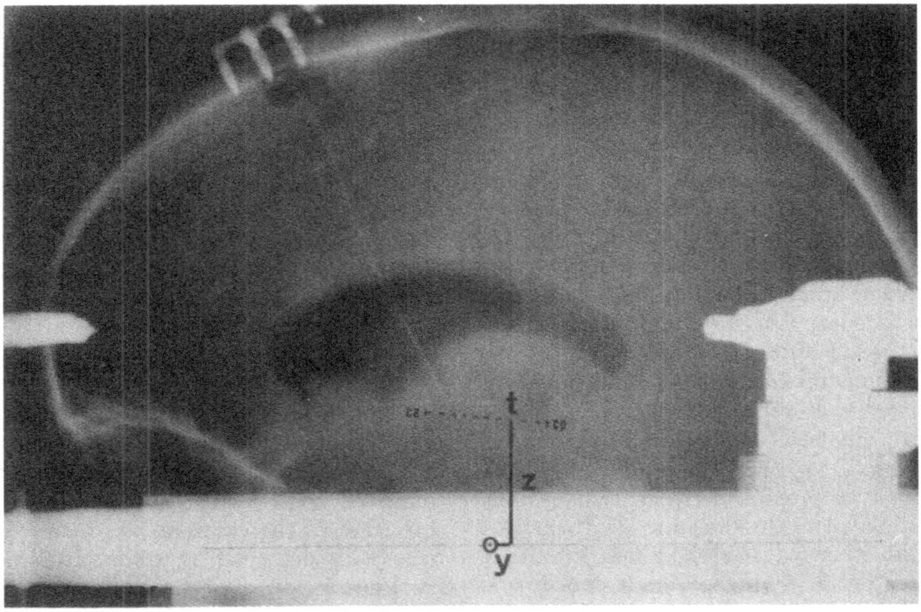

B

FIGURE 7-7. The AP (A) and the lateral (B) ventriculograms show the origin holes (0) of the base ring. The brain target (t), related to ventricular landmarks, is projected onto the X and Y axis of the frame. The stereotactic coordinates, X, Y, and Z are directly measurable using a "corrected" ruler.

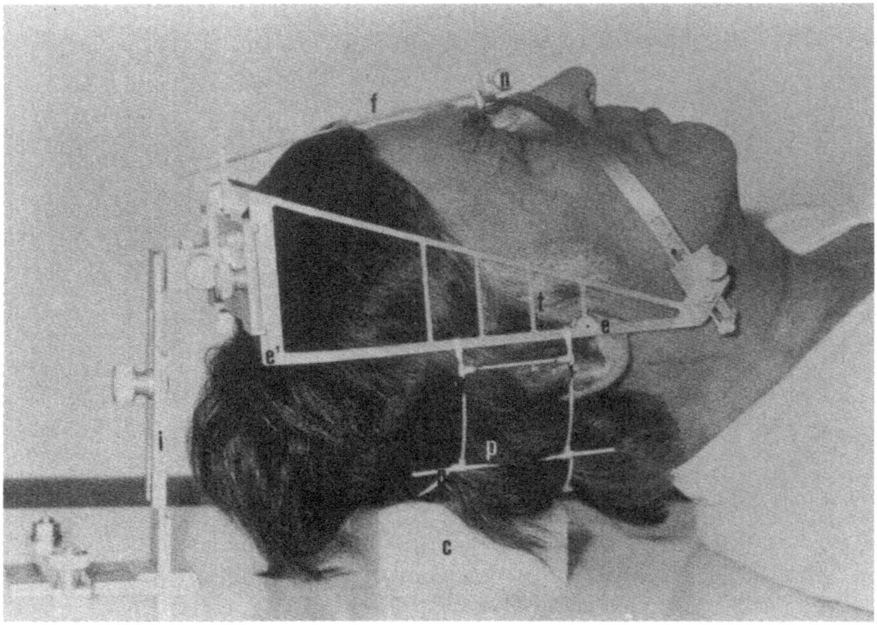

FIGURE 7–8. The CT/MRI adapter mounted to the author's head: f, frontal laterality indicator; n, nasion support; e, ear plug; é–e, posterior ear arm; p, posterior laterality indicator; i, immobilization device; c, plastic cushion.

line; and the third pair at the average level of the hypophysis, amygdala, and dentate nucleus. This arrangement reduces the distance between the most common surgical targets and the nearest reference plane. The distance between two transverse arms, 25 mm, can also be used to verify the accuracy of the longitudinal movements of the CT and MRI tables.

An experimental study in 12 healthy volunteers showed that repeated mountings of the adapter to the head are easily accomplished (A.T. Eriksson, M.I. Hariz, unpublished data). The maximal difference between two mountings extrapolated to the thalamic level was 0.61 mm for the X coordinate, 0.53 mm for the Y coordinate, and 0.96 mm for the Z coordinate. The corresponding mean values were 0.07, 0.16, and 0.17 mm. Although this experimental study showed a very high degree of reproducibility, we recently studied two elderly patients with rigid necks and a shallow nose bridge. During the CT study, their heads rotated around the interaural axis in a retroflexed direction, and the nasion support slipped downwards along the nose. To completely prevent such rotation, we added a rigid band that is strapped between the posterior ear arms and the occiput.

The adapter can be mounted quickly to the head. It is reasonably well tolerated by unsedated patients. Using the CT adapter, only one of 120 patients required that the adapter be removed. This patient had a painful cancer infiltration of the external ear. Sedation with intravenous diazepam is needed in patients with Parkinson's disease who have major tremors of the trunk and head. The adapter can be used for patients of any age. The youngest child we studied was seven years old.

In seven patients who underwent thalamotomy or posteromedial hypothalamotomy, a fairly high correlation was found between the length of the intercommissural line as measured from the ventriculogram and from the CT study [6]. The ventriculography-based measurement produced an intercommissural line slightly longer than did the CT: the mean difference was 0.7 mm, with a range of 0–1.5 mm. The largest discrepancy may have been at least partially due to a dilatation of the ventricle by the insufflated air.

In the same study, a fairly high correlation was also found between the coordinates of the posterior commissure [6]. The mean difference for the Y coordinate was 0.6 mm (range 0–1.5 mm), and for the Z coordinate, 0.6 mm (range 0–3 mm), whereas the X coordinate showed a measurable difference of only 0.5 and 0.25 mm in two of the seven patients. We believe that the current model of the adapter is more accurate than that used in our earlier study [6].

CT Technique

The adapter is mounted to the head with the patient in a sitting position. The ear plugs are pressed against the external auditory canals. The threaded lever at the nasion support is tightened until the ear plugs are pressed steadily against the ear canals so that the adapter can rotate around the interaural axis. To press the nasion support against the nose bridge, the cogwheel screws are wound symmetrically. The cogwheels and the nasion lever are tightened until the adapter remains steady and immobile; stability is confirmed by grasping the adapter at the connector plate and trying to rotate it around the interaural axis. The rigid band is strapped between the posterior ear arms and the occiput after which the posterior "laterality" indicators are mounted at a suitable and symmetrical level. Once the connector plate at the vertex is tightened until the posterior ear arms are fixed against the scalp on both sides, the positions are locked. The positions of the cogwheel cases, the connector plate, and the posterior "laterality" indicators are recorded.

A plastic plate with a head support cushion is placed on the CT table exactly parallel to the long axis of the table. The patient lies down on the table with the occiput resting on the cushion (see figure 7–8). The long axis of the head should be roughly parallel to the long axis of the table. The head should not be forced into such a flexed position that it would tend to extend during the CT scan. The adapter then is locked to the plastic plate.

On a sagittal electronic radiograph (Topogram® or Scoutview®) a cursor line is drawn at the level of, and parallel to, the uppermost transverse arms (figure 7–9, left). If a parallel relationship is obtained, the full length of one or both transverse arms will be visible. During CT-assisted thalamotomy, 2-mm-thick slices are scanned in a ventral direction in 2-mm steps (figure 7–9, right). The height level of the most ventral part of the foramen of Monro is recorded; the anterior commissure lies, on the average, 4 mm below that level. Scanning is resumed until the left and right second transverse arms and the rostral aqueduct have been imaged. The adapter can then be detached.

Magnified images are made of the slices between the level of the foramen of Monro, and the most ventral level scanned. The anterior margin of the posterior commissure is marked with a fine-tipped pen on the film that is most ventral without showing the aqueduct. To verify that the marking corresponds to the posterior commissure and not an anterior part of the aqueduct, the film is superimposed on the next dorsal film on which the posterior wall of the third ventricle is marked; this is done by placing the posterior ear arms on each other. Usually, the anterior and posterior commissures are visible at the same level. If they are not, the angle between the slice and the intercommissural line is measured, after which the length of the intercommissural line can be measured.

The surgical target in the ventrolateral thalamus is marked on the film containing the target level (figure 7–10). The AP target for tremor usually corresponds to a distance that is one-third the length of the intercommissural line anterior to the posterior commissure. Because the lateral site of the target must be chosen in relation to the width of the thalamus, two or three images at and above the target level are superimposed; this technique improves the visualization of the internal capsule. A lateral coordinate 14–15 mm from the midline of the third ventricle is usually correct.

A line is drawn between the anterior lateral

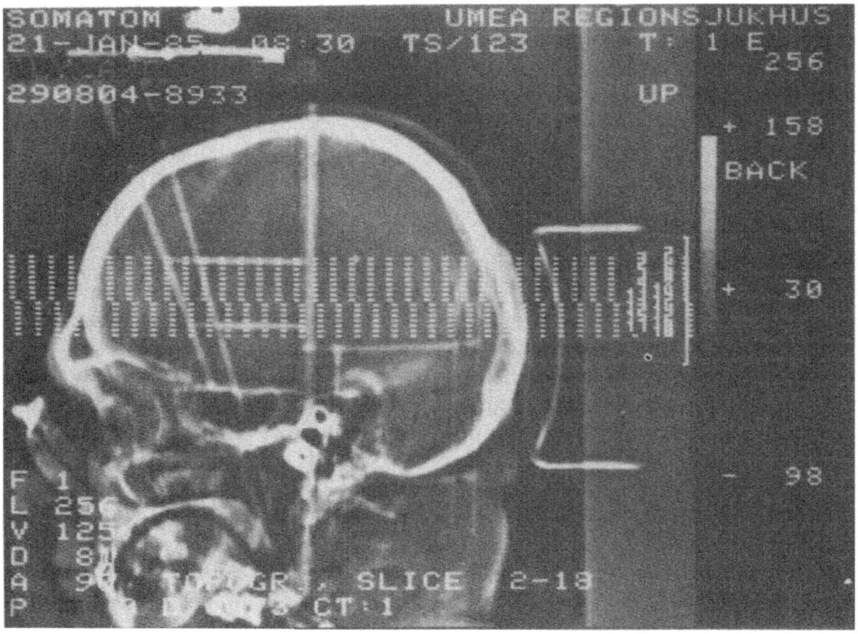

A

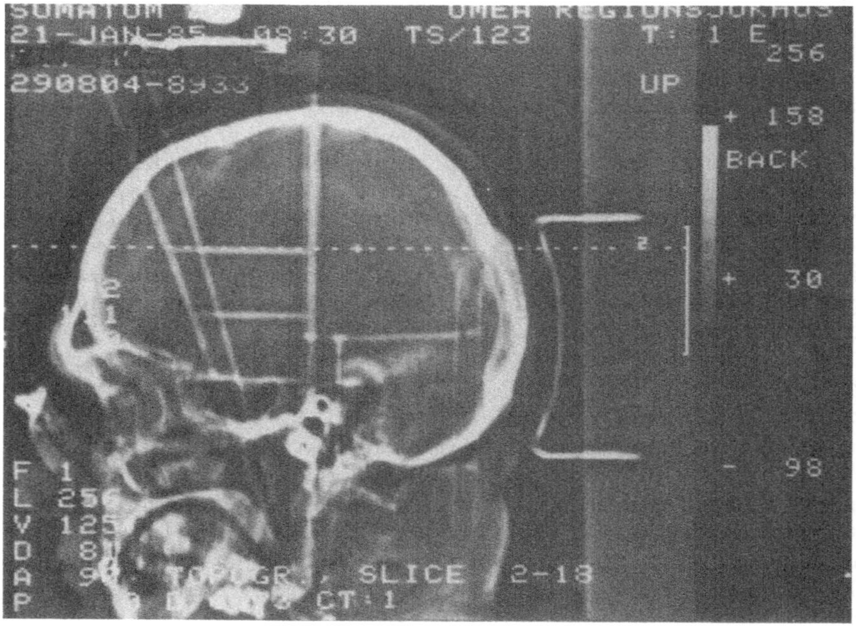

B

FIGURE 7–9. A cursor line drawn at the height of, and parallel to, the uppermost transverse arms (A). For thalamotomy, 2-mm-thick slices are then scanned at 2-mm steps until the second transverse arms and the aqueduct are visible (B).

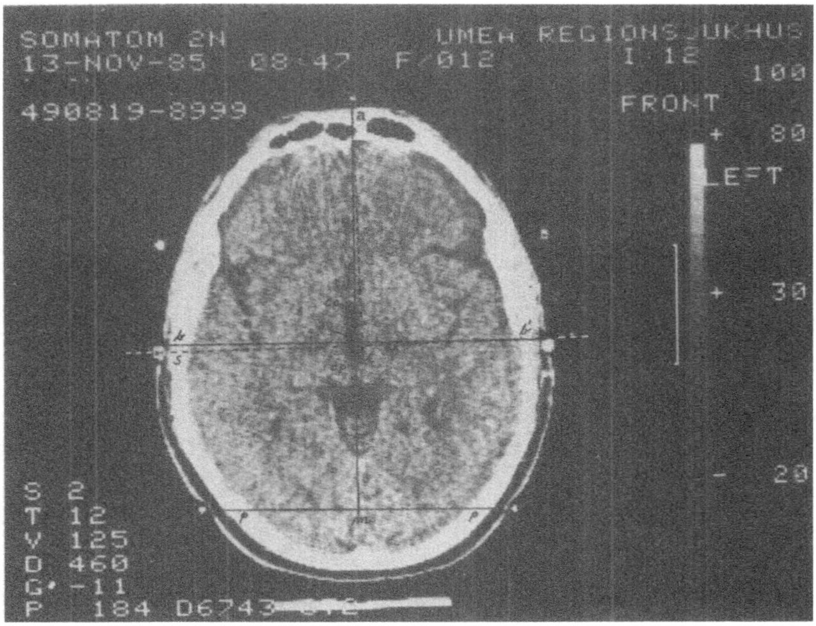

FIGURE 7-10. A slice at the thalamic level. The target (t) has been chosen in relation to the midline of the third ventricle and the anterior and posterior commissures. a–m, midplane of the adapter; b–b̄, binaural plane, s–b, cylinder axis of the Stereoguide; a–d, line perpendicular to s–b̄; a, frontal laterality indicator; p,p, posterior laterality indicators.

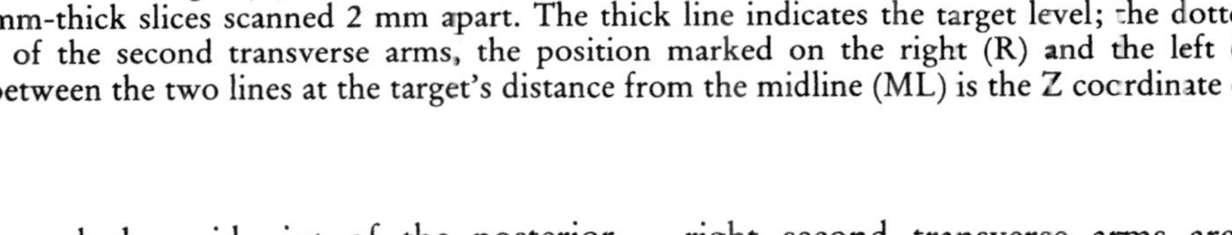

FIGURE 7-11. The height (Z) coordinate is obtained from a chart on which each line represents the midplane of the 2-mm-thick slices scanned 2 mm apart. The thick line indicates the target level; the dotted line shows the plane of the second transverse arms, the position marked on the right (R) and the left (L) side. The distance between the two lines at the target's distance from the midline (ML) is the Z coordinate of the target.

indicator and the midpoint of the posterior lateral indicators. The distance from this line to the target is the lateral coordinate (X). Another line is drawn between the anterior margins of the posterior ear arms. The distance from this line to the target is the AP (Y) coordinate. The ventral coordinate (Z) is measured easily from a chart on which the positions of the left and right second transverse arms are marked in relation to the target level (figure 7-11).

MRI Technique

The same adapter is used for MRI stereotactic surgery. Plastic tubes (2-mm inner diameter) filled with 2 mMol copper sulfate solution are

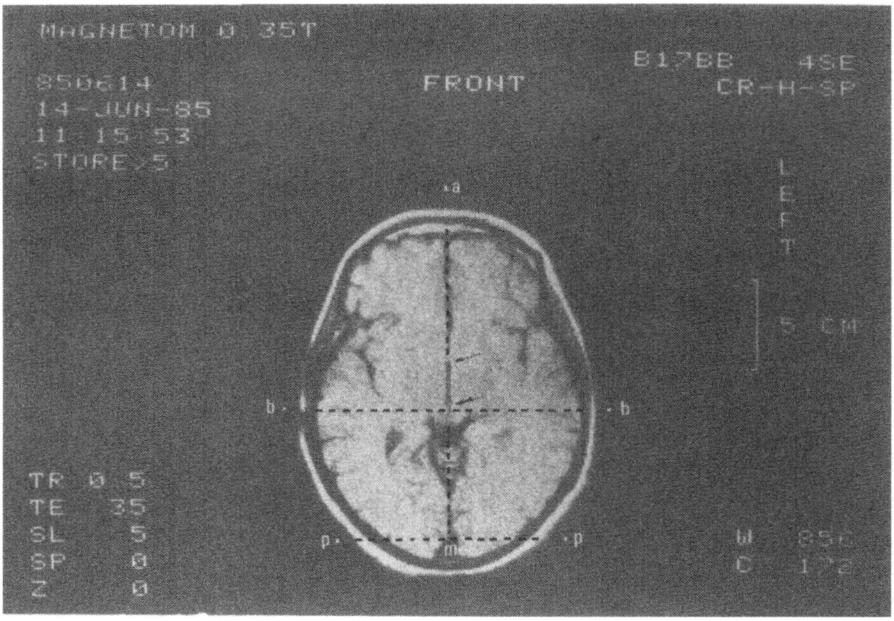

FIGURE 7–12. MRI with the adapter. Determination of the target coordinates is similar to that of a CT study. Fluid-filled plastic tubes attached to the reference structures of the adapter are clearly visible. The arrows indicate the anterior and the posterior commissures.

attached to the reference structures of the adapter. Immobililization of the patient and scanning are carried out as described for the CT technique. The reference structures are visible on the horizontal films (figure 7–12); no reconstructions are needed. For functional stereotaxis, the MRI technique still has some disadvantages relative to the CT technique: the slices are too thick (5 mm), the scanning time is long, and some patients become claustrophobic. However, the resolution of MRI is superior to that of CT. We believe that when the MRI slice thickness is reduced to 2 mm, MRI technique will completely replace the usage of CT, even in functional stereotactic surgery.

The Laitinen stereotactic system permits surgery to be performed at any appropriate time, even months after the CT scan. Because the CT scan already contains all information needed to localize the surgical target, additional radiography may increase possible target errors because of x-ray distortion and magnification. Because some neurosurgeons still prefer to use an x-ray study in the operating room, a description of the method to transfer the CT or MRI coordinates to conventional radiography follows.

Stereotactic Surgery with Radiography

The adapter is remounted to the patient's head as described previously. The Stereoguide is mounted around the adapter and fixed rigidly to the skull after local anesthesia has been administered (figure 7–13). The Stereoguide has neither a contact nor a given relation to the adapter. Instead of the frontal and posterior "laterality" indicators constructed from aluminum pins, similar steel-pin indicators are used to improve visualization on the radiographs.

AP and lateral radiographs show, respectively, the adapter and the base ring of the frame (figure 7–14). The CT target is marked on the radiographs in relation to the three reference planes of the adapter and projected onto the X and Y axes of the frame. The stereotactic X, Y, and Z coordinates thus are obtained directly. The distances measured with a corrected ruler are real. The adapter is detached and the stereotactic procedure is performed.

The position of an electrode is checked with radiography. Additionally, the correct position of an electrode must be confirmed by electrophysiology. Recording the electrical impe-

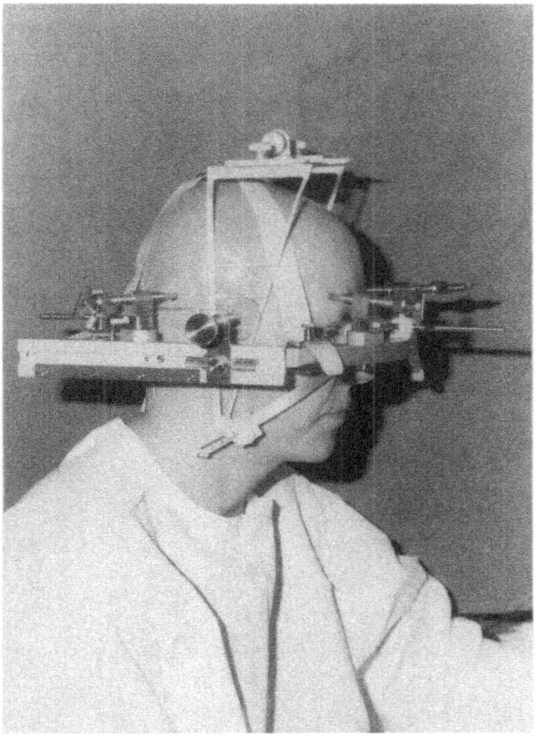

FIGURE 7–13. The adapter and the base ring of the Stereoguide mounted to the patient's head. Note that the patient is in a sitting position and has been given local anesthesia. The adapter and the frame have no contact with each other.

dance of brain tissue is a reliable method [5]. The impedance of gray matter is about 25% less than that of white matter. The impedance of cerebrospinal fluid (CSF) is only 25% that of gray matter. Recordings of spontaneous or evoked cellular activity from the target area are widely used [1] but requires a sophisticated time-consuming technique. We believe that direct electrical stimulation of the target area is simple and very reliable [2]. In patients with Parkinson's disease and tremor, the existing tremor may be aggravated by low-frequency stimulation and stopped by high-frequency stimulation. These responses offer proof that electrocoagulation will stop the tremor. A capsular response, (i.e., flexion contraction in the arm and the face) signifies that the electrode is close to, or in, the internal capsule. Electrical stimulation is also necessary during posteromedial hypothalamotomy, cingulotomy, capsulotomy, and dentatotomy.

Electrocoagulation should be carried out carefully, with continuous observation of both beneficial and harmful effects. If side effects occur, electrocoagulation must be stopped immediately. If necessary, the electrode can be repositioned, and electrocoagulation continued until a desired volume of tissue is destroyed.

Postoperative radiographic assessment of the lesion size usually demonstrates that two to three months elapse before the lesion reaches its final size and shape (figure 7–15). Postoperative radiographic studies are conducted after the adapter has been remounted to the patient's head to confirm the size and the site of the lesion and to demonstrate the accuracy of target localization.

Stereotactic Surgery Without Radiography

Stereotactic surgery can be performed accurately without radiography in the operating room. After remounting the adapter as previously described, the base ring of the Stereoguide is mounted to the skull by means of a hanging brace and a frontal, an occipital, and two lateral supports (see figure 7–13). The base ring must be parallel to the transverse arms of the adapter. It is also important to have lateral and AP symmetry between the base ring and the adapter; this is easily achieved when the transparent plates of the lateral supports are positioned symmetrically on the left and right sides of the adapter. After the area is anesthetized, the four skull screws of the base ring are tightened against the skull.

The patient reclines on the surgical table. The cylinder component is mounted onto the left side of the base ring by means of a cylinder block with an axial steel pin. This steel pin hits the origin of the Y–Z axis of the adapter, that is, the intersection of the second transverse arm and the anterior margin of the posterior ear arm (figure 7–16). The Y and Z positions of the cylinder components are determined. This procedure is repeated on the right side. Some difference between the cylinder positions of the two sides is often noted. The difference between the Y coordinate readings is marked on the CT image containing the target (see figure 7–10), where line (b–b) illustrates the interaural plane of the adapter, and line (s–b) illustrates the cylinder axis of the Stereoguide. A line (a–d) is drawn from the anterior laterality

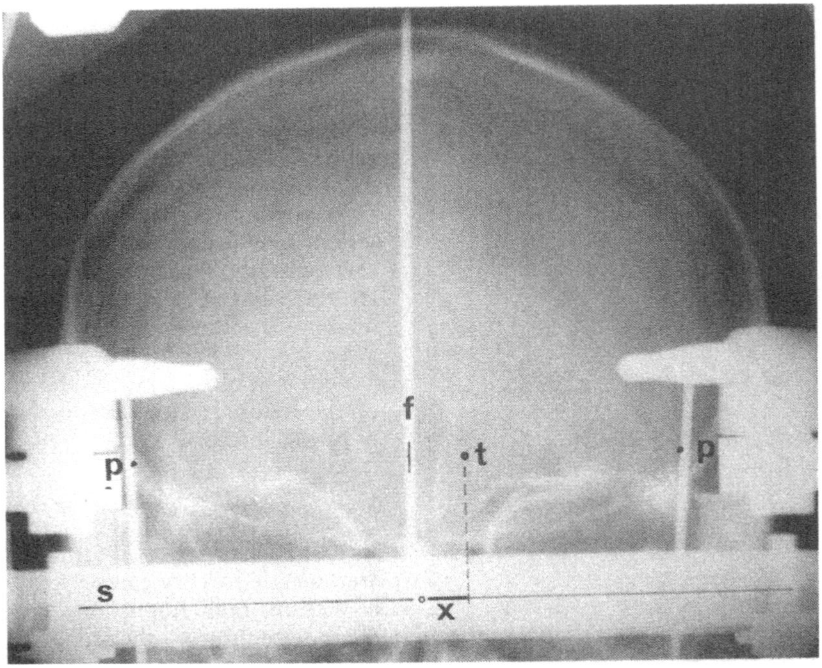

A

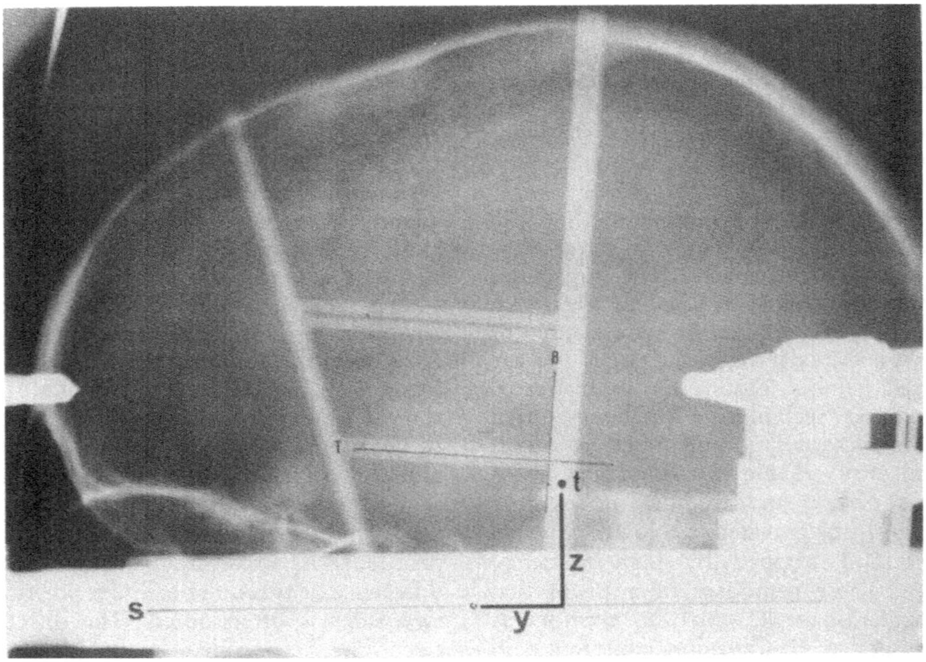

B

FIGURE 7–14. (A and B). Stereotactic surgery with radiography in the operating room. The CT target (t) is marked on the radiograph in relation to the midplane of the adapter (f), the binaural plane (B), and the plane of the second transverse arms (T) and projected onto the X and Y axis of the Stereoguide. The stereotactic coordinates, X, Y, and Z can be read directly with a "corrected" ruler.

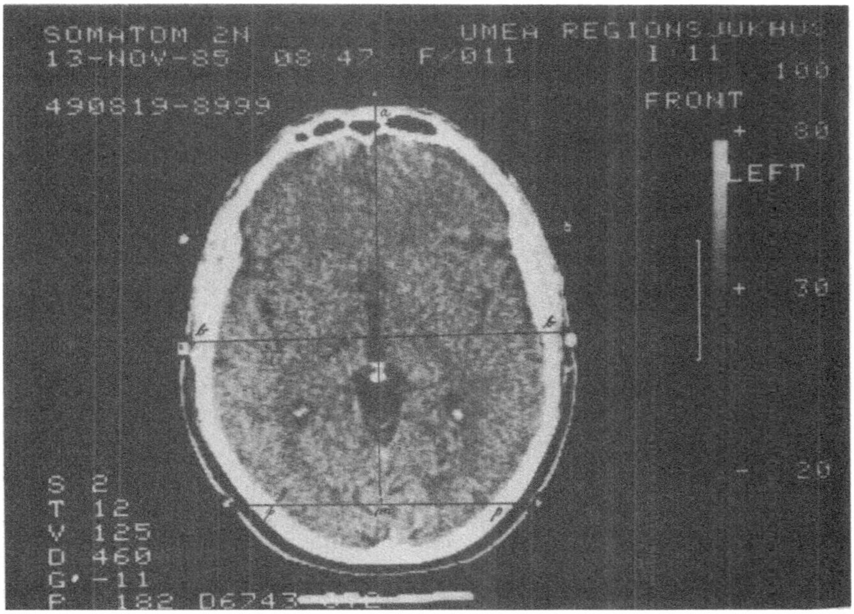

FIGURE 7–15. Postoperative CT study confirms the final size and the site of the lesion as well as the reproducibility of remounting the adapter. The arrow points to a spherical lesion in the ventrolateral nucleus of the thalamus, close to the internal capsule.

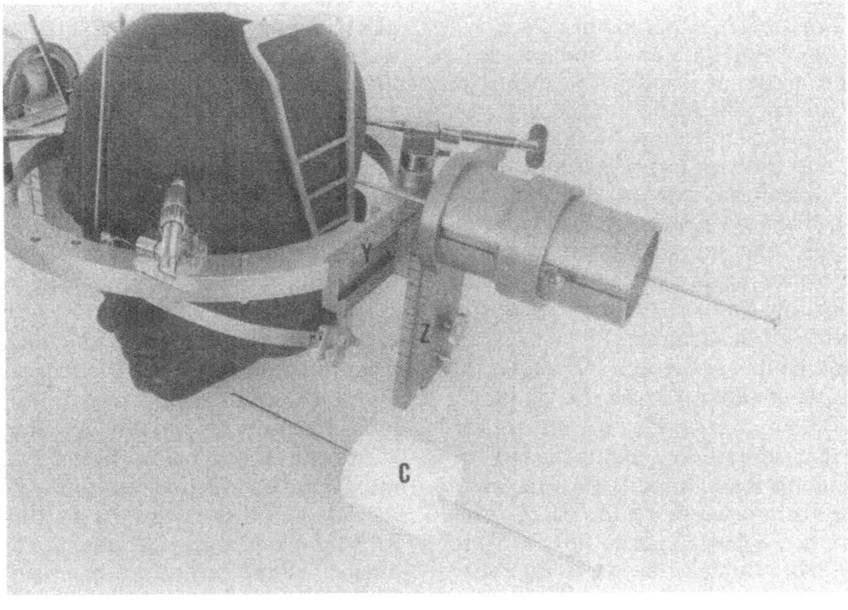

FIGURE 7–16. Stereotactic surgery without radiography in the operating room. The base ring is mounted parallel to the transverse arms of the adapter. By means of a cylinder block (C) with an axial steel pin, the cylinder component is positioned on the base ring so that its axis coincides with the Y–Z origin of the adapter. The position is read on the Y and Z scales of the frame.

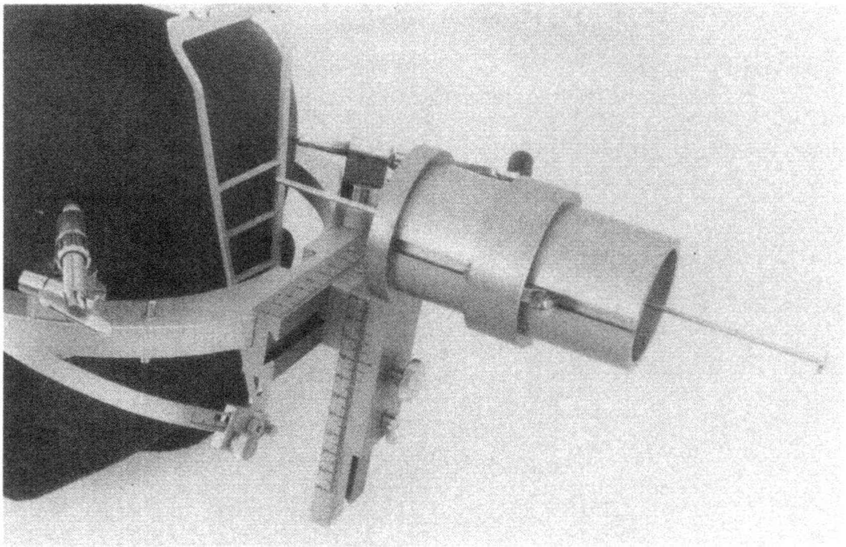

FIGURE 7–17. The Y and Z coordinates from the CT study are added to the Y and Z readings of the frame, respectively, and the cylinder component is positioned accordingly. A similar procedure is performed on the other side of the frame. When the cylinder positions of the two sides have been aligned in relation to the lateral site of the target, the target will lie at the common cylinder axis.

pin perpendicularly to line (s–b). The distance between line (a–d) and the target (t) is the final laterality coordinate (X).

On both sides of the Stereoguide, the CT coordinates Y and Z are added to the mm-scale reading of the origin positions. The means of the readings for coordinates Y and Z indicate, respectively, the final position of the cylinder components, and the surgical target will be located on the common axis of the cylinders (figure 7–17). If the surgical target lies far from the midline (e.g., the amygdala), the laterality must be taken into account; the mean of the left and right readings of the Y and Z coordinates alone will not be accurate.

With the electrode carrier at a 90° angle, the semicircular arc is mounted on the cylinders (figure 7–18). An electrode is introduced through an electrode-guiding cannula, and the arc is moved along the cylinders until the electrode hits the frontal laterality indicator. This position of the arc corresponds to line (a–d) in figure 7–10, from which the final laterality coordinate X, (d–t), is measured. The arc is moved to this position and locked. Now the surgical target is at the midpoint of the spherical system of the Stereoguide and can be reached from any suitable direction.

Stereotactic Angiography

Stereotactic angiography can be conducted on a conventional angiography table, with the CT/MRI adapter mounted to the patient's head. To assess the x-ray magnification of any plane of the brain, a 10-mm-long lead or steel pin is embedded in the ear plugs. A similar pin is attached to the front of the scalp. The patient is immobilized on the angiography table as previously described for CT or MRI imaging. AP angiography is performed with the central x-ray beam at the highest level of the vascular target and parallel to the transverse arms of the adapter (figure 7–19). The x-ray magnification can be calculated for any AP images from the magnification noted on the frontal pin, the ear plug pins, and the posterior laterality indicator pins. Lateral angiography is taken at an angle 90° to the AP exposure (figure 7–20). The central x-ray beam is directed to the Y–Z origin of the adapter that is nearest to the target level. From the lateral angiograms, the Y and Z coordinates of the target are measured. The x-ray magnification for any "laterality" level can be calculated from the distance between two transverse arms on the left and the right side. The actual distance between two arms is 25 mm.

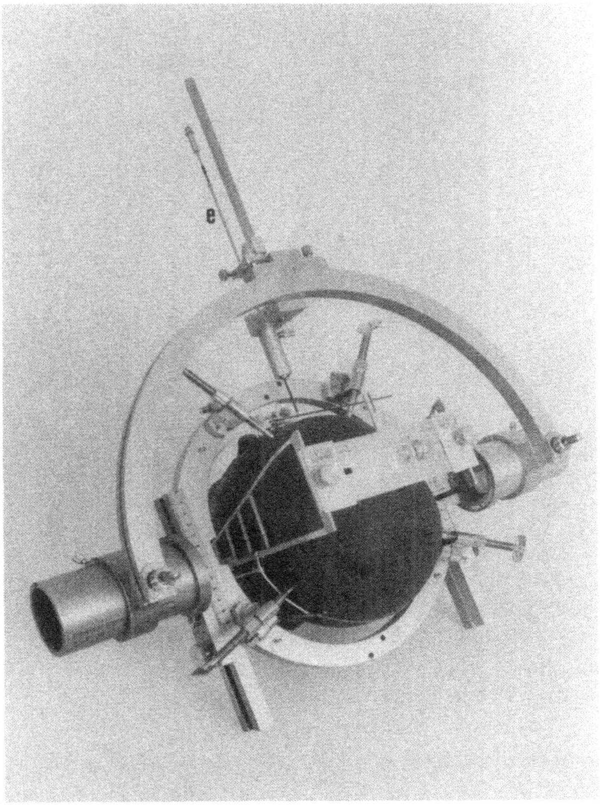

FIGURE 7–18. The semicircular arc with the electrode carrier at a 90° angle is positioned on the cylinders so that an electrode (e) hits the frontal laterality indicator. The position of the arc that is indicated on the cylinders corresponds to line a–d in figure 7–10. From this point, the final laterality of the target (d–t) is measured, and the arc is positioned accordingly. The target lies now at the midpoint of the spherical system of the Stereoguide.

To determine the laterality of the lesion on the AP angiograms, a special chart is used which indicates the actual direction of the lateral and AP central x-ray beams (figure 7–21).

Stereotactic Irradiation with Linear Accelerators

The CT/MRI adapter permits stereotactic irradiation of brain targets with a conventional linear accelerator equipped with a rectilinear horizontal and vertical laser beam system. The movement of the arc-holding beam source and the rectilinear movements of the table must be accurate, yet not all commercial accelerators can ensure the necessary precision.

With the adapter remounted to the head in the position used for the diagnostic procedure, the patient is immobilized on the accelerator table. The table is positioned so that the left laser beams hit the Y–Z origin of the adapter. The Y and the Z coordinates of the table are recorded. The same procedure is repeated on the right side. For a cerebral target in or near the midline of the brain, the means of the left and right Y and Z coordinates are calculated; the values of the diagnostic coordinates Y and Z are added, respectively. The accelerator table is moved to this position. The brain target now corresponds to the common axis of the two lateral laser beams.

To determine the laterality of the target, a chart similar to that used in stereotactic angiography (see figure 7–21) is used. The accelerator table is moved sideways until the sagittal

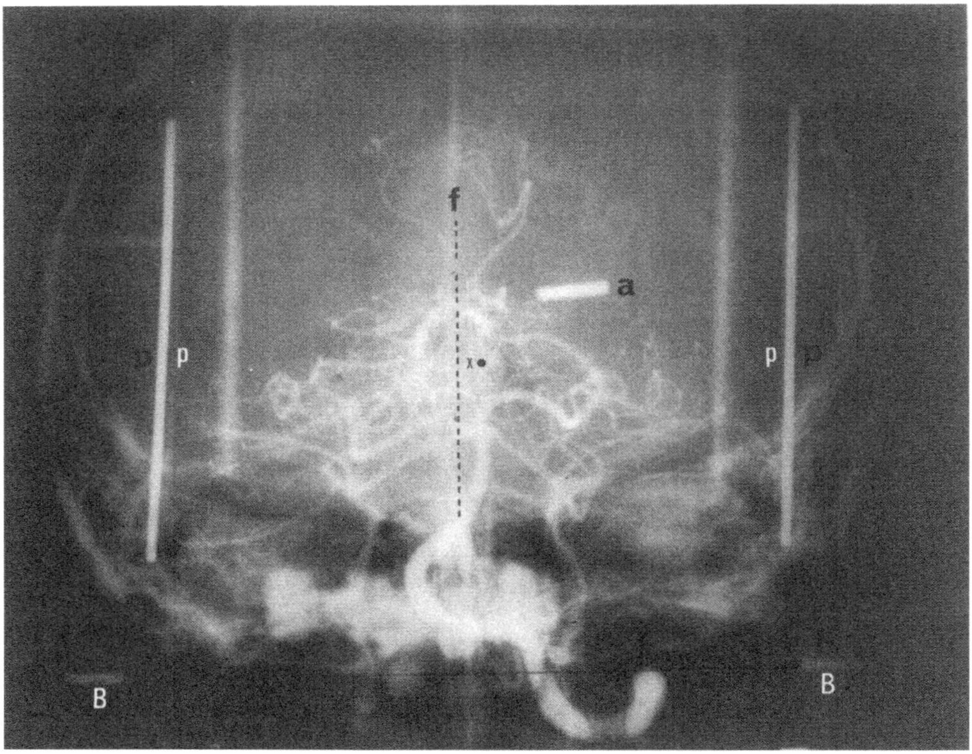

FIGURE 7-19. AP angiogram showing the ear plugs (B), the frontal laterality indicator (f), the frontal magnification pin (a), and the posterior laterality indicators. (p,p).

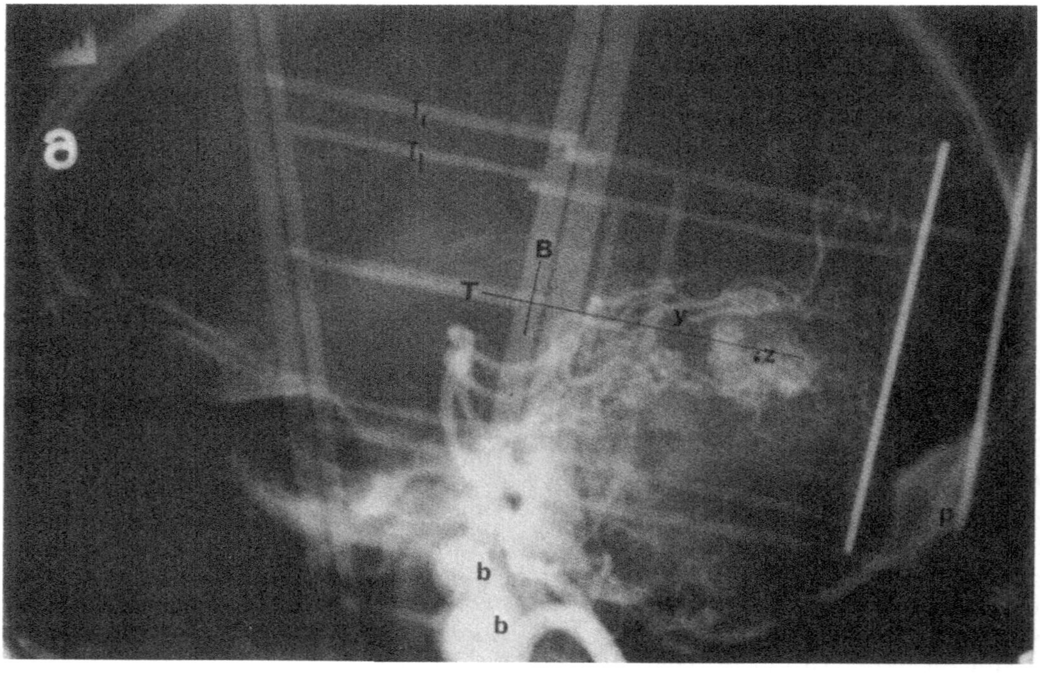

FIGURE 7-20. Lateral angiogram showing the binaural plane (B) and the plane of the second transverse arms (T), to which the vascular target (dot) is related with Y and Z coordinates. The x-ray magnification rate for any laterality level can be measured from the magnifications of the left (T_1) and the right (T_r) transverse arms.

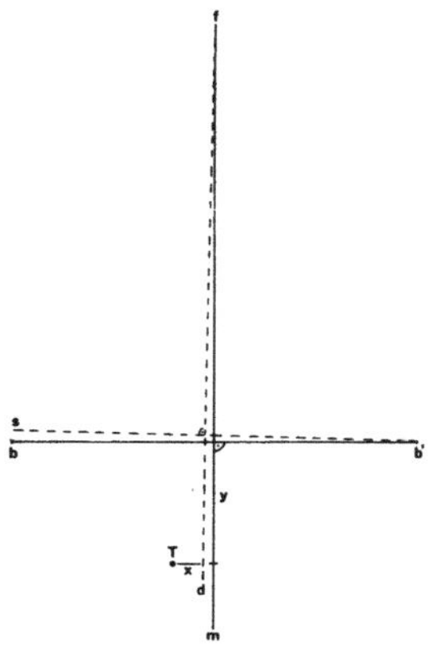

FIGURE 7–21. A chart used for correcting the x-ray beam direction (s/b́) in relation to the binaural plane of the adapter (b–b́). The position of the ear plugs (b,b́) is obtained from the AP angiogram. The dotted line perpendicular to line s–b́ indicates the direction of the central beam of the AP angiogram. The final X coordinate is the laterality distance of the target (T) from line f–d; f, frontal laterality indicator; m, midpoint of b–b́.

vertical laser beam hits the frontal laterality indicator pin. The table is then moved in a lateral direction corresponding to the laterality X coordinate obtained from the chart. The brain target is centered now at the intersection of the three laser beams and can be irradiated from appropriate directions.

Sterotactic Location of Brain Tumors for Open Surgery

The CT/MRI adapter permits accurate location of subcortical brain tumors in relation to the scalp and the skull of the patient. The CT or MRI study is conducted with the adapter mounted to the patient's head as previously described; and the X, Y, and Z coordinates of the center of the tumor are recorded (figure 7–22). The depth of the tumor from the dura is measured also. The adapter is detached and remounted on the day of surgery. The tumor center and its margins are drawn on the scalp in relation to the adapter (figure 7–23), after which the adapter is removed. The skin incision and the craniotomy thus can be placed

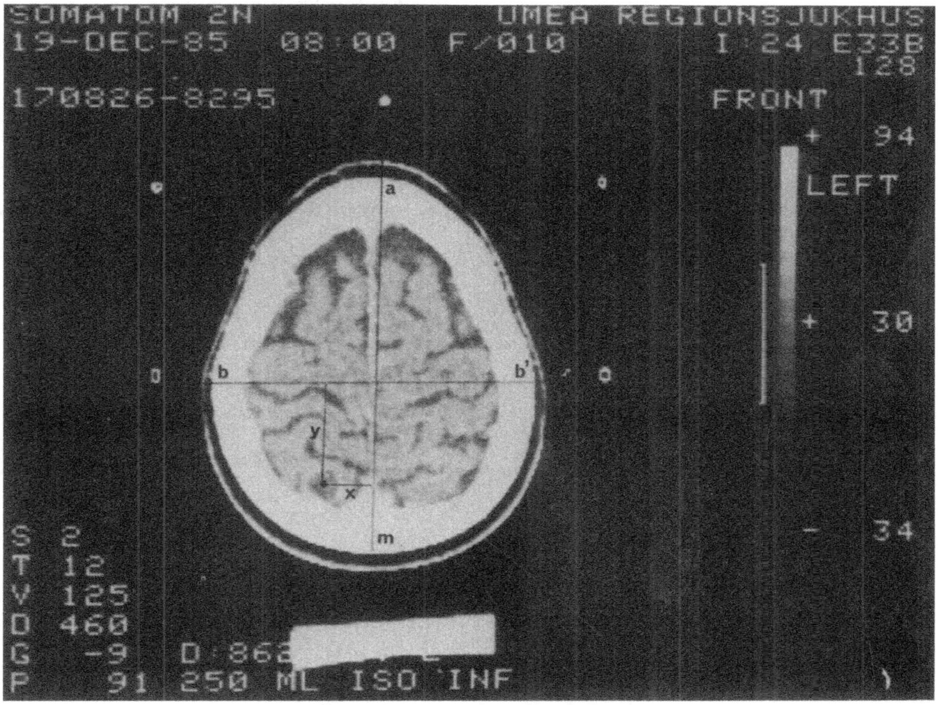

FIGURE 7–22. A small parietal tumor related to the midplane of the adapter (a–m), the binaural plane (b–b́) and the plane of the uppermost transverse arms (not visible).

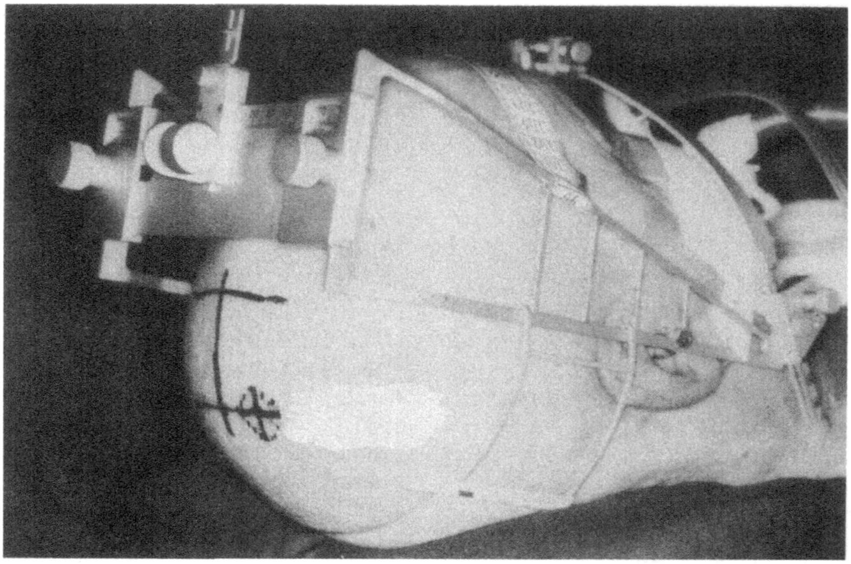

FIGURE 7–23. The tumor coordinates from figure 7–22 have been transferred to the patient's scalp. A minimal skin incision and craniotomy are needed for tumor removal.

accurately. The center of the tumor is marked on the bone, dura, and finally on the cortex. Only a small cortical incision is needed to find the tumor.

References

1. Albe-Fessard D, Arfel G, Guiot G, et al: Dérivations d'activités spontanées et évoquées dans les structures cerebrales profondes de l'homme. *Rev Neurol* (Paris) 106:89–105, 1962
2. Hassler R: Motorische und sensible Effekte umschriebener Reizungen und Ausschaltungen im menschlichen Zwischenhirn. *Dtsch Z Nervenheilk* 183:148–171, 1961
3. Laitinen LV: CT-guided ablative stereotaxis without ventriculography. *Appl Neurophysiol* (in press, 1986)
4. Laitinen LV: A new stereoencephalotome. *Zentralbl Neurochir* 32:67–73, 1971
5. Laitinen LV, Johansson GG, Sipponen P: Impedance and phase angle as locating method in human stereotaxic surgery. *J. Neurosurg* 25:628–633, 1966
6. Laitinen LV, Liliequist B, Fagerlund M, Eriksson AT: An adapter for computed tomography-guided stereotaxis. *Surg Neurol* 23:559–566, 1985

8. THE PATIL SYSTEM

Arun-Angelo Patil

The ability to visualize intracranial structures using computed tomography (CT) has led to the increased popularity of stereotactic procedures among neurosurgeons. Both the adaptation of existing stereotactic systems to the CT scanner and the introduction of entirely new systems have been reported in the literature [1–16]. To make them CT-compatible, most systems have utilized special computer programming.

Principles of the Patil System

As a standard feature, all CT scanners can measure the distance from one point to another on any CT image. This permits measurements of the X coordinate (lateral distance from the midline) and the Y coordinate (posterior-anterior distance) using the cursor of the scanner, if the reference markers of these coordinates are visible on the CT images. Scanners also can identify any given plane of scanning by means of their positioning light. If the plane of the stereotactic system can be aligned with a given plane using the positioning light, the need to calculate or measure the Z coordinate (the distance of the target from the base image) is eliminated. The Patil System has its movable probe carrier mounted on a rotatable arc (figure 8–1) and uses these standard CT-scanner features to obtain coordinate measurements and to place the target at the center of its arc, eliminating the need for calculations or special computer programming.

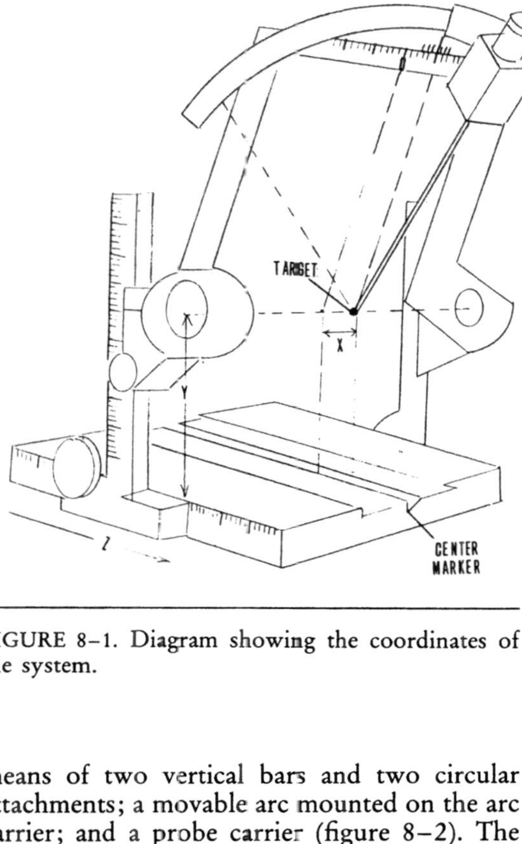

FIGURE 8–1. Diagram showing the coordinates of the system.

The System

The system (Terhorst Technologies, 615 Burdick Expressway East, Minot, ND 58701) has the following components: a base platform; a movable headholder that is mounted on the base platform; a movable and detachable arc carrier that is mounted on the base platform by means of two vertical bars and two circular attachments; a movable arc mounted on the arc carrier; and a probe carrier (figure 8–2). The base platform has a midline groove, one edge of which serves as the center marker for the X coordinate. The top surface of the base platform is the marker for the Y coordinate, which, in this system, is measured from the top of the base platform. The sides of the base platform are marked by indicators. The adjustable vertical bars are mounted on the sides of the base platform. Circular attachments connect the arc carrier to the vertical bars. The top portion of the circular attachment is detach-

L.D. Lunsford (ed.) *MODERN STEREOTACTIC NEUROSURGERY*.

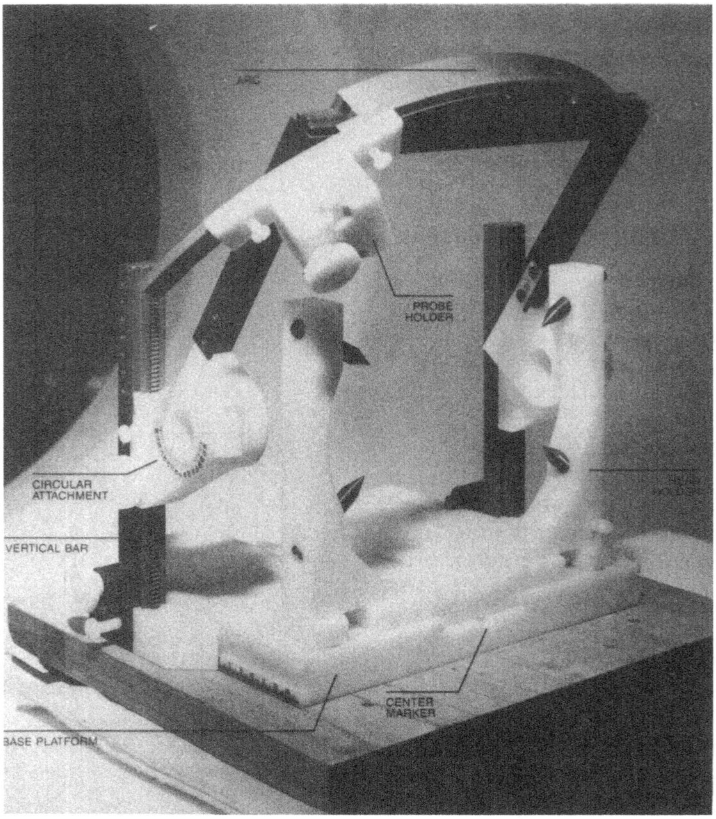

FIGURE 8–2. The stereotactic system.

able, allowing removal of the arc carrier if necessary. The arc carrier rotates around an axis formed by the line joining the centers of the two circular attachments (see figure 8–1). On this axis also lies the center of the arc. The arc can be extended so that even a trajectory of 90° from the vertical is possible.

The movable probe carrier is mounted on the arc. Its inner cylinder has a central hole, and it is interchangeable with cylinders having holes of various diameters, including one cylinder that can accommodate an endoscopic device. The radius of the arc from the top of the probe carrier is 21 cm and requires a probe 21 cm in length. The probe can be moved vertically in the probe holder within a distance of ±1 cm via a rack-and-pinion system (figure 8–3). All other movements of the system also work by rack and pinion. A vernier scale incorporated in the system permits movement in increments of 0.1 mm. The headholder slides along

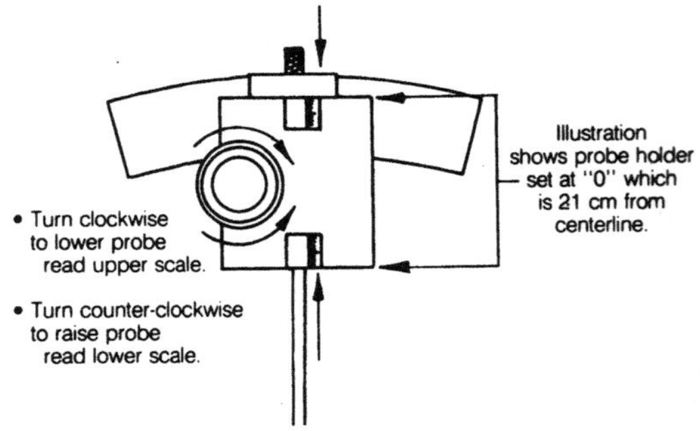

FIGURE 8–3. The fine adjustment of the probe carrier.

the length of the base platform and stops at any required position. Four chromium-plated brass pins are used for head fixation. The headholder, the base platform, the circular attach-

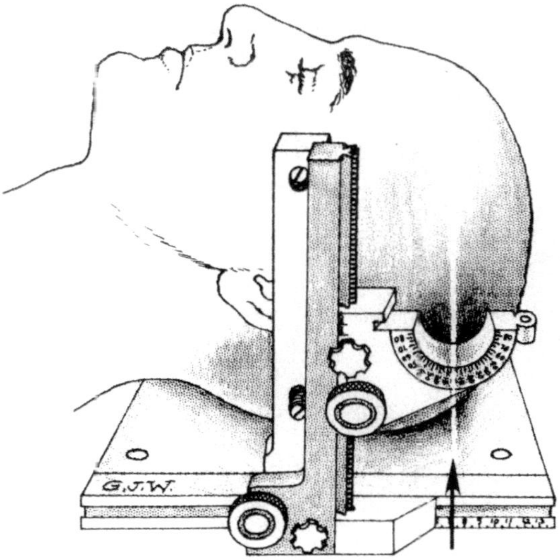

FIGURE 8–4. Alignment of the laser positioning light with the middle of the circular attachment.

ments, and the probe carrier are composed of plastic (acetyl resin). The vertical bars, the arc, and the arc carrier are made of anodized aluminum. The system connects to the scanner with a special table attachment.

Technique for Using the Patil System

After the base platform is fitted on the top of the CT table perfectly parallel to its length, the patient's head is placed in the headholder. CT images are taken with the gantry perfectly vertical in the target region. If the headholder is visible on the CT image in which the target is localized, the headholder is moved to another position to avoid artifact. After the head pins are attached, another image is taken in the CT plane of the target. The laser positioning light is then activated. The circular attachments are moved along the length of the platform by adjusting the vertical bars until the laser positioning light coincides with the vertical line in the middle of the circular attachments (figure 8–4). During this part of the adjustment, the arc (together with the arc carrier) is detached from the system to avoid artifact. The X and Y coordinates are measured from a single image on which the target is localized. Using the cursor of the scanner, the perpendicular distance measured from the center marker of the base to the target is the X coordinate (figure 8–5A), and the distance measured from the top surface of the base platform to the target is the Y coordinate (figure 8–5B). The Y coordinate is adjusted by moving the circular attachment to the required height (figure 8–6A); the X coordinate is adjusted by moving the middle of the arc a distance equal to the X coordinate (figure 8–6B). Next, the arc carrier is reattached to the system, where it can be rotated to any desired angle, and the probe holder on the arc likewise can be rotated to any angle required to reach the target through any point on the skull.

The burr hole can be made before the patient is brought to the CT scan room at any time considered to be safe. The burr hole should be as close as possible to the target. Alternatively, a twist-drill hole can be made in the CT room or after measurements are taken; the patient and the system then can be moved together to the operating room for burr-hole placement. During biopsy, the probe can be moved to different depths to obtain tumor specimens at various levels. For greater accuracy, the smaller diameter of scanning is preferred. Generally a 25-cm scan diameter is best.

HEAD POSITION

Because the coordinates are measured using reference markers on the base platform, the position of the head does not have to be symmetrical. We have performed this procedure with patients' heads in lateral and even prone positions. For occipital and suboccipital approaches, the prone position is required.

TRAJECTORY DETERMINATION

Coronal (figure 8–7A) and sagittal (figure 8–7B) reconstructed images can be used to determine the safest trajectory. The trajectory can be adjusted in the coronal plane by moving the probe carrier on the arc, and in the sagittal plane by adjusting the arc carrier around its axis of rotation.

ACCURACY OF THE SYSTEM

Accuracy of the system depends on the slice thickness of the CT images and the diameter of scanning. The thinner the slice and smaller the diameter of scanning, the greater the accuracy. Using a slice thickness of 1.5 mm and a scan

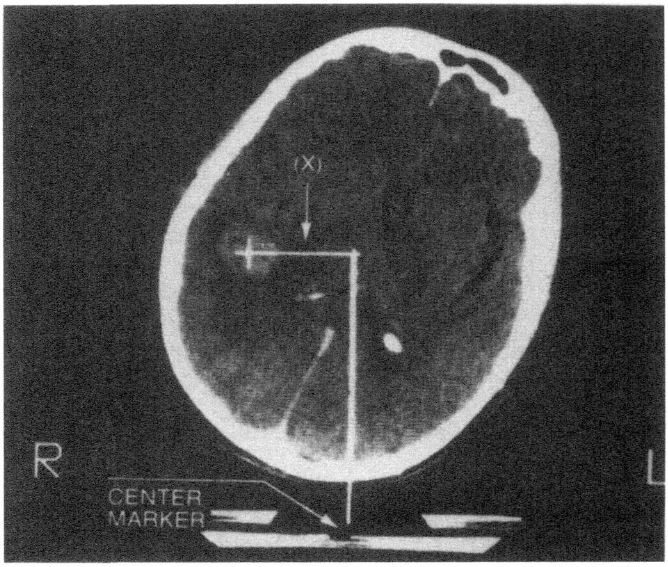

A

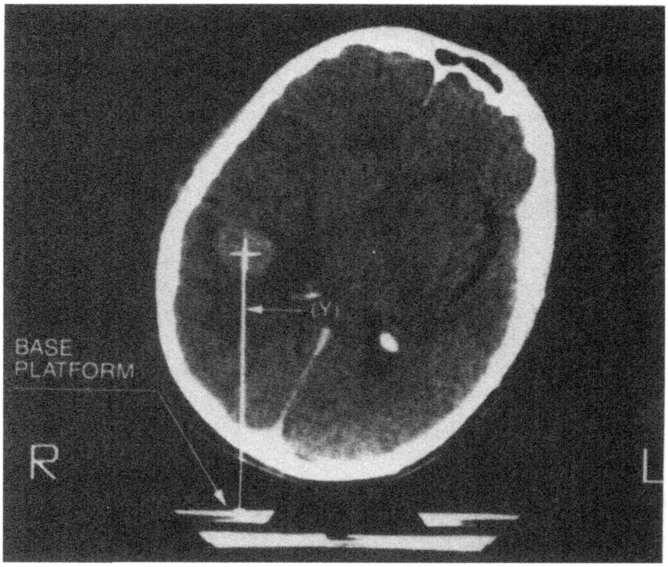

B

FIGURE 8–5. Measurements of the coordinates: X coordinate (A); Y coordinate (B).

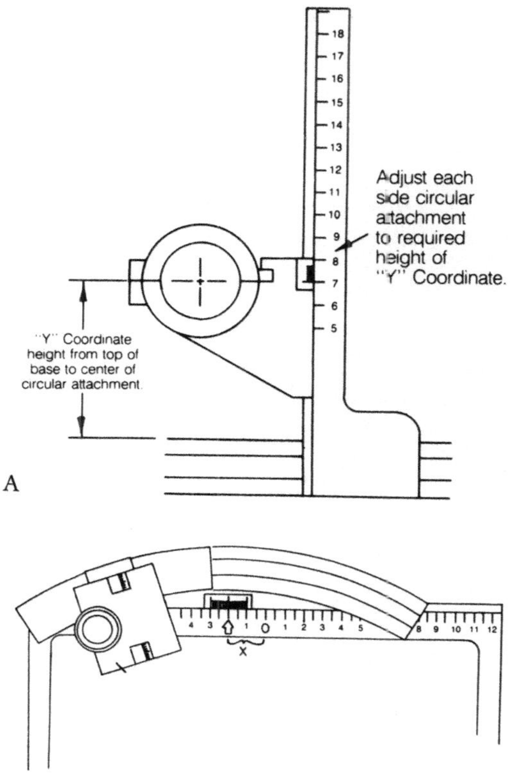

A

B

FIGURE 8-6. Adjustment of the coordinates: Y coordinate (A); X coordinate (B).

diameter of 25 mm, accuracy can be obtained up to 0.3 mm for the X and Y coordinates and up to 0.6 mm for the Z coordinate.

Uses of the Patil System

NUCLEAR MAGNETIC RESONANCE (NMR) SCANNING

Because nonferromagnetic material is used in its construction, the system can be used without any structural modification in the NMR scanner. A thin layer of mineral oil applied to the top surface of the base platform makes the X and Y coordinate markers visible on the scan image and allows direct measurement of these coordinates. The Z coordinate can be measured using the laser positioning light. This light will mark the zero starting point of scanning on the indicators on the sides of the base platform. The distance of the target from this point to the target is determined by multiplying the number of scan images (from the starting image to the image showing the target) by the scan thickness. The middle of the circular attachment then is moved to this point. Another method for determining the zero image plane is to use one surface of the head holder to mark this plane by coating it with oil. This point will be visible on the midsagittal scout picture. The brass head pins do not cause any significant artifact.

FUNCTIONAL NEUROSURGERY

Because this system uses axial images for coordinate measurement, the target must be identified on an axial image. Fortunately, with high-resolution imaging, direct target visualization on the axial scan is possible, especially when the NMR scan shows individual nuclei. In cases in which coordinates still must be defined in relationship to midline intracranial landmarks such as the intercommissural line, the surgeon may first construct a sagittal image, using thin slices (e.g., 5 mm). The target then can be marked directly, using the cursor on this image (figure 8-8A, 8-8B, 8-8C). Next, the distances are measured from the target to both the posterior outer bony surface (figure 8-8D) and the zero starting image (figure 8-8E). The latter distance divided by slice thickness indicates the axial image on which the target is located. The former distance can be measured in the midline on the axial image of the target (figure 8-8F). To mark the target site, lateral distance in the appropriate side is then measured form the central end of this line (figure 8-8G).

INDICATIONS FOR USE

The Patil system can be used for the following purposes:

1. Biopsy of intracranial lesions: brain tumors, inflammatory and parasitic lesions, other unknown lesions
2. Aspiration of cysts
3. Aspiration of brain abscesses and instillation of antibiotics
4. Functional neurosurgery
5. Intracavitary and interstitial irradiation
6. Stereotactic radiosurgery

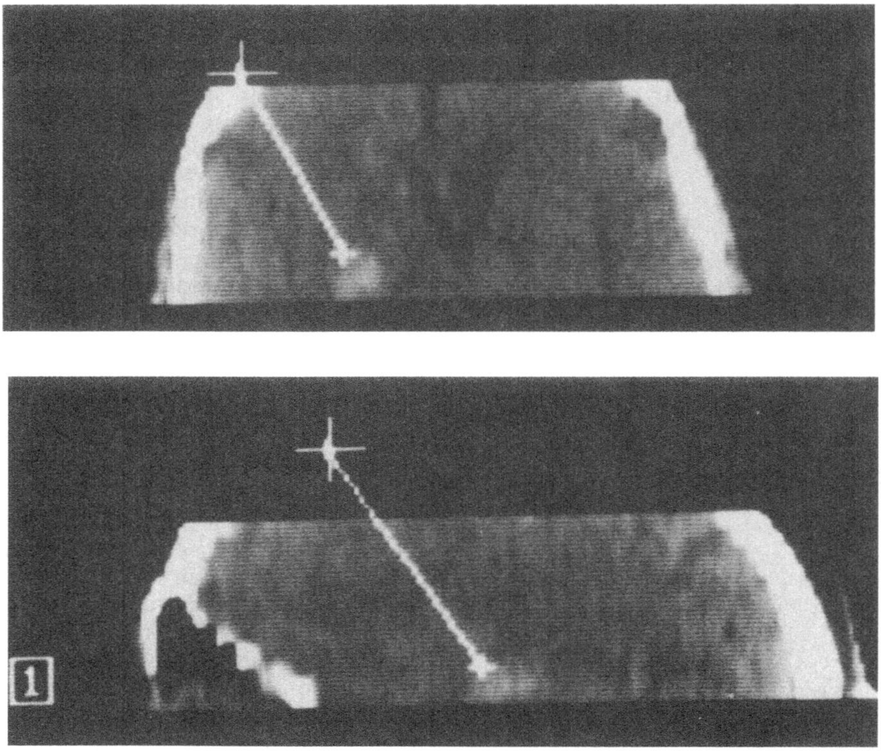

B

FIGURE 8–7. Trajectory in the coronal plane (A). Trajectory in the sagittal plane (B).

7. Stereotactic transsphenoidal chemical hypophysectomy
8. Stereotactic laser microsurgery

Clinical Experience

This system has been employed in more than 60 cases. The most common use has been in diagnosis of deep intracerebral lesions, especially brain tumors, including one case of a brain-stem tumor. In all biopsies the procedure was performed using a 16-gauge needle. If, on gross examination, the removed tissue appeared to be normal, frozen sections were obtained while the patient was still in the system, and, when necessary, another biopsy was performed. A nondiagnostic biopsy on first attempt was usually caused by aspiration of the necrotic center of the tumor. This problem can be overcome by obtaining biopsies at different depths. A 3-ml syringe was used to aspirate the tissue.

We have also used the system for implanting permanent and temporary interstitial radiation sources and for intracavitary irradiation, aspiration of intracranial cysts, stereotactic focal radiation therapy using the linear accelerator, aspiration of intracerebral clots, aspiration of brain abscesses, and instillation of antibiotics. Since we began using this technique, no patients with brain abscesses have needed an open craniotomy.

Unless the patient was restless or uncooperative, only local anesthesia was needed. In the majority of cases, the entire procedure was performed in the CT room, using a twist-drill opening. Some patients were brought to the CT room after a burr hole was made in the operating room. When NMR stereotaxis or stereotactically guided microsurgery was performed, the remainder of the procedure took place outside the CT room, after measurements were obtained in the scanner.

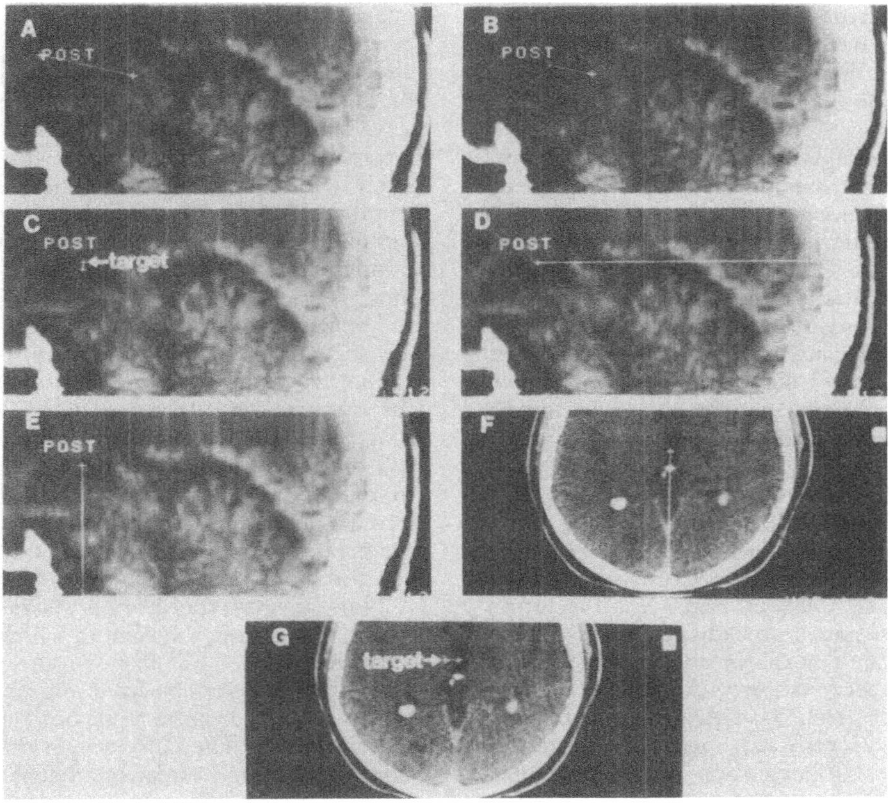

FIGURE 8-8. Marking of the target (thalamotomy for dyskinesia) for functional neurosurgery on an axial image. The target is 11 mm anterior to the posterior commissure and is 2 mm above and 10 mm lateral to the intercommissural (IC) line. (A) The IC line is drawn on the sagittal reconstructed image. (B) A point 11 mm anterior to the posterior commissure is drawn. (C) The target is marked 2 mm above the IC line. (D) The perpendicular distance of the target from the posterior outer surface of the skull is measured. (E) The vertical distance of the target from the base of the image is measured. This distance is divided by the slice thickness of the CT image to find the slice number of the axial image on which the target is located. (F) The axial image of the target. The distance from the target to the posterior surface of the skull is transposed in the midline. (G) The target is marked 10 mm lateral to the midline.

Results

To date, all stereotactic surgical procedures that we have performed using this system have been free of complications. Each biopsy performed with this sytem has resulted in a correct diagnosis.

Comments

The planar image produced by the CT scanner makes it possible to locate the plane of the target using the laser positioning light. Thus, if the target can be approached in this plane, it is necessary only to determine the X and Y coordinates. Based on this principle, simpler stereotactic systems were designed initially [13, 15]. Modifications were then made to allow a center-of-the-arc technique [12, 14]. In the Patil system, the center of the arc coincides with the target as a result of adjusting the X and Y coordinates and bringing the axis of rotation of the arc into the CT plane of the target, using the laser positioning light. With the target thus centered, the target will always be reached with a needle that has a length equal to the radius of the arc, regardless of the position of the probe holder on the arc and regardless of the position of the arc on its axis. An infinite number of trajectories are thus possible, and the surgeon can choose the optimal trajectory.

Because the system is composed of plastic and nonferromagnetic material, it can be used in NMR scanners without modification. Since the head holder is mobile, it is possible to keep it outside the CT plane of the target, eliminating artifact, despite the use of metal head pins. In NMR-guided stereotaxis, the metal head pins do not cause significant artifact. During measurements of the coordinates, only the base platform with the patient's head in the head holder is used, so that no metal parts are in the CT plane of the target, and thus, artifacts are eliminated. The base platform serves as the reference marker both for the X and Y coordinates. With the X coordinate at the center of the base platform, one can perform scans of small diameters, significantly improving the accuracy of the stereotactic procedure. The use of reference markers that can be seen on the CT image allows direct measurments of the X and Y coordinates from a single image without the need for calculations, special computer programming, or integration of the stereotactic system with the scanner. Adjustment of the Z coordinate is simple, because all CT scanners have a positioning light that indicates the different imaging planes. Of course, the accuracy of the Z coordinate depends upon the accuracy of the positioning light. Therefore, it is important that this light be inspected at regular intervals.

Incorporation of a vernier scale and a rack-and-pinion system permits fine, accurate, and quick adjustments of the coordinates. Because the arc itself moves on the arc carrier, laterally placed targets can be reached without using a large arc. This feature also makes the system compact and easy to use. Additionally, an extension system that permits extreme lateral trajectories has been added to the arc; potentially, one can use a trajectory 90° to the vertical. Downward drift of the head end of the table can be a problem, especially when stereotactic systems are attached at the end of the table. To minimize this problem, we have chosen to fix the system on the top of the table.

The thickness of the CT scan slice is an important factor in any stereotactic system. Not only the Z coordinate but also the X and Y coordinates are subject to errors, because the image is a composite picture of a slice of a given thickness. Pixel size is another factor that affects the accuracy of the system. The smaller the diameter of the scan, the smaller the pixel size, and thus the greater the accuracy. Most intracranial lesions can be reached fairly accurately with a 5-mm slice thickness. For targets less than 5 mm in diameter, it is better to use a 2-mm slice thickness. One disadvantage of thinner slices is the extra time needed for scanning.

The Patil system provides the option of placing the burr hole before, during, or after the scanner is used, depending on the preference of the surgeon and the availability of scanner time. The base platform can be lifted very easily from the table, if the patient has to be taken to the operating room. No simulator or intermediate frame for calculation is needed. If the probe is positioned in the CT room, direct confirmation on a CT image can be obtained.

Normally, the trajectory is visible on the CT image when using a system in which the trajectory lies in the CT plane of the target [13]. Using off-axis reconstructed images, it is possible to see the trajectory in both coronal and sagittal planes. The Patil system offers the option of choosing a trajectory visualized in both of these planes.

Summary

The Patil stereotactic system is a relatively simple, accurate, and comparatively inexpensive system with straightforward methodology. The system requires no calculations or special computer programming. It is free of artifact. Laterally placed targets can be reached with ease, and calculations or measurements of the Z coordinate are not necessary. This device needs no intermediate frame or simulator for calculating coordinates and can be used before, during, or after scanning. Direct visualization of the trajectory on CT images is possible. It has the capability of approaching the target from any point on the head, and it is compatible with both NMR and any total body scanner.

References

1. Bergstrom M, Greitz T: Stereotaxic computed tomography. *AJR* 127:167–170, 1976
2. Boethius J, Bergstrom M, Greitz T: Stereotaxic

computerized tomography with a GE 8000 scanner. *J Neurosurg* 52:794–800, 1980
3. Brown RA: A computerized tomography-computer graphics approach to stereotaxic localization. *J Neurosurg* 50:715–720, 1979
4. Brown Ra, Roberts TS, Osborn AG: Simplified CT-guided stereotaxic biopsy. *AJNR* 2:181–184, 1981
5. Colombo F, Angrilli F, Zanardo A, et al: A new method for utilizing CT data in stereotactic surgery: Measurement and transformation technique. *Acta Neurochir* (Wien) 57:195–203, 1981
6. Gildenberg PL, Kaufman HH, Krishna Murthy KS: Calculation of stereotactic coordinates, from the computed tomographic scan. *Neurosurgery* 10:580–586, 1982
7. Goerss S, Kelly PJ, Kall B, et al: A computed tomographic stereotactic adaptation system. *Neurosurgery* 10:375–379, 1982
8. Gouda KI, Freidberg SR, Larsen CR, et al: Modification of the Gouda frame to allow stereotactic biopsy of the brain using the GE 8800 computed tomographic scanner. *Neurosurgery* 13:176–181, 1983
9. Jacques S, Sheldon CH, McCann GD: A computerized microstereotactic method to approach, 3-dimensionally reconstruct, remove and adjuvantly treat small CNS lesions. *Appl Neurophysiol* 43:176–182, 1980
10. Kelly PJ, Alker GJ Jr, Goerss S: Computer-assisted stereotactic laser microsurgery for the treatment of intracranial neoplasms. *Neurosurgery* 10:324–331, 1981
11. Koslow M, Abele MG, Griffith RC, et al: Stereotactic surgical system controlled by computed tomography. *Neurosurgery* 8:72–82, 1981
12. Patil AA: Computed tomography (CT) oriented rotary stereotactic system: A technical note. *Acta Neurochir* (Wien) 68:19–26, 1983
13. Patil AA: Computed tomography-oriented steretoactic system. *Neurosurgery* 10:370–374, 1982
14. Patil AA: Computed tomography plane of the target approach in computed tomographic stereotaxis. *Neurosurgery* 15:410–414, 1984
15. Patil AA: Computed tomography stereotactic head clamp. *Acta Neurochir* (Wien), 60:125–129, 1982
16. Perry JH, Rosenbaum AE, Lunsford LD, et al: Computed tomography-guided stereotactic surgery: Conception and development of a new stereotactic methodology. *Neurosurgery* 7:376–381, 1980

II. MORPHOLOGICAL SURGERY: DIAGNOSIS AND TREATMENT

9. RELIABILITY OF STEREOTACTIC BRAIN TUMOR BIOPSY

Christoph B. Ostertag

Every decision regarding brain tumor therapy, especially radiotherapy, is based on knowing the precise histological type of the tumor. Even the most refined imaging techniques cannot provide a histological diagnosis. In recent years, stereotactic biopsy increasingly has been used to identify the nature of intracranial lesions. With the advancement of computed tomography (CT) and magnetic resonance imaging (MRI), very small tumors and other lesions (less than 5 mm in diameter) can be located precisely, and tissue samples can be obtained from sites inaccessible to open surgery. However, the size and number of stereotactic biopsy samples are limited and require a specialized histopathological approach.

This chapter reviews (1) the technical factors that influence the quality of stereotactic biopsy samples; (2) the processing of samples for cytological (smear) and histological examination; (3) the morphological basis for the interpretation of stereotactic biopsy samples; and (4) the diagnostic potential and the limitations of stereotactic brain tumor biopsies.

CT Stereotactic Biopsy with the Riechert Stereotactic System

CT scans provide a rough indication of the configuration and composition of a tumor. In addition, when the tumor is scanned, target coordinates for stereotactic biopsy can be obtained. To solve the problem of interfacing CT and stereotactic surgery, many different approaches have been proposed within recent years [6, 7, 12, 14, 15, 22–26, 30, 33, 34, 39, 41, 44, 46, 50, 52, 53, 55, 59].

Using standard CT and stereotactic equipment, CT stereotaxy takes advantage of the fact that most stereotactic devices use rectilinear coordinates for indexing. The Riechert stereotactic system (Neuromedix, Umkirch, W. Germany) is used at our institution [48, 49]. Ideally, the axes of the stereotactic frame coincide with the CT-gantry axes, which are represented by cross-hairs on the CT image. The accuracy of target coordinate determination depends on this geometry. In the image containing the target, X and Y coordinates are determined relative to the image cross-hairs and, hence, to the stereotactic frame. Table incrementation defines the Z coordinate, which corresponds to the longitudinal axis of the patient. (For a detailed description, see [6] and [39].) The precision of target coordinates generally is correlated to the image matrix. In the direction perpendicular to the CT image, usually referred to as the Z coordinate, variation is directly related to the thickness of the CT "slice." (The maximum error of Z is approximately equal to the slice thickness.) For the X and Y coordinates, the magnitude of error is related to the pixel size. The prerequisites for accurate target point determination are highly accurate table incrementation and scanner geometry (±0.5 mm). The tools used for the stereotactic intervention (biopsy probes, cannulas, forceps, etc.) are inaccurate by at least 0.5 mm because of their inherent lack of rigidity. Currently, precision greater than 0.5 mm seems impossible to achieve.

Sample Processing

The optimal pathway for serial biopsies usually is selected with computer-reformatted images, which define the shape and geometry of a lesion [17, 58]. Depending on the size and location of the lesion, two to ten tissue samples are

L.D. Lunsford (ed.) *MODERN STEREOTACTIC NEUROSURGERY*.

taken serially at 3- to 10-mm intervals along the puncture tract (hence the term *serial biopsy*). We use two different types of specially designed forceps with shafts 0.8 mm and 1.2 mm in diameter, respectively. The forceps are advanced through an outer cannula [47]. The mouth of the forceps holds tissue samples of approximately 1–4 mm^3 per biopsy site. The extremely small mouth tip yields very small samples, to which the neuropathologist must get accustomed. With this technique, small lesions can be biopsied without pushing or displacing normal anatomical structures, such as the hypothalamus. A smear diagnosis is made immediately by the neuropathologist [5, 21, 37, 40]. The biopsy material, usually three to six specimens, is placed on glass slides, gently spread, and slightly pressed and stained with Loeffler's methylene blue. Loeffler's methylene blue stain is a saturated alcohol solution of methylene blue (30 parts) and potassium hydroxide (1:10,000 aqueous solution, 100 parts). Specimens are stained routinely for two minutes. Microscopic examination of the tissue is performed in the operating room, after which the samples are photographed for documentation. The stereotactic sources of the tissue samples are marked on the slides, which then are embedded in paraffin and processed for routine microscopy. Plastic embedding (Araldite) is used for semithin sections and electron microscopy.

In all cases, the final neuropathological diagnosis is the result of two different diagnostic procedures: intraoperative cytological analysis of smear preparations and postoperative histological examination of the additional paraffin-embedded material. The smear preparations microscopically show features that are different from those of the paraffin preparations. (For detailed descriptions, see [1, 27–29, 43].) When tumors are defined and immediate local interstitial radiotherapy is planned, a therapeutic decision is made on the basis of the smear diagnosis, provided the diagnosis is unequivocal. If the diagnosis is uncertain, the center of the biopsy site is marked with a silver cap, and any therapeutic decision is postponed until the histological diagnosis is available. At our institution, the incidence of transient complications after stereotactic intervention is in the range of 3%, and the mortality is 1% or less (table 9–1).

Tumor Classification and Garding

We use the histological classification of central nervous system (CNS) tumors published by the World Health Organization (WHO) [61]. This scheme has proven to be very useful and

TABLE 9–1. Stereotactic Serial Biopsy: Complications

Author	Year Reported	No. of Cases	Complications (%)	Mortality (%)
Pecker et al. [45]	1979	25	8.0	0.0
Ostertag et al. [43]	1979	302	3.0	2.3
Bosch et al. [9]	1980	100	4.0	2.0
Edner [20]	1981	345	2.3	1.0
Sedan et al. [57]	1981	770	1.4	1.0
Colombo et al. [16]	1982	125	1.6	0.0
Mundinger [41]	1982	582	3.0	1.4
De Divitiis et al. [19]	1983	64	0.0	0.0
Broggi et al. [10]	1984	200	3.0	1.0
Sedan et al. [56]	1984	318	4.5	0.6
Willems et al. [60]	1984	128	0.0	0.0
Apuzzo et al. [3]	1984	100	2.0	0.0
Sceratti et al. [54]	1984	68	2.9	1.4
Kelly et al. [30]	1984	86	0.0	0.0
Coffey and Lunsford [14]*	1985	13	0.0	0.0

* Brain-stem cases only.

has standardized considerably the terminology of CNS tumors. A unified terminology is particularly important when results of various therapeutic measures are compared in multicenter studies. We have adopted the grading system proposed in the WHO classification, becuase the tumor biology as estimated by grading is important in the selection of surgery and adjuvant radiation and/or chemotherapy.

In recent years, considerable progress has been made in the use of immunohistochemical techniques to localize cell and tumor markers [8, 36, 51]. In the nervous system, the presence of glial fibrillary acidic protein (GFAP) has been used to estimate the extent of glial differentiation and to distinguish differentiated gliomas from intracranial nonglial and metastatic tumors [18]. The significance of detecting GFAP in gliomas is, however, severely reduced by the presence of this protein in both reactive and neoplastic astrocytes. In addition, GFAP-positive neoplastic glial cells may possess surface antigens, which can be detected immunohistochemically by monoclonal antibodies [11]. Specific markers have been developed for anaplastic gliomas [13]. Identification of sarcomas and metastatic carcinomas has become possible by the use of monoclonal antibodies to their cytoskeleton proteins [42]. Determination of the replicating cell fraction with an antibody that reacts with a nuclear protein expressed in the G_1, G_2, S_5 and M phases of the cell cycle could become an additional criterion for predicting the biologic behavior of nervous system neoplasms [12]. Future advances in immunohistochemical detection of specific marker proteins will reduce greatly the limitations imposed by the small samples obtained by stereotactic brain tumor biopsies.

Diagnostic Potential and Validity of Stereotactic Brain Tumor Biopsies

From the clinical point of view, is stereotactic biopsy a reliable method? The results of large published series (several hundred cases) indicate that stereotactic biopsy gives pathological information as reliable as that achieved by specimens obtained at craniotomy. This diagnostic potential is illustrated by data derived from a combined series of 1,236 consecutive stereotactic biospy cases performed by the departments of stereotactic neurosurgery at the Universities of Freiburg and Homburg/Saar [2]. This study, which updates previous reports [31, 32, 43] is a retrospective analysis based on autopsy cases, specimens from craniotomies, and, in the majority of cases, patient follow-up studies. The majority of biopsies were taken from supratentorial lesions. Most were in the cerebral hemispheres (52.5%), with a marked predilection for functionally important areas, such as the central region and the speech areas. Lesions were located close to midline structures, such as the basal ganglia in 16.8% of cases, the hypothalamus in 8.2%, the midbrain-pineal region in 9.6% and the pons medulla in 5.4%. Rarely encountered were intraventricular tumors and extracerebral lesions at the base of the skull. There was a distinct prevalence of neuroepithelial tumors (50%), particularly pilocytic (11.3%) and grade II astrocytomas (22.8%); these occurred approximately three times more frequently than in a comparable series of patients treated by open surgery [31]. We noted a relatively high incidence of pineal germinomas (2.5%), whereas meningiomas were rare (1.4%). No cases of neurinomas were diagnosed, as these lesions occured in easily accessible extracranial locations.

Validity of Stereotactic Brain Tumor Biopsies

After combined cytological and histological examination, a definitive tumor diagnosis (including tumor type and approximate grade) was made in 1,008 (81.5%) of 1,236 cases (table 9–2). In 164 cases (13.3%), a clinically suspected neoplastic lesion was excluded by the combination of both procedures. In 41 cases (3.3%), a glioma was diagnosed, but precise grading was not possible. In 23 cases (1.9%), the presence of a tumor was confirmed, but tissue samples were insufficient for histopathological classification.

TABLE 9–2. Results of Stereotactic Serial Tumor Biopsies in 1,236 Cases

Histological Classification	% Cases
Tumor + tumor type + appropoximate grading	81.5
Clinically suspected tumor excluded	13.3
Glioma, no grading possible	3.3
Unclassified tumor	1.9

TABLE 9–3. Accuracy of Stereotactic Diagnosis in 87 Cases

Methods of Assessment	Diagnostic Confirmation	Radiation Necrosis	Diagnostic Discrepancy
Subsequent open surgery	20	1	4[a]
Additional open surgery for recurrent tumor	7	1	2[b]
Additional stereotactic biopsy for recurrent tumor	23	5	3[c]
Autopsy	17	2	2[d]

[a] Necrotic tissue/anaplastic ependymoma; astrocytoma II/astrocytoma III–IV; gliosis, no tumor/craniopharyngioma; oligodendroglioma II/astrocytoma II.
[b] Necrotic tissue/astrocytoma III–IV; astrocytoma II/astrocytoma III–IV.
[c] Necrotic tissue/astrocytoma III; astrocytoma II/astrocytoma III; germinoma/gliosis (first diagnosis was correct).
[d] Pilocytic astrocytoma/cystic necrosis with reactive gliosis and Rosenthal fibers (old hemorrhage); astrocytoma III/metastatic hemangiosarcoma.

Data verified by pathological examination after craniotomy or by autopsy (87 cases) are summarized in table 9–3. In 67 cases, stereotactic diagnoses were confirmed by subsequent craniotomies and resections, by additional biopsies of recurrent tumors, or by autopsies. In nine cases, radiation necrosis was found after interstitial radiotherapy of previously diagnosed neoplastic lesions. Diagnostic discrepancies were found in 11 cases; five were obviously a result of sampling errors, that is, the initial or subsequent stereotactic biopsy had shown only gliosis or necrotic tissue. In three cases, the clinical follow-up revealed a tumor with a higher grade of malignancy; whether this was caused by a sampling error or tumor progression with increasing dedifferentiation and anaplasia is unknown. In three cases, the discrepancy proved to be the result of diagnostic error, mainly because the sample was so small.

To evalute the relative importance of cytological analysis, the diagnoses obtained from smear preparations were correlated with the diagnoses reported with paraffin-embedded sections (table 9–4). The initial cytological diagnosis was confirmed by subsequent histological (paraffin-section) examination of additional samples in 962 cases (77%). The cytological diagnosis was modified in 128 cases (10.5%), of which discrepancies were related to tumor type or grading in 9%. A diagnostic error in smear preparations concerning the presence of tumor tissue occurred in 20 cases (1.6%). In 146 cases (11.8%), histological verification by a single procedure was not possible. This was predominantly because of sampling errors: the biopsy material of one of the two methods employed contained only a border zone of the lesion or consisted of only necrotic or hemorrhagic areas. In these cases, the final diagnosis was usually based on the intraoperative smear preparation.

TABLE 9–4. Correlation of Diagnoses Obtained from Smear Preparations and Paraffin Sections in 1,236 Cases[a]

Confirmation of smear diagnosis by paraffin section diagnosis	
Tumor type and grade confirmed	60.0
Absence of tumor confirmed	10.0
Tumor type confirmed	4.5
Tumor presence confirmed	2.5
Total	77.0
Discrepancy between smear diagnosis and paraffin section diagnosis	
Tumor type discrepancy	5.0
Tumor grade discrepancy	4.0
Tumor presence discrepancy	1.5
Total	10.5
No confirmation by either smear or paraffin section[c]	12.5

[a] From the Universities of Freiburg and Homburg/Saar [2]. Values are given as percentage of cases.
[b] Final diagnosis obtained from smear in 11.5% and from paraffin section in 1.0%.

To achieve a rapid intraoperative diagnosis, supravital staining techniques have been used since 1930 [21]. An alternative to the smear technique is the frozen section technique, which is the most widely used means of obtaining a rapid surgical diagnosis. Large firm pieces of tissue are required for this method, which makes it rather unsuitable for serial stereotactic biopsies. The principal advantages of the smear technique are its technical simplicity, the ease with which multiple tiny tissue probes can be examined, and the distinct cyto-

TABLE 9–5. Stereotactic Serial Biopsy: Overall Diagnostic Accuracy Rate (Cytological Diagnosis and Paraffin Sections)

Author	Year Reported	No. of Cases	Accuracy (%)
Edner [20]	1981	345	91
Colombo et al. [16]	1982	125	70
De Divitiis et al. [19]	1983	64	92
Willems et al. [60]	1984	112	87
Monsaingeon et al. [38]	1984	207	77
Sedan et al. [56]	1984	309	91
Kleihues et al. [32]	1984	600	93
Anagnostopoulos [2]	1986	1,236	95

logical appearance of most tumor entities [35]. The information instantly available from intraoperative smear proparations guides the tissue sampling for paraffin-embedded sections. The final pathological diagnosis results from an analysis of patient data (age, duration of symptoms, lesion location), radiographic findings (CT, MRI, ventriculography, and angiography), intraoperative findings (whether the tumor is cystic, necrotic, solid, calcified, or vital), and the histological examination. Depending on the physiciun's experience, the overall rate of obtaining an accurate diagnosis by stereotactic technique exceeds 90% (table 9–5).

Diagnostic Problems and Limitations

Sample size remains a potential problem in stereotactic biopsy of intracranial neoplasms. The sample volume of 1 mm^3 proved to be sufficient for diagnostic evaluation of tumors that have a homogeneous tissue architecture (pilocytic astrocytomas, grade II astrocytomas, oligodendrogliomas). However, the samll sample size can cause diagnostic errors in tumors with various tissue components (e.g., anaplastic gliomas, craniopharyngiomas, teratoid and metastatic tumors). In cases of large hemispheric gliomas, a larger biopsy sample can be obtained with larger forceps or with other devices, such as the biopsy needles designed by Backlund [4] or Sedan [56].

However, in functionally important deep-seated structures (basal ganglia, hypothalamus, brain stem), the removal of larger samples carries the risk of postoperative neurological deficits. The disadvantages of the small sample size can best be compensated by careful targeting of the biopsy site. To that end, the combination of rapid smear preparations with tissue embedding has proven valuable. Smear preparations often enable the immediate recognition of tumor borders and thus can be used to guide the removal of samples for subsequent paraffin or plastic embedding. We believe that the neuropathologist must be present during the operation.

The distinction between reactive gliosis and the infiltration zone of gliomas presents another difficulty that is not unique to stereotactic samples. The careful estimation of tumor borders is of great importance in calculating tumor volume when interstitial radiotherapy is planned. At present, no reliable morphological criteria can distinguish reactive astrocytes from neoplastic cells in the periphery of a differentiated astrocytoma.

Conclusions

CT-guided stereotactic serial biopsy is an acceptably safe and accurate procedure that avoids major brain trauma. It offers a logical alternative to craniotomies for lesions of neoplastic, developmental, or infectious origin. The primary objective of stereotactic biopsy is to achieve a morphological, as opposed to a radiographic, diagnosis.

With the use of intraoperative smear preparations and routine stains after paraffin embedding, a correct diagnosis is obtained in more than 90% of cases. Errors result from failures to distinguish between infiltrative gliomas and reactive gliosis, from inappropriate grading of inhomogeneously composed tumors, and from sampling errors. Future advances in immunohistochemical staining techniques will further facilitate accurate tumor diagnoses by reducing the impact of small sample size obtained by stereotactic technique.

References

1. Adams JH, Graham DI, Doyle D: *Brain Biopsy: The Smear Technique for Neurosurgical Biopsies*. London: Chapman and Hall, 1981
2. Anagnostopoulos J, Kiessling M, Detmar M, et al: Stereotactic brain tumor biopsy—neuropathological aspects. *Cancer Campaign*, Vol 10. Stuttgart-New York: G Fischer, 1986, (In press)
3. Apuzzo MLJ, Zelman V, Jepson J, et al: Observations with the utilization of the Brown-Roberts-Wells stereotactic system in the management of intracranial mass lesions. *Acta Neurochir [Suppl]* (Wien) 33:261–263, 1984
4. Backlund EO: A new instrument for stereotaxic brain tumor biopsy. *Acta Chir Scand* 137:825–827, 1971
5. Badt B: Mikroskopische Schnelldiagnose bei hirn-chirurgischen Eingriffen. Zentralbl Neurochir 2:123–139, 1937
6. Birg W, Mundinger F: Direct target point determination for stereotactic brain operations from CT data and the calculation of setting parameters for polar-coordinate stereotactic devices. *Appl Neurophysiol* 45:387–395, 1982
7. Böethius J, Bergström M, Greitz T: Stereotaxic computerized tomography with a GE 8800 scanner. *J Neurosurg* 52:794–800, 1980
8. Bonnin JM, Rubinstein LJ: Immunohistochemistry of central nervous system tumors. *J Neurosurg* 60:1121–1133, 1984
9. Bosch DA: Indications for stereotactic biopsy in brain tumors. *Acta Neurochir* (Wien) 54:167–179, 1980
10. Broggi G, Franzini A, Giorgi C, et al: Diagnostic accuracy and multimodal approach in stereotactic biopsies of deep brain tumors. *Acta Neurochir [Suppl]* (Wien) 33:211–212, 1984
11. Bullard DE, Bigner DD: Applications of monoclonal antibodies in the diagnosis and treatment of primary brain tumors. *J Neurosurg* 63:2–16, 1985
12. Burger PC, Shibata T, Kleihues P: The use of the monoclonal antibody Ki-67 in the identification of proliferating cells: Application to surgical neuropathology. *Am J Surg Pathol*, 1986, 10:611–617, 1986.
13. Carrel S, de Tribolet N, Mach JP: Expression of neuroectodermal antigens common to melanomas, gliomas and neuroblastomas. *Acta Neuropathol* (Berl) 57:158–164, 1982
14. Coffey RJ, Lunsford LD: Stereotactic surgery for mass lesions of the midbrain and pons. *Neurosurgery* 17:12–18, 1985
15. Cohadon F, Caille JM, Constant P, et al: Tomodensitometry under stereotaxic conditions. In Bories J (ed): *The Diagnostic Limitations of Computerized Axial Tomography*. Heidelberg, New York, Berlin: Springer, 1978
16. Colombo F, Casentini L, Visona A, et al: Stereotactic biopsy-diagnostic problems: Value of cytological and histological examinations. *Zentralbl Neurochir* 43:309–316, 1982
17. Daumas-Duport C, Monsaingeon V, N'Guyen JP, et al: Some correlations between histological and CT aspects of cerebral gliomas contributing to the choice of significant trajectories for stereotactic biopsies. *Acta Neurochir [Suppl]* (Wien) 33:185–194, 1984
18. Deck JHN, Eng LF, Bigbee J, et al: The role of glial fibrillary acidic protein in the diagnosis of central nervous system tumors. *Acta Neuropathol* (Berl) 42:183–190, 1978
19. De Divitiis E, Spaziante R, Cappabianca P, et al: Reliability of stereotactic biopsy: A model to test the value of diagnoses obtained from small fragments of nervous system tumors. *Appl Neurophysiol* 46:295–303, 1983
20. Edner G: Stereotactic biopsy of intracranial space-occupying lesions. *Acta Neurochir* (Wien) 57:213–234, 1981
21. Eisenhardt L, Cushing H: Diagnosis of intracranial tumors by supravital technique. *Am J Pathol* 6:541–552, 1930
22. Galanda M, Nadvornik P, Sramka M, et al: Stereotactic biopsy of brain stem tumors. *Acta Neurochir [Suppl]* (Wien) 33:213–217, 1984
23. Gildenberg PL, Kaufman HH, Murthy KSK: Calculation of stereotactic coordinates from the computed tomography scan. *Neurosurgery* 10:580–586, 1982
24. Goerss S, Kelly PJ, Kall B, et al: A computed tomographic stereotactic adaptation system. *Neurosurgery* 10:375–379, 1982
25. Huk W, Baer U: A new targeting device for stereotaxic procedures within the CT scanner. *Neuroradiology* 19:13–17, 1980
26. Jacques S, Sheldon CH, McCann GD, et al: Computerized three-dimensional stereotaxic removal of small central nervous system lesions in patients. *J Neurosurg* 53:816–820, 1980
27. Jane JA, Bertrand G: A cytological method for the diagnosis of tumors affecting the central nervous system. *J Neuropathol Exp Neurol* 21:400–409, 1962
28. Jane JA, Yashon D: Cytology of Tumors Affecting the Nervous System. Springfield, IL: Thomas, 1969

29. Kautzky R: Die Schnelldiagnose intracranieller Erkrankungen mit Hilfs des supravital gefarbten Quetschpräparats. *Virchows Arch* [A] 320:495–550, 1951
30. Kelly PJ, Kall BA, Goerss SG: Computer-assisted stereotactic biopsies utilizing CT and digitized arteriographic control. *Acta Neurochir* [*Suppl*] (Wien) 33:233–235, 1984
31. Kiessling M, Anagnostopoulos J, Lombeck G, et al: Diagnostic potential of stereotactic biopsy of brain tumors. A report of 400 cases. In Voth D, Gutjahr P, Langmaid C (eds): *Tumours of the Central Nervous System in Infancy and Childhood*. Berlin, Heidelberg: Springer-Verlag, 1982, pp 247–256
32. Kleihues P, Volk B, Anagnostopoulos J, et al: Morphologic evaluation of stereotactic brain tumor biopsies. *Acta Neurochir* [*Suppl*] (Wien) 33:171–181, 1984
33. Koslow M, Abele MG, Griffith RC, et al: Stereotactic surgical system controlled by computed tomography. *Neurosurgery* 8:72–82, 1981
34. Lewander R, Bergstrom M, Boethius V, et al: Stereotactic computer tomography for biopsy of gliomas. *Acta Radiol* [*Diagn*] (Stockh) 19:867–888, 1978
35. Marshall LF, Adams H, Doyle D, et al: The histological accuracy of the smear technique for neurosurgical biopsies. *J Neurosurg* 39:82–88, 1973
36. McComb RD, Bigner DD: The biology of malignant gliomas—a comprehensive survey. *Clin Neuropathol* 3:93–106, 1984
37. McMenemey WH: An appraisal of smear-diagnosis in neurosurgery. *Am J Clin Pathol* 33:471–479, 1960
38. Monsaingeon V, Daumas-Duport C, Mann M, et al: Stereotactic sampling biopsies in a series of 268 consecutive cases—validity and technical aspects. *Acta Neurochir* [*Suppl*] (Wien) 33:195–200, 1984
39. Moringlane JR, Ostertag CB: La definition spatiale d'une tumeur cerebrale. *Rev Electroencephalogr Neurophysiol Clin*, 17:45–53, 1987.
40. Morris AA: the use of the smear technique in the rapid histological diagnosis of tumors of the central nervous system: Description of a new staining method. *J. Neurosurg* 4:497–504, 1947
41. Mundinger F: CT-stereotactic biopsy of brain tumors. In Voth D, Gutjahr P, Langmaid C, (eds): *Tumors of the Central Nervous System in Infancy and Childhood*. Berlin, Heidelberg: Springer-Verlag, 1982, pp 234–246
42. Osborn M, Weber K: Biology of disease. Tumor diagnosis by intermediate filament typing: A novel tool for surgical pathology. *Lab Invest* 48:372–394, 1983
43. Ostertag CB, Mennel HD, Kiessling M: Stereotactic biopsy of brain tumors. *Surg Neurol* 14:275–283, 1980
44. Patil AA: Computed tomography-oriented stereotactic system. *Neurosurgery* 10:370–374, 1982
45. Pecker J, Scarabin JM, Vallee B, et al: Treatment of tumours of the pineal region: Value of stereotaxic biopsy. *Surg Neurol* 12:341–348, 1979
46. Perry JH, Rosenbaum AE, Lunsford LD, et al: Computed tomography-guided stereotactic surgery: Conception and development of a new stereotactic methodology. *Neurosurgery* 7:376–381, 1980
47. Riechert T, Giesinger MA, Mölbert E: Biopsien während stereotaktischer Operationen beim Parkinson-Syndrom. *Neurochirurgia* (Stuttg) 10:106–110, 1967
48. Riechert T, Wolff M: Die technische Durchführung von gezielten Hirnoperationen. *Arch Psychiatry*. 190:297–316, 1953
49. Riechert T, Wolff M: Ober ein neues Zielgerät zur intrakraniellen elektrischen Ableitung und Ausschaltung. *Arch Psychiatry* 186:225–230, 1951
50. Roberts TS, Brown R: Technical and clinical aspects of CT-directed stereotaxis. *Appl Neurophysiol* 43:171–179, 1980
51. Roessmann U, Velasco ME, Gambetti P, et al: Neuronal and astrocytic differentiation in human neuroepithelial neoplasms: An immunohistochemical study. *J Neuropathol Exp Neurol* 42:113–121, 1983
52. Rushworth RG: Stereotactic-guided biopsy in the computerized tomographic scanner. *Surg Neurol* 14:451–454, 1980
53. Scarabin JM, Pecker J, Brucher JM, et al: Stereotaxic exploration in 200 supratentorial brain tumors: Its value in addition to computerized tomography. *Neuroradiology* 16:591, 1978
54. Sceratti M, Rossi GF: The reliability of stereotactic biopsy. *Acta Neurochir* [*Suppl*] (Wien) 33:201–205, 1984
55. Schlegel W, Scharfenberg H, Sturm V, et al: Direct visualization of intracranial tumors in stereotactic and angiographic films by computer calculation of longitudinal CT sections: A new method for stereotactic localization of tumor outlines. *Acta Neurochir* (Wien) 58:25–27, 1981
56. Sedan R, Peragut JC, Farnarier P, et al: Intraencephalic stereotactic biopsies (309 patients/318 biopsies). *Acta Neurochir* [*Suppl*] (Wien) 33: 207–210, 1984
57. Sedan R, Peragut JC, Farnarier P, et al: Place de la biopsie en condition stereotaxique dans la tactique therapeutique des gliomes malins. *Neurochirurgie* 27:285–286, 1981
58. Unsold R, Ostertag CB, DeGroot J, et al: *Computer Reformations of the Brain and Skull Base*:

Anatomy and Clinical Application. Berlin, Heidelberg, New York: Springer-Verlag, 1982
59. Wester K, Sortland O, Hauglie-Hanssen E: A simple and inexpensive method for CT-guided stereotaxy. *Neuroradiology* 20:255–256, 1981
60. Willems JGMS, Alva-Willems JM: Accuracy of cytologic diagnosis of central nervous system neoplasms in stereotactic biopsies. *Acta Cytol* (Baltimore) 28:243–248, 1984
61. Zulch KJ: *Histological Typing of Tumours of the Central Nervous System*. Geneva: World Health Organization, 1979

10. BIOPSY TECHNIQUES USING THE BROWN-ROBERTS WELLS (BRW) STEREOTACTIC GUIDANCE SYSTEM

M. Peter Heilbrun

Neurosurgeons have been using stereotactic techniques to localize tumors for more than 20 years. Stereotactic systems such as the Talairach frame refined the technique by combining data from angiography and ventriculography. These systems defined tumor location by relating the position of midline brain structures to the position/displacement of major vessels [12, 20, 24].

By 1979, as computerized tomography (CT) scanning revolutionized imaging, compatible stereotactic methods were developed, which could define tumor location by directly transforming two-dimensional CT-image data into three-dimensional stereotactic coordinates [1–4, 6–9, 11, 14–16, 19, 21, 22]. With the improved resolution of magnetic resonance imaging (MRI), stereotactic systems have been adapted to transform MRI data into stereotactic coordinates [9]. The accuracy of CT-guided stereotaxy in defining tumor position for tissue specimens has been widely reported [10, 18, 23]. Stereotactic guidance is the method of choice in the biopsy of small, deep brain lesions [12, 13]. In addition, stereotactic approaches through relatively small skull openings appear to reduce the morbidity associated with the larger craniotomies necessitated by freehand approaches [1, 5, 13]. Stereotactic localization also provides important information about vascular structures so that the surgeon can select approaches that avoid these structures. This technique also permits more precise management of arteriovenous malformations (AVM). Surgical planning for many lesions, regardless of size and depth, benefits from information provided by stereotactic localization [5, 17].

This chapter describes our experience over a five-year period utilizing the Brown-Roberts-Wells (BRW) CT stereotactic guidance systems for applications ranging from a technique of biopsy alone to a localization system enhanced by a wide spectrum of neurosurgical instruments.

Overview of System

The BRW guidance system is described in chapter 5. A unique feature of this system is the independence of its reference plane for the transformation from two to three dimensions. This reference plane is a head ring which is fixed only to the patient's head. No portion of the BRW stereotactic frame attaches to the CT scanner table or gantry. As long as the CT image contains the target lesion along with the images of the nine localizing rods, a hand-held calculator or microcomputer can easily transform the two-dimensional CT-scan data set into the three-dimensional BRW stereotactic coordinate set. Because all patients undergoing stereotactic biopsy have already had a diagnostic CT scan, only 10 to 15 minutes of additional scanner time is required to collect the frame-image data prior to the surgical procedure. Thus, patient discomfort is minimized because rigid fixation to the table is unnecessary, and valuable scanner time is saved. Reduced scanner dependency is important if stereotaxy is to be performed in a hospital with a fully scheduled scanner. The actual surgery is performed in the operating room.

University of Utah Medical Center Experience

From 1979 through 1985 196 stereotactic localization procedures were performed at the University of Utah Medical Center and its affiliated hospitals. By 1984, the majority of surgery for intra-axial brain lesions was performed with stereotactic localization. Moreover, interstitial brachytherapy has accounted for an increasing number of stereotactic procedures over the past two years.

The majority of lesions were tumors; the remainder were infectious, vascular, or degenerative lesions. Lesions were categorized as nondiagnostic when microscopic examination revealed that the tissue was either normal or otherwise unclassifiable, yet the target point of the biopsy was confirmed by postoperative CT. Seven of the 196 cases were classified as nondiagnostic.

Actual false-negative biopsies occurred in an additional seven cases, primarily in lesions that were relatively rigid compared to the normal brain. This disparity occasionally resulted in displacement of the target point by blunt-ended biopsy instruments; the biopsy then excised normal brain tissue that had been moved into the stereotactically defined target. We have learned to minimize this possibility by slightly enlarging the probe track so that the border between normal tissue and the lesion is exposed, after which biopsy tissue is obtained using direct visualization. In our first 100 cases, five biopsies were false-negative. In the following 96 cases, two false-negative biopsies and one false-positive biopsy were obtained. All were related to displacement of the lesion.

Serious complications in the first 100 cases included two deaths, both related to postbiopsy brain swelling associated with malignant tumors. Hemorrhage into the lesion was ruled out in both cases. Moderate morbidity (hemiparesis) occurred in one case when a clot evacuation followed by biopsy of the wall resulted in hemorrhage from an arteriovenous malformation (AVM). Preoperative angiography did not show an AVM, but postoperative angiography enhanced by electronic subtraction and reversal techniques demonstrated a small AVM in the anterior wall of the clot cavity. One patient had an infection. In the subsequent 96 cases, no mortality or serious neurological sequelae occurred; one patient developed aseptic meningitis following a radiation implant.

General Considerations

Once the neurosurgeon decides upon stereotactic localization, several strategies are available: a procedure of closed biopsy alone with either twistdrill or perforator openings, or open biopsy followed by partial or complete resection through a small-to-moderate-sized craniotomy or craniectomy.

Choosing an approach depends on several factors in addition to the location and size of the lesion. The most obvious of these are the structure and apparent cause of the lesion, that is, whether the lesion appears to be circumscribed with a border or infiltrating without demarcation; whether it appears to be heterogeneous with cystic components, enhancing borders, and surrounding edema as with glioblastoma; whether it seems to be homogeneous and of low density or homogeneous and of high density, (e.g., a highly vascular lesion such as a metastatic tumor or a vascular angioma); whether there may be an associated mass effect on the surrounding brain with midline shifts, transtentorial herniation, or ventricular enlargement; and whether the lesion appears to be resectable. Under our protocol, all intra-axial lesions, with the exception of large life-threatening hematomas, are managed with stereotactic localization.

Stereotactic Techniques Using the BRW System

BIOPSY ALONE

The minority of lesions, those judged unresectable because of location, size, or appearance of infiltrative characteristics, are usually considered for biopsy alone, provided that there are no characteristics indicating that hemorrhage might be a problem and there is no significant mass effect suggesting that decompression should be considered. These cases are usually performed under local anesthesia with either a twist-drill or perforator opening.

SMALL CRANIOTOMY

In our experience the majority of patients have lesions that can be potentially resected partially or completely. These lesions are approached through a small craniotomy.

ANTICIPATING HEMORRHAGE

Lesions with a heterogeneous appearance on the CT scan, particularly those with cystic components and enhancing borders, carry a significant risk of hemorrhage. A biopsy performed by targeting the central area of the lesion in an attempt to minimize hemorrhage will often yield necrotic tissue or fluid that will be nondiagnostic even with cytology. To reach an appropriate tissue diagnosis, biopsies of these lesions must include samples of the enhancing border, thus increasing the risk of hemorrhage. The neurosurgeon must be prepared to open the biopsy instrument track to control the bleeding under direct vision in the event that it cannot be controlled with gentle irrigation through the biopsy cannula. Although this more extensive procedure can be done with the patient under local anesthesia, general anesthesia provides time-saving flexibility in the event of hemorrhage.

AVOIDING DISPLACEMENT

Of particular note are lesions that are small, that appear on CT scan to be so firm that they might be displaced by standard biopsy instrumentation, or that lie within or protrude into the ventricular system. These are best handled with a small craniotomy and a modified open approach.

Localization Procedure Using the BRW System

After standard premedication is administered, the patient is transported to a room adjacent to the CT scanner. Both the induction room and the CT scanner suite contain appropriate oxygen, suction, and resuscitation equipment. If general anesthesia will be used for the procedure, the patient must be intubated before the head ring is placed, because the head ring is positioned at nose level to avoid artifact on the scan. Once positioned, the head ring is fixed to the skull by tightening its four stainless steel pins with a standard hex wrench.

Due to the geometry of the BRW system, the head ring does not have to be fixed with exact symmetry; it can be higher either posteriorly or anteriorly or on either side. Thus, the surgeon is free to approach a lateral lesion in a plane parallel to the CT scan image.

Once the head-ring component is fixed, the picket-fence localizer is attached to it, and the patient is positioned centrally in the scanner gantry to ensure that the scan image contains all nine localizing rods. If the scan image containing the target contains artifact from any of the stainless steel fixation pins, the scanner gantry is tilted just enough to eliminate the artifact without affecting the position of the lesion (usually close to the fulcrum of the gantry's tilt).

When the scan is completed, the patient is transported to the operating room, moved to the operating table, and positioned with either the floor stand or the standard Mayfield head-ring adapter. The scalp then is prepared for surgery.

While the patient is moved and prepped, the neurosurgeon reviews the localizing scan. Utilizing the feature of CT scanners that identifies the X and Y coordinates of any pixel, the X and Y coordinates of each of the nine localizing-rod images and any desired number of targets are recorded. This can be done with any scan slice; we generally choose one or two different targets on up to three slices. These data sets then are taken to the operating room.

We enter the data sets into the standard programs of the Epson HX 20 microcomputer, which calculates three-dimensional anteroposterior (AP), lateral (LAT), and vertical (VERT) BRW stereotactic target coordinates. Next, we determine an entry point on the scalp or skull that will provide a safe trajectory to the target. If the target is deep, we choose points on the skull used for standard approaches to the anterior or posterior part of the ventricular system, that is, a coronal or parietooccipital position in a paramedian plane about 2 cm from the midline. These positions are termed *standard* because they traverse relatively silent areas of the cortex through watershed zones away from proximal branches of major vessels.

Determining the stereotactic coordinates of the entry point is simple. We place the BRW arc on the patient's head ring and position a probe at a selected entry point on the skull. AP, LAT, and VERT coordinates are read from the vernier scales and recorded. The appropriate program on the computer is chosen, and the entry-point coordinates are entered. From this information, the computer calculates the four settings for the BRW arc and the distance from a reference point on the arc to the target. Alternatively, the entry point can be chosen from a CT scan image that displays the vertex region of the skull. On this image, a target on the bone can be selected for the entry point, be transformed into a three-dimensional coordinate, and then entered into the computer program. Both of these techniques can be used to derive the BRW coordinates of a known burr hole if the neurosurgeon decides that it would be advantageous to use a prior skull opening for an entry point.

The BRW system can also identify the most efficient probe trajectory to the target within a specific quadrant of the skull. This feature is practical if the target is on or close to the surface of the brain; it eliminates the possibility of choosing an entry point that would result in an inefficient oblique probe trajectory to the target. For example, to obtain frame settings for a lesion in the high right frontal area, the neurosurgeon simply enters into the computer settings that place the arc and the radial slide in the approximate right frontal region. The computer then determines exact arc settings and the shortest path in that quadrant from the probe to the target. This probe track will generally be perpendicular to the target.

Once the arc settings are established by the computer, the accuracy of the computations can be confirmed on the phantom, which allows visualization of the computer targets. Although the phantom is not fundamentally necessary to the procedure, it does provide a reassuring safety check. The concept of using a phantom was developed after our experience with the first BRW prototype. We found that a phantom check significantly increased our confidence in the computed target approach.

Finally, after the scalp has been properly prepared and draped, the arc system is reattached to the head ring. Of the various draping systems available, we prefer a large plastic opaque drape that allows us to isolate but still see the whole head up to the level of the head ring. When the sterilized arc system is attached to the unsterile head ring, any break in the sterile field can be covered easily with a small adhesive plastic drape.

Closed Biopsy Through a Twist-Drill or Perforator Opening

OPENING THE SKULL

The neurosurgeon now is ready to make a scalp incision and skull opening. In the case of a low-density homogeneous lesion with little risk of hemorrhage, a twist-drill opening is appropriate. With the arc in place, standard fittings are utilized. We generally use a 1/4-inch drill bit for the twist-drill opening, because this size opening allows us to see and open the dura and the cortex before advancing the biopsy instrument. Alternatively, a standard perforator opening can be made. The arc system can be pivoted or rotated to the side without breaking sterility. Once the perforator opening is completed and the dura and the cortex opened, the arc is moved back to the appropriate position.

BIOPSY PROCEDURE

We have found two types of instruments to be most useful. The first is a Nashold side-cutting instrument, which provides a core of tissue 10 mm in length and 2 mm in diameter. If we cannot obtain satisfactory tissue for diagnosis with this instrument, we use a 2-mm cup forceps: we place a cannula containing an obturator within a few millimeters proximal to the target site, remove the obturator, and then extract tissue specimens with the cup forceps, which fit through the cannula.

Using both systems, we can obtain tissue at various points along the probe track. In some cases, multiple sampling is important in defining lesion borders.

If bleeding occurs after the biopsy, it is usually seen as a backflow of blood through the cannula of both instruments. A slow flow of blood usually can be controlled with gentle irrigation through the cannula. However, if the bleeding does not stop quickly with irrigation, the twist-drill opening must be enlarged to a small craniotomy to allow direct control.

ULTRASOUND ADAPTATION

In an attempt to develop a real-time monitor, which might aid in the recognition of significant hemorrhage, we placed a second slide onto the BRW arc and attached an ultrasound probe, which fits into a standard perforator opening. An ultrasound probe placed directly on the arc automatically sets the ultrasound-image plane in the plane of the probe trajectory that contains the target. Although this orientation is different than that of the scan plane, it offers an advantage: as the probe travels to the target, one can see changes occur in cyst size as fluid is removed and can monitor potential hemorrhage. To date, this system has been used infrequently because of the poor resolution of compatible ultrasound probes.

Open Biopsy and Resection Through a Small Craniotomy

We generally use a small craniotomy for the skull opening because of the potential for hemorrhage from heterogeneous lesions. The localization technique is the same as for twist-drill openings. Once the central point for the craniotomy is established stereotactically, the arc system can be pivoted away or removed during the craniotomy and then replaced.

At this point, all of the alternatives for operative neurosurgical manipulation are available. First we obtain a biopsy specimen from the target lesion. If we decide to inspect the biopsy area with an endoscope, we use a small cannula with an obturator large enough to accommodate an endoscope 7.5 mm in diameter. Our initial probe track is gradually dilated to the appropriate diameter with soft probes before the endoscope is placed. Dilatation must be extremely gentle; otherwise the brain may be displaced and a false-negative biopsy obtained. Although in low-grade astrocytomas the transition from normal brain to tumor is not visible, the endoscope is useful in higher grade astrocytomas, particularly those with cysts. In such cases, biopsies can be obtained under direct vision, and bleeding generally can be controlled with direct cauterization. In addition, either the argon or neodymium YAG laser can be directed through a fiber-optic cable passed through the endoscope.

If the opening to the lesion is to be larger than 7.5 mm, we prefer to make a cortical incision and to use standard retractor blades rather than a cylindrical cannula, because the blades provide better exposure and seem to result in less brain distortion. All standard retractor blades are attached easily to either the head ring, arc, or special posts that fit into the system. After the lesion is exposed, the tumor can be resected by standard methods.

Recently, we have built special adaptors to attach the operating microscope to the arc if magnification is necessary. In addition, we are trying CO_2 laser tumor resection, utilizing a Sharplan microscan attachment for manual definition of the tumor border and the area of resection. We have also developed a computer software system that emulates the physician's console of the Siemens Somatome CT scanner. We currently utilize this system to redefine tumor borders orthogonal to an identified probe tract and to place parallel catheters and radiation sources for interstitial brachytherapy. This software system should enable neurosurgeons to automatically resect tumors layer by layer along the probe track in a manner similar to that described by Kelly [11, 13].

Case Reports

CASE 1

A 39-year-old woman presented with a two-month history of fatigue, memory loss, blurred vision, and difficulty in writing. Neurological examination revealed a mild right-arm drift and impaired writing ability. A left thalamic lesion thought to be an astrocytoma was apparent on CT scan. Stereotactic biopsy showed inflammatory tissue with no evidence of tumor. A postoperative CT scan 11 months later demonstrated complete resolution of the lesion. Most of her symptoms have cleared (figure 10–1).

Comment. This case demonstrates the importance of tissue diagnosis before undertaking radiotherapy treatment of unresectable deep lesions.

CASE 2

A 58-year-old woman presented with sudden onset of headache, followed by progressive difficulty with short-term memory and "blackout spells" suggestive of seizures. Her neurological examination was normal. A CT scan indicated a heterogeneous lesion deep in the right posterior thalamus, possibly crossing the corpus callosum. CT stereotactic biopsy posterior to the border of the enhancing lesion showed only a few tumor cells. An additional specimen taken at a target 7 mm anterior to the first target contained pleomorphic cells, endothelial proliferation, and necrosis characteristic of a glioblastoma (figure 10–2).

Comment. CT scans exhibiting heterogeneous lesions may indicate the need to sample tissue at several targets in close proximity to obtain a satisfactory diagnosis.

CASE 3

A 67-year-old woman presented with a single seizure and a history of breast carcinoma five

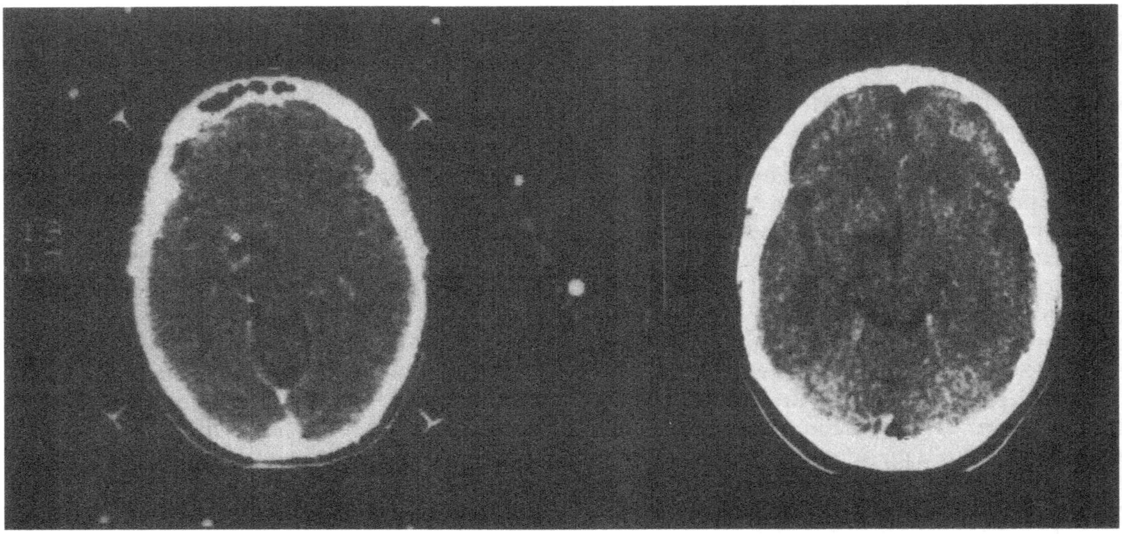

FIGURE 10–1. Localization CT scan demonstrates ring enhancing deep left thalamic lesion (*left*). Eleven months later, CT scan shows resolution of the enhancing area surrounding the lesion (*right*).

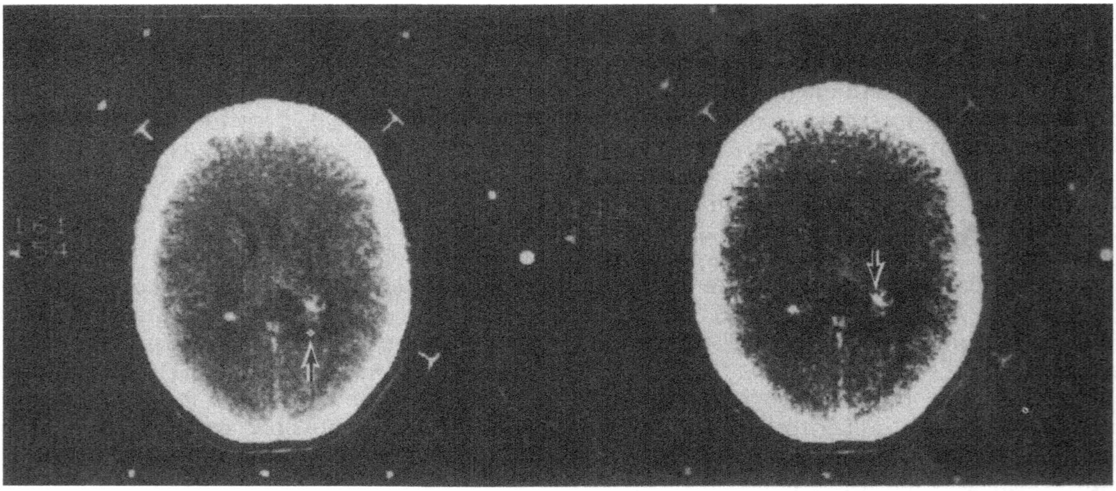

FIGURE 10–2. CT stereotactic biopsy at the posterior contrast-enhancing border of the lesion (*left*) demonstrated a few tumor cells classified as anaplastic astrocytoma (*arrow*). An additional biopsy (*right*) taken 7 mm anterior to the first target (*arrow*) revealed pleomorphic cells, endothelial proliferation, and necrosis characteristic of a glioblastoma.

years earlier, which had been treated with mastectomy and radiation. She had no previous evidence of metastases. A CT scan showed a small surface lesion in the left parietal area, which was thought to be either a metastatic lesion or a meningioma. Following CT stereotactic localization, the meningioma was removed through a small craniotomy. The patient was discharged from the hospital on the first postoperative day (figure 10–3).

Comment. Stereotactic localization of surface lesions allows biopsy and removal through small bone openings slightly larger than the lesion. Small craniotomies may reduce morbidity.

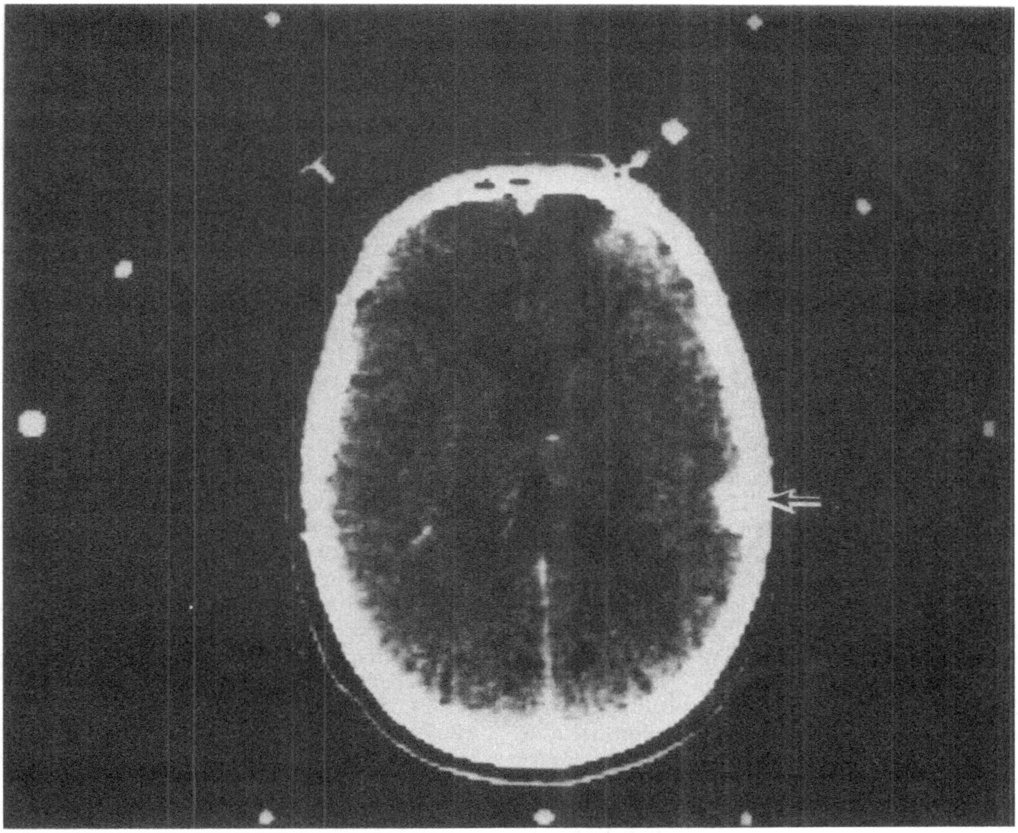

FIGURE 10–3. CT scan localizing the small surface meningioma (*arrow*).

MRI Localization

Early experience suggests that we see structural detail better on MRI than on CT images, particularly with T_1-weighted images. Occasionally, we saw lesions on T_2-weighted images that we did not see on CT scans through the same region. In addition, images can be constructed in the coronal, sagittal, and axial planes. The versatility available with additional coronal and sagittal planes allows the surgeon to establish approaches that may better avoid structures such as the internal capsule. We previously reported our initial experience with a new BRW localizer that allows localization of the target in all three planes [9].

Adapting the BRW system for MRI data required reconstruction with nonferrous materials that would neither degrade nor distort the image. To date, we have found the MRI system useful for localization of lesions in the brain stem and for biopsy of lesions seen only on MRI. The MRI localization system can be combined with CT localization for image comparison. Present limitations of the MRI system are the longer data-acquisition time and the inability to use general anesthesia. However, in certain cases, MRI stereotactic localization is essential.

Summary

Experience in several large series has demonstrated the efficacy and safety of image-guided stereotaxy and the apparent reduction in morbidity in comparison with standard large craniotomies. Although some lesions may be considered, by imaging techniques alone, to be inaccessible, biopsies can be taken before adjunctive radiation and chemotherapy treatments are instituted. Stereotactic biopsy provides a more accurate histological definition of heterogeneous lesions, and stereotactic localization of small subcortical and surface lesions allows complete resections through small skull openings.

References

1. Apuzzo MLJ, Chandrasoma PT, Zelman V, et al: Computed tomographic guidance stereotaxis in the management of lesions of the third ventricular region. *Neurosurgery* 15:502–508, 1984
2. Apuzzo MLJ, Sabshin JK: Computed tomographic guidance stereotaxis in the management of intracranial mass lesions. *Neurosurgery* 12:277–285, 1983
3. Brown RA: A computerized tomography-computer graphics approach to stereotaxic localization. *J Neurosurg* 50:715–720, 1979
4. Brown RA, Roberts TS, Osborn AG: Stereotaxic frame and computer software for CT-directed neurosurgical localization. *Invest Radiol* 15:308–312, 1980
5. Heilbrun MP: Computed tomography-guided stereotactic systems. *Clin Neurosurg* 31:564–581, 1983
6. Heilbrun MP, Brown RA, McDonald PR: Real-time three-dimensional graphics reconstruction using BRW coordinates in a microcomputer environment. *Appl Neurophysiol* (in press)
7. Heilbrun MP, Roberts TS, Apuzzo ML, et al: Preliminary experience with Brown-Roberts-Wells (BRW) computerized tomography stereotaxic guidance system. *J Neurosurg* 59:217–222, 1983
8. Heilbrun MP, Roberts TS, Wells TH, et al: *Technical Manual: Brown-Roberts-Wells (BRW) CT Stereotaxic Guidance System*. Burlington, MA: Radionics, Inc., 1982
9. Heilbrun MP, Sunderland PM, McDonald PR, et al: Brown-Roberts-Wells (BRW) stereotaxic frame modifications to accomplish magnetic resonant image (MRI) guidance in three planes: Axial/coronal/sagittal. Presented at the Annual Meeting of American Association of Neurological Surgeons, Denver Colorado, April, 1986
10. Kelly PJ, Alker GJ: A method for stereotactic laser microsurgery in the treatment of deep-seated CNS neoplasms. *Appl Neurophysiol* 43:210–215, 1980
11. Kelly PJ, Alker GJ, Goerss S: Computer-assisted stereotactic laser microsurgery for treatment of intracranial neoplasms. *Neurosurgery* 10:324–331, 1982
12. Kelly PJ, Alker GJ Jr, Kall B, et al: Method of computed tomography-based stereotaxic biopsy with arteriographic control. *Neurosurgery* 14:172–177, 1984
13. Kelly PJ, Earnest F, Kall BA, et al: Surgical options for patients with deep-seated brain tumors: Computer-assisted stereotactic biopsy. *May. Clin Proc* 60:223–229, 1985
14. Leksell L, Jernberg B: Stereotaxis and tomography. A technical note. *Acta Neurochir* (Wien) 52:1–7, 1980
15. Maroon JC, Bank WO, Drayer BP, et al: Intracranial biopsy assisted by computerized tomography. *J Neurosurg* 46:740–744, 1977
16. Mundinger F, Birg W, Klar M: Computer-assisted stereotactic brain operations by means including computerized axial tomography. *Appl Neurophysiol* 41:169–182, 1978
17. Nauta HJW, Guinto FC, Pisharodi M: Arterial bolus contrast medium enhancement for computed tomographically guided stereotactic biopsy. *Surg Neurol* 22:559–564, 1984
18. Ostertag CB, Mennel HD, Kiessling M: Stereotactic biopsy of brain tumors. *Surg Neurol* 14:275–283, 1980
19. Perry JH, Rosenbaum AE, Lunsford LD, et al: Computed tomography-guided stereotactic surgery: Conception and development of a new stereotactic methodology. *Neurosurg* 7:376–381, 1980
20. Scerrati M, Fiorentino A, Fiorentino M, et al: Stereotaxic device for polar approaches in orthogonal systems: Technical note. *J Neurosurg* 61:1146–1147, 1984
21. Sheldon CH, McCann G, Jacques S, et al: Development of a computerized microstereotaxic method for localization and removal of minute CNS lesions under direct 3-D vision. *J Neurosurg* 52:21–27, 1980
22. Spiegel EA, Wycis HT, Marks M, et al: Stereotaxic apparatus for operations on the human brain. *Science* 106:349–350, 1947
23. Storrs BB, Walker ML: Use of a CT-guided stereotaxic apparatus in pediatric neurosurgery. *Concepts Pediatr Neurosurg* 5:214–223, 1985
24. Talairach J, Bancaud J, Szikla G, et al: Approche nouvelle de la neurochirurgie de l'epilepsie. *Neurochirurgie* 20(Suppl 1):1–98, 1974

11. DIAGNOSIS AND TREATMENT OF MASS LESIONS USING THE LEKSELL STEREOTACTIC SYSTEM

L. Dade Lunsford

The Role of Stereotactic Surgery

Because of the increasing number of patients harboring small or critically located intracranial mass lesions, and because frequently such lesions are revealed relatively soon in the course of disease by noninvasive imaging methods, modern neurosurgeons have established stereotactic surgery as a prominent technique in the diagnosis and treatment of neurological disease. Stereotactic surgery has become a standard tool in neurosurgery in the same way as the ultrasonic aspirator, the laser, and (in microsurgery) the operating microscope. In some centers, stereotactic technique has been used in as many as 30% of all patients with intracranial mass lesions. The choice of a particular stereotactic device has reflected the training, goals, and experience of the individual surgeon. This chapter details our experience using the Leksell stereotactic system at the University of Pittsburgh and Presbyterian-University Hospital between February 1981 and January 1986.

Table 11–1 demonstrates the indications for stereotactic surgery at our center. Despite the major advances in neurological diagnosis provided by advanced imaging devices such as computed tomography (CT) and magnetic resonance imaging (MRI), histological diagnosis has remained mandatory. In a prior review of our first 102 stereotactic cases, we found that in 26% of the cases, stereotactic surgery resulted in a new diagnosis that was either not considered or considered unlikely based on preoperative clinical, laboratory, or radiological testing [14]. In other published series, stereotactic surgery resulted in an accurate diagnosis in between 91%–96% of cases and often led to major changes in postoperative treatment [14].

When precise treatment is mandatory, for example, when a patient is undergoing intracavitary irradiation or interstitial brachytherapy for tumor, therapeutic stereotactic surgery is required [3, 6]. No other technique permits 1-mm precision. In other cases, such as brain abscesses, stereotactic aspiration with or without catheter drainage has proven to be a superior method of treatment, obviating the need for craniotomy and major surgical resection [16]. We advocate stereotactic surgery when brain lesions are small, deep, or multiple, or when lesions are located in critical brain structures and thus not amenable to surgical resection. In the treatment of malignant cerebral gliomas, we reserve major cytoreductive surgery for those lesions located in the poles of the cerebral hemispheres or for patients whose neurological

TABLE 11–1. Indications for Stereotactic Surgery

Why?
1. Accurate histological diagnosis is mandatory
2. Precise treatment is planned

When?
1. Lesions are small, deep, multiple, or not amenable to surgery
2. Despite lesion size, patient's symptoms or signs are insignificant or likely to be exacerbated by conventional craniotomy or resection
3. Lesions are multiple
4. Adverse medical conditions or advanced patient age exist

Where? Lesions of the cerebrum, brain stem, or cerebellum

L.D. Lunsford (ed.) *MODERN STEREOTACTIC NEUROSURGERY*.

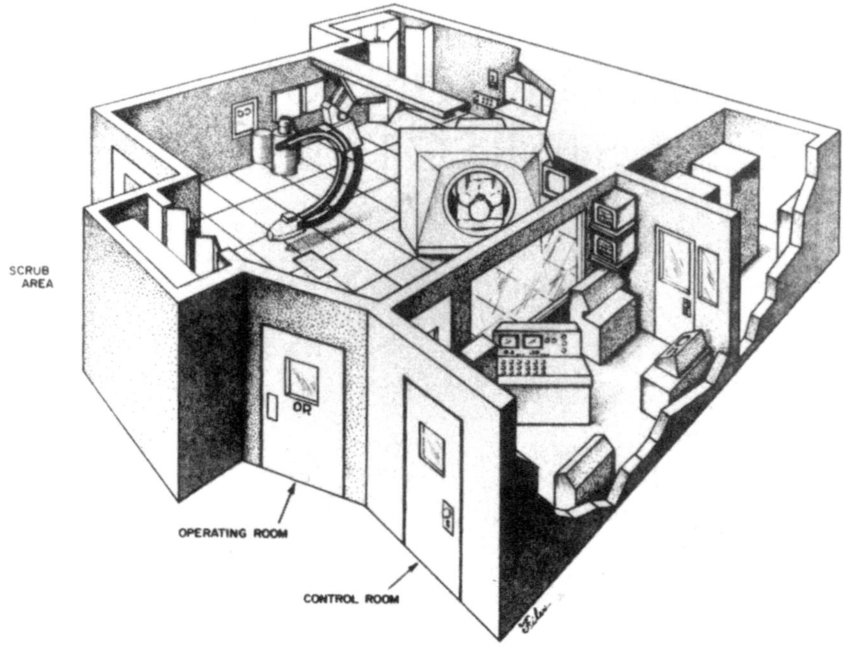

A

FIGURE 11–1. Architectual drawing (A) of the stereotactic operating suite at Presbyterian-University Hospital, Pittsburgh, PA. The scanner is reversed from its normal position in a radiological imaging suite to allow wide access to the head. (Reprinted with permission from *Neurosurgery* 15: 559–561, 1984.) The operating suite (B) is equipped with a high-resolution CT scanner (GE 8800, General Electric Medical Systems, Milwaukee, WI) and an integrated C-arm fluoroscopic imaging intensifier with 100-mm angiographic capabilities (Phillips Medical Systems). (Reprinted with permission from *Surg Neurol* 22:222–230, 1984.)

symptoms resulting from major mass effect might render them unable to undergo postoperative adjuvant therapies such as radiation and chemotherapy. In some patients, radiological imaging will disclose a lesion of considerable size, yet these patients exhibit few significant clinical signs or symptoms. In cases in which conventional craniotomy and resection are deemed likely to induce unacceptable postoperative neurological deficits, stereotactic surgery achieves diagnosis and guides postoperative treatment. When multiple lesions are present, usually due to central nervous system (CNS) infection or tumors, or when adverse medical illness or advanced age exists, stereotactic surgery is valuable. Lesions of the cerebrum, cerebellum, and brain stem are all amenable to stereotactic intervention.

Safety of Stereotactic Surgery

In contrast to the adverse outcomes reported after brain biopsies were performed in an era when imaging tools were less sophisticated, recent series of stereotactic surgery have demonstrated the remarkable safety of this procedure. Mortality after stereotactic surgery has been reduced to between 0% and 3%, and morbidity to between 5% and 10% [14].

The Site for Stereotactic Surgery

Stereotactic surgery dependent upon advanced imaging methods can be performed in several ways. First, stereotactic localization can take place in a diagnostic CT or MRI radiological suite after which surgery itself is conducted in

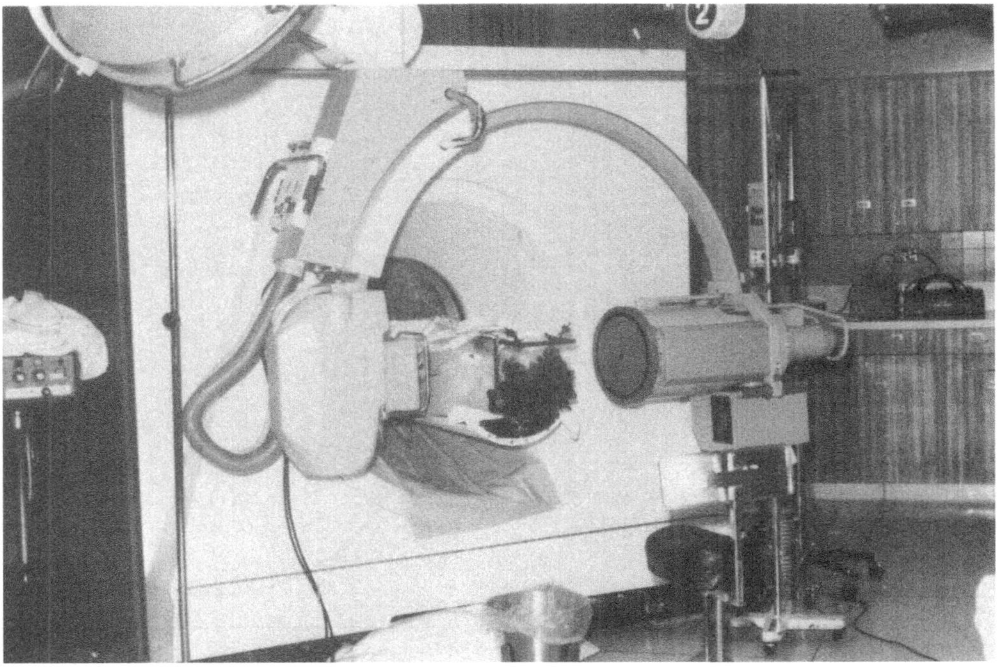

B
FIGURE 11–1 (cont.)

a conventional neurosurgical operating room [13]. Second, both the imaging and surgical portions of the procedure can be performed in a radiological suite equipped with appropriate anesthesia life support systems, if the appropriate sterile environment is maintained [19]. At Presbyterian-University Hospital and the University of Pittsburgh we have chosen a third possibility: the installation of a dedicated resolution CT scanner in the operating room itself (figure 11–1) [8, 9, 17, 18, 20].

Procedures and Techniques

Between 1981 and 1985, 322 patients had stereotactic surgery at Presbyterian-University Hospital. The number of stereotactic procedures has continued to increase each year (figure 11–2). Owing to the nature of our referral pattern and the needs of our community, 240 cases (74.5%) underwent diagnostic brain biopsy or aspiration of various brain lesions (figure 11–3). In 40 cases (12.4%), specific therapeutic intervention was performed. In an additional 42 cases (13%) functional neurosurgical intervention was performed using CT stereotactic technique alone (figure 11–4). Functional neurosurgical procedures included thalamotomy for movement disorders, placement of deep brain electrodes for deep brain stimulation recording or in epileptic patients, internal capsulotomy for pain or affective disorders, and pituitary alcohol injection.

DIAGNOSTIC SURGERY TECHNIQUE

In elective cases, the patient was seen the evening before surgery by the surgeon and the anesthesiologist. A hexachlorophene shampoo was performed that evening. Immediately prior to surgery, the patient was premedicated with an anxiolytic agent (i.e., hydroxyzine, 50–100 mg), an anticholinergic, and a boost in corticosteroids as indicated. Whenever possible, the patient sat in a chair during application of the stereotactic frame. A supplemental intravenous narcotic (fentanyl) was administered under the direction of the anesthetist in attendance. After the entire head was prepped with isopropyl alcohol, the frame was centered on the head by means of ear bars placed into the unanesthetized external auditory canals. Steel sleeves were inserted through the scalp after local scalp infiltration with 1% lidocaine.

The position of the pins was selected in ad-

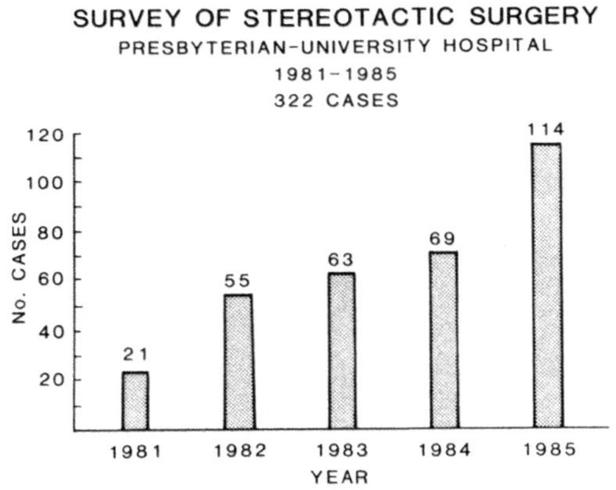

FIGURE 11-2. The role of stereotactic surgery at Presbyterian University Hospital, Pittsburgh, PA, has increased each year between 1981 and 1985.

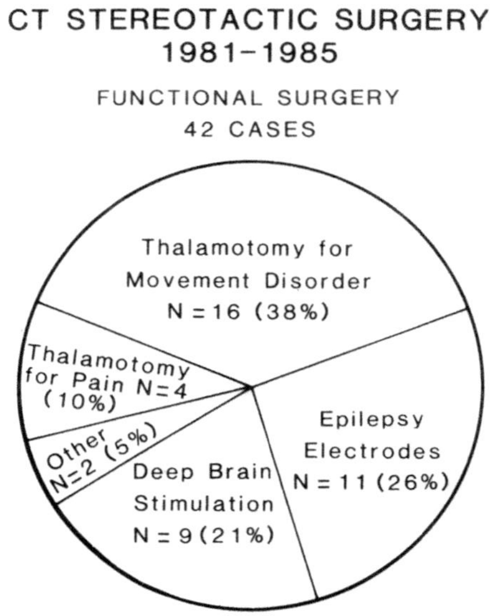

FIGURE 11-4. The usage of CT stereotactic technique in functional neurosurgical cases at Presbyterian-University Hospital, Pittsburgh, PA.

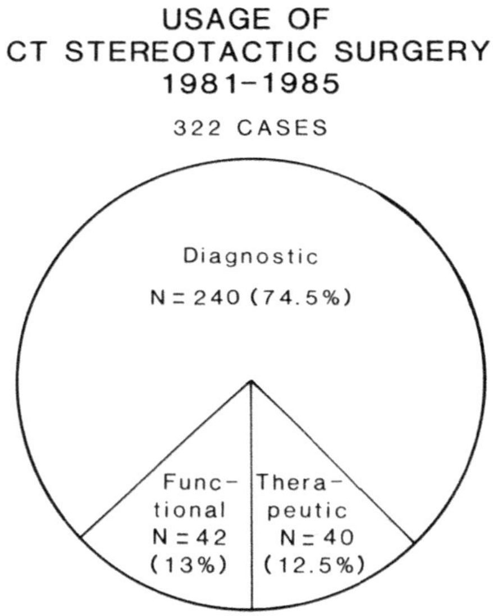

FIGURE 11-3. Usage of CT stereotactic technique in 322 cases that underwent surgery at Presbyterian-University Hospital between 1981 and 1985.

vance, after the preoperative CT or MRI was reviewed. For skull base or posterior fossa lesions, all four pins were placed high (two in the posterior and two in the anterior vertex of the skull). For mesencephalic or diencephalic lesions, the posterior pins were set low in the suboccipital area, and the anterior pins were placed high in the frontal region. For lesions in the cerebral hemispheres above the level of the third ventricle, all four pins were placed as low as possible in the supraorbital and suboccipital regions. During CT imaging, this technique tended to minimize image artifacts produced by the plastic pin holders and the carbon-fiber pins. For MRI, specific location of the pins was not critical, as neither the frame nor pins have a nuclear magnetic resonance signal. The MRI fiberglass pins had to be very short so that the entire coordinate frame fit within the MRI radiofrequency coil.

Distortion of the frame on the ear canal bars caused some patients to experience discomfort during frame application. This problem was reduced by inserting the ear bars less deeply within the ear canals and by supporting the frame during placement and as the pins were drilled. Application of the coordinate frame took approximately five minutes. The patient then rested supine upon the CT scanner pallet with the head coordinate frame fixed to the magnetic coordinate frame adapter, which, in turn, was attached precisely to the CT scanner. Intravenous contrast enhancement was performed during the application of the frame. Patients with a known iodine allergy were premedicated with corticosteroids, thereby eliminating significant contrast reactions in our series. Our radiological technique consisted of serial axial CT images performed parallel to the coordinate frame base. The location of the axial images was selected from the electronically generated lateral skull radiograph (Scoutview®). For most mass lesions, serial 5-mm-thick slices scanned in 5-mm increments (by table movement) provided more than adequate accuracy and delineation. For smaller lesions we used 5-mm-thick slices imaged at 3-mm table intervals by table movement (figure 11–5). The use of very narrow slices (1.5 mm) was reserved for functional neurosurgical intervention, because this time-consuming technique increased spatial resolution at the expense of contrast resolution and increased radiation exposure [7, 10]. Stereotactic coordinates for the target were chosen by one of the three methods outlined in chapter 3. Reformatted CT imaging in coronal, sagittal, or paraxial images proved valuable in depicting probe trajectories. Usage of special software for the GE 8800 CT scanner to determine targets and preselect probe trajectories was also advantageous.

After radiological imaging was complete, the scalp was shaved surrounding the selected entry point for the probe. The entire head, hair, and coordinate frame were prepped again with alcohol. More than 90% of our operations were performed using local anesthesia supplemented by intravenous sedation, provided by the the anesthetist in attendance. We reserved general anesthesia for patients who are extremely anxious or who were undergoing transsphenoidal or occipital approaches to the cerebellum or brain stem in the prone position. Target trajectories were selected in advance and were designed to avoid the most critical functional areas of the brain and to enable serial stereotactic biopsies to be made throughout the tumor volume (figure 11–6). Frontal, supraorbital, lateral, vertex, occipital, and suboccipital transcerebellar approaches were selected according to the location of the lesion [5, 9]. We now perform transcerebellar stereotactic surgery with the patient in the semisitting position, after moving the patient from the CT scanner pallet to a standard operating-room table; immediate postoperative CT imaging takes place after the patient has been returned to the CT scanner pallet. Open stereotactic approaches are performed after conventional burr-hole placement, opening of the dura, and inspection of the pial surface, if the probe trajectory seems likely to pass near or through important vascular pial structures. Percutaneous twist-drill approaches with the stereotactic arc are used preferentially when suboccipital, occipital, frontal, or coronal probe entry sites are selected. In general, we have continued to place burr holes followed by inspection of the pial surface when planning lateral trajectories through the temporal lobe or trajectories through the sylvian fissure or parietal lobe.

Immediately after completing the procedure, postoperative CT images are performed. If the lesion is evacuated (e.g., colloid cysts, brain abscesses, or hematomas), intraoperative CT imaging is obtained. A probe-guide holder is used to secure the probe at the target site, and then the stereotactic arc is removed [11]. The probe-guide holder is attached to the vertex of the frame and permits virtually artifact-free imaging of the brain while the probe actually is at the target site. This device also has a vernier stop, which allows advancement or retraction of the probe in the preselected trajectory after the arc has been removed and during intraoperative CT imaging.

DIAGNOSTIC SURGERY RESULTS

Of 240 patients undergoing diagnostic stereotactic surgery, a diagnosis was achieved in 230 (95.8%) (table 11–2). In three patients, a histological diagnosis was reached after a second stereotactic biopsy procedure. Glial neoplasms were identified in 129 cases (53.8%). Seventy cases (29.1%) had histological criteria (marked anaplasia, mitoses, necrosis, and vascular endothelial proliferation) that confirmed a diagnosis of glioblastoma; 34 cases had anaplastic astrocytomas. In all procedures, CT was used as the primary localization method. More recently, we have also used MRI in a select group of patients to define the tumor and to attempt to accurately assess tumor volume [15]. Such a case is demonstrated in figure 11–7. Although MRI provided graphic delineation of the neoplasm and offered contrast resolution superior to CT, variation in relaxation time emphases (T_1 and T_2) failed to correlate significantly with histological samples obtained at specified sites within the tumor. In both malignant gliomas

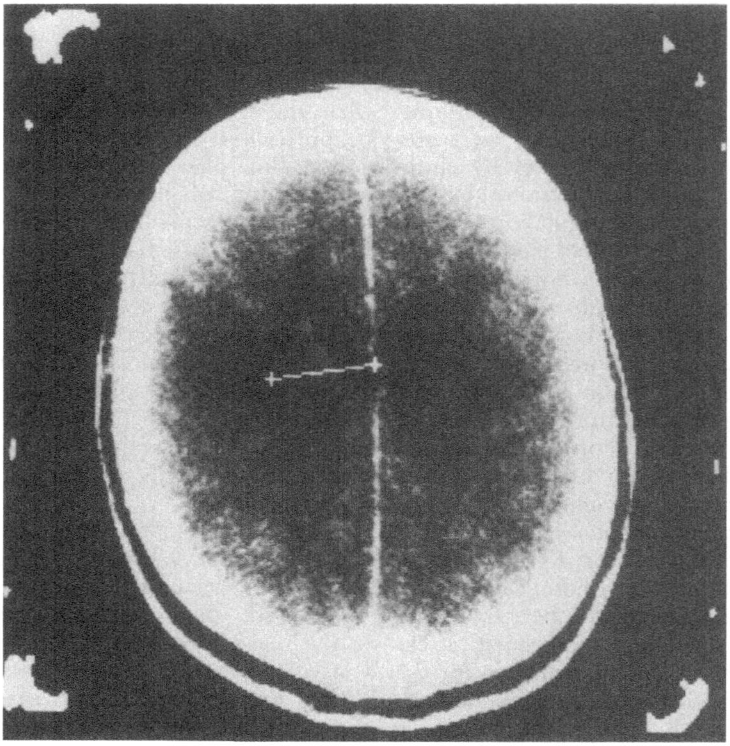

A

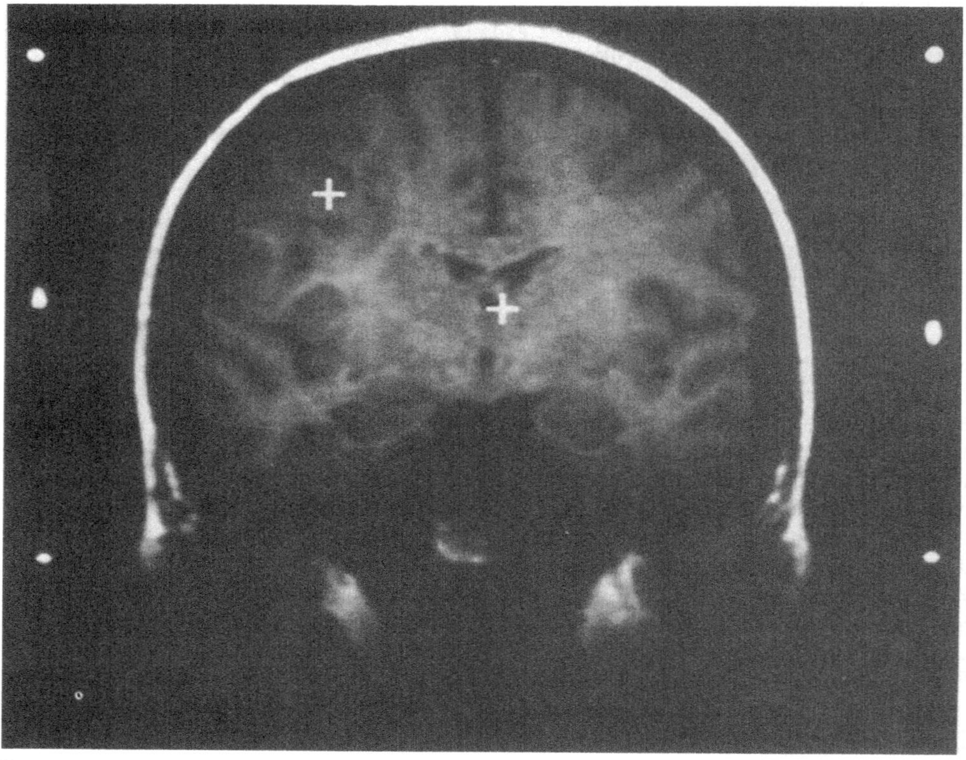

B

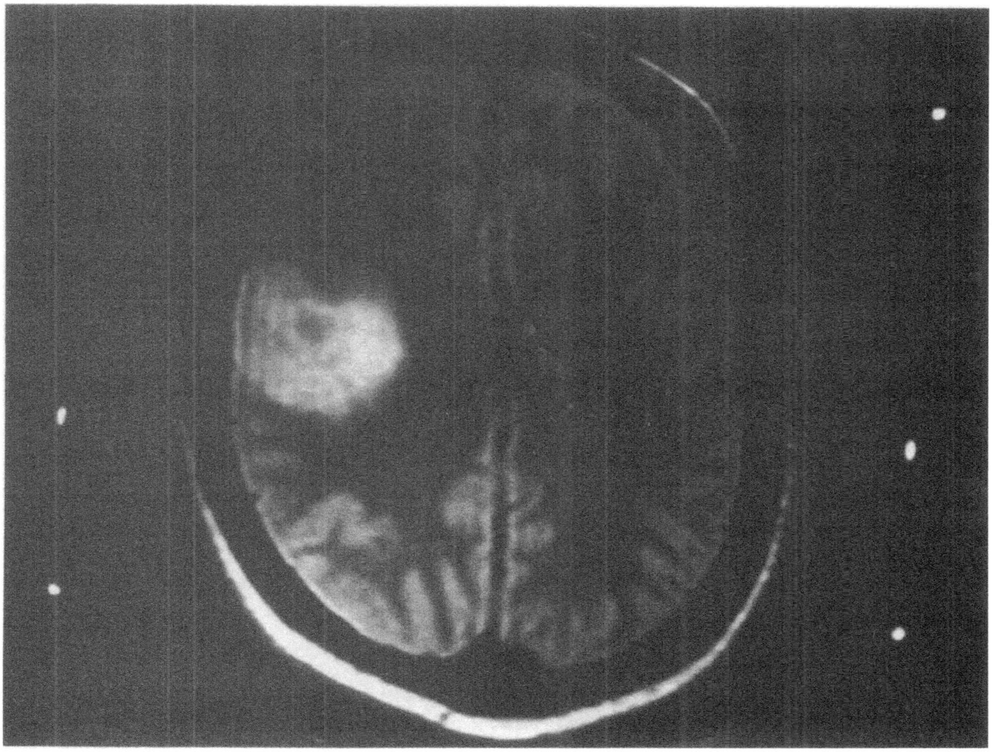

C

FIGURE 11–5. Intraoperative CT scan (A) demonstrating a low-attenuation mass in the right frontal region of a 33-year-old woman with seizures. The center of the frame and target are identified. A stereotactic coronal MRI (T_1-weighted) (B) demonstrates the lesion and surrounding brain No artifacts from the frame are identified. The frame center and target are identified. Stereotactic axial MRI (T_2-weighted) (C) demonstrates a much larger lesion than CT. CT- and MRI-derived targets are identical.

and well-differentiated astrocytomas, we identified neoplastic cells in the periphery of lesions well beyond the mass delineated by either CT or MRI. Histological sampling remains the only way to validate actual tumor margins, especially in preparation for subsequent adjuvant treatments such as intersitial brachytherapy.

Preoperative confusion resulting from the similar appearance of glial neoplasms and metastatic tumors was resolved by stereotactic surgery. We confirmed metastatic cancer in 22 patients (9.1%) in our series, the majority of whom had no known primary source for the tumor. Conversely, a number of patients with "multiple lesions" on CT scans proved to have malignant gliomas. Detailed intraoperative imaging usually disclosed that the lesions were contiguous, although portions of the tumor were not enhanced significantly.

Primary (CNS) lymphomas were identified in 16 patients, all of whom subsequently were treated with external-beam radiation therapy. The CT appearance of primary CNS lymphomas frequently mimicked that of malignant gliomas, but the pattern of contrast enhancement tended to be substantially more uniform and much denser in lymphoma cases. CNS lymphomas frequently involved the corpus callosum and were spread diffusely throughout the brain. Clinical symptomatology often seemed quite insignificant in comparison to the extensive evidence of disease demonstrated by CT.

Stereotactic biopsy and aspiration of brain abscesses were performed in 14 patients; eight also had catheter drainage of the abscess for a period of two to four days. All patients recovered after prolonged (two to four weeks) intravenous antibiotic treatment; no patient required multiple drainage procedures. In three patients who had germinomas, postoperative radiation therapy was used as the primary treatment following stereotactic biopsy; no patient subsequently required craniotomy.

Neuroepithelial cysts of the thalamus and

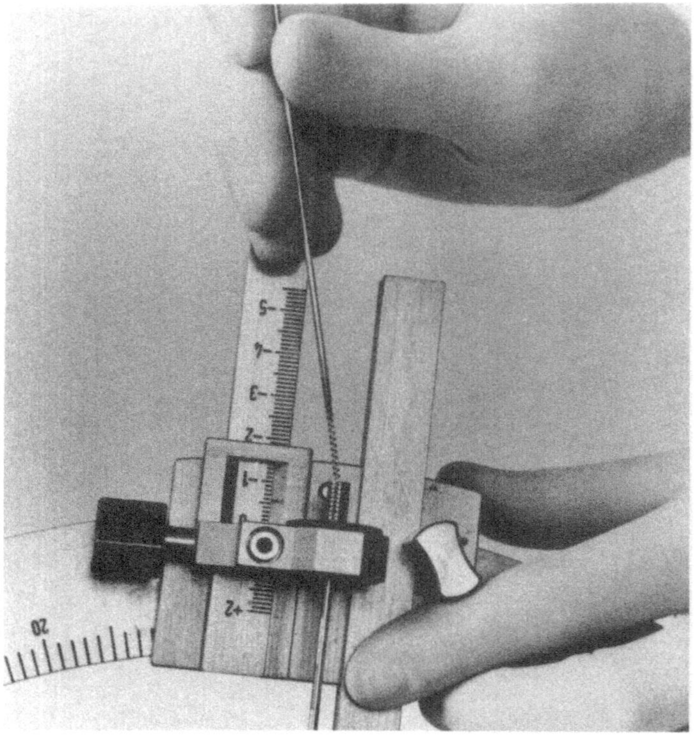

A

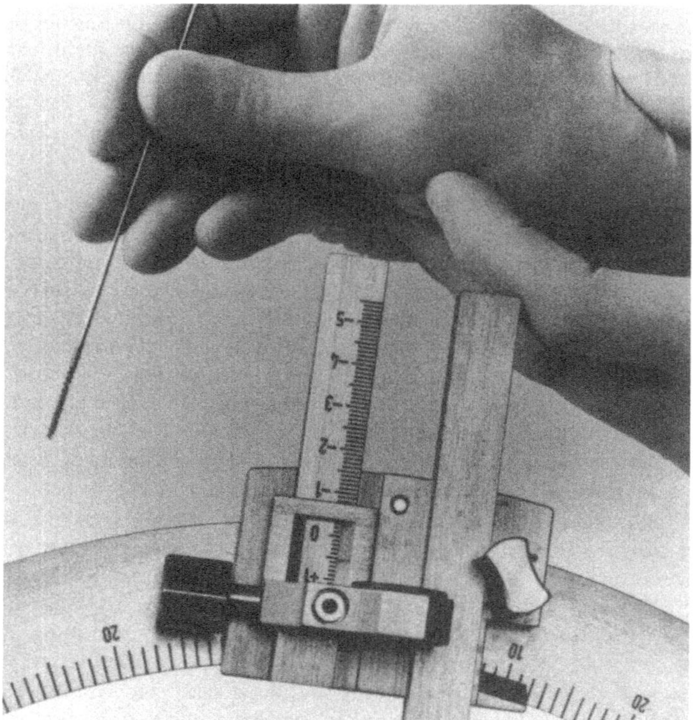

B

FIGURE 11-6. Precise stereotactic biopsies are obtained using the Backlund Spiral (A). This instrument retrieves a "core" specimen (B) by rotating the spiral between the thumb and forefinger (C) until the specimen is extruded on the thumb or forefinger (D).

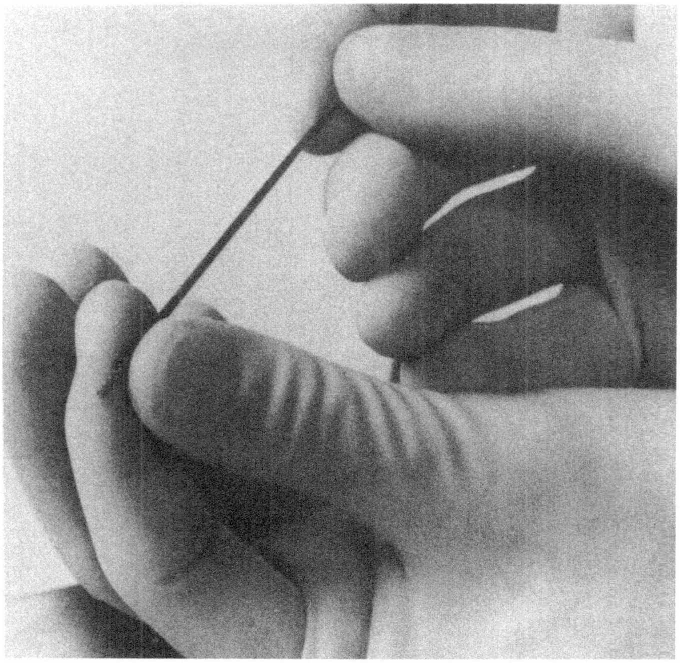

C

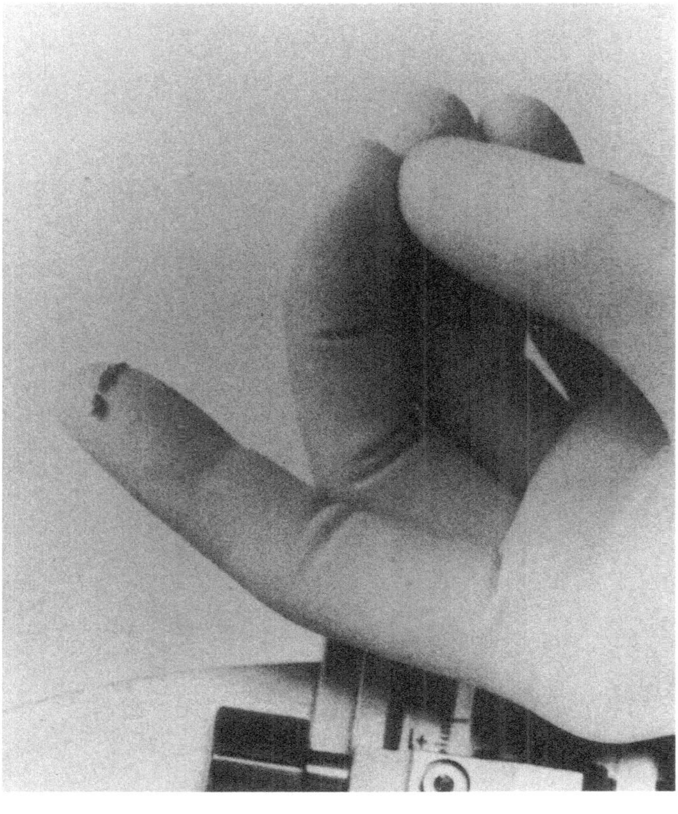

D

FIGURE 11–6. (cont.)

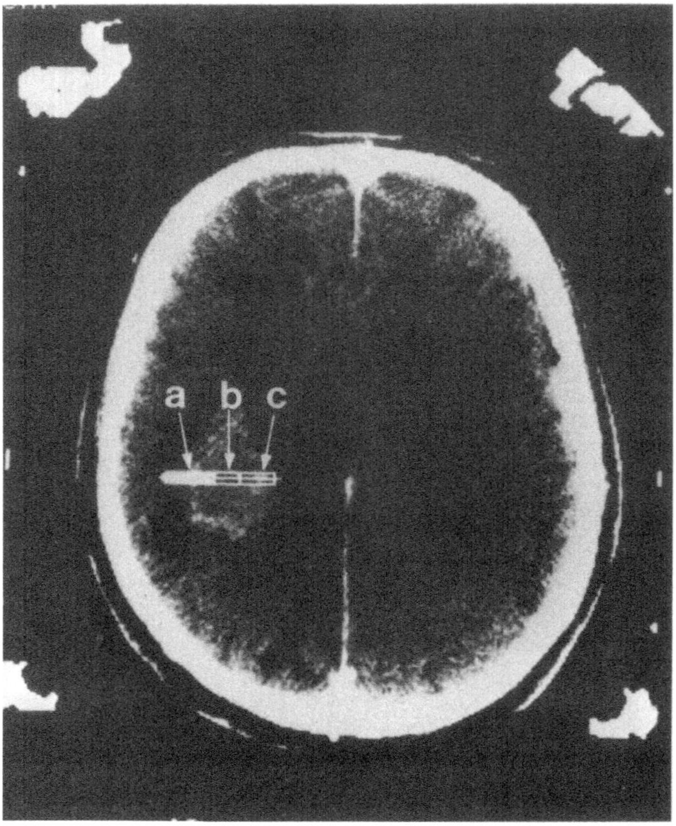

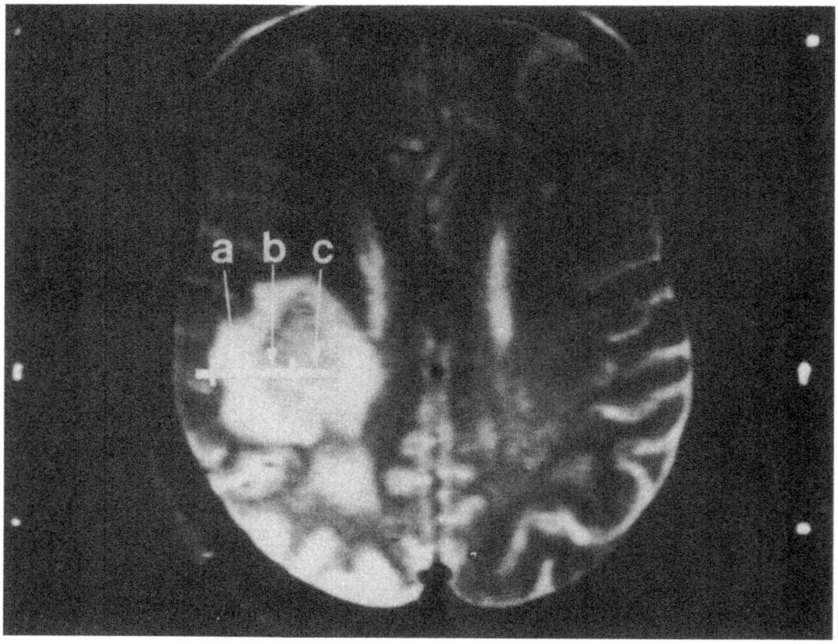

B

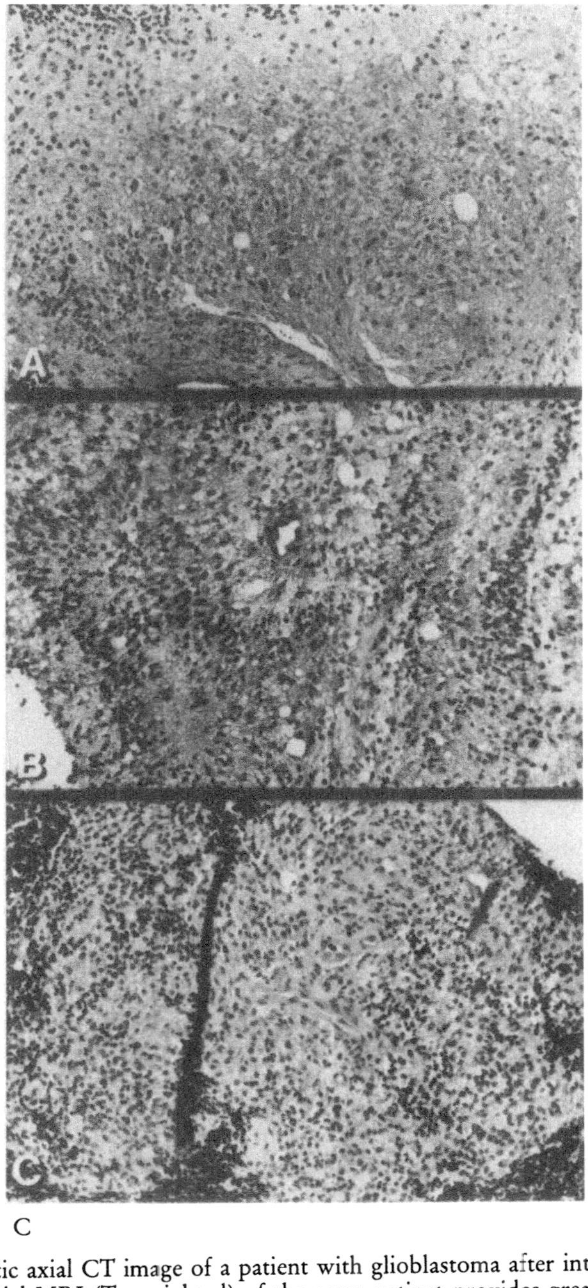

C

FIGURE 11–7. Stereotactic axial CT image of a patient with glioblastoma after intravenous contrast enhancement (A). Stereotactic axial MRI (T_2-weighted) of the same patient provides greater detail of the tumor and surrounding brain as well as reduced artifact (B). Histological sampling revealed anaplastic astrocytoma in the low-attenuation area on CT; glioblastoma is identified in the contrast-enhancing margin and centrally (C).

TABLE 11–2. CT Stereotactic Surgery at Presbyterian-University Hospital, Pittsburgh, PA: Survey of Diagnoses Obtained in 240 Cases

Diagnosis	No. Cases	Percentage
Glioblastoma	70	29.1
Anaplastic astrocytoma	34	14.1
Astrocytoma	25	10.4
Metatastic tumor	22	9.1
Lymphoma	16	6.7
Brain abscess[a]	14	5.8
Hematoma	9	3.8
Encephalitis	7	2.9
Vascular malformation	6	2.5
Colloid cyst	5	2.1
Germinoma	4	1.7
Neuroepithelial cyst	4	1.7
Degenerative disease	4	1.7
Epidermoid tumor	3	1.3
Other[b]	7	2.9
Nondiagnostic	10	4.2
Total	240	100

[a] Eight cases had catheter drainage; three cases had acquired immune deficiency syndrome (AIDS).
[b] Includes one case each of infarct, porencephaly, leukoencephalopathy, neurosarcoid, vasculitis, granuloma and progressive multifocal leukoencephalopathy.

TABLE 11–3. CT Stereotactic Surgery at Presbyterian-University Hospital, Pittsburgh, PA, 1981–1985: Diagnostic Surgery in 240 Cases

Lesion Location	No. Cases	Percentage
Cerebral hemisphere	149	62
Basal ganglia	27	11
Thalamus	12	5
Third ventricle	11	5
Corpus callosum	10	4.1
Pons	10	4.1
Pineal region	7	2.9
Cerebellum	5	2.1
Midbrain	4	1.7
Suprasellar	4	1.7
Intrasellar	1	0.4
Total	240	100

midbrain are low-attenuation lesions associated with local mass effect but no surrounding cerebral edema [1]. These thin-walled cysts frequently were not recognizable by histological technique but were identified by the lack of any evidence of neoplastic tissue in the biopsy specimen. Injection of metrizamide into the neuroepithelial cyst delineated the entire structure and confirmed the absence of communication with the ventricular system. These benign cysts were decompressed by simple aspiration; no patient with a diagnosis of a neuroepithelial cyst required more than a single aspiration to achieve long-term remission symptoms.

The vast majority of lesions in our series (table 11–3) were located in the cerebral hemispheres, usually subcortically (149 cases, 62%). Lesions primarily were within the basal ganglia in 27 cases (11%) or the thalamus in 12 cases (5%). Corpus callosum lesions proved to be either malignant gliomas (eight cases) or primary CNS lymphomas (two cases).

Five patients underwent stereotactic procedures for mass lesions in the cerebellum; ten patients had masses in the pons, and four had them in the midbrain. Our technique for stereotactic surgery of the midbrain and pontine lesions has been described [5]. We used a transcerebellar route to the pons when the lesion was located at the level of, or slightly inferior to, the middle cerebellar peduncle. Midbrain lesions were reached through a transfrontal, transventricular approach along the long axts of the brain stem. In small lesions of the brain stem such as these, fine-needle aspiration was used as the primary technique, because large samples frequently were impossible or too risky to obtain. Transcerebellar approaches were performed under general anesthesia with the patient either in the prone position on the CT scanner table or in the semisitting position on a separate operating-room table. Plastic plates that supported the occiput in normal positions were removed, and the frame was attached by tape to the magnetic footplates to achieve fixation with the patient in the prone position. Intraoperative imaging was performed during or after the procedure without obtaining a new localizing scan, because the relationship of the frame to the scanner table remained the same in both the prone and supine positions. Postoperative CT imaging was performed in all patients; those patients undergoing surgery in a sitting position were returned to the CT scanner table in the operating room.

Histopathological specimens were obtained

by either of two techniques, both described by Backlund [2]. Serial 10-mm spiral corkscrew biopsies were performed by inserting a needle 2.1 mm in outer diameter through the lesion at sampling sites that included: tissue surrounding the contrast-enhancing portion of the tumor, the contrast-enhancing portion itself; and the center of the tumor, whether of low attenuation or not. These sampling sites were marked on the CT images for subsequent demonstration to the neuropathologist (figure 11–8). In addition, at least one aspiration or biopsy was performed by advancing and retracting a sharp-tipped needle 1.9 mm in diameter into the lesion to a depth of 10 mm, while 2.5 ml of gentle suction was applied with a syringe.

If at any time bleeding occurred from the needle, no additional biopsy specimens were obtained. The biopsy needle was left at the site of bleeding, and the stylette was replaced intermittently to eliminate occlusion of the needle and to allow blood to egress. At the conclusion of the procedure, the biopsy needle was placed at the deepest biopsy point and then gradually withdrawn, while the surgeon ascertained that there was no further bleeding from the needle. If bleeding was noted at any point, the needle was kept there until bleeding ceased.

Each histological specimen was immediately placed in a 10% buffered formalin solution. Frozen-section diagnoses were not performed, except in cases of suspected brain abscess or encephalitis [9, 14]. We have found that a frozen-section diagnosis of either primary or metastatic tumors may be unreliable and unnecessary, occasionally leading to frustration on the part of both the neuropathologists and the surgeons [9]. This frustration leads to an attempt to extract larger amounts of tissue, sometimes at the expense of producing a brain hemorrhage. We decided that a negative biopsy was preferable to an operative complication. All specimens were collected from the operating room by the neuropathology technician. On the day following the stereotactic procedure, the surgeon and the neuropathologist reviewed the permanently stained biopsy specimens in conjunction with the intraopearative CT or MRI. Such an approach led to a nonpressured, amiable relationship between neurosurgeons and neuropathologists and fostered a very acceptable diagnostic rate (95.2%).

Because only small samples were obtained by stereotactic technique, histological diagnosis was occasionally difficult. We found that formalin-fixed preparations, subsequently stained by hematoxylin and eosin (H&E) or other appropriate stains, provided the greatest chance of reaching an accurate diagnosis. Other centers have used a smear technique for cytological preparations. Obtaining a highly positive biopsy rate required the skill of neuropathologists with experience in the technique as well as skilled histological technicians capable of dealing with very small tissue fragments. Clinical and radiographic features of the lesion were often indispensable in reaching a correct diagnosis. Nondiagnostic or equivocal biopsies were obtained in several situations: (1) when the histological samples were minute, a feature which usually occurred when the lesions themselves were small or were located in critically important brain areas; (2) when cystic lesions had thin walls (the cyst collapsed after puncture, changing the stereotactic target); the cyst wall itself often was millimeters thick; and (3) when the preoperative differential diagnosis was excessive or a variety of clinical possibilities existed, any one of which could have explained the patient's illness. In such instances, brain biopsy occasionally failed to provide the answer [14].

THERAPEUTIC SURGERY

Increasingly, the goals of stereotactic surgery reflect the importance of therapeutic intervention rather than simply diagnosis of brain lesions. CT stereotactic surgery was performed solely for therapeutic intervention in 40 cases at our center (figure 11–9). In four cases, ventricular drains were placed for periodic cyst aspirations or for external ventricular drainage in patients with "slit" ventricles. Figure 11–9 does not include our patients with brain abscesses or intracerebral hematomas, all of whom also underwent diagnostic brain biopsy at the time of evacuation or drainage of the lesion. Stereotactic craniotomy with lesion resection was performed in three cases with the Leksell stereotactic device and in seven additional cases, with a CT-compatible head holder designed for intraoperative imaging.

Interstitial Brachytherapy

Long used in European centers for the treatment of both well-differentiated and malignant astrocytomas [4], interstitial brachytherapy has

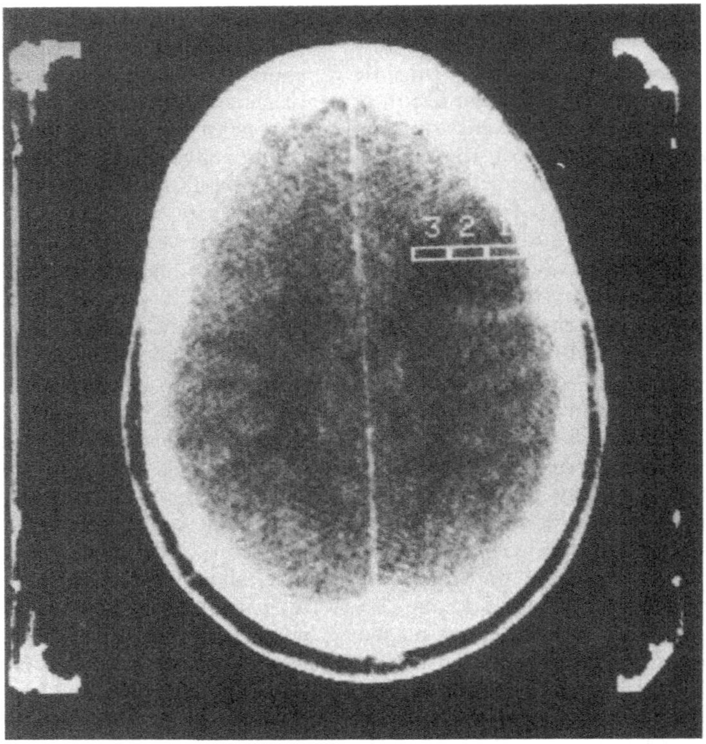

A

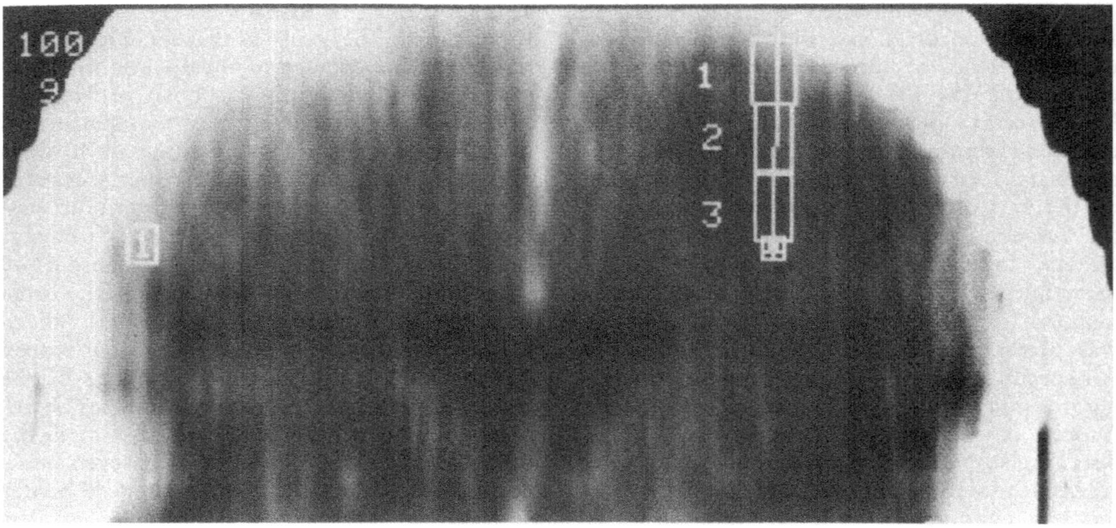

B

FIGURE 11–8. Axial (A) and coronal reformatted (B) stereotactic CT images display the pathway of a probe through the tumor. The targets can be displayed on coronal magnetic resonance (C, T_1-weighted) and axial magnetic resonance images (D, T_2-weighted). These sites are correlated with the histology during review with the neuropathologist.

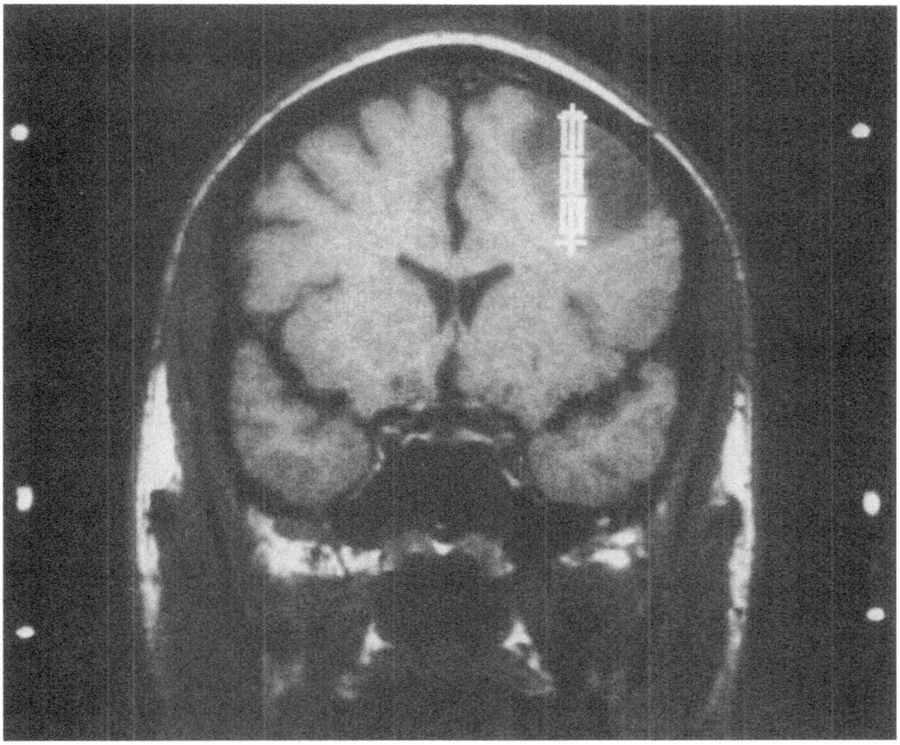

C

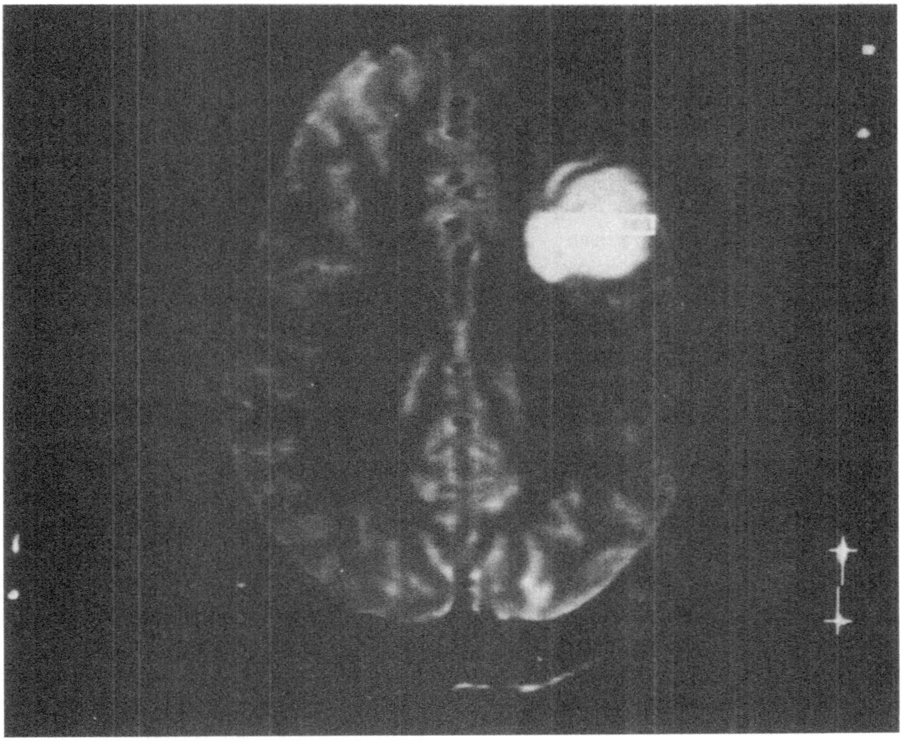

D

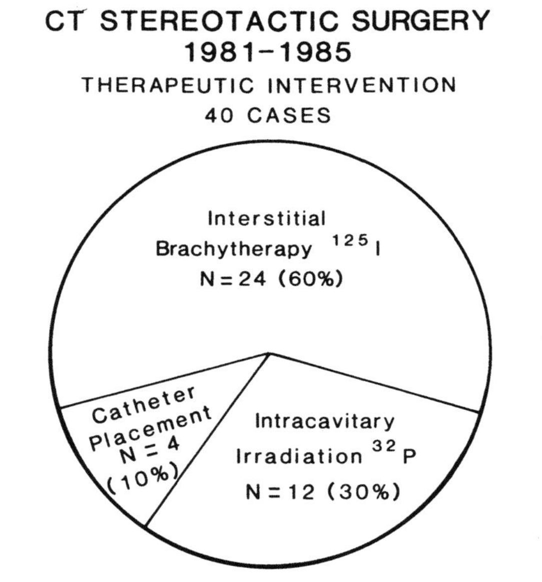

FIGURE 11–9. CT stereotactic therapeutic surgery was performed in 40 cases at Presbyterian-University Hospital, Pittsburgh, Pennsylvania, between 1981 and 1985.

undergone cautious clinical trials in the United States. Gutin and co-workers performed therapeutic implants using iodine-125 in more than 100 cases. Gutin's reports have indicated a trend towards improved survival and an increase in the symptom-free interval after implantation [6]. Many questions remain about the role of interstitial brachytherapy in the treatment of malignant gliomas: What is the proper target? What is the proper dose? Who is the proper patient? What grade of neoplasm should be treated? How does it compare to other multimodality treatments such as chemotherapy?

Our technique of interstitial brachytherapy was essentially similar to Gutin's [6]. As of January 1, 1986, 24 patients were treated. Our primary group of patients (previously untreated) had a clinical diagnosis of glioblastoma or anaplastic astrocytoma. We used the enhancing margin of the tumor, demonstrated by CT scan, as the target volume; it received 5,000–6,000 cGy by afterloading technique over a 5-to-6-day period (figure 11–10).

Reports of multimodality therapy indicate that approximately 50% of patients with malignant gliomas survive one year and 25% survive 18 months [21]. It should be recalled that to be eligible for a randomized study designed to evalute multimodality therapies a patient must have a sufficient performance scale (Karnovsky) rating. Furthermore, significant variables, such as the patient's age at time of diagnosis and the extent of surgical resection, have not been well controlled in previous studies. It is probable that the actual results of treating glioblastoma and anaplastic astrocytoma are far worse than published results. The confounding variables have been well defined by Shapiro [21].

Our results (median postdiagnosis survival rate) for interstitial brachytherapy (glioblastomas and anaplastic astrocytomas treated without adjunctive chemotherapy) equaled or surpassed published results for multimodality treatment that included chemotherapy. We consider these findings preliminary but promising, warranting further investigation in multicenter, randomized, controlled trials. No patient undergoing interstitial brachytherapy developed an increased neurological deficit or postoperative hematoma; one patient had a superficial burr-hole infection. Since we switched to a twist-drill percutaneous insertion technique, we have had no patient with subsequent infection even though the catheters were left implanted through the skin for five to seven days. Postimplantation, cerebral swelling and/or radiation necrosis occurred in approximately 30% of all cases. Three patients subsequently required a craniotomy, "debulking" of the necrotic tumor mass, and a prolonged course of corticosteroid medication. Histological samples taken at the time of cytoreductive surgery following interstitial brachytherapy revealed features of both radiation necrosis and continued tumor growth, indicating the need for further efforts in the treatment of malignant gliomas.

INTRACAVITARY IRRADIATION

Cystic neoplasms of the brain were treated with intracavitary implantation of a beta-emitting isotope designed to provide a lethal radiation dose to the secreting cells of the cyst wall. Since 1971, this approach has been advocated by Backlund [3], who has treated more than 100 cases of solitary or multicystic craniopharyngiomas. Backlund's results surpassed those reported for conventional irradiation

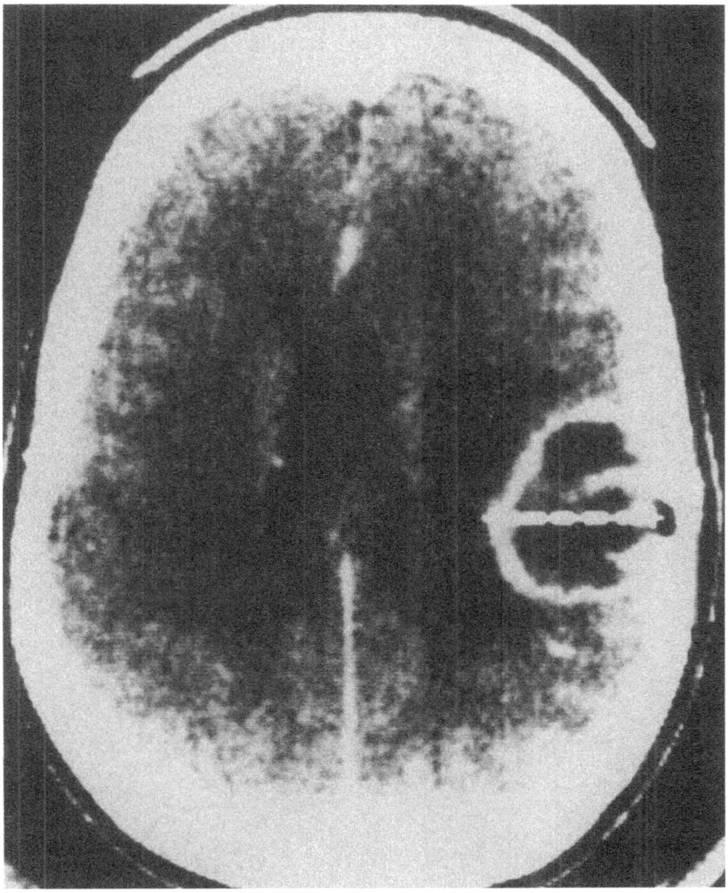

A

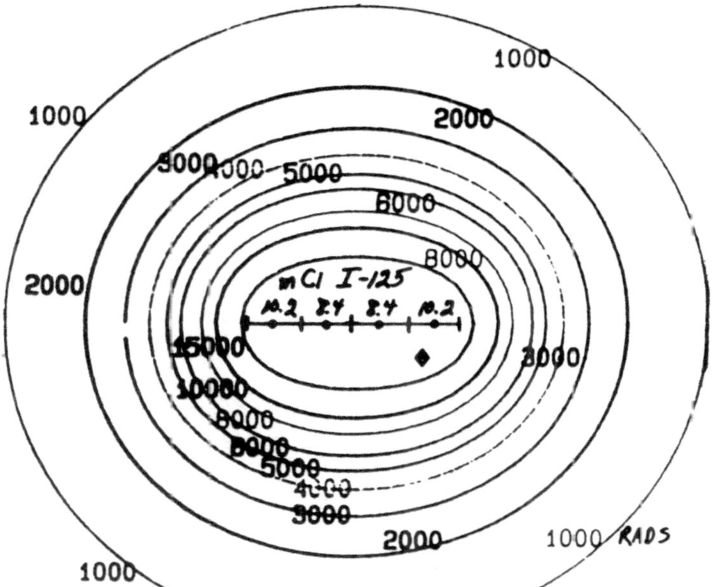

B

FIGURE 11–10. Intraoperative CT scan of a patient undergoing implantation of ^{125}Iodine seeds for brachytherapy (A). Brachytherapy dosimetry (B) for a solitary catheter implanted from a left temporoparietal trajectory. Four ^{125}I seeds were implanted (total mCi = 37.2) 1,000 cGy per day were delivered to the enhanced tumor margin. Postoperative CT scan 11 months after ^{125}I brachytherapy (C).

C

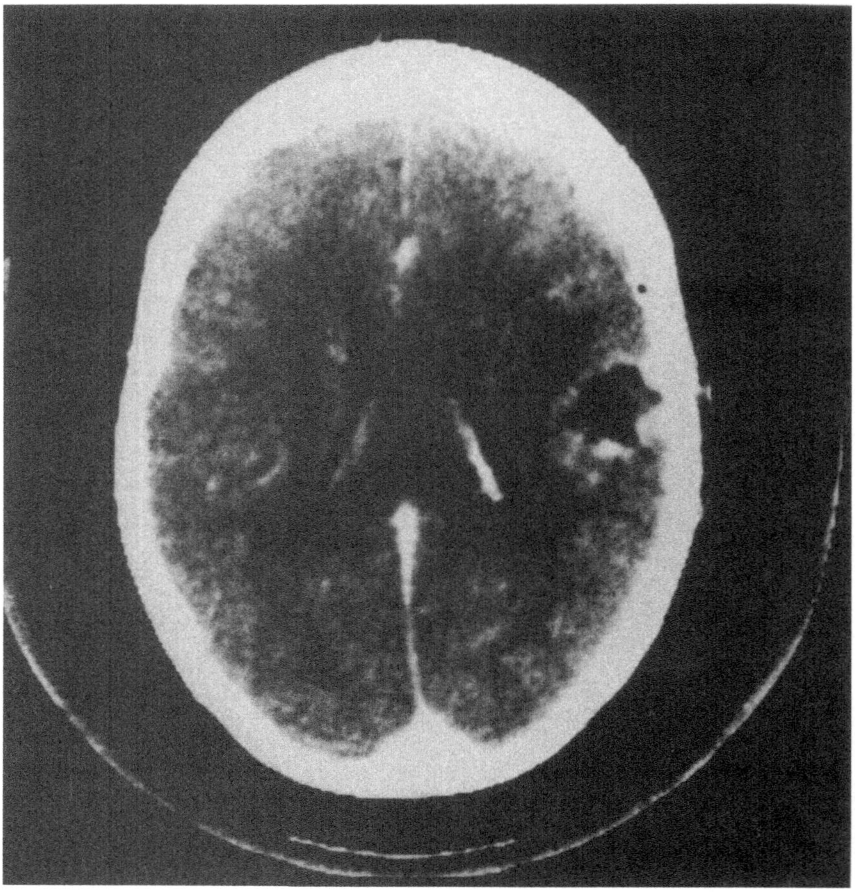

FIGURE 11–10. (cont.)

and/or surgical resection. Beta-emitting isotopes used for intracavitary irradiation include yttrium-90 rhenium-186 and phosphorous-32 (^{32}P). In the United States, only ^{32}P chromic phosphate in colloidal suspension is available for intracavitary irradiation.

The dosage of ^{32}P was calculated to provide a total cyst-wall dosage of 25,000 cGy administered over five half-lives of the isotope (70.2 days). Because the half-value tissue penetration of the beta-emitting energy of ^{32}P is 1.1 mm, the radiation effects virtually were limited to the cyst wall. Accurate calculation of the cyst volume was mandatory for dosimetry. We used two techniques for volume calculations and performed an experimental analysis of both. The technique reported by Backlund [3], who used intracystic technetium-^{99}m to measure cyst volume, remains the bench mark. More recently, we have used CT scanning alone; the standard computer software of the CT scanner has enabled us to measure the area of the cyst on each slice in square centimeters and to multiply the summed areas by the slice thickness to obtain the volume. We found no significant variation in cyst-volume estimation or dosimetry when we compared the isotope dilution technique described by Backlund with the CT technique [12].

After the stereotactic frame was applied, we performed high-resolution CT imaging of the brain to measure the cyst volume. The cyst was punctured by a 0.9-mm sharp needle designed to make the smallest possible hole in the cyst. Because the cyst had to kept at its preoperative volume, we removed only enough fluid to allow the introduction of the ^{32}P. The minimal amount of aspirated cyst fluid was sent for a microscopic analysis that included an examination for the presence of cholesterol crystals.

All nine patients with solitary cystic craniopharyngiomas demonstrated cyst regression, stabilization of preexisting endocrinological deficits, and stabilization or improvement in visual field defects (figure 11–11). Three patients with cystic glial neoplasms were treated. Cyst regression occurred in all cases, but subsequent growth of the solid portions of the tumor ultimately resulted in the death of all three patients. Stereotactic implantation of intracavitary irradiation with a beta-emitting isotope should be the primary treatment of solitary cystic or multicystic craniopharyngiomas. We believe that microsurgical resection should be limited to patients with solid craniophayrngiomas.

Complications and Concerns: Diagnostic and Therapeutic Stereotactic Surgery

POSTOPERATIVE COMPLICATIONS

Postoperative complications in our 240 patients are summarized in table 11–4. Cerebral hematomas occurred in eight patients. In three patients (1.3%), postoperative CT scans demonstrated either an intratumoral hematoma (one case) or an intraventricular hemorrhage (two cases of lesions involving the choroid plexus). Five additional patients had major intracerebral hematomas that required craniotomy and evacuation; none suffered an operative mortality because the hematomas were evacuated promptly. However, all five patients who required hematoma evacuations had increased neurological deficits in comparison to their preoperative status. Only one patient with a malignant glioma suffered an intracerebral hematoma. Postoperative hematomas occurred in two patients with brain abscesses, both of whom had very large abscesses that were vigorously drained by stereotactic technique. Brain abscesses are friable lesions with extensive neovascularization and blood vessel fragility. Based on these two complications, we recognized that minimal aspiration (followed by catheter drainage in large abscesses) was sufficient for clinical cure when coupled with appropriate long-term intravenous antibiotic therapy.

In one patient with a pontine CNS lymphoma, a postoperative cerebellar hematoma developed six hours after surgery; this patient had an unrecognized bleeding diathesis. One patient developed a frontal lobe hematoma at the site of a biopsy performed in the course of an evaluation for dementia. This patient had poorly controlled hypertension during surgery. Of the eight cases of hematoma, six were recognized on the immediate postoperative CT scan; three required immediate craniotomy and evacuation.

Two patients developed wound infections at the site of the burr hole, and one developed a wound seroma in the incision site. Preoperative vigilance for possible clotting abnormalities, strict control of systemic hypertension both during and after surgery, and avoiding vigorous drainage of brain abscesses would have prevented most of these complications.

Among our patients, we identified no correlation between the contrast-enhancement pattern or the preoperative angiographic demonstration of tumor vascularity and the risk of postoperative hemorrhage. Two patients with glial neoplasms developed postoperative hematomas, one of whom required a craniotomy and evacuation. The source of bleeding in this latter patient was found to be a small laceration of a subcortical artery.

Concerns and Cautions

Stereotactic biopsy and therapy are safe and effective techniques to diagnose and to treat lesions throughout the brain. Although it has been used advantageously to eliminate diagnostic confusion, stereotactic surgery still must be regarded as a potentially risky procedure. When the preoperative differential diagnosis is extensive, brain biopsy may not answer the clinical question and should not precede a thorough and extensive evaluation for possible systemic causes of a brain lesion. We do not advocate stereotactic biopsy in cases of dementia unless an appropriate lesion can be identified by CT or MRI. In the evaluation of an apparent brain metastasis, we perform a brief

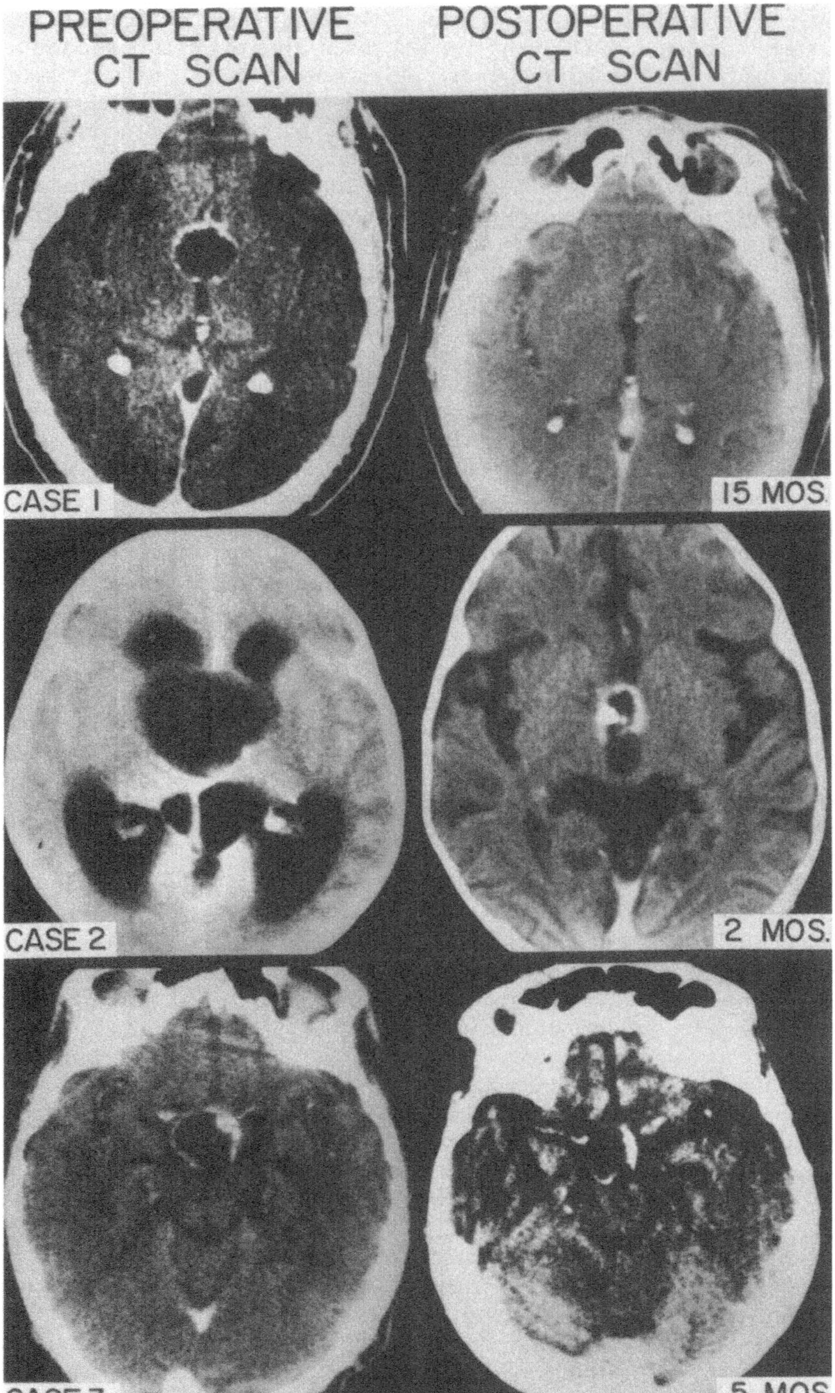

A

FIGURE 11–11. (A, B, and C) Preoperative and postoperative CT images of nine cases with intracranial cystic neoplasms, all of whom underwent stereotactic ^{32}P placement. Cyst repression was observed in all cases. (Reprinted with permission from *Appl Neurophysiol* 48:146–150, 1985.)

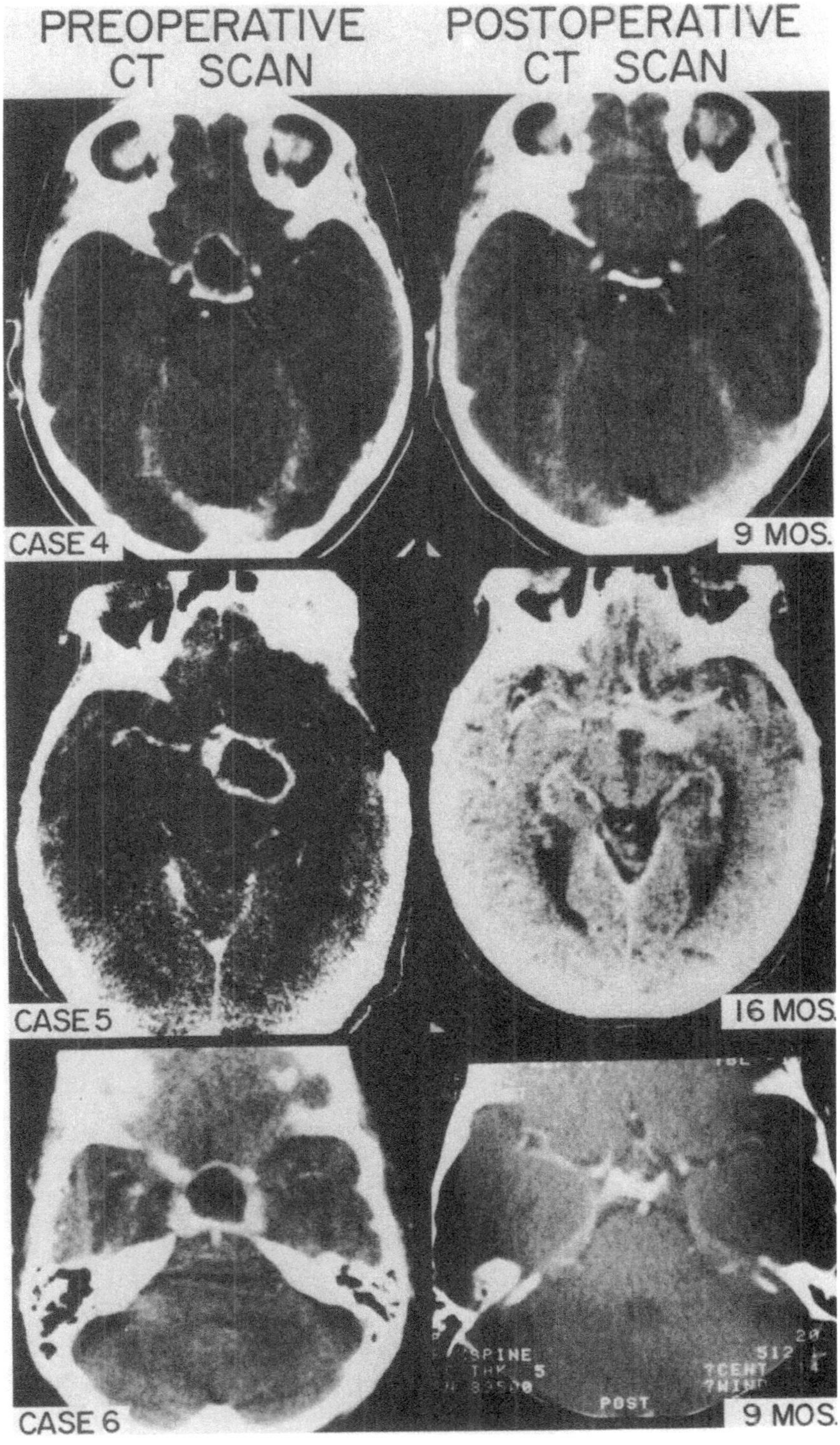

B

FIGURE 11–11. (cont.)

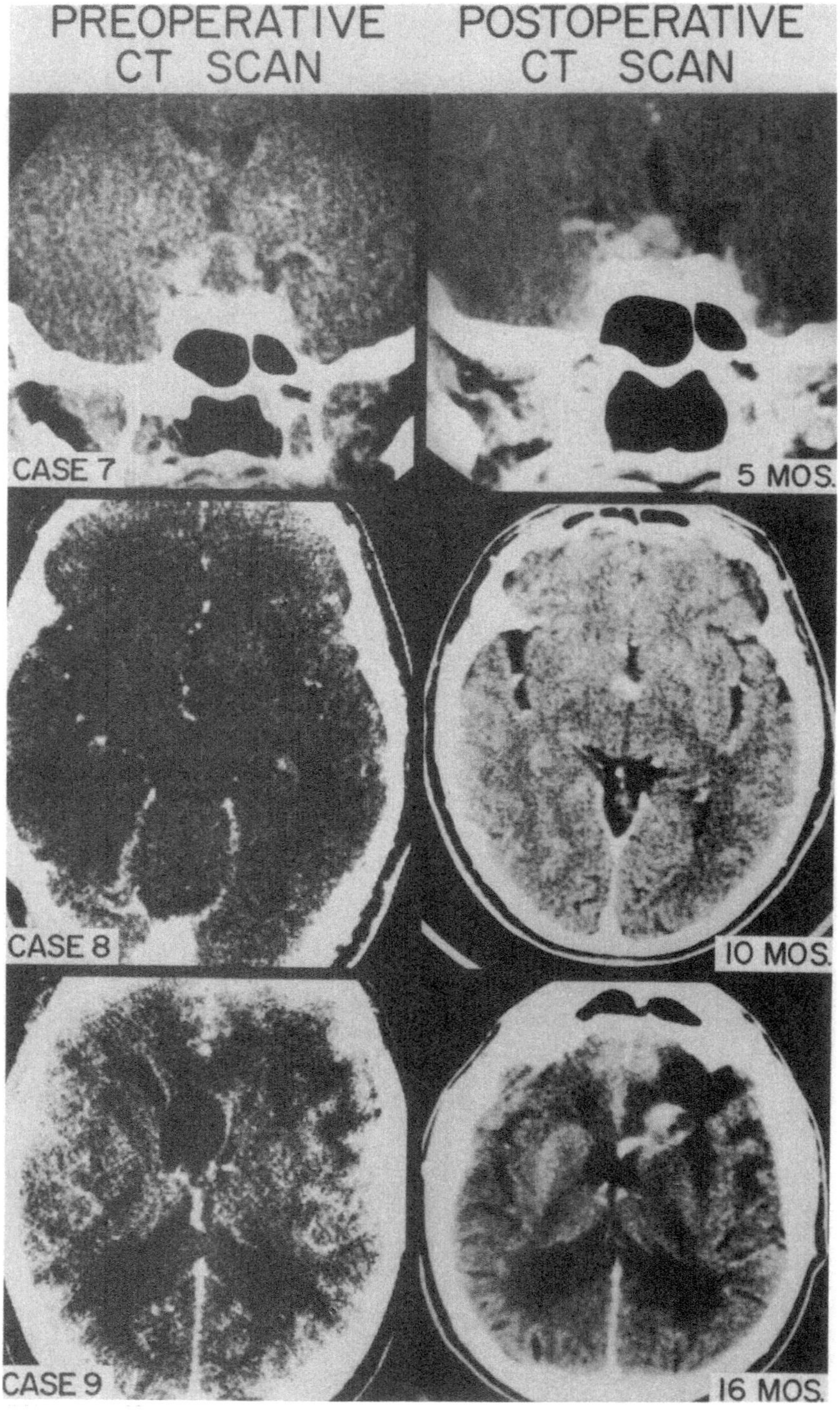

C

FIGURE 11–11. (cont.)

TABLE 11-4. CT Stereotactic Surgery at Presbyterian-University Hospital, Pittsburgh, PA, 1981-1985: Postoperative Complications in 240 Diagnostic Cases

Complication	No. Cases	Percentage
Mortality	0	0
Intracerebral hematoma		
With clinical symptomatology[a]	5	2.1
Without clinical symptomatology[b]	3	1.3
Wound		
Infection (burr-hole site)	2	0.8
Seroma	1	0.4
Total	11	4.6

[a] Required craniotomy and evacuation.
[b] Demonstrated by postoperative CT scan.

series of screening tests to search for a primary lesion before proceeding directly to stereotactic biopsy. These tests include a chest x-ray and CT scans of the chest and abdomen.

Because of the risk of contamination of the stereotactic instruments and the subsequent need for extensive sterilization procedures involving hypochlorite solutions, we do not perform stereotactic biopsies in cases of suspected slow viral infections. Despite the advances in both CT and MRI radiological techniques, we currently do not believe that either technique provides a sensitive indication of actual histological tumor margins; thus, these tools should be carefully assessed as a means to determine subsequent interstitial brachytherapy dose planning.

Our experience with the Leksell stereotactic system has demontrated that it is a versatile, practical, and simple device for the diagnosis and treatment of lesions located throughout the brain and brain stem. Stereotactic surgery is integrated firmly within the field of modern neurosurgery.

References

1. Andrews BT, Halks-Miller M, Berger MS, et al: Neuro-epithelial cysts of the posterior fossa: Pathogenesis and report of two cases. *Neurosurgery* 15:91-95, 1984
2. Backlund EO: A new instrument for stereotaxic brain tumor biopsy. *Acta Neurol Scand* 137:825-827, 1971
3. Backlund EO: Studies in craniopharyngioma. Stereotaxic treatment with intracystic yttrium 90. *Acta Chir Scand* 139:237-247, 1973
4. Bernstein M, Gutin PH: Interstitial irradiation of brain tumors. A review. *Neurosurgery* 9:741-750, 1981
5. Coffey RJ, Lunsford LD: Stereotactic surgery for mass lesions of the midbrain and pons. *Neurosurgery* 17:12-18, 1985
6. Gutin PH, Phillips TL, Wara WM, et al: Brachytherapy of recurrent malignant brain tumors with removable high-activity iodine-125 sources. *J Neurosurg* 60:61-68, 1984
7. Latchaw RE, Lunsford LD, Kennedy WH: Reformatted imaging to define the intercommissural line for CT-guided stereotactic functional neurosurgery *AJNR* 6:429-433, 1985
8. Lunsford LD: A dedicated CT-system for the stereotactic operating room. *Appl Neurophysiol* 45:374-378, 1982
9. Lunsford LD: The role of CT-guided stereotaxy in morphologic and functional surgery of the human brain. In Latchaw RE (ed): *Computed Tomography of the Head, Neck, and Spine*. Chicago: Yearbook, 1984, pp 743-764
10. Lunsford LD, Latchaw RE, Vries J: Stereotaxic implantation of deep brain electrodes using computed tomography. *Neurosurgery* 13:280-286, 1983
11. Lunsford LD, Leksell L, Jernberg B: Probe holder for stereotactic surgery in the CT scanner: A technical note. *Acta Neurochir* (Wien) 69:297-304, 1983
12. Lunsford LD, Levine G, Gumerman LW: A comparison of computed tomographic and radionuclide methods to determine intracranial cystic tumor volumes. *J Neurosurg* 63:740-744, 1985
13. Lunsford LD, Maroon JC: CT localization and biopsy of intracranial lesions. In Schmidek HD, Sweet WH (eds): *Current Techniques in Operative Neurosurgery* (2nd ed). Orlando, FL: Grune & Stratton, 1982, pp 403-418
14. Lunsford LD, Martinez AJ: Stereotactic exploration of the brain in the CT era. *Surg Neurol* 22:222-230, 1984
15. Lunsford LD, Martinez AJ, Latchaw RE: Stereotaxic surgery with a magnetic resonance and computerized tomography compatible system. *J Neurosurg* 16: , 1986
16. Lunsford LD, Nelson PB, Rosenbaum AE: Stereotactic aspiration of a brain abscess using the therapeutic CT scanner: Case report. *Acta Neurchir* (Wien) 62:25-29, 1982
17. Lunsford LD, Parrish R, Albright L: Intraoperative imaging with a therapeutic CT scanner. Technical note. *Neurosurgery* 15:559-561, 1984
18. Lunsford LD, Perry JE, Rosenbaum AE: Stereotactic surgery using the therapeutic CT scanner. *Surg Neurol* 18:116-122, 1982

19. Perry JH, Rosenbaum AE, Lunsford LD: Computed tomography–guided stereotactic surgery: Conception and development of a new stereotactic methodology. *Neurosurgery* 7:376–378, 1980
20. Rosenbaum AE, Lunsford LD, Perry JH: Computerized tomography–guided stereotaxis: A new approach. *Appl Neurophysiol* 43:172–173, 1980
21. Shapiro WR: Multimodality therapy of malignant gliomas. *Barrow Neurological Institute Quarterly* 1:48–52, 1985

12. VOLUMETRIC STEREOTAXIS AND COMPUTER-ASSISTED STEREOTACTIC RESECTION OF SUBCORTICAL LESIONS

Patrick J. Kelly

Intracranial tumor volume can be defined in stereotactic space by computed tomography (CT), magnetic resonance imaging (MRI), or serial stereotactic biopsies [2, 18, 21]. The defined volume can be treated by stereotactically implanted interstitial radionuclide sources, which create a therapeutic isodose configuration geometrically fitted to the defined tumor volume [24, 26, 27]. Alternatively, the tumor volume can be interactively resected by the computer-assisted stereotactic laser procedure described in this chapter [14, 17, 25].

System Development

Volume stereotaxis was first utilized in attempts to more accurately plan interstitial radionuclide source placements in deep-seated neoplasms. Life-sized clay models of the lesions were built from contour templates derived from enlarged CT axial images and reconstructions. These models could be sliced perpendicularly to the intended implantation angles. Simulated radionuclide sources and resultant isodose contours were superimposed to derive an optimal placement of the sources, which delivered a lethal dose of radiation to the global tumor volume while maintaining safe radiation levels in surrounding brain tissue.

Many lesions were too complex geometrically to permit fitting to the lesional volume a precise isodose configuration produced by a finite number of radionuclide sources. Other lesions were too large to consider interstitial irradiation as a safe therapeutic option. In addition, some tumors grew so rapidly that they were too large to be successfully treated by acceptable amounts of radiation by the time the therapeutic dose level had been accumulated [9]. Therefore, some other means of reducing tumor burden had to be developed.

Unfortunately, the deep location of most of the subcortical tumors in our patients precluded conventional surgical resection because of localization problems during an open operation: a surgeon risked getting lost while attempting to find a subcortical tumor. This risk was increased the deeper the procedure extended below the cortical surface. Therefore, to localize these subcortical tumors, stereotactic techniques were incorporated into conventional craniotomies.

We performed our first stereotactic craniotomies using a standard Todd-Wells frame, an operating microscope, and a carbon dioxide laser directed from a microslad on the microscope [15, 16]. Tumor targets were represented as a series of contours on anteroposterior (AP) and lateral stereotactic teleradiographs, and the progress of these procedures was monitored by serial radiographs. However, intraoperatively defining tumor margins from edematous brain tissue and maintaining orientation within complex three-dimensional tumor volumes remained a problem.

Independently, we had begun using an operating-room computer system to model and display a computer-resident stereotactic atlas during functional stereotactic surgery [5, 13, 22]. Digitized outlines of the atlas substruc-

L.D. Lunsford (ed.) *MODERN STEREOTACTIC NEUROSURGERY*.

tures, suspended in a three-dimensional computer-image matrix, could be displayed along any arbitrary plane usually parallel or orthogonal to a probe trajectory. Tumor outlines also could be digitized from contiguous CT slices, suspended in the same image matrix, and similarly reformatted.

In our initial system, atlases and tumor section images were transferred by data link to a microprocessor (Apple II with Tektronix simulator board) in the operating room. The stereotactic head holder was modified for CT compatibility, and a localization system for the Todd-Wells stereotactic frame was developed [6, 17]. The reference marks created by the localization system and multiple points around the boundary of the lesion on each CT image were digitized manually with a digitizing tablet. A computer program interpolated a tumor volume and calculated the mechanical adjustments on the Todd-Wells frame, which centered the interpolated volume in its focal point. Next, we attempted to relate the position of the surgical laser beam to the reformatted tumor outlines.

A 400-mm-radius arc quadrant holding the operating microscope was constructed. This mounted on the base unit of the standard Todd-Wells frame such that the focal points of the 400-mm and the standard 135-mm arc quadrant were the same. The carbon dioxide laser beam, delivered to a manipulator box (microslad) on the operating microscope, was deflected into the surgical field by a mirror controlled by a joystick. A double-gimballed attachment, fitted onto the joystick, transmitted the joystick's movements to potentiometers mounted on the X and Y axles of the gimbals. The potentiometers converted the joystick's movements to voltages, which were transferred to the game-paddle ports of the Apple II microprocessor; the microprocessor then positioned a cursor on the display screen in calibrated relationship to the position of the laser in the surgical field [17]. This was displayed along with the tumor outlines generated by the computer. Thus, the surgeon received real-time feedback on the spatial position of the surgical instrument (laser) in relationship to the stereotactically positioned target volume [24].

Many changes in hardware and software and refinements in methodology have taken place since the development of these first interactive surgical procedures. The stereotactic frame was modified significantly, and the software was expanded to increase the efficiency and accuracy of data input and surgical interaction [12]. MRI and digital angiography are now incorporated into the surgical data base [14, 25].

As technology evolved, clinical experience with a variety of subcortical and deep-seated lesions was gathered. This chapter describes the current instrumentation and methodology for computer-assisted stereotactic laser microsurgery and summarizes clinical experience with the procedure at the Mayo Medical School.

Instrumentation

STEREOTACTIC FRAME

The instrument currently used for computer-assisted stereotactic laser microsurgery is described in chapter 6 and elsewhere [12, 23, 28]. A servomotor-controlled three-dimensional slide system positions an intracranial target point into the focal point of the arc quadrants attached to the instrument's base plate. A 400-mm-radius arc quadrant indexes into position when stereotactic control is required during a craniotomy. Smaller arc quadrants (135-mm and 160-mm radii) are used to direct intracranial biopsy probes and to hold the stereotactic retractors through which tumors are exposed and removed (figure 12–1).

A microscope and laser-manipulator apparatus (microslad) travel per-pendicular to a tangent to the 400-mm arc quadrant and are thus directed to the focal point of the arc quadrant, regardless of the arc or collar angles selected. The focal distances of the microscope and microslad from the focal point of the arc quadrant are controlled by a servomotorized drive system on the carriage. Optical encoders (Bausch & Lomb Acu-Rite II, Rochester, NY) on the microscope/microslad carriage and on the three-axis slide system record the distances of the microscope and laser foci from the focal points of the arc quadrant and the X, Y, and Z stereotactic coordinates, respectively, and relay this information to digital display units on the control panel. The microscope/microslad drive system is controlled by foot pedal; the X, Y, and Z frame coordinates are set by switches on the control panel, which is operated by a technician.

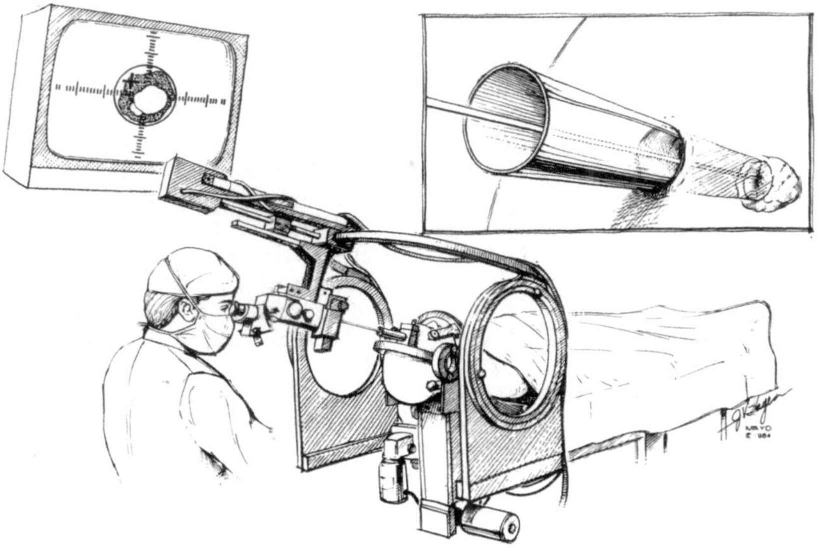

FIGURE 12–1. Instrumentation for computer-assisted stereotactic laser microsurgery: The operating microscope and microslad are suspended from a 400-mm arc quadrant; the stereotactic retractor is directed to the tumor by internal arc quadrant. A computer display terminal shows slices of tumor volume defined by CT and MRI at the level of retractor insertion. The laser's position in the surgical field is indicated by a cursor on screen.

MICROSLAD

The carbon dioxide laser and HE-NE aiming beam are delivered to the microslad from a Sharplan 743 surgical laser (Sharplan 743, Laser Industries, Tel-Aviv, Israel) by an articulated optical arm. The beams pass through a variable focus lens system (which changes the focal length and thus the spot size) and then are reflected by two mirrors which ultimately direct the laser beams into the surgical field. These mirrors are mounted on the shafts of galvanometers which have a pitch related to a voltage supplied by the digital-to-analog (DAC) board of the operating-room computer system. Specific voltages supplied by the DAC to the galvanometers deflect the laser beam in a precise and reproducible manner at a given focal length in the surgical field.

A joystick, controlled by the surgeon, transmits the desired positions of the laser beam in the surgical field to the computer system by optical encoders within the joystick assembly. The digital pulses from the encoders are instantaneously converted to voltages related to galvanometers in the microslad; these galvanometers position the laser beam at the required location in the surgical field. On an operating room display monitor, the cursor displays the position of the laser beam in an X–Y grid centered on the surgical viewline. Reconstruction of the CT and MRI-defined tumor volumes, scanned perpendicular to the viewline at the focus levels of the microscope and laser, are also displayed on the monitor in relationship to this grid. In addition, the computer can supply voltages to the microslad galvanometers by preset patterning programs for automatic sweeping of the laser beam during tumor vaporization.

STEREOTACTIC RETRACTORS

Cylindrical retractors attach to the 135-mm or 160-mm arc quadrants and are secured by a collet. Retractors 140-mm long and 1, 2, or 3 cm in diameter are available. During surgery, the depth of stereotactic insertion is calculated by measuring the length of the retractor portion extending outside its mounting bracket on the arc quadrant. The following equation is used: depth = 140 − (M − R), where *depth* is the distance of the retractor along the surgical viewline to or beyond the focal point of the arc quadrant, M is the distance measured between the retractor mount on the arc and the extending end of the retractor, and R is the radius of the arc quadrant used.

During surgery, a dilator, inserted through the retractor, separates a subcortical incision made by the laser. After this, the retractor may be advanced over the dilator to a deeper location.

ACCESSORY INSTRUMENTS

When stereotactic retractors are used, extra-long bipolar forceps (Radionics Inc., Burlington, MA) with a shaft length of 150-mm are required to control bleeding in the surgical field. Suctions, tips, dissectors, and alligator scissors 150- to 160-mm long are also used.

Database Acquisition

Patients undergo stereotactic CT scanning or MRI with their heads secured in the CT/MRI-compatible head holders [6, 12, 14, 17–25]. Slices 5-mm thick are gathered through the target lesion with the use of medium body format on the General Electric 8800 CT scanning unit. Axial magnetic resonance images 5-mm thick are obtained on the Picker resistive system or the General Electric 2 Tesla system.

Stereotactic stereoscopic cerebral angiography is also performed on General Electric DF 3000 or 5000 digital angiographic systems. To localize major sulci, the deep vessel segments (apparent on the stereoscopic view) are marked on the orthogonal arterial and venous phases of the stereotactic angiogram [30].

Tumor Volume Interpolation

The archived data tapes from the CT and MRI examinations are transferred to the operating-room computer system. (Independent Physician's Diagnostic Console [IPDC] for General Electric 8800 CT Scanning Unit, General Electric Medical Systems Division, New Berlin, WI.) The surgeon views each of the CT and magnetic resonance images that demonstrate the target lesion, then digitizes the boundary of each on contiguous CT and magnetic resonance images, using the display unit's cursor, trackball subsystem, and deposit key, as described in chapter 7. In addition, a point in the approximate geographical center of the lesion on one of the CT images is digitized as the reference target point. The interpolated CT and MRI-defined volumes will be constructed about this point, and calculations will be given that center this point in the focal point of the stereotactic arc-quadrant frame. The CT- and MRI-defined volumes may then be sliced perpendicular to any specified viewline that is expressed in arc and collar angles on the stereotactic instrument. This data also will be reformatted for any desired surgical position and expressed as patient rotation (0 = supine, 90° = right shoulder down, lateral decubitus, 180° = prone, etc.). The actual numbers for patient rotation and arc and collar angles are determined from surgical planning.

Surgical Planning

Ideally, tumors should be approached from the closest possible cranial entry point along the long axis of the lesion, with a trajectory that traverses nonessential brain tissue in a direction parallel to major white-matter projections. This approach trajectory or viewline is specified to the computer as arc and collar angle settings on the stereotactic instrument.

However, in many instances, not all of these conditions are possible, and the selected approach will be a compromise designed to preserve the patient's neurological function by preventing injury to essential neurological tissue. Thus, the stereotactic relationship of important neural and vascular structures to the tumor volume must be established, and the surgical approach planned to circumvent them. For instance, the precentral convolution cannot be traversed if a neurological deficit is to be avoided. Therefore, deep precentral lesions are approached anteriorly through a microsurgically split precentral sulcus. Posterior approaches are used for lesions located behind the central sulcus. On the other hand, lesions that extend to within a few millimeters of the cortical surface can be approached directly with an incision in the crown of the overlying an nonviable gyrus.

Anterior thalamic lesions are exposed by a retracted incision through the anterior limb of the internal capsule; unilateral lesions should be well tolerated. Posterior thalamic lesions are approached through a transcortical incision at the temporal occipital junction, with the patient prone (180° rotation) or semiprone (135° rotation for left-sided lesions, 225° for right-sided lesions). Dorsal thalamic lesions are exposed and resected through the lateral ventricular floor.

Midline posterior fossa lesions are exposed through the vermis; lateral lesions are exposed through the cerebellar hemisphere. Midline pontine lesions that elevate and extend to the floor of the fourth ventricle are resected through a midline incision in the floor of the ventricle. In these cases, the head holder is rotated 30° on the receiving yoke of the base unit toward the surgeon to provide a comfortable working situation; an arc angle of 30° returns the surgical approach to the midline. Computer software recalculates the target point for any patient rotation so that the derived frame adjustments continue to place the target point in the focal point.

Lateral pontine lesions are exposed through the middle cerebellar peduncle. In this case, the patient is prone (180° rotation) and the arc angle is approximately 30° to 40° on the side of the lesion.

As is evident, the surgical approach is expressed in terms of patient rotation (which depends on the working position most comfortable for the surgeon) and arc and collar angles (which depend on the safest line of attack to the lesion). It is advisable to simulate the arc and collar settings on an arc quadrant after the patient is positioned in the stereotactic frame. This will ensure that the determined angles provide the best working situation. During the surgical procedure, the computer continuously displays the patient rotation, the arc and collar angles, and the stereotactic frame settings, along with the image displays (figure 12–2A, B).

Surgical Procedure

The patient is given general endotracheal anesthesia, and the stereotactic head frame is replaced; the pin placements and micrometer settings used during the data acquisition phase are again utilized. The patient is positioned in the stereotactic frame such that index marks on the receiving yoke line up with the marks on the headholder that indicate the desired rotation. After the head is prepped and draped, the 135-mm-radius arc quadrant is installed, and the patient's head is moved to position the target point onto the focal point. The arc and collar angles are selected and secured.

To monitor possible intracranial shifts in the tumor after the skull and dura are opened, the following procedure is recommended: The skull is opened with a stereotactically directed 1/8-inch drill, and the tumor is traversed with a biopsy cannula. A series of stainless steel balls (0.5-mm in diameter) are deposited at 5-mm intervals along the viewline (figure 12–3). The position of these markers on AP and lateral stereotactic teleradiographs provide reference points for any subsequent intracranial shifts that are detected. If a shift of the reference markers is detected (which is extremely uncommon in our experience), the position of the tumor volume is shifted in the computer image matrix in order to take this into account in the subsequent image displays. Next, the scalp is opened with a linear incision, and the skull is opened with a 1½ to 2-inch cranial trephine centered on the twist-drill hole through which the reference balls were deposited. The dura is opened in a cruciate fashion. At this point, the procedure varies depending on whether the lesion is superficial or deep.

SUPERFICIAL LESIONS

The computer displays the configuration of the trephine in relationship to the reformatted tumor outlines (see figure 12–2A). This keeps the surgeon oriented during removal of the tumor. A section of the cortex the same size and configuration as the most superficial tumor image is removed with bipolar forceps and scissors. A plane is then created around the tumor with bipolar forceps or stereotactically directed laser. The surgeon should refer frequently to the computer monitor during the resection while isolating the lesion from surrounding brain tissue. With this technique, high-grade gliomas can be removed intact. A plane of dissection is *always* found around these tumors corresponding to the contrast-enhancing margin on CT scan. After the specimen is removed, the "tumor bed" appears to be edematous white matter, which a biopsy will confirm. Unfortunately, biopsies also disclose isolated tumor cells within this edematous white matter.

DEEP TUMORS

The display monitor shows the position of the cylindrical retractor as a circle on the CT image

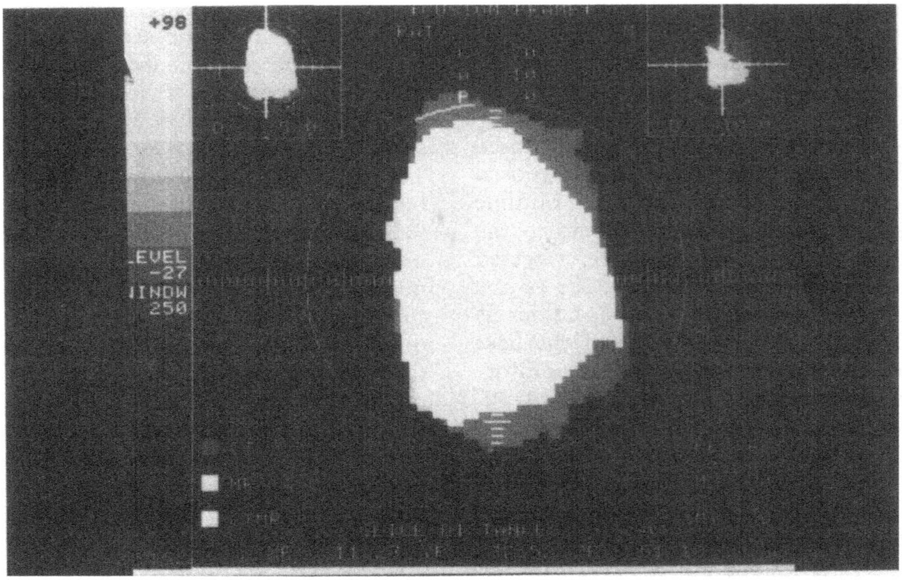

A

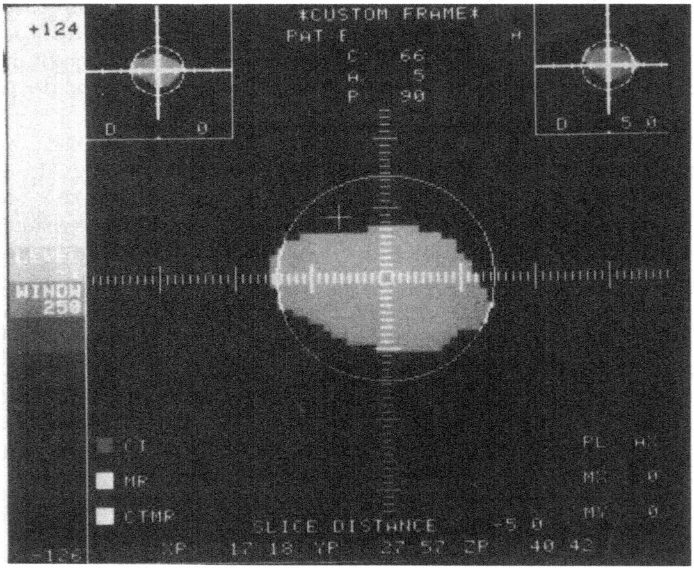

B

FIGURE 12–2. (A) The computer displays the configuration of a 5-cm trephine superimposed on reformatted slices of superficial tumor sliced perpendicular to viewline. Different gray levels indicate CT and MRI-defined limits. A "lookahead" sequence displays serial tumor sections at specified intervals. The circle indicates the position of the cylindrical retractor. (B) Computer displays arc and collar settings; patient rotation; and the X, Y, and Z frame settings corresponding to the surgical situation displayed on the screen.

of the tumor. The surgical laser position is shown by the cursor. A "lookahead" option displays deeper tumor images along the viewline so that the surgeon can anticipate the configuration of the tumor as it will be encountered during the procedure (see figure 12–2A). Using the computer display as a guide, the surgeon creates a plane of dissection around

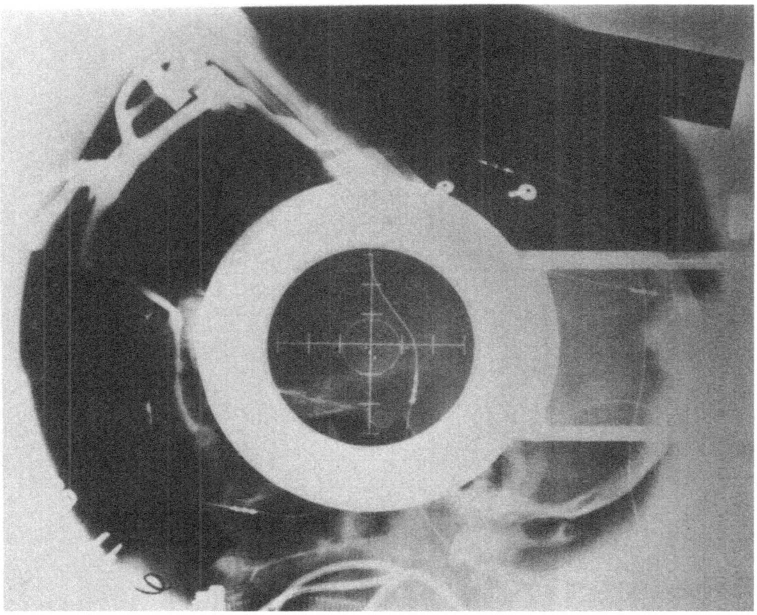

FIGURE 12–3. A lateral teleradiograph documents the position of stainless steel reference balls that have been deposited stereotactically along surgical viewline.

the lesion with the laser, advances the retractor, and deepens the incision circumscribing the tumor. Tumor within the retractor is then removed with 65–85 watts of defocused laser power in either the manual or automatic mode. (In the automatic mode, the computer sweeps the laser beam by specified programmed sequence, based on the CT- or MRI-defined tumor limits.) Thus, the tumor is removed slice by slice, from the most superficial to the deepest. The surgeon monitors the surgical field view through the operating microscope, as well as the display screen, which indicates the locations of the laser and retractor relative to the CT- and MRI-defined tumor boundaries. AP and lateral teleradiographs are obtained to document the progress of the procedure and record possible movements of the reference balls (which are removed as they are encountered during the procedure) (figure 12–4). Hemostasis is achieved with the extra-long-bipolar forceps.

Results

Since 1980, 146 computer-assisted stereotactic craniotomies have been performed on 140 patients. Five patients underwent repeat procedures for residual (three patients) and recurrent (two patients) tumors, and one of these patients underwent a third procedure for recurrent tumor. Patients ranged in age from 2 to 78 years, with an average age of 46.8 years. Lesion locations are illustrated in figure 12–5, and histologies are listed in table 12–1. In neurological examinations performed one week after the procedure, 67 patients had improved neurologically, and 59 patients were neurologically unchanged (39 had been normal preoperatively and remained normal postoperatively; 20 patients had preoperative neurological deficits that did not improve postoperatively).

Seventeen patients were neurologically worse: seven patients developed superior-quadrant visual-field deficits following posterior temporal approaches to medial temporal or thalamic lesions, one patient had a complete homonymous hemianopia following an occipital approach to a posterior thalamic lesion, and nine patients experienced worsening of neurological deficits noted preoperatively. Three deaths occurred within one month after surgery: one from massive brain-stem edema following removal of a ventral thalamic astrocytoma with brain-stem infiltration apparent on MRI, one from a ventricular infection after

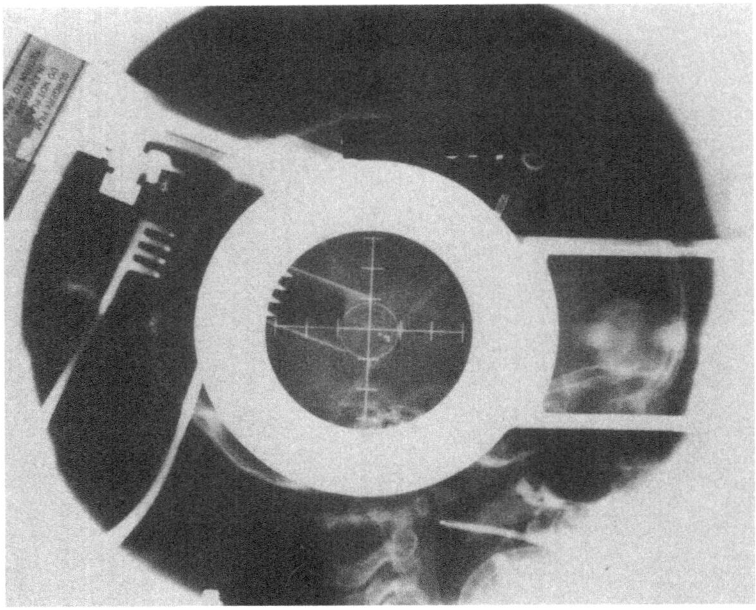

FIGURE 12–4. Lateral teleradiograph shows retractor position during resection of posterior thalamic astrocytoma.

TABLE 12–1. Tumor Histology in 140 Patients Undergoing Computer-Assisted Stereotactic Resections

Type of Lesion	No. of Patients
Astrocytoma grade IV	32
Astrocytoma grade III	12
Astrocytoma grade II	23
Metastatic	38
Oligodendroglioma	9
Vascular	14
Miscellaneous*	12
Total	140

* Lymphoma (2), Tuberous Sclerosis (2), Meningioma (3), Abscess (1), Choroid Plexis Papilloma (1), Colloid Cyst (1), Ganglioglioma (2).

resection of a previously irradiated teratoma from the third ventricle, and one from a massive pulmonary embolus two weeks after resection of a thalamic cavernous hemangioma.

From this overall experience, we have been able to draw some conclusions about the expedience of computer-assisted stereotactic laser microsurgery in specific lesions. In addition, we have derived certain technical maneuvers that are useful in the stereotactic removal of various lesions, depending on histology and anatomical location.

High-Grade Glial Tumors

Computer-assisted stereotactic resection can remove all CT-defined contrast-enhancing portions of glioblastomas from neurologically important subcortical areas, with acceptable levels of mortality and morbidity (figure 12–6). However, the mean postoperative survival of our patients harboring grade IV astrocytomas and treated with postoperative external-beam radiation therapy was only 38 weeks [23]. Even though postoperative CT studies in our series demonstrated the absence of contrast enhancement around the surgical defect, new areas of contrast enhancement developed within low-density areas close to and remote from the surgical defect within six to nine months after the procedure. Death in the majority of these cases was therefore due to tumor "recurrence" and progression.

Nevertheless, the survival times in our patients who had tumors in central and deep-seated locations (historically associated with poor survival and high surgical morbidity and

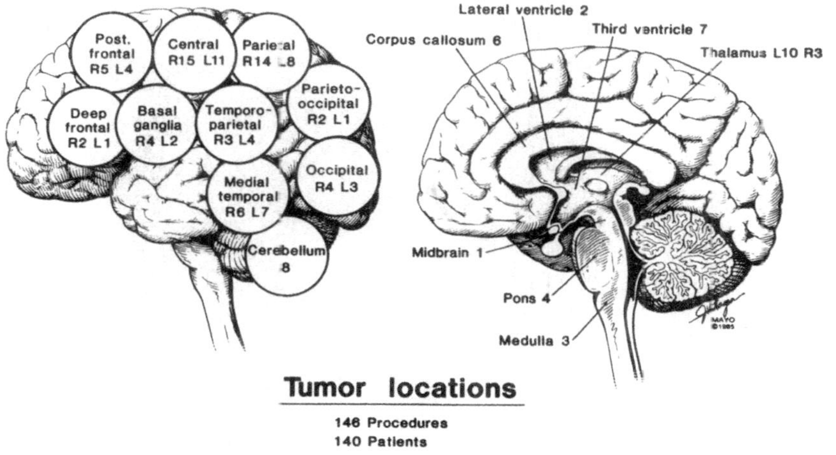

FIGURE 12-5. Tumor location in 146 computer-assisted stereotactic laser craniotomies.

mortality) [4, 8] is similar to those quoted in other series [3, 4, 8, 10, 11, 29, 31]. It should be noted, however, that a high percentage of the patients in these series had lesions in the frontal and temporal lobes, which are more amenable to radical surgical resection by lobectomy.

Preoperative stereotactic MRI (especially the T2-weighted image) always demonstrated much larger areas of abnormality than were indicated by CT scanning. It is likely that resection of the MRI-defined volume (technically feasible with our instrumentation) would remove a much more significant portion of the neoplasm, thereby increasing survival. However, examination of specimens from regions of CT contrast enhancement and CT hypodensity in patients with high-grade gliomas revealed that a large area of intact edematous brain parenchyma infiltrated by aggressive isolated tumor cells surrounds the mass of tumor tissue represented by CT contrast enhancement [1, 2, 18]. This edematous, infiltrated parenchyma appears to extend as far as the area of signal-prolongation abnormality on the T2-weighted MRI [18]. Theoretically, resection of the volume defined by the MRI abnormality would prolong postoperative survival [9]. However, unacceptable neurological deficits would result from removal of the intact, although infiltrated, parenchyma. Therefore, computer-assisted stereotactic resection of the volume of tissue defined by contrast enhancement on a CT scan permits reducing the tumor burden as aggressively as possible while still preserving neurological function in the majority of patients with grade IV astrocytomas.

A similar problem exists for patients with grade III astrocytomas and oligodendrogliomas. Although these tumors do not grow as rapidly as glioblastomas, isolated tumor cells infiltrate intact and surrounding edematous parenchyma [18]. Computer-assisted stereotactic resection does not cure these patients; tumors recur later in the patient's postoperative course than with glioblastomas, but generally in the same spatial pattern. However, as with glioblastomas, the procedure can remove all of the solid tumor tissue component of the neoplasm, which is defined by the contrast-enhancing volume on stereotactic CT scanning [23]. The surrounding low density on CT scans, and regions of prolonged signal abnormality on MRI again represent infiltrated, edematous but intact parenchyma [18].

Low-Grade Astrocytomas

The resectability of these tumors depends on the degree of histological circumscription. In adults, the tumor usually is manifested by an area of low density on the CT image and prolongation of signal on MRI. Stereotactic serial biopsy studies of these so-called fibrillary astrocytomas reveal that the tumor is composed almost entirely of infiltrated intact parenchyma, with little tumor tissue proper

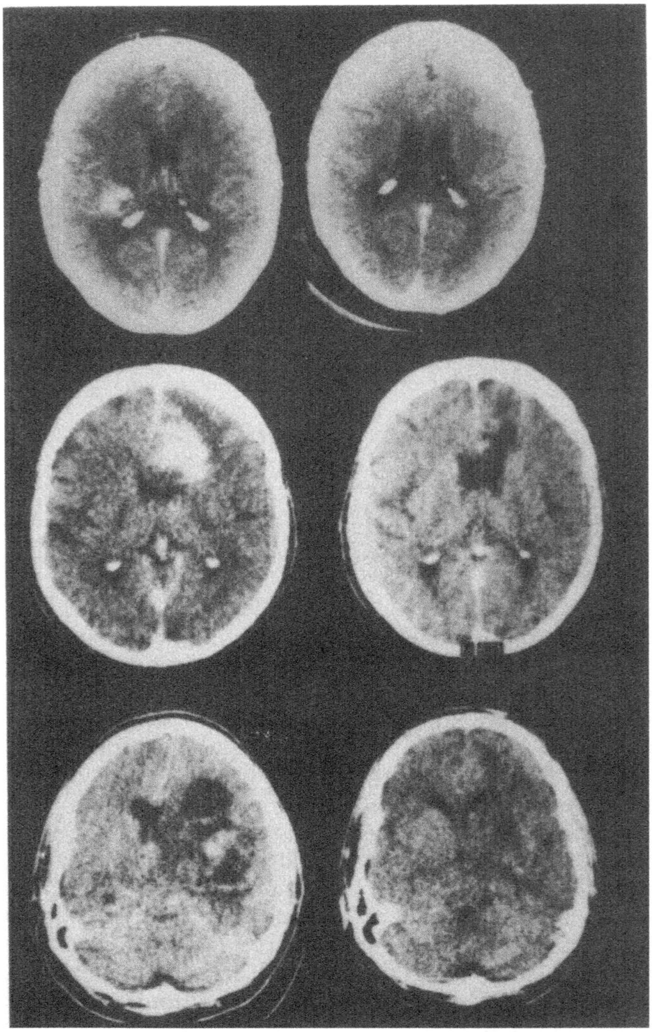

FIGURE 12–6. Preoperative and postoperative CT scans in three patients who underwent computer-assisted stereotactic laser resections: top—grade IV astrocytoma, deep-right parietal area; middle—grade IV astrocytoma in corpus callosum; bottom—grade III astrocytoma in basal ganglia.

[2, 18]. Therefore, resecting the tumor by stereotactic craniotomy involves resecting intact but infiltrated parenchyma, defined by the low-density areas on CT images and signal prolongation on MRI. In important brain areas, this results in a postoperative neurological deficit [14, 23].

On the other hand, pilocytic astrocytomas, which tend to occur in children in spite of the fact that many are located in the thalamus, are histologically circumscribed. They can be completely resected by computer-assisted stereotactic technique with excellent postoperative results (figure 12–7) [23]. The borders of these lesions are accurately defined by contrast enhancement on CT images [2, 18]. Occasionally, adults may develop pilocytic astrocytomas, but this is so unusual that we generally perform a confirmatory stereotactic biopsy before considering the patient for computer-assisted stereotactic laser resection.

Pontine astrocytomas are usually fibrillary and not well circumscribed. However, radiation therapy seems to demarcate these lesions from pontine parenchyma, creating a zone of neovascularity between the central necrotic

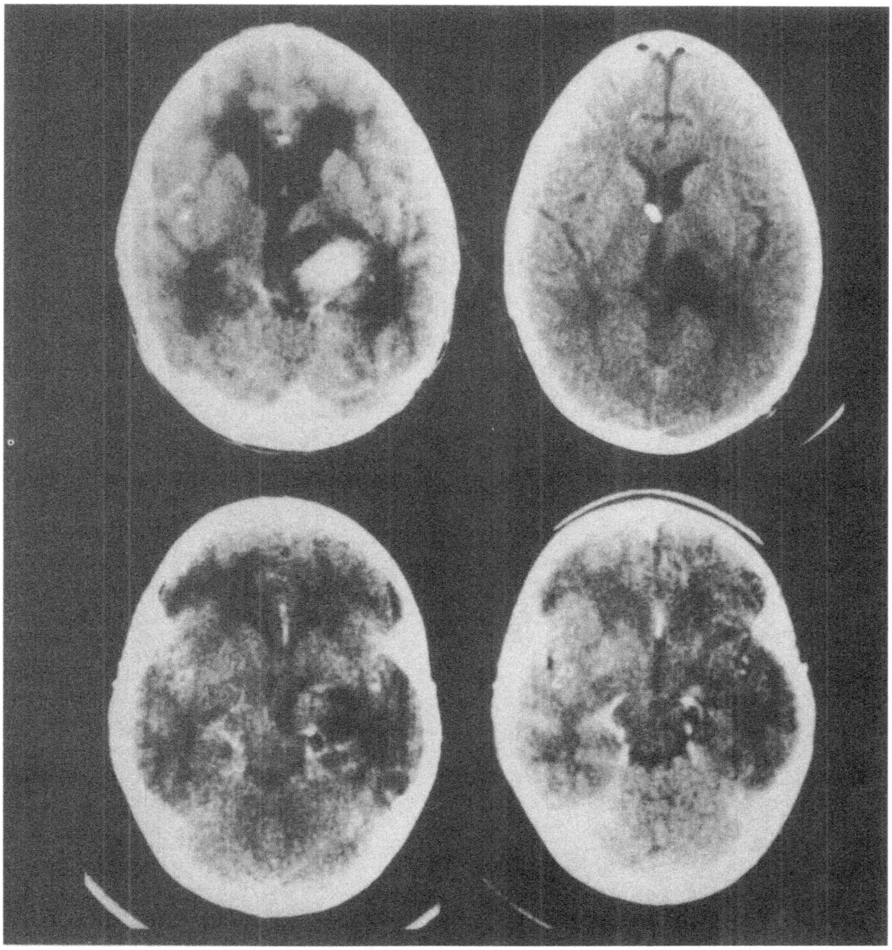

FIGURE 12–7. Preoperative and postoperative contrast-enhanced CT scan in a five-year-old girl with a pilocytic astrocytoma in the left thalamus, removed from the posterior approach (*top*). CT scan of an eight-year-old boy with a pilocytic astrocytoma resected by the anterior approach (*bottom*).

tumor and the peripheral edematous (usually infiltrated) parenchyma. The area of central necrosis can be resected stereotactically without inherent neurological risk, if the zone of contrast enhancement on CT images extends to the floor of the fourth ventricle or far laterally into the middle cerebellar peduncle, either of which will facilitate the approach (figure 12–8).

Metastatic Tumors

Metastatic tumors are usually located in the gray-white junction subcortically. They can occur at the crown of a gyrus superficially. On the other hand, they can lie at the gray-white junction in the depths of a deep sulcus and seem quite deep and difficult to find during a conventional craniotomy. Most surgeons have had the unsettling experience of trying to locate deep subcortical metastatic lesions during a conventional craniotomy. In addition, the tumor may be deep to the insular cortex, deep to the mesial occipital cortex, or under the cortex of the interhemispheric fissure.

Solitary metastases in patients with stable disease can be completely resected stereotactically, with more favorable levels of postoperative morbidity than are associated with conventional craniotomy for these lesions [7, 28]. Metastatic tumors are histologically circumscribed and can be completely resected (figure

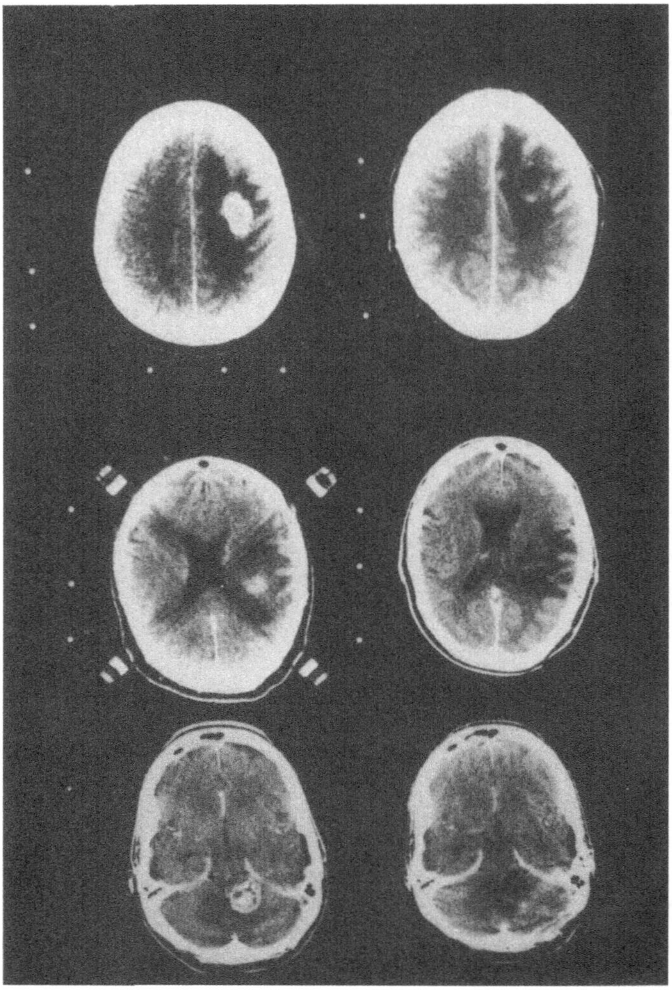

FIGURE 12–8. Metastatic tumors: top—left precentral tumor (approached through the precentral sulcus); middle—left subinsular tumor (resected through the sylvian fissure); bottom—left middle cerebellar peduncle (transcerebellar approach).

12–9). Nevertheless, in all of our patients, surgery has been followed by external-beam radiation therapy to treat possible microscopic metastatic lesions not visible on CT images. In our six-year experience with computer-assisted stereotactic resection of intracranial metastases, there has not been a single local recurrence of the tumor. However, one patient with adenocarcinoma (lung) developed a second metastatic lesion in the other hemisphere four years after stereotactic resection of the first.

Stereotactic technique can be advantageous in resecting superficial as well as deeply situated lesions. Stereotactic localization helps center small cranial trephines directly over superficial lesions (the trephine need be no larger than the cross-sectional area of the neoplasm). The approach is therefore selective, direct, and exposes no more brain than is absolutely necessary.

Postoperative neurological deficits can arise from damage to cortical and subcortical white matter during the *approach* to deep-seated lesions. The surgical results, thus depend on knowledge of the tumor's relationship to the overlying cortex and on a well-planned surgical approach.

We have found the following technical

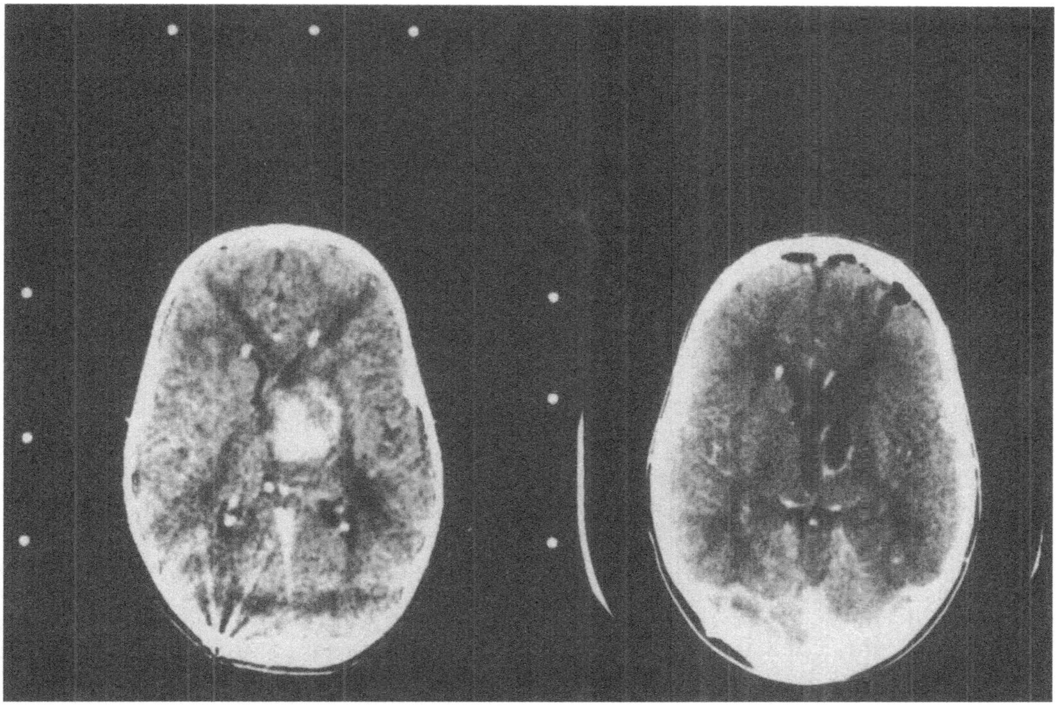

FIGURE 12–9. Preoperative and postoperative CT scans in a left thalamic mass with associated hemorrhage.

points useful: lesions located in the subcortical tissue at the depths of a sulcus are best approached by first microsurgically splitting the sulcus and then gently retracting the adjacent gyri to insert the stereotactic retractor. Medially located lesions should be approached through the interhemispheric fissure; the cortical incision is made in the mesial cortex directly over the lesion. In this situation, stereotactic placement of reference balls prior to trephine craniotomy, as described previously, is advisable. Subsequent radiographs thus can detect movement of the tumor that could occur during retraction of the hemisphere. Subinsular tumors can be approached by splitting the sylvian fissure directly over the neoplasm, inserting the stereotactic retractor, and making a vertical incision in the cortex to expose the tumor.

The smallest trephine necessary to remove the metastasis is used, so that a minimal amount of brain tissue is exposed. The trephine is placed in order to approach the tumor by a preplanned oblique trajectory that passes through a sulcus; the position of the sulcus can be established by stereoscopic stereotactic arteriography during the data-acquisition phase. The computer display provides the surgeon with useful information on the global configuration of the neoplasm when the margins between neoplasm and brain tissue are unclear. Thus, complete resection always can be achieved.

Vascular Malformations

The surgeon should be reluctant to perform a biopsy of superficial or deep-seated circumscribed lesions that demonstrate intense contrast enhancement on CT images. Although arteriograms may not demonstrate vascularity consistent with an arteriovenous malformation (AVM), postoperative hemorrhage could occur if the biopsy revealed a cryptic AVM or cavernous hemangioma. Certainly, the clinician could observe the lesion with serial CT scans to exclude malignant astrocytomas and oligodendrogliomas, which would enlarge with time.

Computer-assisted stereotactic microsurgical resection provides an alternative to either closed stereotactic biopsy or observation.

Cryptic AVM and cavernous hemangioma are well-circumscribed lesions that can be completely removed stereotactically with relatively low risk. A by-product of establishing the histology is that seizures, when present, usually stop or diminish significantly.

The following procedure is employed for the resection of these lesions: The three-dimensional configuration of the lesion is established by stereotactic CT scanning. Guided by the displayed reformatted slices, the surgeon cuts around the lesion with a slightly defocused, stereotactically directed, and computer-monitored carbon dioxide laser. Alternatively, the lesion can be resected through the stereotactic retractor with the use of extra-long aspirators and bipolar forceps.

Small, deep-seated active AVM's can also be resected by similar techniques. The positions of the feeding vessels are established in the three-dimensional surgical-planning matrix and approached and clipped or coagulated before the remainder of the lesion is dissected from the surrounding parenchyma.

Intraventricular Lesions

Many surgeons operate on lesions within the lateral ventricles without utilizing stereotactic control. Instead they use intraventricular landmarks to maintain orientation while trying to locate the lesion. This is usually a satisfactory method in patients with large lateral ventricles; however, small or normal sized ventricles may present difficulty in locating the lesion and maintaining orientation. A more limited but direct approach to intraventricular lesions can be made stereotactically. Brain and ventricular incisions need to be just large enough to remove the lesion. A 1.5-inch trephine and 1-cm or 2-cm cylindrical retractors are used (figure 12–10).

Lesions of the third ventricle are approached through the right lateral ventricle. One fornix is incised to extend the stereotactic retractor into the lesion. An internal decompression of the lesion is performed with the laser until only a thin rim of the capsule remains. The computer display of the cross-sections of the digitized tumor volume are extremely useful during this phase; the surgeon can be quite aggressive within the tumor, with no risk of extending through the capsule and damaging the ventricle walls. Next, the retractor is withdrawn to the level of the ventricle roof, and the capsule is carefully dissected from the ventricle walls. The tumor capsule can be contracted with the defocused laser, which facilitates the dissection of the capsule from the wall of the third ventricle.

Large Lesions

Deep-seated tumors 5 cm in diameter or larger can be removed with the technique and instrumentation just described, even though the largest retractor is only 3 cm in diameter. The surgeon approaches and removes different parts of the tumor sequentially as they are positioned in the focal point of the stereotactic frame where they are under the retractor opening. First, the cross-sectional image of the tumor on the display screen is translated so that the current target lies within the circle designating the cylindrical retractor as viewed by the surgeon. The computer calculates new frame coordinates, which are then duplicated on the frame. A technician activates the switches that control the servomotors of the three-dimensional slide system until the desired coordinates appear on the digital display panel. Thus a new target point is positioned in the focal point of the stereotactic arc-quadrant system.

In resecting large lesions, a plane of dissection is developed around the borders of the tumor to isolate it from surrounding brain tissue before any of the lesion is removed. This maneuver prevents shifting of the neoplasm within the intracranial compartment caused by tumor decompression, which could render the stereotactic coordinates inaccurate. Very large lesions can be resected at two, or in some cases more, successive operations (see figure 12–10). Repeat procedures are performed easily after acquisition of a new database that represents the tumor volume (reduced after the first procedure) as a new target volume in space. The skin and trephine cranial openings and the white matter incision to the lesion that were made during the initial procedure are utilized for the second procedure.

Conclusion

Computer-assisted stereotactic laser microsurgery is used to maintain a surgeon's three-dimensional orientation during the approach to

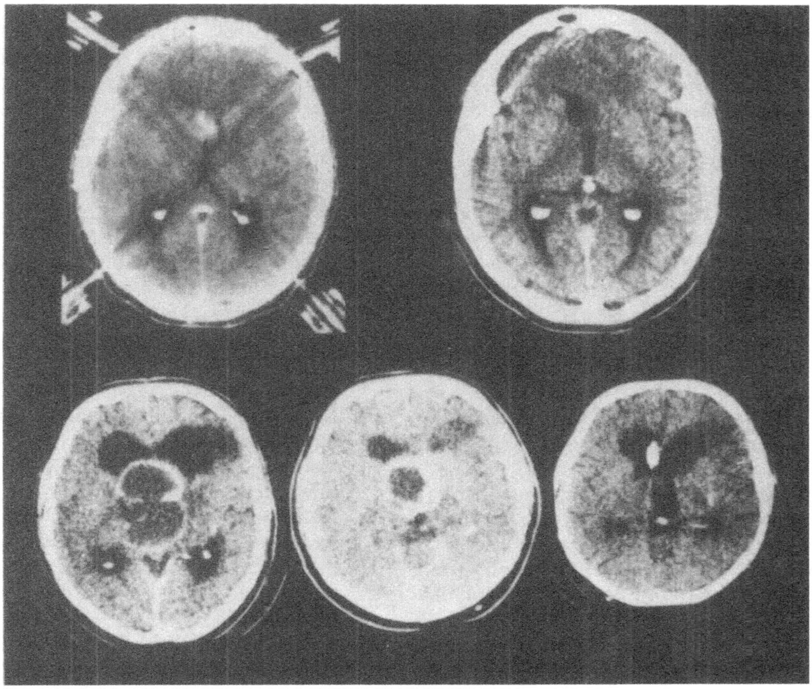

FIGURE 12–10. Preoperative and postoperative CT scans in intraventricular lesions: top—meningioma; bottom—large ganglioglioma removed in two stages.

intracranial lesions of the subcortex. In addition, computer reconstruction and interoperative display of CT and MRI data provide orientation to the global lesional volume and precise feedback regarding the location of surgical instruments (stereotactic retractor and carbon dioxide laser) in relationship to planar contours of the lesion displayed on a monitor in the operating room. With this method and instrumentation, aggressive resection of subcortical lesions with minimal damage to surrounding brain tissue is possible. Thus, lesions can be resected from neurologically important areas with acceptable levels of morbidity and mortality [14, 23, 24].

The procedure described in this chapter more clearly benefits patients who have histologically circumscribed lesions, such as pilocytic astrocytomas, metastatic tumors, intraventricular lesions, and vascular lesions [23]. Postoperative results have depended more on the degree of histological circumscription than on the location of the lesions. For patients with high-degree glial neoplasms, gains in long-term survival appear small when compared with the results of more conventional surgical methods. However, for centrally located and deep-seated lesions, a maximal reduction of tumor burden and better postoperative neurological results can be achieved with computer-assisted stereotactic resection than with conventional procedures.

References

1. Burger PC, DuBois PJ, Schold SC, et al: Computerized tomographic and pathological studies of the untreated, quiescent, and recurrent glioblastoma multiforme. *Neurosurgery* 58:159–169, 1983
2. Daumas-Duport C, Monsaingeon V, Szenthe L, et al: Serial stereotactic biopsies: A double histological code of gliomas according to malignancy and 3-D configuration, as an aid to therapeutic decision and assessment of results. *Appl Neurophysiol* 45:431–437, 1982
3. Frankel SA, German WJ: Glioblastoma multiforme: Review of 219 cases with regard to natural history, diagnostic methods and treatment. *J Neurosurg* 15:489–503, 1958
4. Gehan EA, Walker MD: Prognostic factors for

patients with brain tumors. *Natl Cancer Inst Monogr* 46:189–195, 1977
5. Giorgi C, Kelly PJ: A study of the three-dimensional distribution of somatosensory evoked responses in human thalamus to aid the placement of chronic stimulating electrodes for treatment of pain. *Acta Neurochir* (Wien) 30:279–287, 1980
6. Goerss SJ, Kelly PJ, Kall BA, et al: A computed tomographic stereotactic adaptation system. *Neurosurgery* 10:375–379, 1982
7. Haar F, Patterson RH Jr: Surgery for metastatic intracranial neoplasm. *Cancer* 30:1241–1245, 1972
8. Hitchcock E, Sato F: Treatment of malignant gliomata. *Neurosurg* 21:497–505, 1964
9. Hoshino T, Barker M, Wilson CB, et al: Cell kinetics of human gliomas. *Neurosurg* 37:15–26, 1972
10. Jelsma R, Bucy PC: Glioblastoma multiforme: Its treatment and some factors affecting survival. *Arch Neurol* 20:161–171, 1969
11. Jelsma R, Bucy PC: The treatment of glioblastoma multiforme of the brain. *Neurosurg* 27:388–400, 1967
12. Kall BA, Kelly PJ, Goerss SJ: Interactive stereotactic surgical system for the removal of intracranial tumors utilizing the CO_2 laser and CT-derived database. *IEEE Trans Biomed Eng* 32:112–116, 1985
13. Kall BA, Kelly PJ, Goerss SJ, et al: Methodology and clinical experience with computed tomography and a computer-resident stereotactic atlas. *Neurosurg* 17:400–407, 1985
14. Kelly PJ: The biopsy and treatment of subcortical intracranial masses-stereotactic methods. In press
15. Kelly PJ, Alker GJ Jr: A method for stereotactic laser microsurgery in the treatment of deep-seated CNS neoplasms. *Appl Neurophysiol* 43:210–215, 1980
16. Kelly PJ, Alker GJ Jr: A stereotactic approach to deep-seated central nervous system neoplasms using the carbon dioxide laser. *Surg Neurol* 15:331–335, 1981
17. Kelly PJ, Alker GJ Jr, Goerss SJ: Computer-assisted stereotactic laser microsurgery for the treatment of intracranial neoplasms. *Neurosurg* 110:324–331, 1982
18. Kelly PJ, Daumas-Duport C, Kispert DB, et al: The histologic concomitants of computed tomographic and magnetic resonance imaging abnormalities in glial neoplasms studied by CT and MRI based stereotactic serial biopsies. In preparation.
19. Kelly PJ, Earnest F, Kall BA, et al: Surgical options for patients with deep-seated brain tumors: Computer-assisted stereotactic biopsy. *Mayo Clin Proc* 6:223–229, 1985
20. Kelly PJ, Kall BA, Goerss SJ: Computer simulation for the stereotactic placement of interstitial radionuclide sources into CT defined tumor volumes: Technical note. *Neurosurgery* 14:442–448, 1984
21. Kelly PJ, Kall BA, Goerss SJ: Transposition of volumetric information derived from computed tomography scanning into stereotactic space. *Surg Neurol* 21:465–471, 1984
22. Kelly PJ, Kall B, Goerss SJ, et al: A method of CT-based stereotactic biopsy with arteriographic control. *Neurosurg* 14:172–177, 1984
23. Kelly PJ, Kall BA, Goerss SJ, et al: Methodology for and clinical experience with computer-assisted stereotactic laser resection of intra-axial brain neoplasms. *J Neurosurg* 1986, In press
24. Kelly PJ, Kall BA, Goerss SJ, et al: Precision resection of intra-axial CNS lesions by CT-based stereotactic craniotomy and computer-monitored CO_2 laser. *Acta Neurochir* (Wien) 68:1–9, 1983
25. Kelly PJ, Kall BA, Goerss SJ, et al: Results of computer-assisted stereotactic laser resection of deep-seated intracranial lesions. *Mayo Clin Proc* 61:20–27, 1986
26. Kelly PJ, Olson MH, Wright AE: Stereotactic implantation of iridium^{192} into CNS neoplasm. *Surg Neurol* 10:349–354, 1978
27. Kelly PJ, Olson MH, Wright AE, et al: CT localization and stereotactic implantation of Ir^{192} into CNS neoplasms. In Szikla G (ed): Amsterdam: Elsevier/North Holland Biomedical Press, 1979, pp 123–128
28. MacGee EE: Surgical treatment of cerebral metastases from lung cancer: The effect on quality and duration of survival. *Neurosurg* 35:416–420, 1971
29. Salcman M: Survival in glioblastoma: Historical perspective. *Neurosurg* 7:435–439, 1980
30. Szikla G, Bouvier G, Hori T, et al: Three-dimensional angiography for stereotactic localization of normal and pathological cortical structures. Presented at the Annual Meeting of the European Society of Stereotactic and Functional Neurosurgery, Paris, 1979
31. Walker M, Green SB, Byar DP, et al: Randomized comparisons of radiotherapy and nitrosources for the treatment of malignant glioma after surgery. *N Engl J Med* 303:1323–1329, 1980

13. COMPUTERIZED MICROSTEREOTACTIC NEUROSURGICAL ENDOSCOPY UNDER DIRECT THREE-DIMENSIONAL VISION

Skip Jacques
C. Hunter Shelden
Harold R. Lutes

Computerized tomography (CT) and magnetic resonance imaging (MRI) have given neurosurgeons the opportunity to visualize intracranial lesions much earlier than was heretofore possible with more invasive techniques. Continued improvement in image resolution has led to the diagnosis of intracranial lesions that are too small to be located and removed by conventional methods. In this chapter, we describe our stereotactic method, including carbon dioxide laser vaporization, for the removal of small central nervous system (CNS) lesions under three-dimensional visual control.

With the development and refinement of CT and MRI, small CNS lesions can be detected by noninvasive scanning methods that incorporate computer-processing of the data. In conjunction with engineers at the California Institute of Technology, multiple computer programs have been developed to enhance regions of interest on CT and MRI scans by magnification, digital processing, and three-dimensional color reconstruction techniques [4]. These data are then used to calculate a stereotactic approach. A new head-fixation system enables information transfer from a CT or MRI scan to a stereotactic surgical system [2, 4]. Newly developed instruments are mounted on a micromanipulator for guidance at the operative site.

Description of Instrumentation

The tumor "resectoscope," available in various sizes, consists of a tubular piece of aluminum alloy; the distal end is tapered and has tulip-like blades which can be opened and closed (figure 13–1). Side vents allow easy entry for newly designed roto-dissector instruments (figure 13–2). Other instruments, including microforceps and instruments for hemostasis, also can be inserted through this side port. Initial entry is obtained with specially designed tissue expanders, which are of similar shape and sized sequentially to approximate the size of the tulip-sized resectoscope. The resectoscope subsequently is introduced into the brain with the tulip-like blades closed (see figure 13–1, right). After following the precalibrated Z-axis target, the blades are opened, exposing the lesion. The blades are activated by an inner tubular sleevelike mechanism which, when moved distally, separates the blades. A newly designed plastic tip for the larger resectoscope now makes the entire distal portion of the apparatus disposable (figure 13–3). Opening the blade expands the tissue and stretches surrounding tissue sufficiently to prevent bleeding into the air-filled cavity. As the resectoscope is opened, the optical system moves distally along the sleeve as the blades open. When the blades

L.D. Lunsford (ed.) *MODERN STEREOTACTIC NEUROSURGERY*.

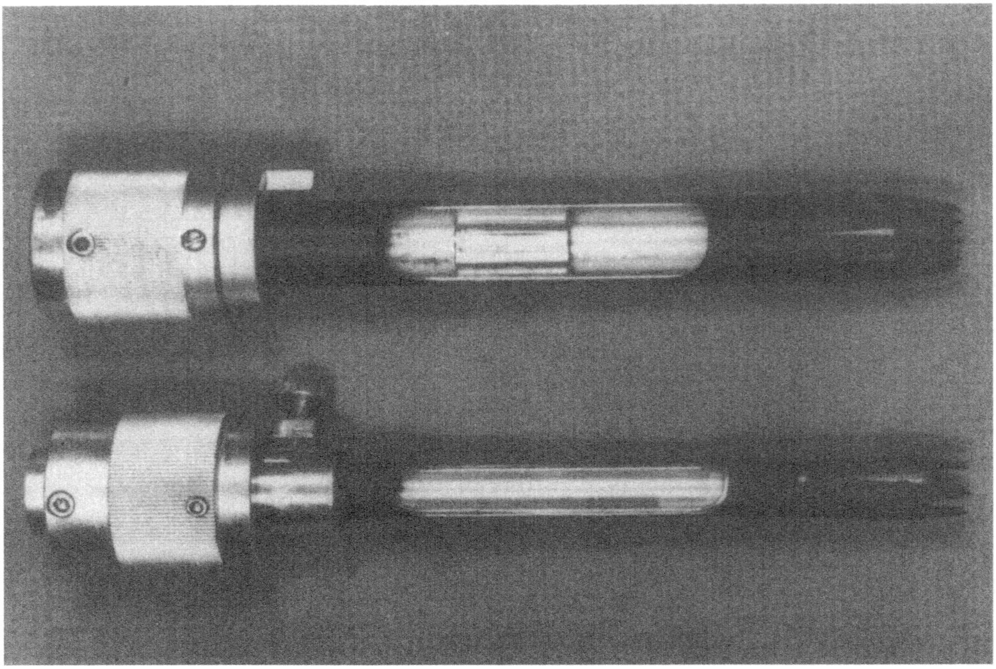

A

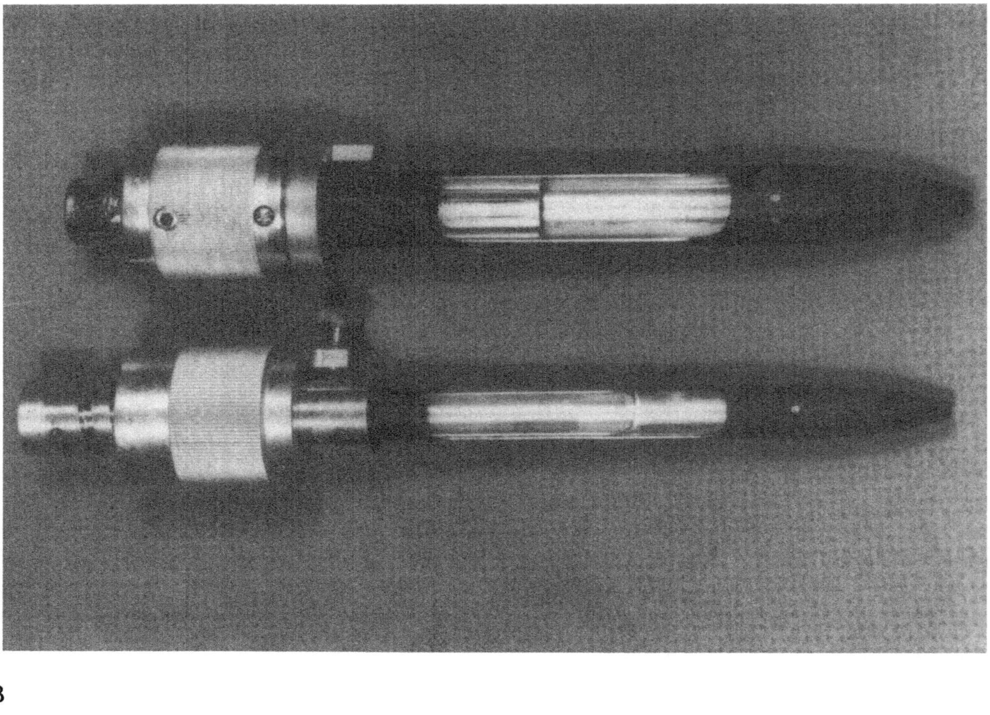

B

FIGURE 13–1. Standard (top) and small-sized tumorscopes; tulip is in open position (A). Tulip is in closed position (B).

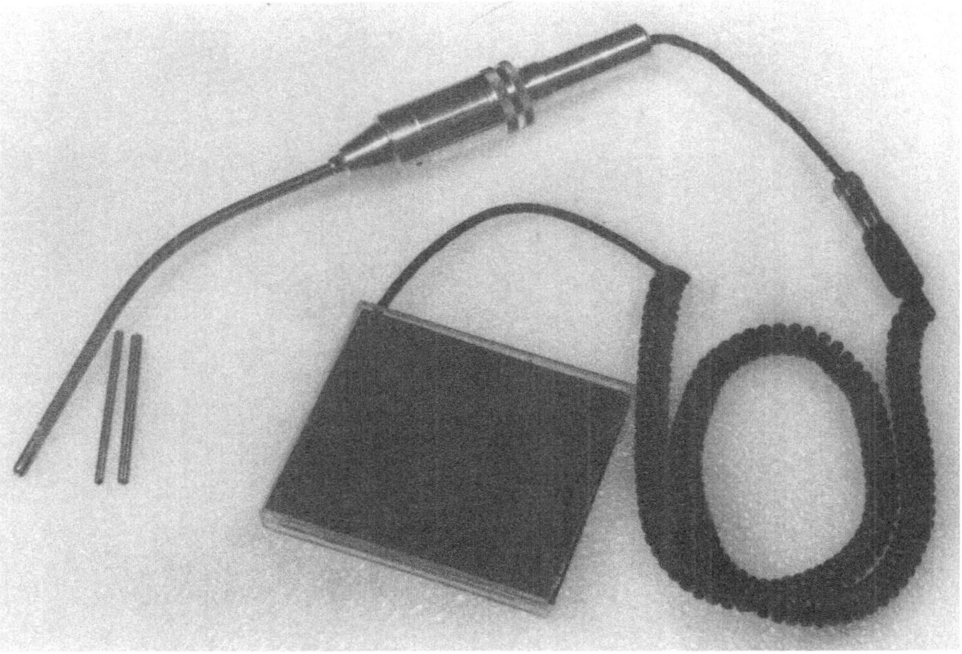

FIGURE 13–2. Roto-resector for use with Shelden tumorscope is battery operated.

are fully opened, the tip of the optical system is moved distally to a point that corresponds to the focal length of the lens system.

The original design provided for visulization of lesions through a monocular scope; however, it soon became apparent that three-dimensional vision was essential for accurate dissection of small lesions deep in the brain. Because no such system was commercially available at the time, the following binocular system was designed.

Optical System

Modern-day endoscopy has been highly refined for use in many body cavities having an air-filled or fluid-filled opening, such as the bladder, knee, or intestines. Because neurosurgery involves brain tissue, the requirements are quite different.

When an endoscope is inserted into brain tissue, both light and vision are blocked as soft tissue gathers in front of the instrument. We found it essential to provide some means of forming a cavity around the area of interest, in this case, a small tumor. It further became apparent that monocular vision was inadequate for this application because of the lack of landmarks and other monocular clues. An authority on stereoscopic vision, imaging, and photography developed our optical system; he felt that a three-dimensional stereoscopic system must be developed as an essential part of surgical endoscopy. Requirements for such an instrument include these factors:

1. Small size
2. Short focal-length optics
3. High resolution
4. Self-contained fiberoptic illumination
5. Wide angle of view
6. Stereoscopic view with normal convergence
7. Parallel optics of rod lens
8. A method of retracting tissue to form an air- or fluid-filled chamber in front of the objective lenses.

We wanted to be able to work through an average-sized burr hole (approximately ½–⅝-inch diameter). We tested several endoscopes and found the Storz Pediatric Endoscope to be the smallest instrument of good optical quality. It has both a superior optical system and a good fiberoptic illumination system. The endo-

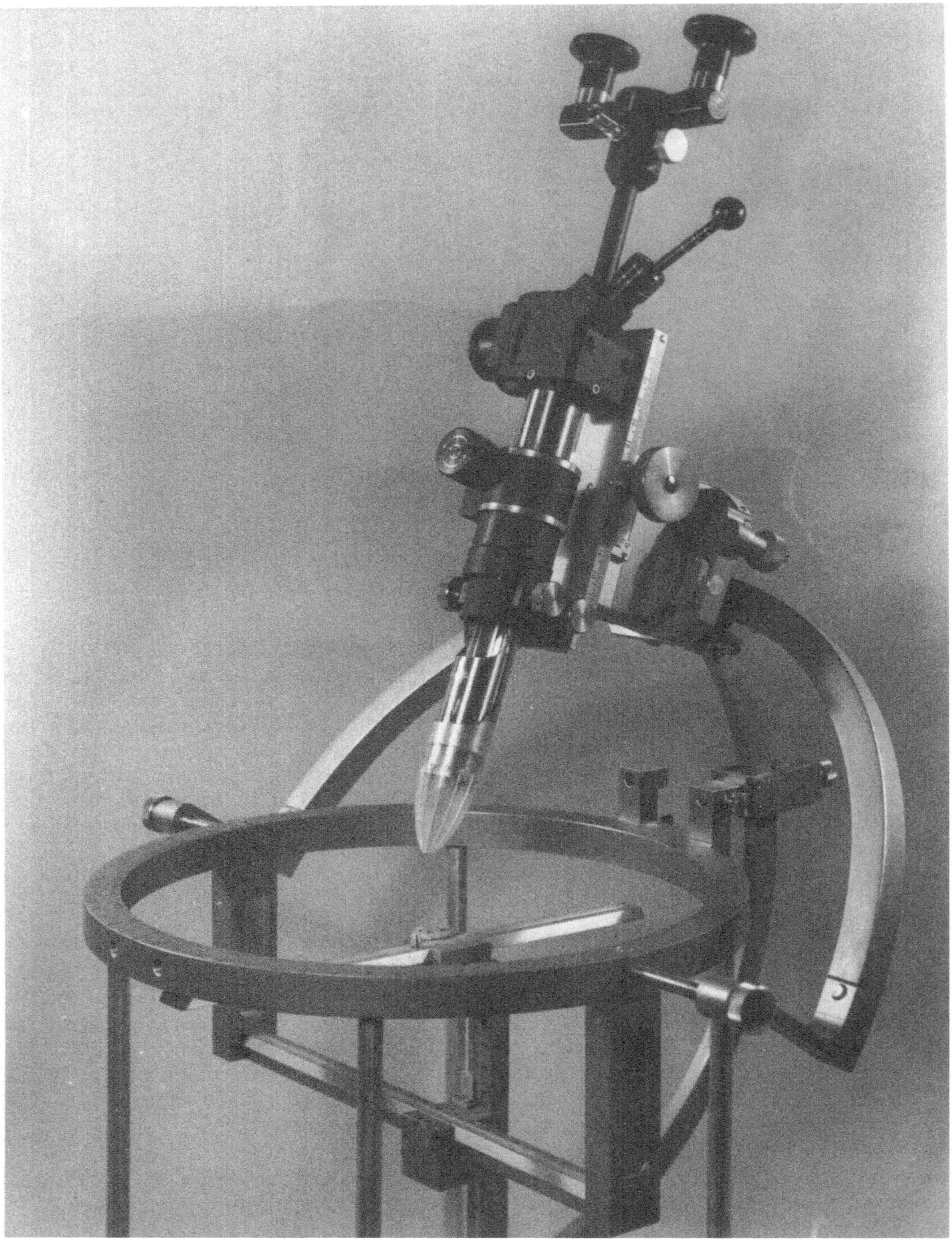

FIGURE 13–3. Large Shelden-Jacques tumorscope for laser adaptation, mounted on phantom ring with stereo endoscope in place.

scope has a focal length of 20 mm and, therefore, has nearly universal focus (from infinity to about 2 mm) in front of the objective lens face. This provides a very versatile system: objects at 20 mm appear normal in size; at 10 mm they are magnified by a factor of two; and at 5 mm, by a factor of four. This would appear to be a very convenient way to obtain magnification; unfortunately, an object of unknown size at an unknown distance from the lens has no basis for size comparison. Because size is a function of distance, and distance is not precisely known or controllable, the surgeon is likely to become confused. These limitations do not occur with endoscopy in other parts of the body. Although our initial proposal for stereoscopic presentation was met with skepticism, we procured two identical endoscopes and designed a special device to hold the tubes so that they would be at the same angle of convergence and so that the surgeon's eyes would have about 9 inches working or viewing distance when the object of regard was exactly 20 mm from the entrance pupil of the objective lens.

Thus, a stereoscopic or three-dimensional view of the object is produced 2.1 in size, and the object is visible despite the "window effect" created by the lens tubes. If the object is moved nearer, it becomes magnified and appears to project through the window toward the viewer. If the object is moved away, it becomes smaller and appears behind the window. This provides a precise method for judging size. In addition, objects or instruments used during surgery can be placed on the visual target with full control with the use of stereopsis, the highest form of visual distance judgment. As with any other stereoscopic device, this technique requires that the viewer have normal binocular stereoscopic vision.

With a monocular instrument, depth and distance can be judged only by secondary clues (known size and distance, texture, overlapping contours, parallax, apparent motion of an object, etc.). We believe that the development of stereoscopic endoscopy permits the control and visulization necessary to minimize tissue damage during surgery for small brain tumors and opens the possibilities of precise enhanced vision to many other fields of surgical endeavor.

A basic principle of illumination states that front or flat lighting (in which all shadow areas are filled with light) causes an object to appear to have very little texture and roundness. Side lighting produces increased texture and contour. The illuminating system of an endoscope provides flat front light, so the object is brightly illuminated but has little texture, except that provided by color contrast of tissues. Stereoscopic vision provides all the benefits of a monocular system with the outstanding advantages of normal two-eyed viewing: a more natural view and less visual fatigue.

A complete design drawing was submitted to the Karl Storz Endoscopy Company for manufacture and eventually a unit was developed (figure 13–4). It consists of a dual stereoscopic system with parallel optics of Hopkins rod lenses, which have 3.5-mm interaxial separation and a working distance of 20-mm focal length. Eyepieces are adjustable for interocular distances of 55–68 mm. The convergence required is equal to that needed for an object at 16 inches working distance with normal vision, and the object of regard appears normal size at 20 mm from the distal end of the scope. When an object is moved to 10 mm, it is magnified by a factor of two; at 40 mm, an object appears half its size. Thus, linear perspective changes rapidly at a very high angle. A 4:1 size change is equal to an object at 8 inches being moved to 32 inches. To become accustomed to this unusual ratio, some practice is necessary. Close-up viewing of stereo pictures in a hand-held stereoscopic viewer offers good practical training.

A tissue-dilating, expandable tulip-shaped unit was developed to complete the Shelden-Jacques tumorscope (see figure 13–1). This unit houses the stereo endoscope and provides a means of attachment to the stereotactic support system as well as a side port for introducting special surgical instruments (figure 13–5). During stereoscopic viewing, the blades create a plane of reference causing the tumor to appear as if through a window. Objects appear to be in front of, even with, or behind the window plane. Objects which appear even with the window or blades are doubled in size, providing a ready size control.

The ability to perceive size, texture, and perspective in stereoscopic relief reduces the possibilities for errors of visual judgment by enabling the surgeon to use binocular vision during placement of dissecting instruments. Precision of placement is thus improved.

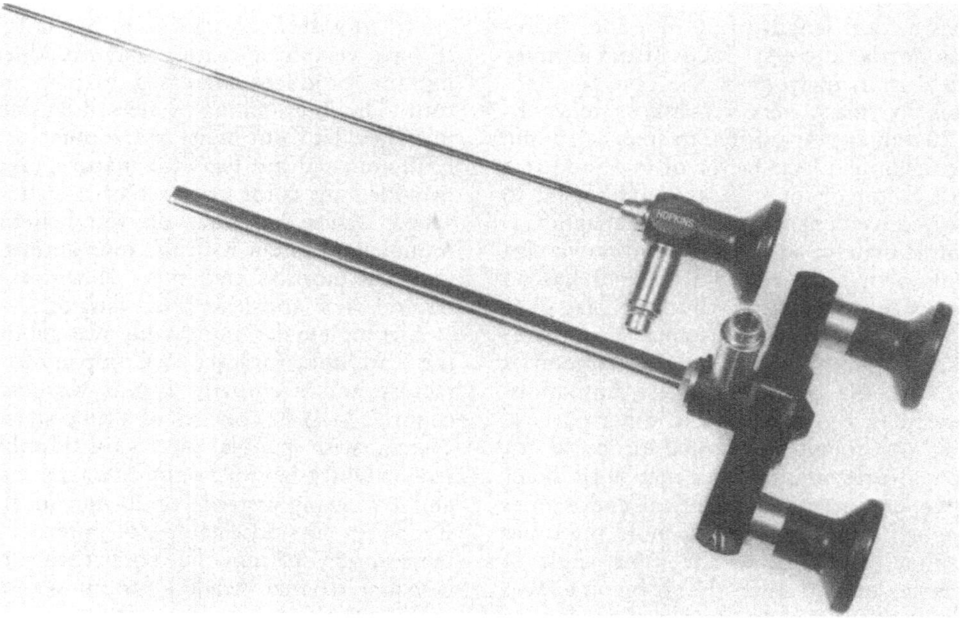

FIGURE 13-4. Monocular pediatric scope (top) and stereo endoscope.

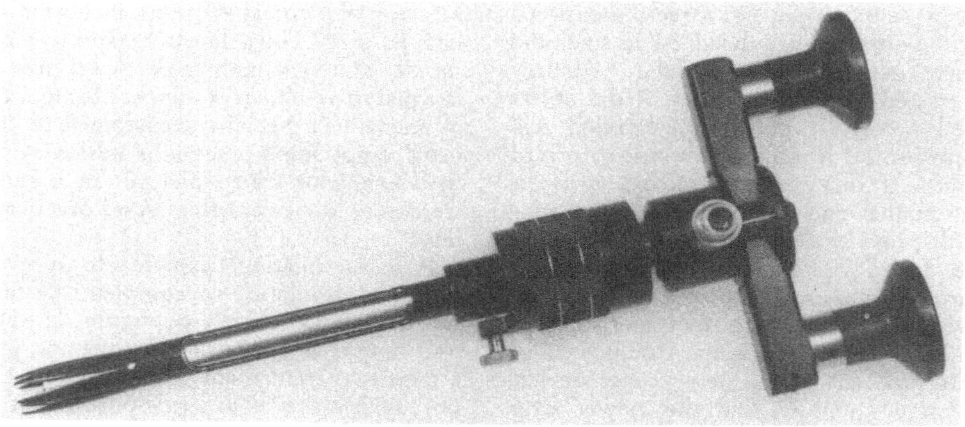

FIGURE 13-5. Small tumorscope tulip in open operating position with stereo endoscope in place.

Currently, we are using three tumorscope sizes (see figure 13-1): standard (15.5 mm in diameter), large (25 mm in diameter), and small (10.2 mm in diameter).

Any neurosurgical endoscope should have:

1. A tubular shaft, 14 mm maximum diameter, containing a binocular scope.
2. Tulip-like blades at the distal end that can be opened when the target is reached along the Z axis. Proper tension of the blades on brain tissue stretches tiny vessels and prevents bleeding from the brain area exposed between the open blades. The working distance between tips should be 10 mm.
3. An air-filled cavity between the end of the optical system and the tumor.
4. A side port for introducing instruments, suction, and carbon dioxide laser. The laser greatly improves the precision of tumor re-

moval (see figure 13–3). In the future, when specialized markers are available, a minute area of tumor tissue will be identified during surgery by hematoporphyrin derivatives, which emit red light when excited by ultraviolet light.

5. A fiberoptic system containing six Hopkins units in each parallel unit; such a system provides adequate distance from the skull to allow freedom of movement for the surgeon. An additional set of quartz fibers is required to excite porphyrin derivatives for tumor indentification or to excite other substances for photoradiation and lysis of the lesion.

The "tulip system" provides a virtually bloodless field in which to operate, particularly since the recent addition of the carbon dioxide laser. Binocular vision affords the capability of modified microdissection in the controlled environment of the system. The effectiveness of this or any other stereotactic system, of course, depends upon the accuracy with which the target point can be reached. At our institution, information for the stereotactic coordinates is obtained from General Electric 8800 or 9800 CT scanners and/or a Diasonics MR imager. The major problem has been determining the Z axis, which we believe must have an accuracy of ±1 mm. We have redesigned a Riechert-Mundinger system to help in determination of the X, Y, and Z axes [4]. The steel patient ring was replaced with one made of aluminum to minimize artifacts on the scan, and the skeletal attachment was replaced with pins passing through the plane of the ring itself, thus eliminating further distortion especially on the CT scan (figure 13–6).

The X and Y axes can be determined accurately by algorithms developed at our institution in conjunction with engineers at the California Institute of Technology. The Z axis is determined directly from CT or MR imaging data. CT and MR scanners at our institution provide magnetic tapes with reconstructed image data, which are decoded and placed on a high-speed mass-storage disk. The images are then viewed on high-resolution display monitors. The computer manipulates the intensity map and the function memory of the frame buffer, thus altering the gray-scale mean and range. Contrast in the middle-to-white range is further enhanced by incorporation of the gamma exponent correction for cathode ray displays into the intensity map determined for the desired gray scale. The computer program allows use of the line printer connected to the computer to obtain a hard copy of the scan image or any subsection of the image.

Magnification programs have been developed also. Regions of interests are marked with a tracking pen on a magnetic tablet, and the outlined area is then redisplayed, occupying the full screen. Magnification is performed without filtering, which allows very high magnification of minute areas of images without blurring. In this manner, contour boundaries of small structures can be determined more accurately.

Localization of Tumors

The coordinate axes for locating the tumor are determined from an aluminum ring, which is mounted on the patient. Four pins are placed at 0°, 90°, 180°, and 270° on the ring. The locations of the pins are transferred to the computer with the tracking pen. The equation of the circle of the ring is approximated in pixel coordinates. The center of the ring is estimated as the center of the mass of the four points, and the radius of the circle is the averaged radii from the center of the mass to each point. Conventional stereotactic coordinates are defined such that the positive X axis is to the patient's right and the positive Y axis is anterior. The origin is defined as the absolute center of the ring along the X, Y, and Z axes.

To determine the Z coordinate (figure 13–6), a set of pins is mounted on the aluminum ring in each of the four quadrants perpendicular to the plane of the patient ring; each set consists of four pins which are 14 mm, 12 mm, 10 mm, and 8 mm in height, respectively. The longest pin in each set is positioned at integral multiples of 90° along the ring. The remaining pins descend in height counterclockwise. The ring is mounted on the skull and then clamped to a base which, in turn, attaches to the CT gantry and thus holds the ring parallel to the scanning plane. The accuracy of coordinate determination is dependent upon this geometry. Accuracy is confirmed by obtaining an image immediately past the tips of the four shortest pins; none of these pins should appear in any image that does not contain all four.

The number of pins seen on each scan is

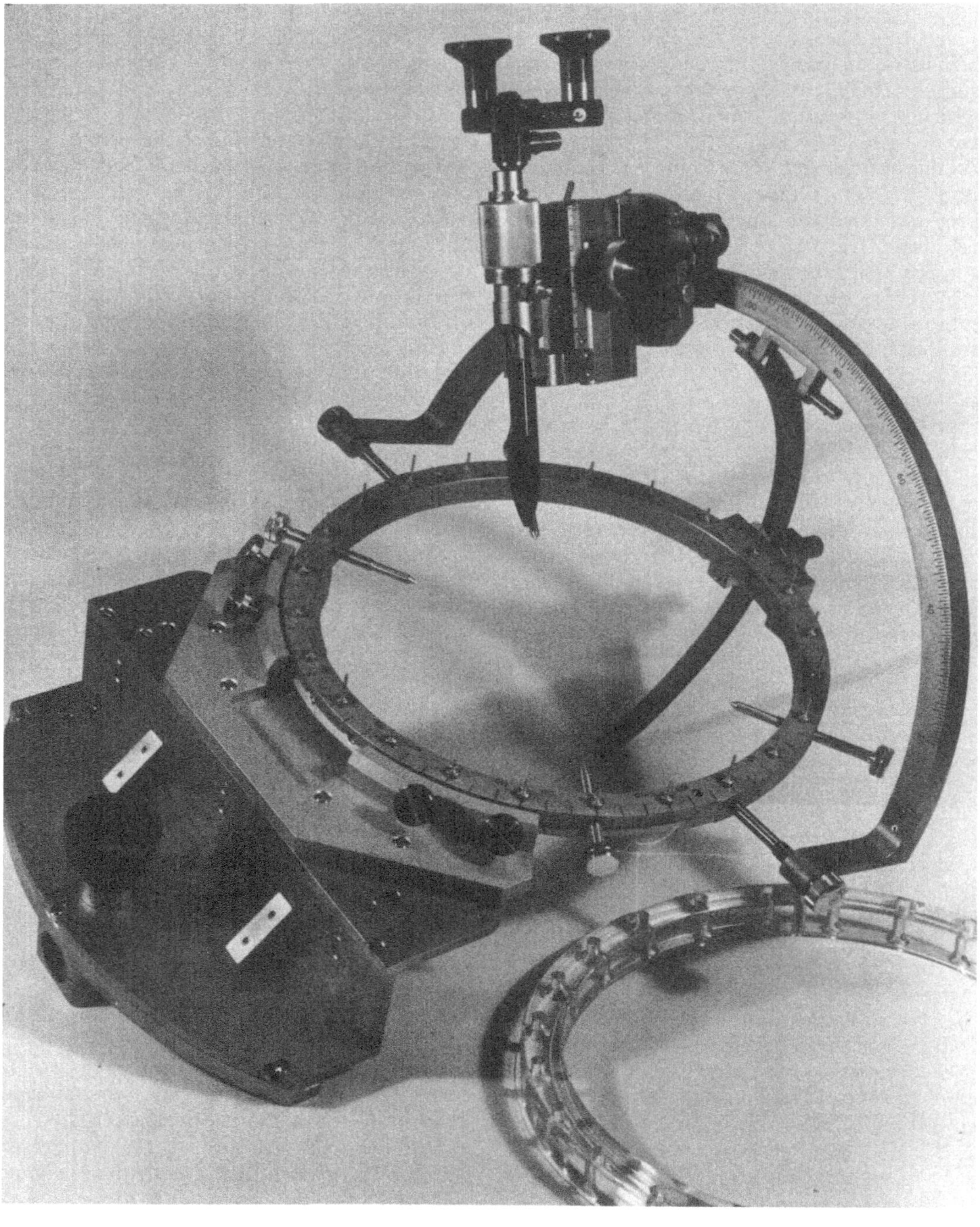

FIGURE 13-6. Patient ring with vertical pins used for Z coordinate calculations.

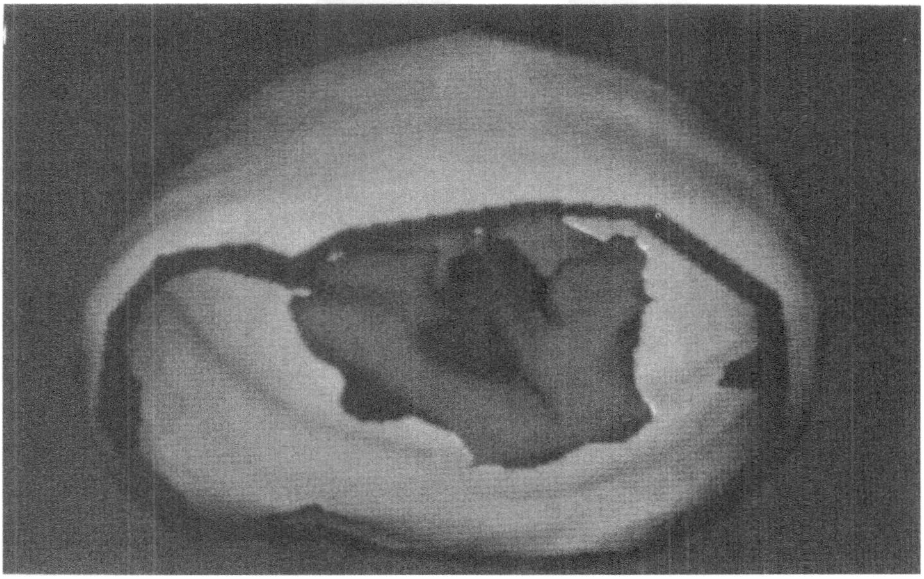

FIGURE 13–7. Three-dimensional reconstruction of a brain tumor with surrounding edema.

entered into the computer. When the pin count changes between consecutive scans, the Z coordinate can be estimated: an average is taken of the heights of the shortest pin still appearing and the pin that disappeared; to this is added one-half the height of the ring. As the increment between the pins is 2 mm, the center of the ring along the Z axis is thus located with an accuracy of ±1 mm. (Further computer-program refinements using volume-averaging artifacts actually makes Z axis localization accurate to within a few tenths of a millimeter.) The tracking pin on the magnetic tablet is used to locate the center of the tumor. The actual X and Y coordinates are calculated by multiplying the difference in pixel coordinates from the center of the ring to the center of the tumor by pixel size. The position of the Z axis is determined directly as the difference between the scan depth and the center of the ring. The location of the tumor in "ring coordinates" is then transferred to the surgical phantom apparatus for plotting of the most ideal angle of attack.

Aside from aiding in Z axis determination, advanced computer programs (Jet Propulsion Laboratory and the California Institute of Technology) provide valuable information concerning the microanalysis of these lesions. Three-dimensional image reconstruction techniques allow the surgeon to visualize the surface contour of the tumor prior to actual operation (figure 13–7). Computer "removal" of the tumor by software manipulation makes possible 360° inspection of the lesion and of the surface of the underlying edema contiguous to the tumor. This is very important in light of new adjuvant immunotherapeutic techniques [1, 3].

Summary

We have described a unique method of localizing and removing minute CNS tumors under binocular vision. Intracerebral tumor resection by dual xenon-arc illumination under direct binocular three-dimensional vision has been practical in treating many patients to date. The stereotactic guidance system utilizes coordinates obtainable directly from CT and/or MRI scan data.

Although this system originally was designed to remove small CNS brain tumors, it is adaptable to intracerebral lesions of larger size and various pathologies. The system has also proven useful for evacuation of small intracerebral hematomas and metastatic tumors. The neurosurgeon is able to cope with the most minute lesions that can be seen with modern imaging techniques and can be much more productive than is possible with more routine stereotactic-guided biopsy system. These improvements are important in modern treatment of CNS neoplasia, because smaller residual tumor burdens increase the potential effectiveness of adjuvant therapeutic techniques, particularly given this new ability to find and remove minute lesions.

References

1. Ingram M. Shelden CH, Jacques S, et al: Development and successful trial of immunotherapy for malignant glioma in the dog. *Neurol Res* (In press)
2. Jacques S, Shelden CH, McCann GD, et al: Computerized three-dimensional microstereotactic removal of small central nervous system lesions in patients: Case reports. *J Neurosurg* 53:816–820, 1980
3. Shelden CH, Ingram M, Jacques S, et al: Apparent destruction of spontaneous glioblastoma in a dog by autologous lymphocytes. *Pulse* (J So Cal Vet Med Assoc) 26:13–14, 1984
4. Shelden CH, McCann G, Jacques S, et al: Development of a computerized microstereotaxic method for localization and removal of minute CNS lesions under direct 3-D vision: Technical report. *J Neurosurg* 52:21–27, 1980

14. STEREOTACTIC POSITRON EMISSION TOMOGRAPHY IMAGING FOR TUMOR DIAGNOSIS

Hans Von Holst
Kaj Ericson
Mats Bergström
Georg Norén

Computed tomography (CT) of intracranial tumors, especially when used in combination with stereotaxis, has been of great value to the neurosurgeon in obtaining an accurate diagnosis and assessing tumor margins. For benign tumors such as meningiomas and neurinomas, correlation between appearance on CT and neuropathology usually is consistent. However, for gliomas, the distribution of abnormality as defined by CT images often does not correlate well with the pathologist's findings. In many cases, CT cannot differentiate clearly between normal brain and glioma tissue. We believe that neurodiagnostic parameters that directly evaluate cell metabolism and cell function allow a better discrimination between normal and pathological tissue.

Positron emission tomography (PET) is a powerful diagnostic nuclear medicine research tool. The biochemical processes of the human brain can be localized precisely and measured quantitatively with PET. The measurement of regional tissue function by PET technique requires the incorporation of a radioactive isotope into a molecule that traces the physiological pathways of interest. Numerous metabolically active substances are labeled with short-lived positron-emitting isotopes so that their distribution can be studied with noninvasive tomographic instruments [3, 12, 13]. The amount of radioactivity in different regions is calculated and seen as images that define absolute concentrations of the tracers within cross-sections of the brain. Images showing distribution of the tracers in the brain can reveal pathological alterations useful in the diagnosis and classification of brain tumors. The radioactive tracers used in tumor diagnosis are 11-C-D-methionine and L-methionine for the evaluation of amino acid utilization, 11-C-D-glucose for the study of tissue energy metabolism, and gallium-68-ethylenediaminetetraacetic acid (^{68}Ga-EDTA) for the detection of blood-tumor-barrier (BTB) defects. Regional blood flow and blood-volume oxygen use and oxygen extraction fractions also can be measured. Several different receptor systems within the brain have been studied in vivo. Because of the new type of information obtainable with PET, and the complementary properties of CT and PET, techniques have been developed for stereotactic PET investigations and for the transfer of spatial information between CT and PET [1].

Head Fixation

Patients with intracranial tumors verified by CT are studied after being fitted with a custom-made head-positioning device, which allows us accurate patient transfer between CT and PET imaging procedures. Reusable fixation is achieved by molding a fiberglass mesh, hardened by ultraviolet light, around the patient's head. This mold contains four aluminum plates, which can be attached rigidly to a base plate with several attachment knobs and holes (figure 14–1). The purpose of this base plate is twofold: to provide external mechanical reference points to which diagnostic and therapeutic

L.D. Lunsford (ed.) *MODERN STEREOTACTIC NEUROSURGERY*.
Martinus Nijhoff Publishing. Boston/Dordrecht/Lancaster.

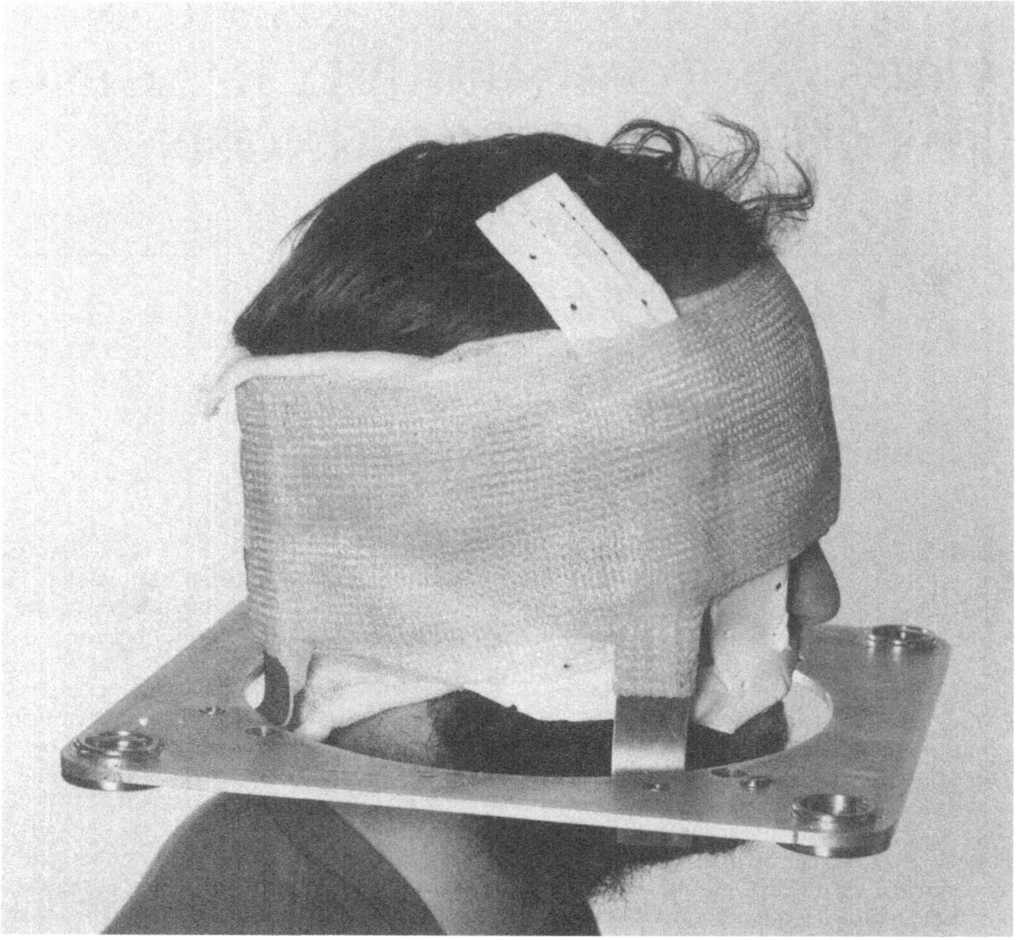

FIGURE 14-1. Fiberglass mold and base plate fixed to patient's head.

devices can be attached, and to conveniently secure the patient's head to the examination table. No imaging artifacts are created using this fixation. The fiberglass mold can be reapplied in order to duplicate the images during subsequent stereotactic biopsy procedures to facilitate repeated radiation treatment. Accuracy in the reapplication of the mold is greater than 3 mm [6].

After the head-positioning device is applied, a special diagnostic localization frame is attached to the base plate (figure 14-2). To eliminate artifacts, it is constructed of plastic and aluminum. It is applied easily and locked to the base plate. The frame is small enough to allow its structures to be included in the reconstruction field.

The examination tables of both the CT and PET scanners are equipped with a head holder to which the base plate and the attached helmet can be fastened (figure 14-3). For the CT examinations, a GE (General Electric Medical Systems, Milwaukee, WI) CT/T scanner is used. Scans are obtained before and after administration of an intravenous contrast agent. We inject a bolus dose (1-1.5 ml/kg body weight) of nonionic contrast medium. The slice spacing (13.5 mm) is chosen to correspond to that of the PET scanner.

PET studies are performed with a Scanditronix (Uppsala, Sweden) PC-384B camera with four detector rings for the simultaneous measurement of seven slices. C-11-Methionine, C-11-glucose, and ^{68}Ga-EDTA are used as

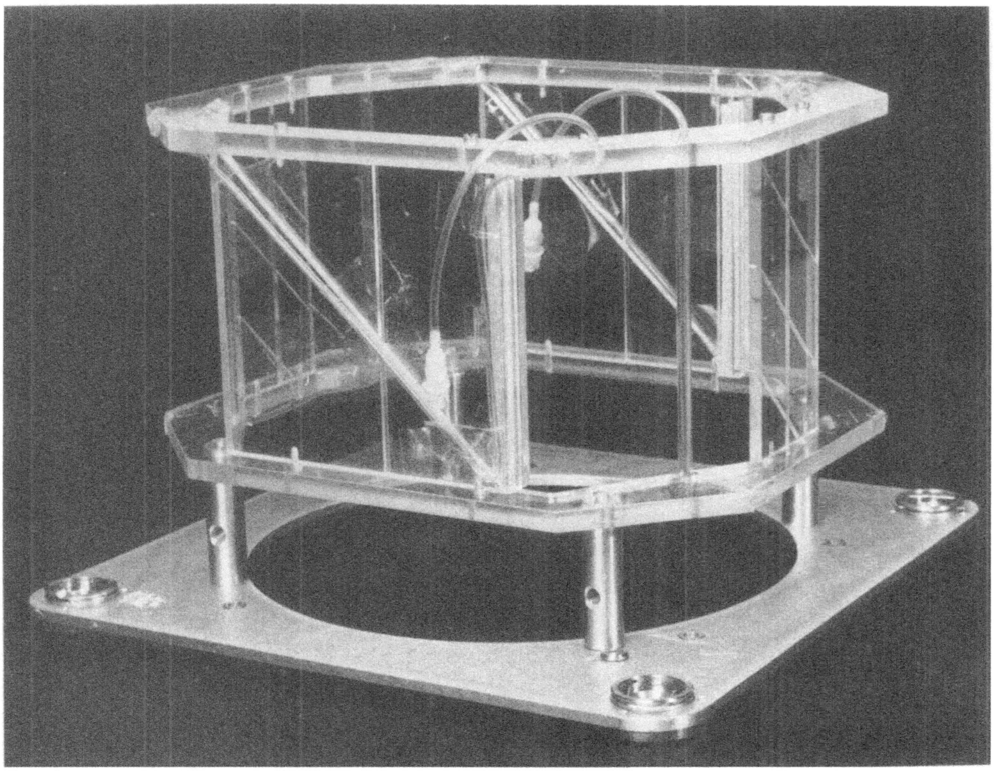

FIGURE 14-2. Localization frame made of plastic with embedded aluminum strips. The two diagonal structures are used to find the image level. The corner of the angle is at the zero reference plane. A thin plastic tube is attached to the frame along the structures used for localization. A solution containing positron-emitting radionuclides can be injected into the tube.

tracers in doses of 200, 600, and 300 MBq, respectively. The tracers are injected as rapid bolus doses and the measurements begin immediately afterwards. During a total examination time of 50–60 minutes, a series of data sets are collected for later analysis of the dynamics of the tracer accumulation. At the end of the PET study, a localizing box is attached to the base plate. This box is similar in design to that used for CT, but instead of aluminum strips, thin plastic tubes filled with a solution containing ^{68}Ga-EDTA are used to define the reference structures on the PET scan (see figure 14–3).

With the head-fixation device, we can obtain CT and PET images that have the same orientation. Structures or targets for biopsy can be transferred easily from one modality to the other. With morphological information from CT, the exact location of areas with a pathological isotope accumulation can be determined. The head-fixation device also can be used during angiography, an advantage when the target is close to the large intracranial vessels. The selected target for biopsy can be transferred to the stereotactic angiography and adjusted if necessary. In a few cases, this technique has been used to avoid puncture of the pericallosal and internal carotid arteries. Biopsies have been obtained 5 mm from these vessels without problems.

Target Calculation

After the tumor has been identified on the CT images, a suitable target for stereotactic biopsy is chosen, and the stereotactic coordinates of the target are calculated. The image level (the Y coordinate) is determined first. This coordinate is defined as the distance between the chosen

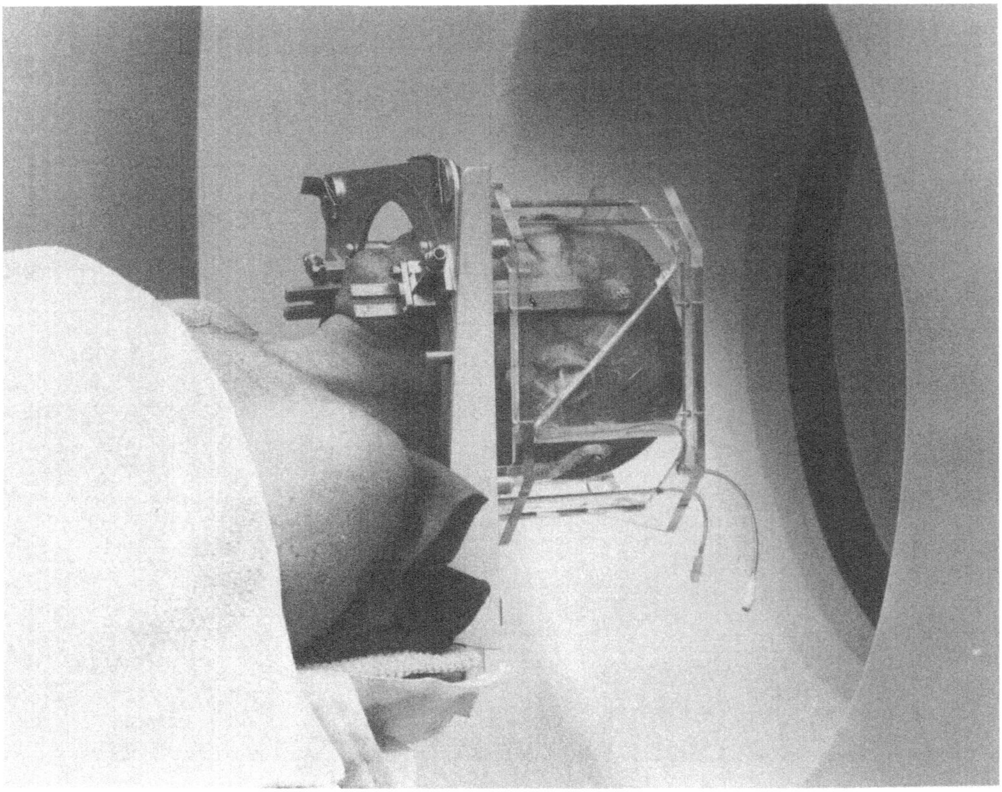

FIGURE 14–3. Patient positioned in the scanner. A special head holder supports the base plate. The thin tube on the localization frame is filled with ^{68}Ga-EDTA in water.

image and a reference plane, the stereotactic Y coordinate of which is zero. The localization frame contains two aluminum strips at 90° and 45° angles to the reference plane (see figure 14–2). These strips are used to determine the Y coordinate. The origin of the coordinate system must be defined to calculate two remaining coordinates in the scanning plane (X and Z). Two perpendicular lines are drawn between indentations in the middle of the plastic structures. The intersection of the two lines indicates the center of the reference frame, which is also the center of the stereotactic system. With standard CT software, a cursor is used to mark the target and the origin of the coordinate system, which causes the X and Y target coordinates to appear on the computer screen. A similar localization frame is used during PET studies; it has thin tubes filled with a solution containing ^{68}Ga a generator-produced, positron-emitting isotope. A computer program automatically searches for the bright spots in the image produced by these tubes, and the coordinate system is shown on the screen (figure 14–4). Using a cursor, the neurosurgeon can plan a stereotactic biopsy site on the computer screen, and all relevant instrument settings will be displayed. The coordinates also can be determined more conventionally, as with CT.

After the stereotactic coordinates for the target are calculated, the stereotactic biopsy is performed in the operating room with the Leksell coordinate frame (AB Elekta, Stockholm, Sweden). During surgery, the patient receives premedication and local anesthesia. The head-positioning device is fixed to the operating table (figure 14–5) and an opening in the fiberglass mold is created easily to perform skull trephination at the selected site of surgical intervention. Next, the Leksell frame is fixed to the base plate, and the coordinates are set. Usually, the entry point is chosen in a horizontal plane corresponding with the CT and PET

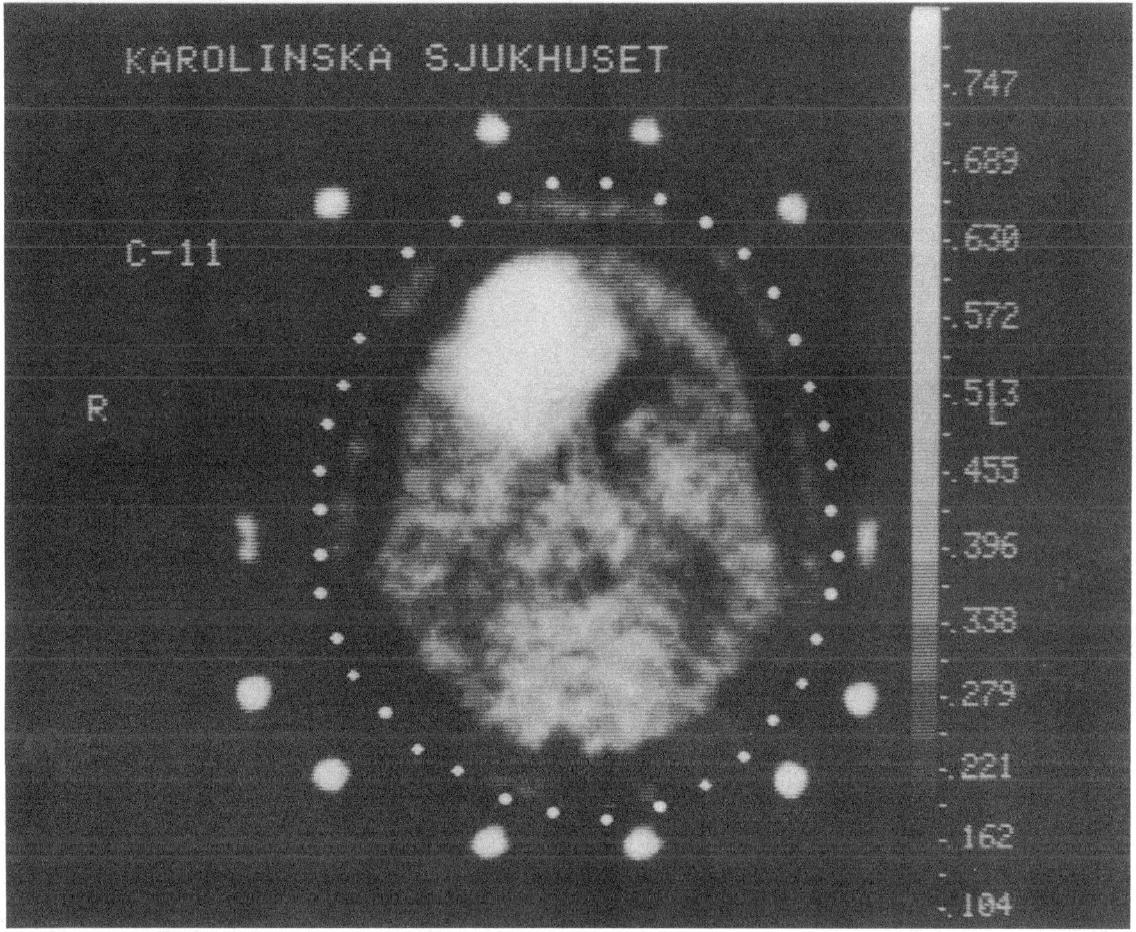

A

FIGURE 14–4. Marked methionine accumulation in a grade II astrocytoma. (A) The spots around the skull are produced by tubes in the localizing box containing ^{68}Ga. To determine the center of the stereotactic system, two intersecting diagonal lines are drawn between structures in this box. (B) By drawing a line on the image from the center of the stereotactic system to the selected target, the coordinates for each end of the line are obtained. The stereotactic coordinates are obtained by subtracting these two sets of values. (C) The distance between the target and the reference level is determined by measuring the distance between a reference point and a structure angled at 45°.

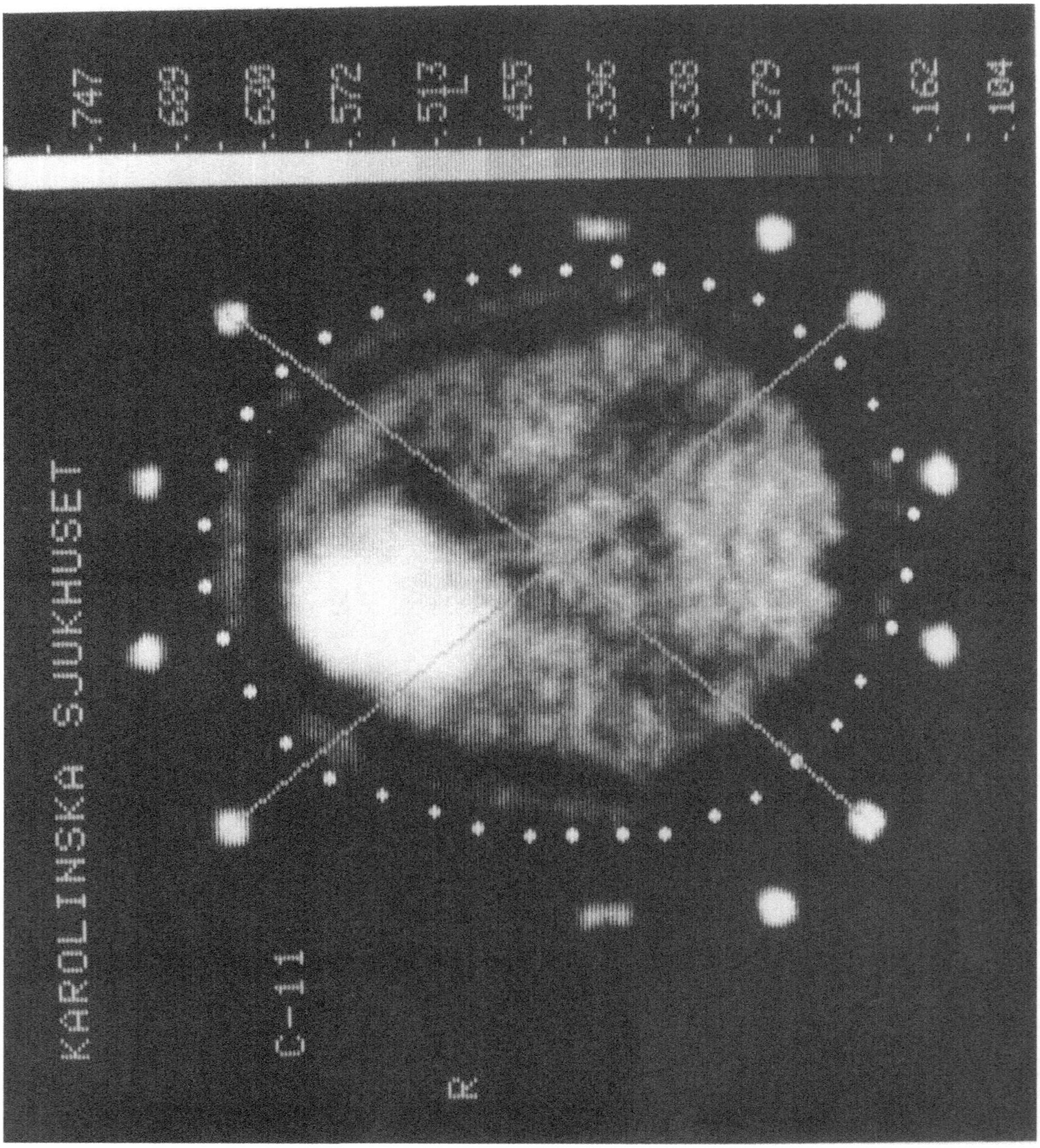

B FIGURE 14–4. (cont.)

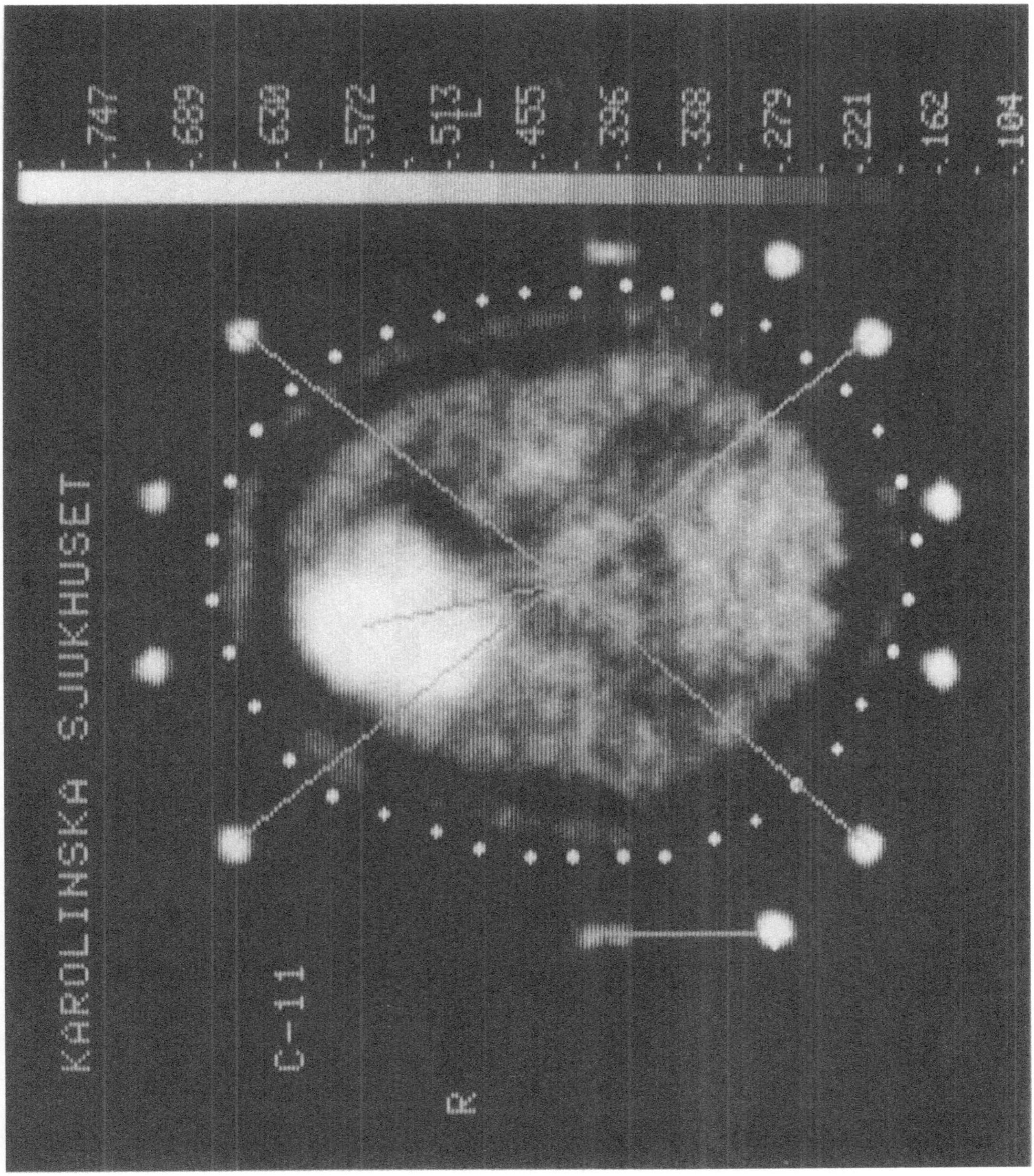

C

FIGURE 14–4. (cont.)

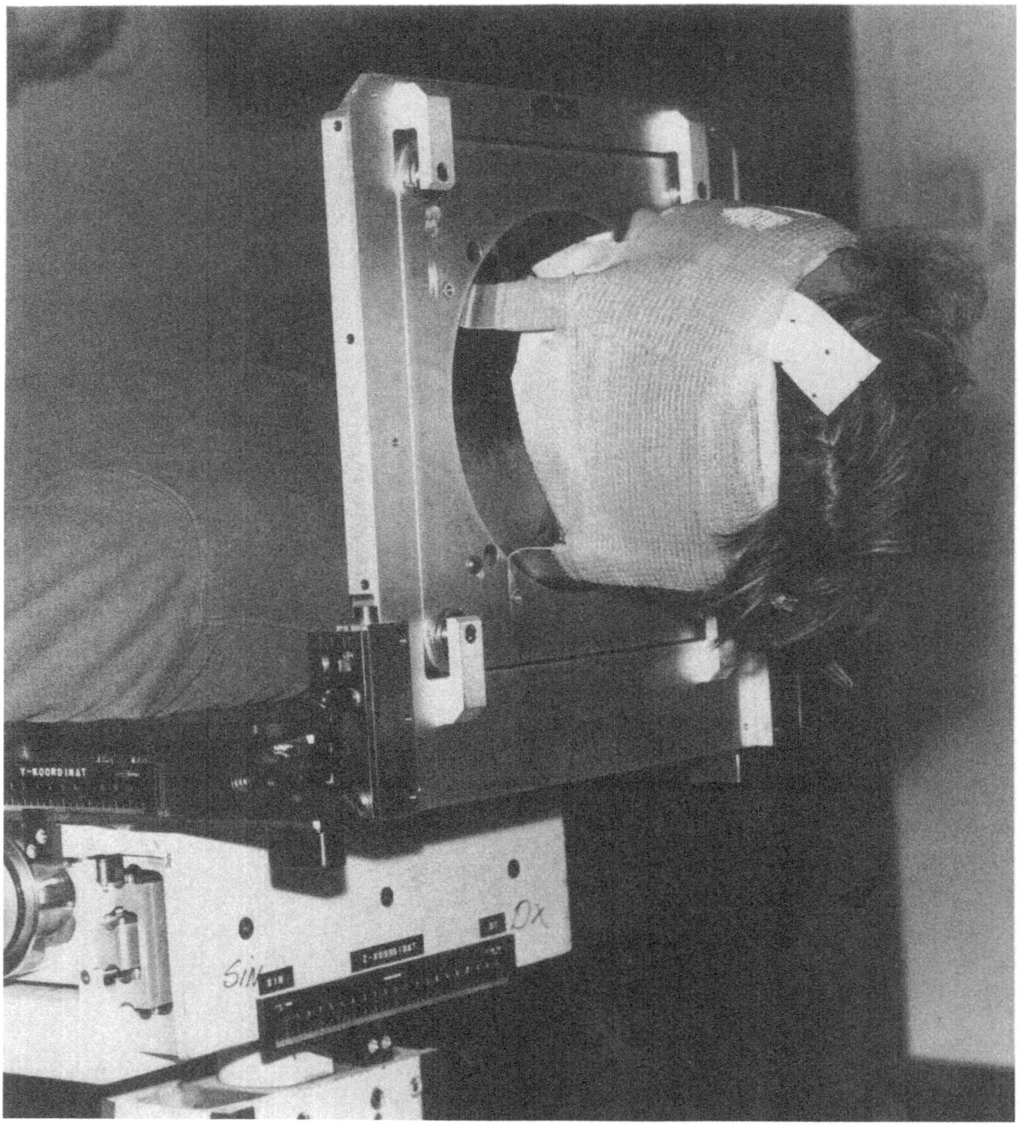

FIGURE 14–5. The head-positioning device has special head holders for attaching it to the operating table.

images. This facilitates comparison of the neuropathological and neuroradiological findings at the various biopsy sites. In most cases, multiple biopsies are performed. A Backlund spiral biopsy (AB Elekta, Stockholm, Sweden) is used to obtain cylindrical samples 10 mm long and 2 mm wide. Several biopsies are taken along the needle trajectory, starting in edematous or normal brain tissue surrounding the tumor, continuing through the tumor, and preferably extending distally. Special care should be taken to obtain one biopsy sample that transverses the tumor margin.

Results

We have used PET imaging to investigate astrocytomas (grade II, according to the World Health Organization), mixed gliomas, anaplastic astrocytomas, and meningiomas. The following is a summary of our results.

ASTROCYTOMAS (NINE PATIENTS)

On CT images, grade II astrocytomas appeared as more or less ill-defined low-attenuation regions. Minimal contrast enhancement was seen in part of one tumor, but in the other tumors there were no signs of a BTB disruption. On PET scans, six patients showed a greater accumulation of methionine in what was believed to be tumor tissue than in normal brain tissue (see figure 14–4); in two patients, the concentration was comparatively reduced in parts of the tumor. In three patients, the methionine uptake was greatly less at least in part of the tumor than in normal brain. Glucose accumulation was lower in five of nine astrocytomas. In the remaining four, the accumulation of glucose did not differ significantly from that of normal brain tissue, but all showed an increased absorption of L-methionine. Eight patients had no signs of a BTB defect as measured with ^{68}Ga-EDTA. In one patient, gallium collected in a small part of the tumor, although the whole tumor displayed a marked accumulation of methionine and reduced glucose uptake. One patient examined with ^{68}Ga-EDTA three months after earlier PET scans exhibited no signs of a defective BTB. Findings by PET examination with ^{68}Ga-EDTA corresponded well with those by contrast-enhanced CT.

MIXED GLIOMAS (OLIGOASTROCYTOMAS, THREE PATIENTS)

As with the astrocytomas, CT demonstrated somewhat ill-defined low attenuation regions without signs of contrast-medium extravasation through the BTB. All tumors showed a marked concentration of methionine and reduced accumulation of glucose. One patient had a faint uptake of gallium but no contrast enhancement on CT. A patient examined with ^{68}Ga-EDTA had a small region of gallium accumulation within a large tumor, although no enhancement was seen on CT. A series of CT examinations 16 months later showed no evidence of significant tumor growth since the earlier PET scan.

ANAPLASTIC ASTROCYTOMA (TWO PATIENTS)

A significantly increased accumulation of gallium, glucose, and methionine as well as a distinct contrast enhancement on CT were seen in portions of an anaplastic astrocytoma in one patient. However, the greater part of the tumor appeared on the methionine scan as an area of increased tracer accumulation. The other patient with an anaplastic astrocytoma had a lesion that was seen on CT as a low-attenuation region with slight contrast enhancement in a small, peripheral part. Considerable methionine uptake was noted in a region much larger than the enhnacing area on CT. The regions of CT contrast enhancement and the PET maximal methionine concentration did not correspond. The glucose accumulation was similar to that of normal brain tissue. An area of increased gallium uptake in a small part of the tumor corresponded to a similar area of CT contrast enhancement.

MENINGIOMAS (TWO PATIENTS)

Both patients with meningiomas demonstrated an increased accumulation of all tracers used for PET examinations as well as a marked contrast enhancement on CT. The dimensions of both tumors appeared similar with PET and CT.

Discussion

Significant differences were found in the degree of regional glucose and methionine accumulation in the intra-axial tumors; these changes paralleled similar attenuation changes seen by CT. The tumor size was approximately the same on methionine scan and on CT in six of 16 patients; in four of these six patients, the lesions appeared much smaller on the glucose examination; and in two patients, the lesion could not be discerned at all on the glucose scan. In three patients, the tumor was larger on the methionine scan than on CT. When compared with CT studies, the glucose examinations of these patients indicated a smaller lesion on CT in two patients and a similar size lesion in two; in three patients, the tumors could not be detected. Both cases of anaplastic astrocytoma were detected convincingly with methionine but not with glucose, ^{68}Ga-EDTA, or CT. Peritumoral edema sometimes was encountered and verified by stereotactic biopsies. These areas were low-attenuation by CT and also showed a decreased glucose accumulation. The methionine uptake in these areas did not differ significantly from that of normal brain tissue.

Although CT is very valuable in the detection of many brain tumors and in the analysis of their differential diagnosis, exact delineation and grading of gliomas are not possible by this method [7, 8, 10]. Moreover, in many cases, CT cannot correctly differentiate between tumor and edema; in some cases, neoplastic areas are not identified at all by CT. In most of our cases, there were definite differences between the areas of increased methionine uptake on PET scan and the pathological areas shown by CT. In all our cases, the pathology depicted by PET using methionine was confirmed by the biopsy samples. We believe that CT should be supplemented with a methionine PET study when an accurate assessment of the tumor size is desirable.

The reaons that the C-11-methionine accumulates are not known. The radionuclide is absorbed by tumors and in normal brain tissue in a continuous linear fashion throughout the whole examination period [9]. Possible mechanisms include the incorporation of methionine into proteins or the donation of the labeled methyl group, which is used in a wide spectrum of other biochemical processes. Possibly, methionine is transported very slowly into the site of protein synthesis and subsequently slowly refluxed with a turnover time that lasts longer than the examination. Regardless of the factors involved, the end result is a marked trapping of the tracer in the tissue.

The accumulation of the enantiomers L-methionine and D-methionine has been investigated in an additional five patients who had astrocytomas. One was anaplastic, and the rest were low-grade astrocytomas. Only one patient had a small region of disrupted blood-brain barrier. The rate of tracer accumulation in tumor tissue was 2.5 times higher with L-methionine than with D-methionine. In normal brain, the ratio was 2.8. The rate, but not the degree, of accumulation was the same in normal brain and in tumor tissue. This suggests that the transport mechanism of L-methionine in tumor tissue is stereospecific with the same dynamics as in normal brain tissue, where it is known to be a carrier-mediated transport.

In a prior study, we examined several patients who received L-methionine with and without the simultaneous infusion of unlabeled amino acids. The methionine accumulation in the tumor and in normal brain was reduced by a factor of 150%–250% when amino acids were infused, unless massive barrier damage existed, in which case tumor uptake was not affected. Thus, the absorption of C-11-methionine is influenced by competition with other amino acids which are known to use the same carrier system in normal brain. This is a further indication that tumor uptake is governed by a carrier-mediated transport across the BTB.

Fluorine-18-fluorodeoxyglucose (F-18-FDG) has been used more widely than either C-11-methionine or C-11-glucose to estimate brain tumor metabolism [2]. This tracer is reportedly more accurate than CT in predicting the histological grading of astrocytomas [10]. PET with F-18-FDG also has been used to differentiate between tumor recurrence and radiation necrosis of the brain [11]. Because only two patients with anaplastic astrocytomas (and no glioblastomas) are included in our investigation, our results with C-11-glucose cannot be compared directly with the results of Patronas [10].

PET scanning with ^{68}Ga-EDTA surpasses contrast-enhanced CT in detecting disruption of the blood-brain barrier [4], at least with the doses of iodinated contrast used in our CT studies. Ilsen and colleagues reported that accumulation of gallium occurred in all of nine low-grade astrocytomas [5]. PET with ^{68}Ga-EDTA proved to be slightly superior to contrast-enhanced CT in enabling recognition.

Conclusion

PET enables us to visualize and determine in vivo functional and metabolic features of intracranial tumors. These factors have been shown to provide valuable information in the diagnosis of these tumors.

PET scanning with C-11-L-methionine often reveals solid tumor tissue in areas that appear normal on CT images. It is also obvious that some tumors extend beyond the area of abnormal methionine uptake. Therefore, we have found that CT and PET along with histological confirmation by stereotactic biopsy are immensely useful. Only through studies like these can the potential of old and new diagnostic modalities be assessed accurately.

Whether gliomas should be regarded as generalized or local tumors is controversial. However, localized treatment such as surgery, radiation therapy, and brachytherapy undoubtedly will continue to be performed. In such cases the determination of the margins is desirable.

Because PET has the potential to trace biochemical properties, its role is greater than just evaluation of tumor extent. PET can be used to characterize functional properties of a tumor in vivo to monitor rapid effects of new types of treatment. Effects on cell function always must precede effects on tumor volume and gross density changes. Finally, the ability of PET to measure receptor interaction potentially can be used for more accurate histological evaluation.

References

1. Bergström M, Boëthius J, Eriksson L, et al: Head fixation device for reproducible position alignment in transmission CT and positron emission tomography: Technical note. *J Comput Assist Tomogr* 5:136–141, 1981
2. DiChiro G, Brooks RA, Patronas NJ, et al: Issues in the in vivo measurement of glucose metabolism of human central nervous system tumors. Ann Neurol 15:138–146, 1984
3. Ehrin E, Westman E, Nilsson SO, et al: A convenient method for the production of C-11-labelled glucose. *J Label Compd Radiopharmacol* 17:453–461, 1980
4. Ericson K, Bergström M, Eriksson L, et al: Positron emission tomography with 68-Ga-EDTA compared with transmission computed tomography in the evaluation of brain infarcts. *Acta Radiol* [*Diagn*] (Stockh) 22:385–398, 1981
5. Ilsen HW, Sato M, Pawlik G, et al: 68-Ga-EDTA positron emission tomography in the diagnosis of brain tumors. *Neuroradiology* 26:393–398, 1984
6. Kingsley DPE, Bergström M, Berggren BM: A critical evaluation of two methods of head fixation. *Neuroradiology* 19:1–6, 1980
7. Lilja A, Bergström M, Hartwig P, et al: Dynamic study of supratentorial gliomas with L-(methyl-11-C-)-methionine and positron emission tomography (PET). *AJNR* (In Press)
8. Lilja A, Bergström M, Spannare B, et al: Reliability of computed tomography in assessing histopathological features of malignant supratentorial gliomas. *J Comput Assist Tomogr* 5:625–636, 1981
9. Patlak CS, Blasberg RG, Fenstermacher JD: Graphical evaluation of blood-to-brain transfer constants from multiple-time uptake data. *J Cereb Blood Flow Metab* 3:1–7, 1983
10. Patronas NJ, Brooks RA, De La Paz RL, et al: Glycolytic rate (PET) and contrast enhancement (CT) in human cerebral gliomas. *AJNR* 4:533–535, 1983.
11. Patronas NJ, DiChiro G, Brooks RA, et al: 18-Fluorodeoxyglucose and positron emission tomography in the evaluation of radiation necrosis of the brain. *Radiology* 144:885–889, 1982
12. Phelps ME, Mazziotta JC, Huang SC: Review: Study of cerebral function with positron emission tomography. *J Cereb Blood Flow Metab* 2:113–162, 1982
13. Stone-Elander S, Nilson JLG, Blomquist G, et al: 11-C-2-Deoxyglucose: Synthesis and preliminary comparison with 11-C-D-Glucose as a tracer for cerebral energy metabolism in PET studies. *Eur J Nucl Med* 10:481–486, 1985

15. STEREOTACTIC TREATMENT OF COLLOID CYSTS OF THE THIRD VENTRICLE

L. Dade Lunsford
Walter A. Hall

Colloid cysts of the third ventricle represent 0.3%–2.0% of all brain tumors [10]. Despite their rarity, these lesions have fascinated neurosurgeons since the first was removed successfully through a pineal approach by Dandy in 1921 [3]. The interest in colloid cysts developed because of their surgical accessibility, their benign histology, and their occasionally disastrous sequelae when left untreated [4, 16]. However, their clinical behavior frequently is not benign. Although most patients (85%–96%) present with headaches, fluctuating or progressive dementia, seizures also are describe [18]. Even recently, sudden unconsciousness followed by death, possibly secondary to acute hydrocephalus leading to herniation, has been associated with colloid cysts [16].

Since the development of computed tomography (CT), and more recently, magnetic resonance imaging (MRI), colloid cysts of the third ventricle are now recognized earlier and more often. The location, volume, and CT attentuation factors (e.g., hyper, iso-, or hypodensity) have been described [5]. These lesions are readily identifiable on multiplanar MRI; they usually demonstrate high signal on both T_1- and T_2-weighted images because of the high protein content of the viscous material [8].

Various surgical approaches have been developed to remove colloid cysts. Surgical intervention has been directed at removing the cyst and opening the cerebrospinal fluid (CSF) pathways. Conservative management in the form of bilateral ventriculoperitoneal shunting has been advocated, but this treatment requires and accurate preoperative diagnosis of the lesion and can be disastrous if shunt occlusion later occurs. The third ventricle can be reached by transfrontal, transcallosal, and transventricular-subchoroidal surgical approaches [1, 9, 17]. The transcallosal approach is tolerated well by patients who do not have significant hydrocephalus [1, 17]. In 1978, Bosch and co-workers reported on the treatment of colloid cysts by stereotactic aspiration [3]. No recurrences were seen in four patients up to seven years after surgery. Other authors since have described CT stereotactic aspiration [2], catheter removal techniques [6], and endoscopic removal of colloid cysts [14].

Between January 1976 and December 1985, at the University Health Center of Pittsburgh, 17 patients underwent surgery for colloid cysts. Seven patients had stereotactic aspiration performed as the initial procedure. This chapter describes the technique and results of stereotactic aspiration in the context of our overall experience with colloid cysts and the clinical problems and concerns that these histologically benign but potentially dangerous lesions present.

Clinical Summary

Table 15–1 demonstrates the clinical and radiographic findings in the 17 patients who were referred to our center for treatment (ten men and seven women, aged 19–63 years). Fifteen patients had headaches; eight (47%) demonstrated signs of increased intracranial

L.D. Lunsford (ed.) *MODERN STEREOTACTIC NEUROSURGERY*.

TABLE 15–1. Clinical and Radiographic Findings in 17 Patients with Colloid Cysts of the Third Ventricle, 1975–1985*

Finding	No. of Patients	Percentage
Clinical symptoms		
Headache	15	88
Nausea/vomiting	8	47
Altered vision	7	41
Weakness	6	35
Numbness	4	23
Tinnitus	3	18
Neck stiffness	3	18
Seizures	3	18
Neurological examination		
Papilledema	7	41
Dementia	4	23
Upgaze palsy	3	18
Herniation	1	6
Computed tomography		
Hydrocephalus	17	100
Precontrast		
High attenuation (hyperdense)	12	72
Brain attenuation (isodense)	3	18
Low attenuation (hypodense)	1	6
No mass	1	6
Postcontrast		
No Enhancement	15	88
Enhancement	2	12
Angiography		
Hydrocephalus	6	35
Elevation of internal cerebral vein	6	35
Avascular mass at the foramen of Monro	5	30
Normal	5	30
Not performed	3	18

* 13 patients had craniotomy and cyst removal; seven had attempted stereotactic aspiration.

pressure, including nausea and vomiting; and seven (41%) had visual difficulties. Neurological evaluation disclosed papilledema in seven patients, paresis of upward gaze (three patients), and dementia (four patients). One patient presented with an acute herniation syndrome.

CT revealed a dilated ventricular system (hydrocephalus) in each of the 17 patients. CT performed without contrast enhancement revealed a high-attenuation (hyperdense) mass in 12 patients (72%), a brain-attenuation (isodense) mass in three patients (18%), and a low-attenuation (hypodense) mass in one patient (6%). In one patient, no mass was identified by an early-generation CT scanner. Only two patients demonstrated enhancement of the colloid cyst after intravenous contrast was given. Cerebral angiography, performed on 14 patients, confirmed hydrocephalus in six (35%) and elevation of the internal cerebral vein in six (35%). An avascular mass at the foramen of Monro was found in five patients (30%), but the results of angiography were interpreted as normal in five patients (30%).

Since the introduction of CT-compatible stereotactic instrumentation at our center, we have chosen to perform stereotactic aspiration as the initial procedure in seven patients (figure 15–1). In all patients, mass lesions at the foramen of Monro were identified by CT scans. The preoperative estimation of tumor volume ranged from 0.5–5 ml. We performed cerebral angiography preoperatively in all stereotactic cases to assess the relationship of the internal cerebral and thalamostriate veins to the iden-

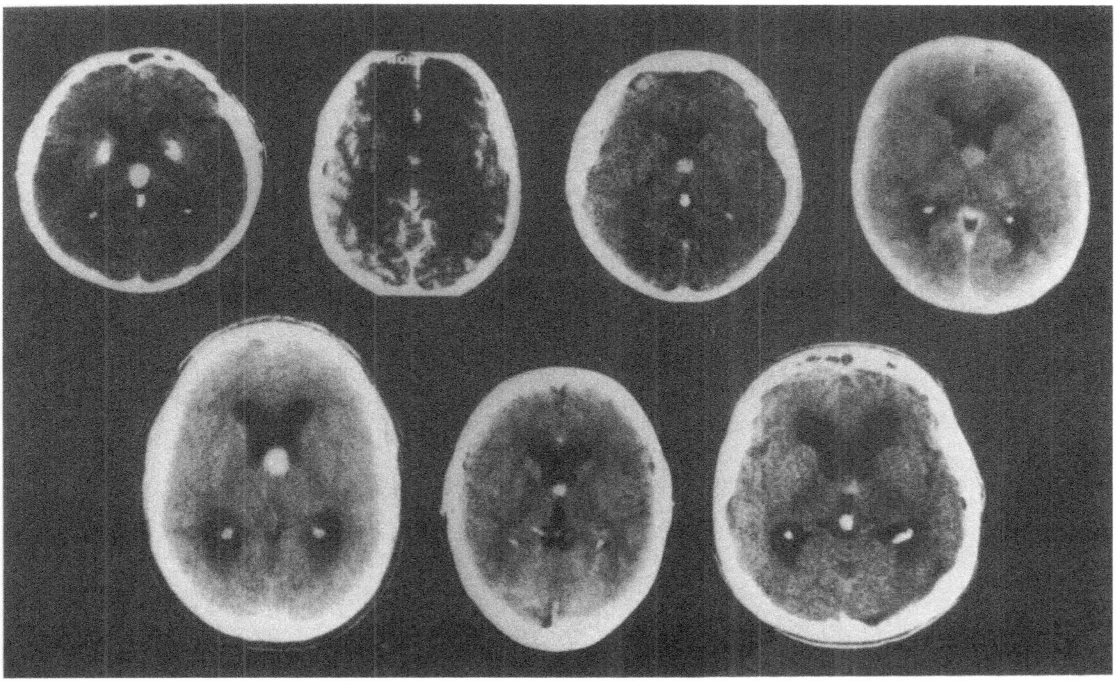

FIGURE 15–1. Preoperative CT scans demonstrating colloid cysts of the third ventricle in seven patients who had stereotactic aspiration as the initial surgical treatment.

tified mass. A transfrontal-transcortical stereotactic approach was used each time.

Surgical Approach

All seven patients underwent stereotactic aspiration in an operating room equipped with an advanced-generation CT scanner (GE 8800) [13]. After the administration of local anesthesia (1% lidocaine) supplemented by intravenous sedation, the Leksell stereotactic head frame was applied to the patient's head. The patient rested supine upon the CT scanner table for initial intraoperative imaging. After intravenous contrast enhancement was given, 5-mm-thick axial CT images were obtained in the region of the third and lateral ventricles. Multiplanar reformatted imaging of the lesion was performed to help determine its location and size (figure 15–2). The volume of the lesions was estimated with the cursor trackball and region-of-interest (ROI) technique [12].

Stereotactic coordinates of the target were obtained from the CT scan (chapter 3). The right frontal region was then shaved and prepped in a limited area surrounding the coronal suture. A percutaneous twist-drill approach was used for four patients, and a burr hole was placed at the coronal suture for three. After opening or puncturing the dura with the needle, the probe (1.8 mm outer diameter) was advanced through the ventricular system to the target site. Because the probe often displaced the colloid cyst, the needle was advanced 3–5 mm beneath the actual target site. In most patients, the surgeon felt a slight resistance as the needle entered the cyst; penetration of the cyst was confirmed by the absence of CSF flow from the needle after the stylet was removed.

To perform the initial aspiration, a 10-ml syringe was attached to the stopcock on the needle. To aspirate the tumor, 6–8 ml of suction was applied to the syringe, and the needle was retracted and advanced a distance of approximately 5 mm. Significant resistance was often felt, and the amount of suction needed to withdraw the colloid material from the cyst was usually greater than expected. If the colloid material was aspirated successfully with the 1.8-mm needle, the needle was left in position. If not, a 2.1-mm outer-diameter probe was then inserted at the target site. From 10

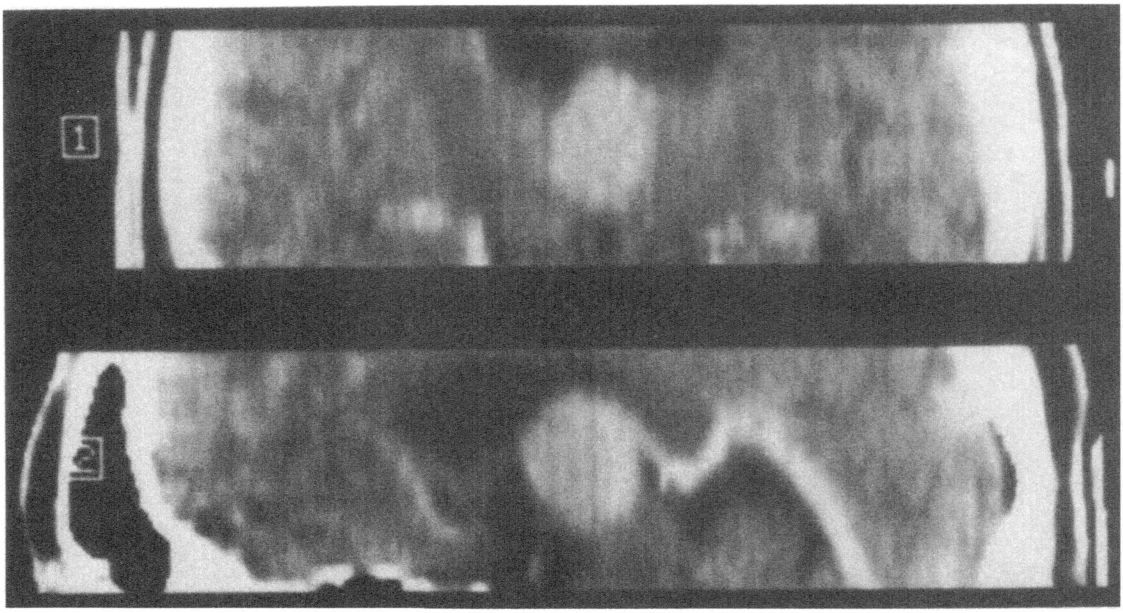

FIGURE 15–2. CT multiplanar reformatted image of a colloid cyst of the third ventricle obtained at the time of stereotactic aspiration. Volume estimation was performed also.

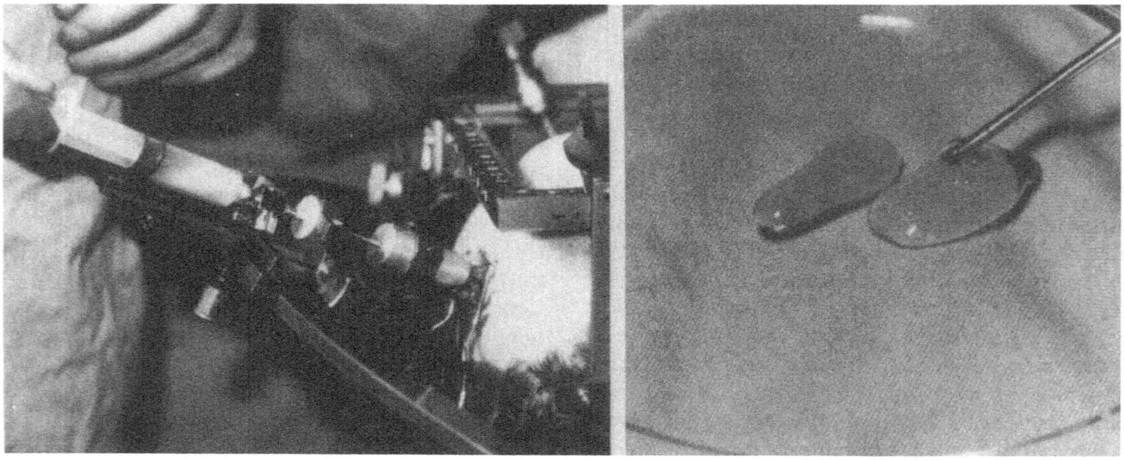

FIGURE 15–3. (*Left*) Intraoperative aspiration of colloid cyst. All patients were awake. The probe guide attaches to the frame and permits low artifact CT imaging. (*Right*) Evacuation of viscous colloid material. If the material is of greater viscosity (cheese-like), aspiration is impossible.

mm above the target site, a corkscrew spiral biopsy was performed in an attempt to fenestrate the cyst. The specimen thus obtained was sent for histological review. The surgeon removed the spiral biopsy stylet and again employed suction to aspirate the cyst, using the larger needle. Aspiration was continued until the withdrawn colloid material reached approximately the volume estimated preoperatively from the CT image (figure 15–3).

The Leksell stereotactic arc then was removed, and the probe was fixed to the frame

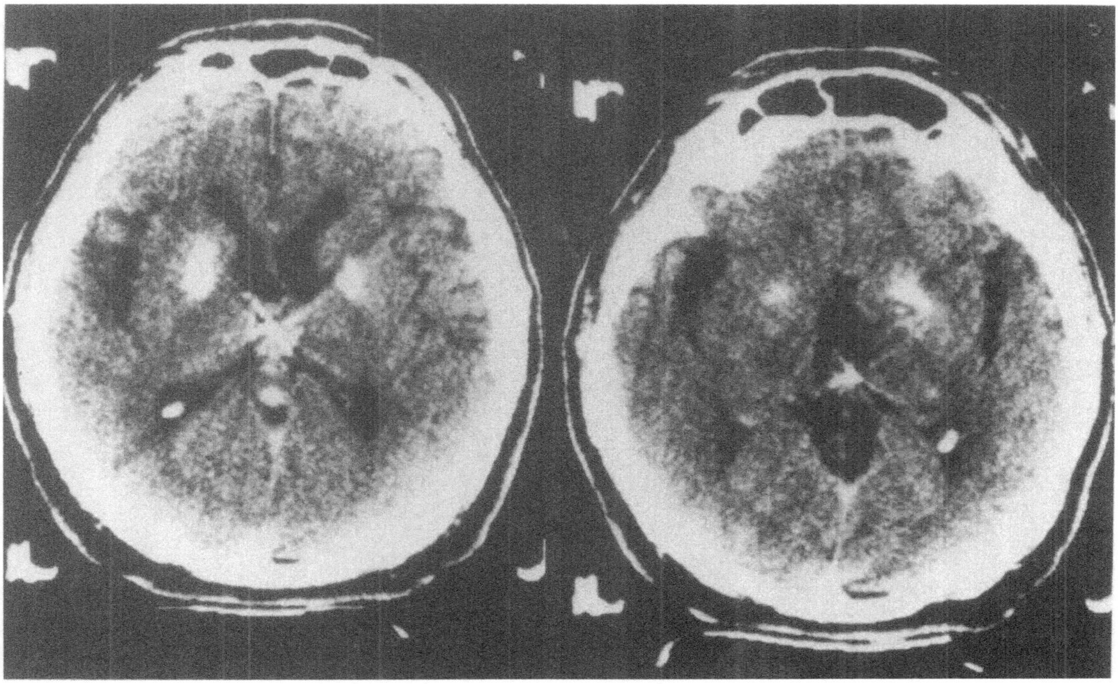

FIGURE 15-4. (*Left*) Intraoperative CT scan demonstrating the position of the stereotactic probe in the colloid cyst. (*Right*) Postaspiration CT scan demonstrating evacuation of the colloid cyst.

with a percutaneous probe holder that permitted intraoperative imaging [11]. The patient and frame were returned to the CT aperture, and repeat CT images of the colloid cyst were obtained (figure 15-4). The position of the needle tip within the remnant of the cyst was confirmed by CT. If residual colloid material was demonstrated, a repeat aspiration was performed. In two patients it was necessary to reposition the needle because colloid material was noted posterior to the position of the needle, as seen on the intraoperative CT image. The cyst then was reaspirated in an attempt to remove as much material as possible.

After aspiration, several CT images of the area were obtained to exclude postoperative complications, including intraventricular hemorrhage; that complication was not identified in this series of cases. Intraoperative CT ventriculography was performed next by the instillation of 1-2 ml of 170 mg iodine per milliliter of metrizamide into the lateral ventricle. The patient's head was gently rocked back and forth in an attempt to disperse the contrast agent within the ventricular system. Repeat CT images were obtained, starting at the level of the fourth ventricle, to assess postoperative patency of the ventricular system (figure 15-5). The probe and probe holder were removed, and the wound was closed. After surgery, our patients were monitored overnight in a neurosurgical continuous-care unit.

Results of Stereotactic Treatment

Table 15-2 demonstrates the results of preoperative, operative, and postoperative treatment of seven patients who underwent stereotactic aspiration. In five patients, incomplete aspiration was demonstrated by intraoperative, and postoperative CT scans. One patient had an initial subtotal aspiration of colloid material volume, but complete evacuation was accomplished by reaspiration five months after the first procedure. One patient achieved complete aspiration of a 2-ml colloid cyst. Follow-up duration ranged from eight to 46 months. Patient 1 subsequently required a ventriculoperitoneal shunt for persistent hydrocephalus, despite adequate aspiration. Patients 3, 4, and 5 later underwent craniotomy for removal of the cyst because of persistent symptoms secon-

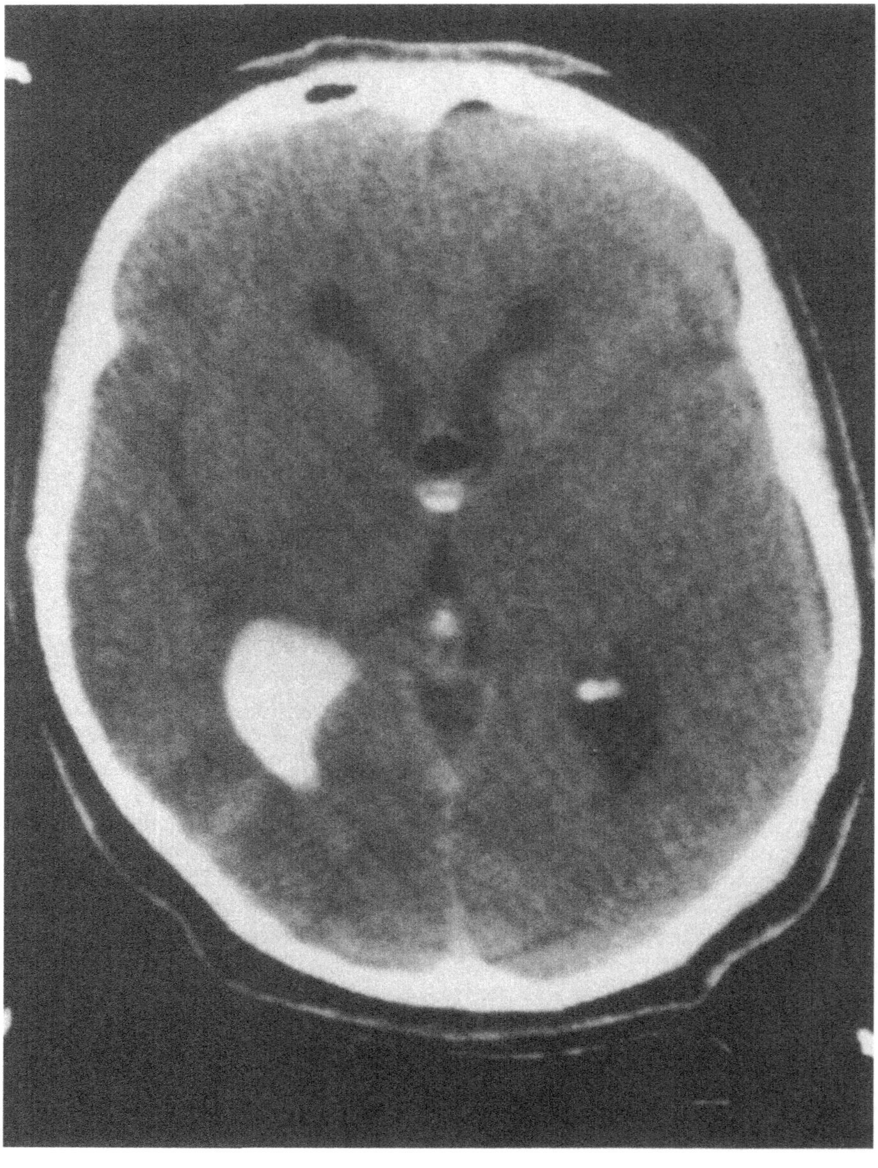

FIGURE 15-5. After aspiration, 1–2 ml of 170 mg iodine/ml metrizamide was placed within the lateral ventricle to confirm patency of the ventricular system.

dary to incomplete aspiration. Patient 6, who had a ventriculoperitoneal shunt placed prior to referral, required no postoperative treatment after aspiration. Our detailed intraoperative and postoperative studies revealed that two patients achieved complete aspiration, three patients partial aspiration, and two patients could not be aspirated (table 15–3).

Intraoperative CT ventriculography after aspiration revealed a patent ventricular system in five of the six patients studied. No operative complications occurred after stereotactic surgery, and no new neurological deficits were noted. One patient (No. 2) had intracystic filling by the ventricular contrast material, which flowed from the lateral ventricle into the fenestrated portion of the cyst. Because the contrast agent was isoosmotic, we chose to

TABLE 15–2. Results of Stereotactic Aspiration in Seven Patients

Patient No.	Age/Sex	Clinical Presentation	Preoperative Treatment	Size of Cyst	Degree of Aspiration	Postoperative Treatment	Follow-up Duration (months)	Follow-up Status
1	60/M	Headache; dementia		2 ml	Incomplete	Ventriculoperitoneal shunt	22	Intermittent headache; normal
2	63/M	Dementia; headache		5 ml	Complete*	Reaspiration 5 mos. later	23	Improved; mildly demented
3	48/M	Headache; blurred vision; seizure		1.5 ml	Incomplete	Transfrontal craniotomy	26	Normal
4	36/F	Headache; nausea/ vomiting blurred; vision		2.5 ml	Incomplete	Transcallosal craniotomy	67	Normal
5	26/F	Headache		1 ml	Incomplete	Transcallosal craniotomy	16	Hemiparetic (venous infarct after craniotomy)
6	29/M	Headache; herniation	Ventriculo-peritoneal shunt	0.5 ml	Incomplete	Nonc	8	Normal
7	41/F	Headache		2 ml	Complete	None	46	Normal

* Required two procedures.

TABLE 15-3. Postoperative Results in Seven Patients

Operative findings (N = 7)	
Completely aspirated	2[a]
Partially aspirated	3
Unable to be aspirated	2
Intraoperative CT ventriculography after aspiration (N = 6)	
Ventricular system patent	5
Ventricular system obstructed	1[b]
Operative complications	
Mortality	0
New neurological deficit	0
Retained intracystic water-soluble contrast agent	1
Seizures	0

[a] One patient required two procedures; removed by repeat stereotactic aspiration.
[b] Required transfrontal craniotomy for persistent headache.

observe this patient rather than attempt to remove the intracystic contrast material immediately. CT scan performed three and five days after surgery demonstrated that the contrast material continued to fill the cyst, and repeat stereotactic aspiration was performed subsequently to evacuate this material.

Discussion

Modern neurodiagnostic imaging tools, including CT and MRI, are the procedures of choice for identifying colloid cysts of the third ventricle (figure 15-6). These techniques facilitate determination of ventricular size, cyst size, and the location of the cyst in relationship to the third ventricle. These imaging tools also help to exclude the different diagnostic possibilities of other anterior third ventricular masses: basilar artery aneurysm, third ventricular meningioma, hypothalamic glioma, ependymoma, choroid plexus papilloma, xanthogranuloma, cysticercosis, teratoid tumor, tuberous sclerosis, noncommunicating cysts of the septum pellucidum, craniopharyngioma, and pituitary adenoma [15]. The earlier recognition of such third

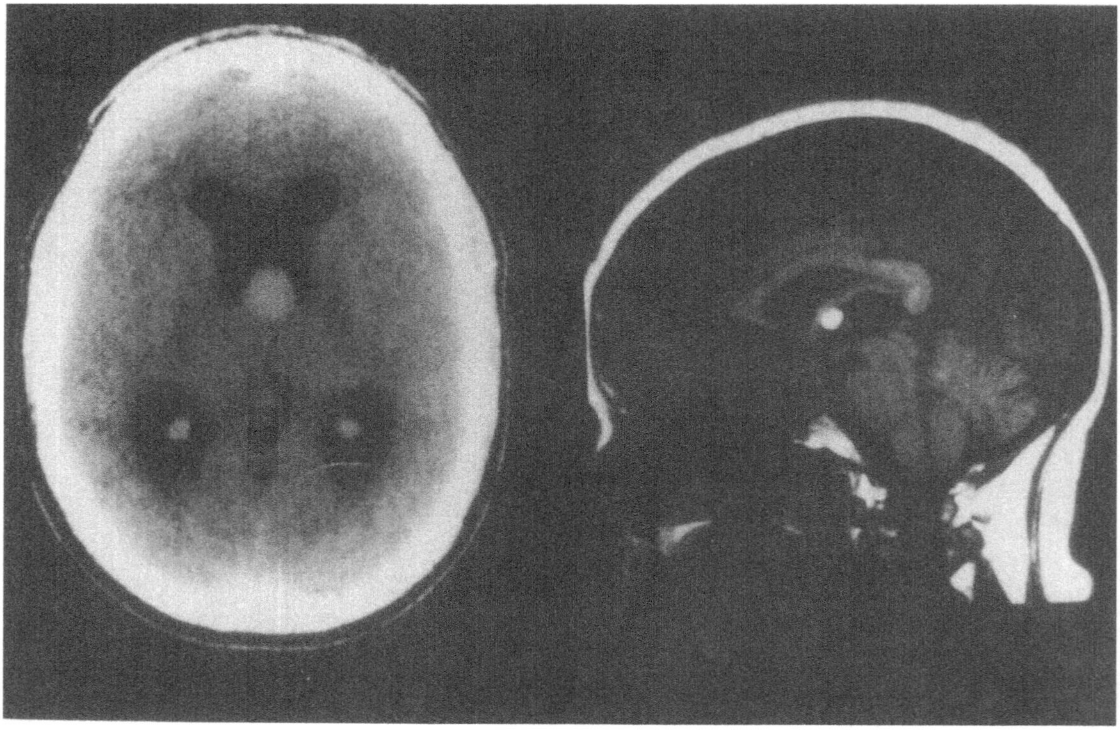

FIGURE 15-6. (*Left*) Axial CT scan illustrating a colloid cyst of the third ventricle. (*Right*) Midsagittal MRI (T_1-weighted) demonstrating the high signal of the colloid cyst due to the protein content of the viscous material.

ventricular lesions has prompted the introduction of potentially efficacious and certainly less invasive techniques such as stereotactic aspiration [2, 3, 15].

The seven cases reported here demonstrate both the feasibility and difficulties of stereotactic aspiration. Although we have performed CT stereotactic surgery as the initial procedure for such lesions since 1981, we have come to realize that stereotactic aspiration alone may not be sufficient in many cases. More definitive surgery, such as transcallosal or transventricular removal, continues to be required. Even successful aspiration (or even complete removal) does not always restore the ventricular system to normal size, and persistent hydrocephalus, when present, may require postoperative spinal fluid diversion by ventriculoperitoneal shunting.

We found three reasons for the failure of stereotactic aspiration. First, the consistency of the viscous material within the colloid cyst ranges from soft, mucoid, and gelatinous (easy to aspirate) to firm, inspissated, dense, and cheesy material that is impossible to aspirate with a needle 2.1 mm in diameter. We have been unable to determine by preoperative imaging studies which lesions can be aspirated. We found no correlation between the attenuation pattern seen on CT images and the subsequent ability to aspirate a colloid cyst. Second, the colloid cyst may be displaced from the needle tip as the needle is advanced to the target, changing the target location, and rendering penetration of the cyst wall difficult and potentially hazardous. Third, the dense fibrocollagenous connective tissue and epithelium that form the cyst itself may be impossible to puncture.

Stereotactic aspiration does not remove the outer lining of the cyst, but simple aspiration of the colloid material has led to long-term symptomatic relief without recurrence in the four patients reported to date [3]. It is important to confirm that the ventricular system is patent after either complete or incomplete aspiration, or symptoms will persist.

To compare our results of stereotactic surgery with those of craniotomy, we also reviewed the results of conventional surgery for colloid cysts at our institution. Between 1975 and 1986, five patients underwent transfrontal craniotomy and removal of colloid cysts, three of whom had preoperative ventriculoperitoneal shunts. Although one patient developed bilateral subdural collections which required evacuation, all five patients ultimately achieved satisfactory neurological outcomes. Of eight patients who underwent transcallosal craniotomy and removal, two suffered postoperative venous infarctions resulting in major neurological deficits (hemiparesis). One patient acquired an infection of the bone flap and meningitis, and another patient required bilateral postoperative shunts for intermittent headaches. In contrast to craniotomy and direct surgical removal, stereotactic surgery was associated with no complications but with a high rate of incomplete aspiration.

In addition to stereotactic aspiration, a freehand puncture and catheter aspiration technique guided by intraoperative CT has been described by Gutierrez-Lara and co-workers [6]. A transventricular endoscopic removal has been advocated by Apuzzo and associates [2]. Stereotactic ventricular endoscopic surgery combines precise localization of the lesion with a technique that enables opening and evacuation of the cyst under direct vision. At present, endoscopic surgery requires a large diameter probe or bilateral ventricular access to allow positioning the stereotactic probe from one side and the endoscope from another. We are currently exploring the benefit of stereotactic endoscopy or laser resection, as advocated by Kelly and colleaques [7]. We endorse stereotactic surgery as the initial treatment of choice. If clinical symptoms remain or radiographic evidence of persistent or recurrent cyst formation is demonstrated, definitive surgical exploration of the third ventricle by craniotomy should be performed. Even after complete removal, however, persistent hydrocephalus and clinical symptomatology may subsequently require spinal fluid diversion. Colloid cysts continue to be a fascinating problem, and while histologically benign, they remain potentially treacherous. As smaller, perhaps even asymptomatic colloid cysts of the brain are identified, stereotactic surgery will be used to identify and remove such lesions.

References

1. Antunes JL, Louis KM, Ganti SR: Colloid cysts of the third ventricle. *Neurosurgery* 7:450–455, 1980
2. Apuzzo MLJ, Chandrasoma PT, Zelman V, et

al: Computed tomographic guidance stereotaxis in the management of lesions of the third ventricular region. *Neurosurgery* 15:502–508, 1984
3. Bosch DA, Rahn T, Backlund EO: Treatment of colloid cysts of the third ventricle by stereotactic aspiration. *Surg Neurol* 9:15–18, 1978
4. Chan RC, Thompson GB: Third ventricular colloid cysts presenting with acute neurological deterioration. *Surg Neurol* 19:358–362, 1983
5. Ganti SR, Antunes JL, Louis KM, et al: Computed tomography in the diagnosis of colloid cysts of the third ventricle. *Radiology* 138:385–391, 1981
6. Gutierrez-Lara F, Pantino R, Hakim S: Treatment of tumors of the third ventricle: A new and simple technique. *Surg Neurol* 3:323–325, 1975
7. Kelly PJ, Kall BA, Goerss S, et al: Computer-assisted stereotactic laser resection of intra-axial brain neoplasms. *J Neurosurg* 64:427–439, 1986
8. Kjos BO, Brant-Zawadzki M, Kucharczyk W, et al: Cystic intracranial lesions: Magnetic resonance imaging. *Radiology* 155:363–369, 1985
9. Lavyne MH, Patterson RN: Subchoroidal trans-velum interpositum approach to mid-third ventricular tumors. *Neurosurgery* 12:86–94, 1983
10. Little JR, MacCarty CS: Colloid cysts of the third ventricle. *J Neurosurg* 39:230–235, 1974
11. Lunsford LD, Leksell L, Jernberg B: Probe holder for stereotactic surgery in the CT scanner: A technical note. *Acta Neurochir* (Wien) 69:297–304, 1983
12. Lunsford LD, Levine G, Gumerman LW: Comparison of computerized tomographic and radionuclide methods in determining intracranial cystic tumor volumes. *J Neurosurg* 63:740–744, 1985
13. Lunsford LD, Martinez AJ: Stereotactic exploration of the brain in the era of computed tomography. *Surg Neurol* 22:222–230, 1984
14. Powell MP, Torrens MJ, Thomson JLG, et al: Isodense colloid cysts of the third ventricle: A diagnostic and therapeutic problem resolved by ventriculoscopy. *Neurosurgery* 13:234–237, 1983
15. Rivas JJ, Lobato RD: CT-assisted stereotactic aspiration of colloid cysts of the third ventricle. *J Neurosurg* 62:238–242, 1985
16. Ryder JW, Kleinschmidt-DeMasters BK, Keller TS: Sudden deterioration and death in patients with benign tumors of the third ventricle area. *J Neurosurg* 64:216–223, 1986
17. Shucart WA, Stein BM: Transcallosal approach to the anterior ventricular system. *Neurosurgery* 3:339–343, 1978
18. Yenermen MH, Bowerman CI, Haymaker W: Colloid cysts of the third ventricle: A clinical study of 54 cases in the light of previous publications. *Acta Neuroveg* 17:211–277, 1958

16. STEREOTACTIC EVACUATION OF INTRACEREBRAL HEMATOMA

Alfred C. Higgins
Blaine S. Nashold

Brain hemorrhages have been recognized and recorded in medical literature for more than a century. Today they are classified by type, including primary (spontaneous) hemorrhage, posttraumatic hemorrhage, and hemorrhage secondary to various disease states. Causes of secondary hemorrhage include brain tumors, vascular anomalies such as aneurysmal defects and arteriovenous malformations (AVM), angiopathies, and coagulopathies. Brain hemorrhages also are classified by location: cerebral or supratentorial, cerebellar, and brain stem. Supratentorial hemorrhages may be further divided into either lobular or deep (in the region of the basal ganglia, the internal capsule, and the thalamus). Parenchymal hemorrhage may be accompanied by dissection of blood into the ventricular system (figure 16–1).

Early clinical studies considered the mortality rate for cerebral hemorrhage to approach 80%–90%. Even when survival statistics are revised by computed tomography (CT) studies of stroke patients, the mortality rate for spontaneous intracerebral hemorrhage remains in the 60%–70% range [13, 34]. Yet their appropriate treatment remains controversial. Advances in both diagnostic and therapeutic capabilities have led to a more aggressive approach to the treatment of brain hemorrhages of all types and in all locations. Reviews of the epidemiology, pathophysiology, and historical evolution of treating spontaneous intracerebral hemorrhages are provided by Cahill [10] and Higgins [18]. This chapter addresses the stereotactic approach to the evacuation of spontaneous or so-called primary intracerebral hemorrhages.

The Evolution of Stereotactic Instruments for Hematoma Evacuation

In 1978, Backlund introduced a new stereotactic instrument for mechanical evacuation of intracerebral hematomas [4]. This technological advance proved to be superior to simple needle aspiration. A postoperative cranial CT scan of one patient undergoing hematoma evacuation by this technique showed subtotal evacuation of copious amounts of acute hematoma coagulum.

In 1980, we adopted Backlund's technique, demonstrating in three patients that this method can adequately evacuate acute brain hemorrhages without the necessity for open craniotomy [18]. We subsequently modified Backlund's original device, incorporating a vented cannula in a tandem arrangement adjacent to the original helical cutting mandrel (figure 16–2) [17]. In 1981, this device was refined further to incorporate both aspiration and venting cannulas within the same polished outer housing (figure 16–3) [19].

In 1982, Broseta published results of a study of 16 patients who underwent stereotactic evacuation of deep-seated intracerebral hematomas via the Backlund technique [9]. CT scan follow-up was employed to assess the extent of hematoma evacuation and the occurrence of rebleeding. The findings demonstrated that this was a satisfactory mechanical technique for removing acute coagulated clot from deep hematomas.

Hondo (in 1983) [21] and Matsumoto (in

L.D. Lunsford (ed.) *MODERN STEREOTACTIC NEUROSURGERY*.

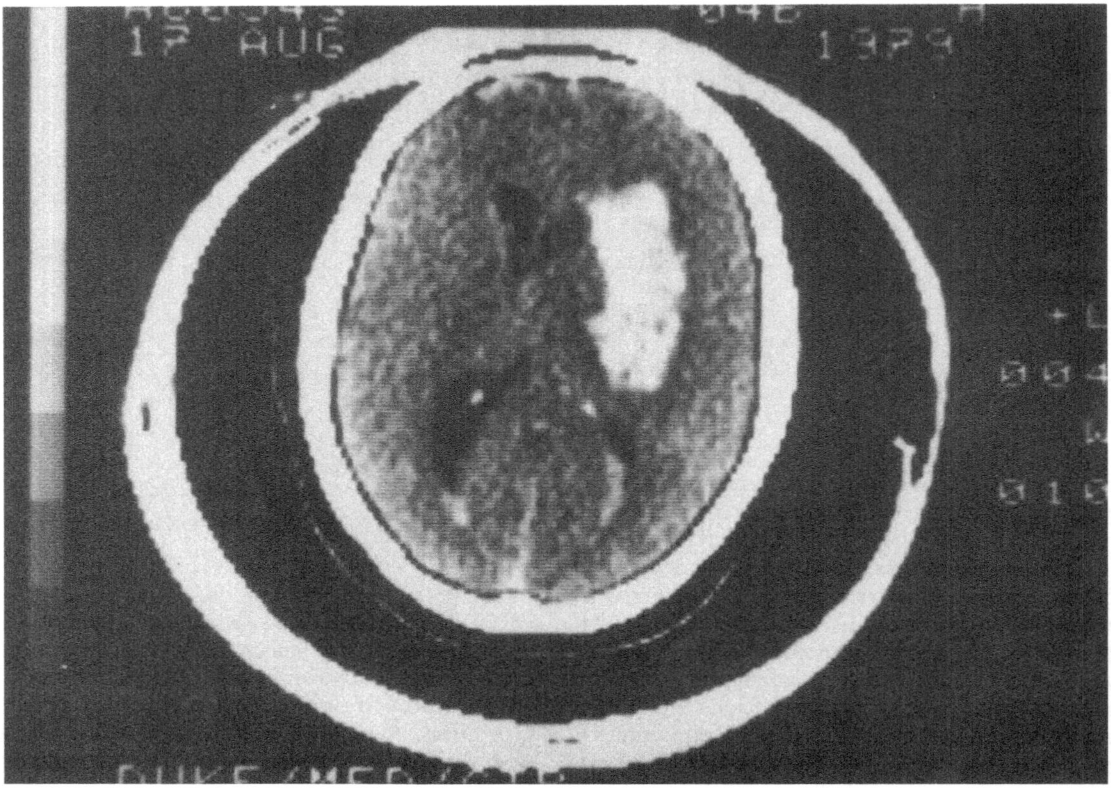

FIGURE 16–1. Cranial CT scan demonstrating hemorrhage in the region of the left basal ganglia.

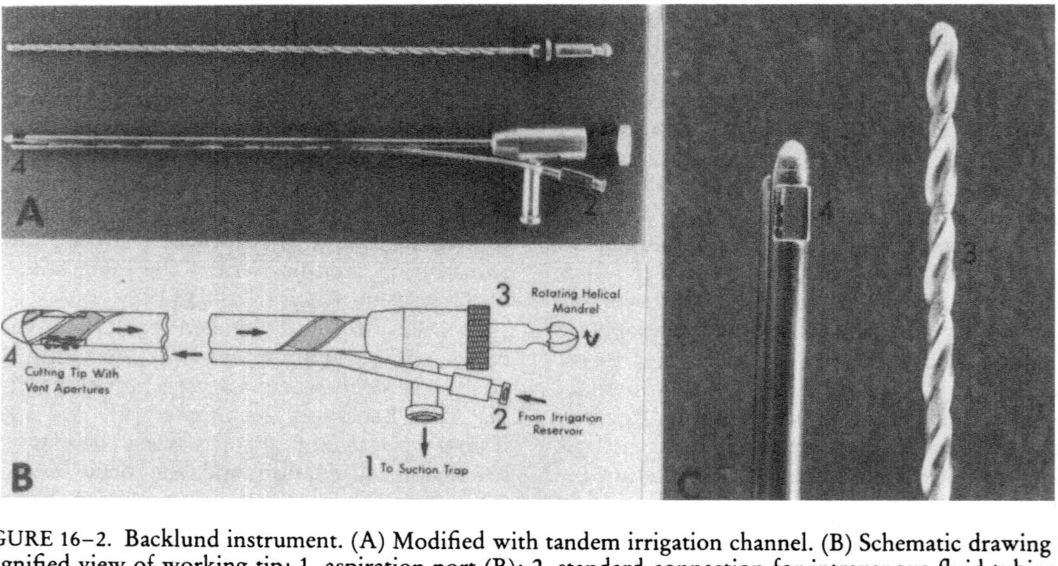

FIGURE 16–2. Backlund instrument. (A) Modified with tandem irrigation channel. (B) Schematic drawing (C) Magnified view of working tip: 1. aspiration port (B); 2. standard connection for intravenous fluid tubing on irrigation channel (A and B); 3. manually operated helical mandrel (A, B, and C); 4. cutting tip with side ports (A, B, and C).

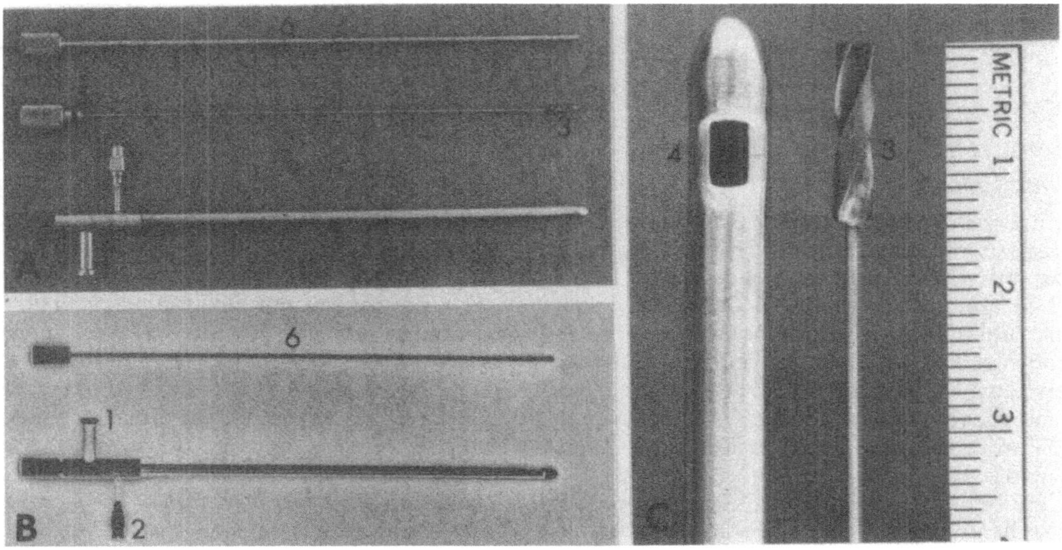

FIGURE 16–3. (A) Higgins-Nashold instrument. (B) Radiograph of instrument with mandrel in place. (C) Magnified view: 1. aspiration port (A and B); 2. standard connection for intravenous fluid tubing on irrigation channel (A and B); 3. helical cutting mandrel (A and C); 4. side cutting port (C); 5. O-ring seal (A); 6. Obturator (A and B).

1984) [29] reported on a somewhat different stereotactic approach. They used freehand, CT-guided flexible catheterization of deep-seated hematomas for evacuation of acute liquefied blood and for repeated irrigation and aspiration of the hematoma cavity over the course of several days. This technique differs from those described previously in that instillation of urokinase for enzymatic degradation of the solidified clot replaced the need for direct mechanical agitation and fragmentation. As with previous trials of stereotactic hematoma evacuation, their patients were evaluated with CT before and after surgical intervention; the CT images indicated satisfactory dissolution and resolution of the hematoma cavity. Some would deny that Hondo's method is truly a stereotactic technique because of the freehand puncture of the hematoma cavity [3]. However, regardless of the mechanism for penetrating the hematoma, the use of urokinase for liquefying the solid components of an intracerebral hemorrhage must be regarded as an innovation in hematoma therapy [1].

Further modification of Backlund's technique was reported by Kandel in 1985 [23]. This method used a motor-driven helical mandrel contained in a device very similar to Backlund's original cannula. Kandel's work is important for several reasons, including the high-speed mechanical fragmentation of solid blood coagulum by a motor-driven helical mandrel and the postoperative insertion of a flexible balloon-tip catheter for postoperative tamponade of the hematoma cavity.

Successful evacuation of brain-stem hemorrhages by stereotactic needle aspiration also was reported in 1983 by Beatty and Zervas [5] and in 1985 by Bosch and Beute [7].

Overall, the experience of surgeons with various techniques of stereotactic evacuation for brain hemorrhages has been extremely limited. Reasons for this include the overall poor prognosis for patients sustaining large brain hemorrhages, the lack of definition of clinical and radiodiagnostic criteria to indicate which patients might benefit from surgical evacuation, and a lag in the enthusiasm of the neurosurgical community for the use of stereotactic approaches. Given the renaissance of stereotaxy in conjunction with the use of CT and computer-guidance systems, the obstacles may be overcome [2, 12, 27].

Diagnosis of Intracerebral Hematoma and Indications for Evacuation

Before the development of CT, establishing the diagnosis of primary intracerebral hemorrhage was very difficult and time-consuming. Today, CT imaging of the brain has become the standard and accepted method for diagnosing this problem. The sensitivity of current CT scanners enables the physician to detect small hemorrhages (approximately 5 mm in diameter, 0.07 ml in volume), which makes it possible to diagnose hemorrhage in virtually any portion of the brain or brain stem. Often, the location of a hemorrhage is sufficiently diagnostic to obviate the need for cerebral arteriography. This is particularly true of small localized hemorrhages within the basal ganglia or thalamus, the parenchyma of the cerebellum, or the pons, all common locations of primary hemorrhages. At other times, the magnitude or location of the hemorrhage may leave in question the origin of the bleeding. In such cases, cerebral arteriography should be performed to identify vascular lesions such as aneurysms, AVM, venous angiomas, or highly vascular tumors. Electroencephalography may be helpful but is unnecessary in the acute state. Lumbar puncture for this diagnosis has become obsolete and is virtually contraindicated in this setting. Finally, intracranial pressure (ICP) monitoring may help to identify patients developing pressure waves or continuously elevated ICP.

In addition to providing more rapid and accurate diagnosis, CT has better defined the evolution of spontaneous hemorrhage and has helped to establish objective criteria for surgical evacuation. To some extent, the reduction of overall mortality figures noted previously may be attributed to the fact that smaller foci of hemorrhages are now dectectable and are classified correctly, rather than being misdiagnosed as ischemic strokes. For deep hemorrhages involving the basal ganglia, the internal capsule, and the thalamus, hematoma volumes of 25 ml or less are rarely associated with mortality. This somewhat arbitrary volume corresponds to a diameter of approximately 3 cm in each axis of measurement. Volume alone cannot entirely explain the widely differing clinical pictures presented by patients with deep brain hemorrhages [25]. The direction of spread or dissection of these hematomas is also very important in a patient's prognosis. When dissection occurs rostrally or laterally, patients may demonstrate unilateral symptoms, including hemiparesis or hemiplegia. When dissection occurs caudally into the midbrain structures, even patients with small hematomas may develop progressive obtundation or coma directly associated with the destructive forces and mass effect of the hemorrhage at the brain stem. Typically, patients with small hemorrhages located in the region of the basal ganglia and internal capsule recover satisfactorily over a course of several months, concomitant with reabsorption of the hematoma. Those who develop hemorrhages greater than 25 ml and demonstrate a progressive deterioration in level of consciousness should be considered for surgical evacuation, because these findings are associated with a much worse prognosis than exists for those patients maintaining higher levels of consciousness [6, 8, 11, 14–16, 22, 25, 30–37].

More superficial or so-called lobar hemorrhages are quite amenable to standard surgical evacuation, often with an excellent prognosis [10, 26, 28, 33]. The lobar location of a primary cerebral hemorrhage should not contraindicate the use of stereotactic technique. Direct surgical approach and visualization of the hematoma cavity in this setting, however, provides the advantages of complete evacuation of the hemorrhage focus, visualization of residual points of hemorrhage for hemostasis, and the opportunity for biopsy of brain substance adjacent to the hematoma cavity for further pathological diagnosis [20].

Patients with deep hematomas measuring 25–85 ml by CT scan definition, tend to have a high rate of mortality and morbidity. It is within this group that surgical evacuation can improve both mortality rates and the quality of life for survivors [24, 25, 33, 35].

In patients with hemorrhages greater than 85 ml within the deep brain structures, prognosis for survival is extremely poor, regardless of intensive medical therapy or surgical evacuation. Most likely, these hemorrhages already have irreversibly damaged the upper brain stem, leading to permanent coma. Deeply comatose patients who demonstrate deep intracerebral hemorrhages greater than 85 ml or whose hemorrhages clearly involve extensive areas of the brain stem probably are not candidates for any type of surgical evacuation procedure. Some also feel that patients with hemorrhages involving the thalamus are poor candidates for surgical evacuation because of the primary destruction of important thalamic cellular elements [10]. Patients with hemorrhages sufficiently small to be confined to the thalamus may be candidates for needle aspiration procedures comparable to those used for evacuating brain-stem hemorrhages. Extensive thalamic hemorrhages are prone to extend either into the ventricular system or more laterally into the internal capsule region, making strict anatomical classification difficult.

Patients with parenchymal cerebellar hemorrhages may be deeply comatose from acute mass effect within the posterior fossa rather than from direct destruction of the brain stem. These patients routinely should be considered for urgent or emergent surgical evacuation. Lobar cerebellar hemorrhage is a neurosurgical emergency and prompt treatment frequently results in satisfactory to excellent recovery [10].

Finally, patients who have limited focal hemorrhage within the upper brain stem may be considered candidates for conventional or stereotactic surgery when these lesions are relatively small (1 cm in diameter) and have not resulted in profound coma. In these cases, a stereotactic approach is likely to be much less hazardous than craniotomy and exploration of the brain stem by direct visualization.

Once the diagnosis of primary intracerebral hemorrhage is established, medical intensive therapy should be implemented immediately. Treatment should include rigorous control of systemic blood pressure, corticosteroid therapy, and consideration of the use of osmotic diuretics to control ICP. Ventricular drainage may be necessary to relieve acute hydrocephalus or hematocephalus. Patients who are drowsy or obtunded should be considered for placement of ICP monitors and for possible surgical hematoma evacuation by either craniotomy or stereotactic technique. The choice of method lies with the surgeon and depends partially on the patient's age and general health with regard to the advisability of a general anesthetic. The surgeon also must choose the most expedient technique, given time requirements, equipment availability, and the experience of the operating surgeon with the technique.

Timing of Surgery

Stereotactic evacuation of a deep brain hemorrhage may be applied any time following the ictus. The decision for surgical intervention is based chiefly on the development and extent of neurological impairment. The deterioration of a patient's clinical condition directly attributable to intracerebral hemorrhage usually occurs within the first 72 hours after hemorrhage. Beyond that time, morbidity and mortality risks gradually increase because of secondary effects, such as debilitation, respiratory compromise, pneumonia, systemic sepsis, and pulmonary embolus. Some advocate very early operation for intracerebral hemorrhage, even within the first six hours after ictus [23, 24, 35]. This approach is more physiological than is delayed operation. Thus far, the ischemic effects of local tissue compression have not been well documented or identified. However, recent investigations indicate that the margins of the hematoma cavity are affected adversely by prolonged mechanical pressure and by exposure to the by-products of blood decomposition [36].

Technical Considerations

Because surgically dedicated CT equipment is scarce, evacuation usually must be performed in an operating room remote from a CT scanner. In such cases, CT coordinates for the extreme dimensions of the hematoma must be translated into coordinates for use by the stereotactic device. The target for cannulation, whether by a flexible catheter or a surgical instrument, should be the central portion of the hematoma. Penetration of the hematoma cavity often results in immediate release of liquefied blood or serum. Gentle aspiration can be used to evacuate soft coagulated blood. At this juncture, the technique reported by Hondo employs the instillation of approximately 6,000 units of urokinase [21]. Subsequent aspiration of liquefied hematoma and reinstillation of urokinase is repeated at intervals of approximately six to eight hours. With the

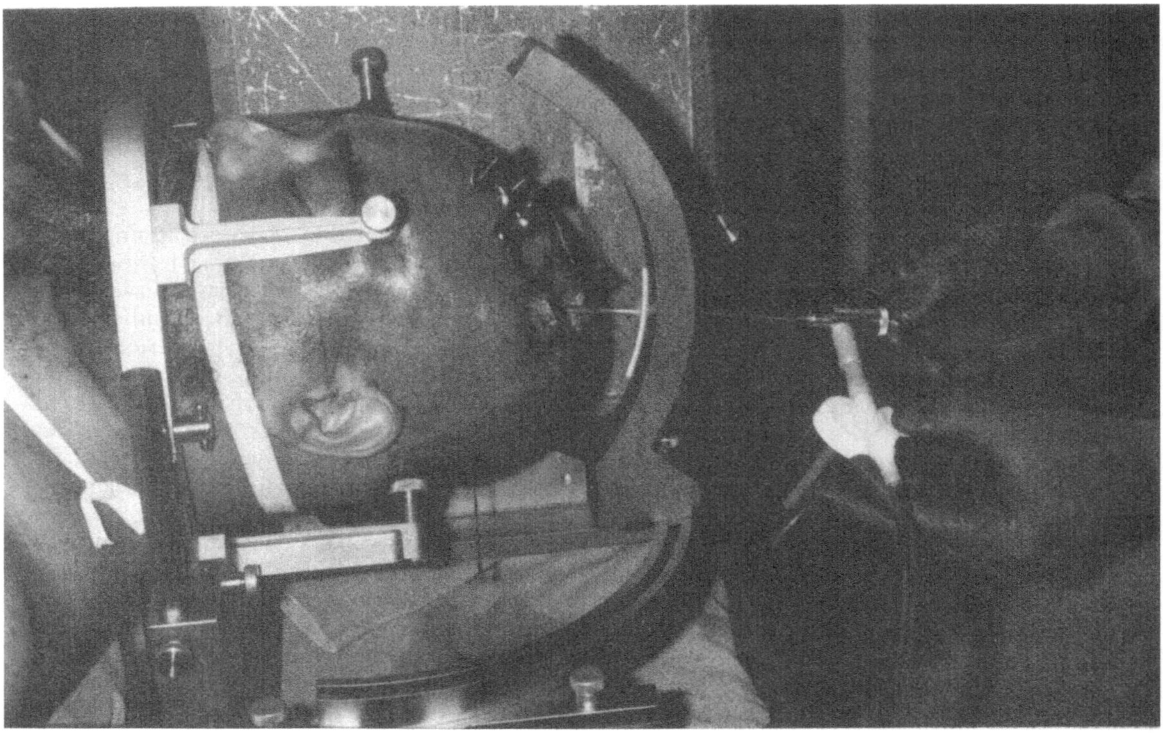

FIGURE 16-4. Stereotactic evacuation of intracerebral hematoma. Note the disposable, graduated suction trap in the surgeon's left hand.

appropriate sterile technique, this procedure can be repeated for several days after implantation of the catheter. This method requires considerable time and therefore may not be the most expedient procedure for acute decompression or reduction of mass effect.

Procedural considerations are more complex with any of the stereotactic instruments described by Backlund, Higgins, or Kandel [4, 19, 23]. Once the operating portion of the cannula has been placed in the center of the hematoma cavity, suction applied to the evacuator in conjunction with gentle rotation and agitation of the helical mandrel causes fragmentation and aspiration of pieces of solid coagulum. Vigorous vacuum aspiration (0.2 atmospheres or less) may be needed to evacuate more tenacious clot [23]. It should be emphasized that aspiration vacuum pressures measured at the hub of the instrument are not transmitted diffusely to intracranial contents because of the frictional effects of coagulum entering the shaft of the device. Saline irrigation through the tandem port of the Higgins-Nashold instrument or intermittent removal and direct mechanical cleaning of the helical mandrel of the Backlund instrument may be required for continued clot evacuation. If the procedure is performed under direct CT guidance, it may be possible to obtain direct assessment of the progress of the hematoma evacuation. Otherwise, strict volumetric measurement of the evacuated portion should be used to estimate completion of the procedure. A small, graduated suction trap is extremely helpful in this situation (figure 16-4). For hematomas with an unusually long axis of dissection, multiple penetrations of the cavity may be advisable to evacuate the extreme limbs of the hematoma. Care should be taken to observe for aspiration of brain tissue through the cannula, an indication that the working portion of the cannula is in contact with the cerebral wall of the hematoma cavity.

Evacuation of a small brain-stem hematoma requires only a hollow-needle-type cannula with an outside diameter of less than 3 mm. Larger instruments have no place in evacuating hemorrhages within the brain stem. The stereotactic approaches used by Beatty and Bosch incorporate a frontal-vertex trephination and a trajectory that traverses the midbrain. Although such a trajectory is used routinely for other functional stereotactic procedures, large-diameter instruments can injure brainstem structures.

Although complete evacuation of deep intracerebral hematomas with these techniques has been reported, it is doubtful that this truly can be achieved by stereotactic approach. The primary goal of such surgery should be to decompress the mass effect created hy the hematoma. Hematomas measuring up to 25 ml can spontaneously lyse and reabsorb, resulting in excellent clinical improvement. Therefore, it seems unnecessary to attempt total removal of the hematoma via stereotaxis.

Postoperative tamponade within the hematoma cavity by a balloon-tip catheter, as described by Kandel [23], may be of some benefit in preventing postoperative hemorrhage. It is not entirely clear how this technique by tamponade alone results in satisfactory hemostasis; immediate refilling of a noncollapsing cavity is a possible explanation. Placement of an ICP-monitoring device prior to surgery or following evacuation may be helpful in monitoring the postoperative course of patients undergoing this surgery. However, many of these devices measure only diffuse ICP and not compartmental pressure within the confines of the meninges. Indwelling cannulation of the hematoma cavity may be of greater value, first for assessing local compartmental pressure and second for repeated drainage of residual air or fluid from the hematoma cavity. Currently, postoperative cranial CT scanning is the method of choice for evaluating both the extent of successful evacuation and the recurrence of acute hemorrhage within the operative site. It is therefore recommended that CT scanning be performed on each surgical patient within one to two hours after completing the evacuation procedure.

Complications

As with any other type of surgical approach, stereotactic evacuation of intracerebral hemorrhage carries with it the usual possible complications of hemorrhage, infection, worsening neurological deficit, and death.

Hemorrhages may take the form of subdural accumulation of blood, new intracerebral hemorrhage from the passage of an instrument through the brain tissue, or, more likely, recurrent bleeding within the evacuated hematoma cavity. For this reason, it is extremely important to evacuate the hematoma from its central coordinates. Designated stereotactic instruments such as those of Backlund and of Higgins should never be used freehand. These instruments are designed to be rigidly supported in a stereotactic frame that allows for accurate placement within the hematoma and prevents uncontrolled wandering of the operating tip of the instrument. The greatest hazard in using these instruments is aspiration and avulsion of the leptomeninges of the cerebral sulci or major fissures or of larger arterial vessels. These structures are often pushed aside by the advancement of the enlarging hematoma; strict observance of the boundaries of the hematoma cavity should prevent such occurrences. Freehand use of the instruments or careless positioning of the instrument tip outside the hematoma cavity can cause severe hemorrhage.

Following mechanical evacuation of larger hematomas, it is not unusual to find a residual, air-filled cavity on the postoperative CT study. The pneumocephalus is probably caused by the failure of surrounding compressed cerebral tissues to obliterate immediately the evacuated hematoma cavity. No serious consequences of this complication have been reported, but under certain circumstances, entrapped air could expand and contribute to focal compartmental pressure or more diffuse elevation of ICP. Ordinarily, this form of pneumocephalus absorbs over the course of several days. The postevacuation placement of a flexible indwelling catheter can aid in monitoring compartmental pressure or subsequent evacuation of residual air or fluid from the hematoma cavity.

Results

Since Backlund's initial report of subtotal evacuation of a supratentorial basal ganglia region hemorrhage by stereotactic approach, fewer than 150 stereotactic cases have been reported, most by Broseta, Hondo and Matsmoto, and Kandel (table 16–1) [9, 21, 23, 29]. The remainder have been individual cases or small groups of patients [1–3, 5, 7, 12, 18]. Although the authors of the larger series have compared their results in using stereotaxis with both the

TABLE 16–1. Reported Stereotactic Hematoma Evacuations

Surgeon	Technique[a]	No. of Cases	Supratentorial/ Infratentorial	Cases of Mortality (%)	Cases of Rebleeding
Acampora	1, 3	NA	NA	NA	NA
Apuzzo	2	4	NA	NA	NA
Backlund	2	1	1/0	0	0
Beatty	1	1	0/1	0	0
Bosch	1	1	0/1	0	0
Broseta	2	16	16/0	13 (81%)	2
Colombo		1	0/1	1 (100%)	0
Higgins	2	3	3/0	1 (33%)	1
Hondo	3	51	48/3	7 (14%)	2
Kandel	2	32	32/0	7 (22%)	5

[a] 1 = Simple suction aspiration; 2 = suction/mechanical fragmentation; 3 = suction/urokinase.
NA = Not available

statistics for nonsurgical management of intracerebral hematomas and those for standard craniotomy approaches, the case numbers available are not satisfactory for direct statistical comparison.

Another problem in analyzing the outcome of stereotactic operative cases is a direct consequence of the inherent severity of brain hemorrhage. Earlier surgeons who operated for cerebral hemorrhage could not benefit from cumulative data acquired by years of CT examination of patients developing cerebral hemorrhage. Both Higgins and Broseta performed stereotactic evacuation for patients who were not expected to survive without surgical intervention and who tended to be extremely poor candidates for general anesthesia and standard craniotomy techniques. Given the limited number of patients and the lack of direct comparison with patients randomized to other forms of therapy, it is difficult to ascertain whether stereotactic evacuation actually influenced patient outcome. However, these studies demonstrate the technical capabilities of stereotactic approach.

Backlund's original patient developed a primary intracerebral hematoma, estimated to be at least 100 ml in volume and located lateral to the thalamus and basal ganglia of the right cerebral hemisphere [3]. The hematoma was evacuated successfully, and the patient returned to his former occupation approximately ten months after surgery.

We previously described three patients who developed deep-seated intracerebral hemorrhages that presumably originated in the basal ganglia but were sufficiently large to dissect throughout multiple anatomical structures [18]. One patient died in the postoperative period from multiple complications of prolonged coma, and two patients survived with disabling neurological deficits. One of the surviving patients developed the reaccumulation of blood within the hematoma cavity.

Broseta's group of 16 patients included ten with basal ganglia hemorrhages and six with subcortical lobar-type hemorrhages with estimated volumes varying from 25–180 ml [9]. The overall mortality rate for this group was 81%; however, when analyzed by level of consciousness, comatose patients who were totally unresponsive experienced a mortality rate of 85%–100%. Three patients ultimately returned to a normal life with intact intellectual function. There were two cases of postoperative rebleeding.

Apuzzo has reported the successful evacuation of four intracerebral hematomas, but he has not given details of their location and volume nor of patient conditions before and after surgery [2].

Stereotactic evacuation of a 10-ml cerebellar hematoma by transtentorial trajectory has been reported by Colombo, but he did not give the neurological outcome. The patient died postoperatively from pneumonia [12]. Two cases of successful stereotactic aspiration of brain-stem hematomas have been reported by Beatty and

Bosch, each with relatively successful functional outcome despite demonstrable residual neurological impairment on detailed examination [5, 7].

To date, the most detailed analysis of surgical results from stereotactic evacuation of intracerebral hematomas has been compiled by Hondo and Matsumoto [21, 29]. Their series included 51 patients whose lesions were divided by anatomical location: basal ganglia (34 cases, 12.9–135 ml), subcortical or lobar type (11 cases, 17–69 ml), thalamic (three cases, 17–42 ml), and cerebellar (three cases, 18–22 ml). This study is valued for its laboriously compiled, detailed statistics regarding patients' age and sex, their preoperative neurological state, the interval between onset of hemorrhage and operation, CT classification, estimated hematoma volume, initial volume aspiration at the time of surgery, and eventual outcome following surgery. Such data are necessary for a sound assessment of results.

Significant findings from this study are categorized both technically and functionally. From a technical standpoint, it was found that aspiration vacuum pressures of approximately 0.1 atmosphere (70 cm Hg) were required to aspirate solid coagulum. Even so, only 30% of the estimated volume could be extracted on the initial penetration of the hematoma cavity. With repeated instillation of urokinase (6,000 IU), excellent resolution of intracerebral hematomas was achieved. This technique does not completely prevent the recurrence of intracerebral bleeding; rebleeding was reported in two of these cases. Operative mortality and quality of survival for these patients compare favorably with those for a similar group who underwent craniotomy for evacuation of hemorrhages under direct visualization. These authors concluded that patients with rapidly developing symptoms, including progressive obtundity and evidence of compartmental herniation or brain-stem dysfunction, might better be treated by craniotomy with one-step evacuation. Mortality figures for this group of patients who showed signs of compartmental herniation or profound coma reached 50%–93%, regardless of the treatment administered. Postoperative survival quality also was considered to be poor for the majority of patients with severe preoperative neurological impairment. Those with hemorrhages in excess of 85–90 ml originating in the basal ganglia also showed the poorest recovery after intervention.

The only other sizable series of patients treated for intracranial hemorrhage by stereotactic evacuation is reported by Kandel [23]. This report described mechanical evacuation and aspiration of 32 intracerebral hematomas classified as basal ganglia (16 cases) or combined basal ganglia and lateral structures (14 cases). By clinical criteria, all of these patients were severely comatose or semicomatose at the time of surgery. Hematoma volumes were estimated to range from 24–115 ml. Virtually complete evacuation of hematoma cavities were confirmed by CT in all but four cases. Repeat hemorrhages developed in five patients, and death resulted from recurrent hemorrhage in three. Overall mortality in this series was 22% or seven patients. Of the survivors, only two were said to be severely debilitated.

An important technical consideration in this study was the use of a motor-driven mechanical aspirator of the screw type mentioned previously. This instrument differs from those of Backlund and Higgins in that aspiration occurs in a straight line from the tip of the instrument, rather than through a side port in the cannula. In addition, the postoperative placement of a saline-inflated balloon catheter in the hematoma cavity is believed to reduce recurrent hemorrhage by providing a graded and controlled means for collapsing the hematoma cavity after evacuation. A multilumen cather may also allow for monitoring intracavitary pressure and for postoperative evacuation of intracavitary air or fluid.

Kandel noted that two of his patients suffered from intracerebral hemorrhage secondary to structural vascular abnormaliites. One experienced rupture of a cerebral artery aneurysm, and the other developed bleeding from rupture of AVM. Venous angiomas of the brain stem also presumably were responsible for spontaneous hemorrhage in the cases reported by Beatty and by Bosch. Despite these successful evacuations, it is doubtful that stereotactic evacuation will play a significant role in treatment of hemorrhages secondary to aneurysm or AVM in surgically accessible locations. Craniotomy for primary evacuation of hemorrhage and for microsurgical aneurysm ligation or extirpation of the AVM offers a more controlled and expeditious method for dealing with these particular vascular entities.

Conclusion

Available data from multiple sources are not yet sufficiently extensive to draw rigorous statistical conclusions about the efficacy of stereotactic hematoma evacuation. The more extensive and recent experiences published by Hondo and by Kandel provide valuable information and clinical data supporting the role of stereotactic techniques as a viable treatment modality, comparable in results to those obtained by standard craniotomy techniques. For cases of focal brain-stem hemorrhages, stereotactic evacuation ultimately may prove to be the optimal therapy by minimizing the hazards of open exploration.

References

1. Acampora S, Profeta G: Stereotaxic evacuation of hematomas (letter). *J Neurosurg* 62:460, 1985
2. Apuzzo LJ, Sabshin JK: Computed tomographic guidance stereotaxis in the management of intracranial mass lesions. *Neurosurgery* 12:277–285, 1983
3. Backlund EO: Stereotaxic evacuation of hematomas (letter). *J Neurosurg* 62:460–461, 1985
4. Backlund EO, Holst H von: Controlled subtotal evacuation of intracerebral hematomas by stereotactic technique. *Surg Neurol* 9:99–101, 1978
5. Beatty RM, Zervas NT: Stereotactic aspiration of a brain stem hematoma. *Neurosurgery* 13:204–207, 1983
6. Bolander HG, Kourtopoulous H, Liliequist B, et al: Treatment of spontaneous intracerebral hemorrhage: A retrospective analysis of 74 consecutive cases with special reference to computer tomographic data. *Acta Neurochir* (Wien) 67:19–28, 1983
7. Bosch DA, Beute GN: Successful stereotaxic evacuation of an acute pontomedullary hematoma: Case report. *J Neurosurg* 62:153–156, 1985
8. Brambilla GL, Rodriguez Y, Baena R, et al: Spontaneous intracerebral hemorrhage: Medical or surgical treatment. *J Neurosurg Sci* 27:95–101, 1983
9. Broseta J, Gonzalez-Darder J, Barcia-Salorio JL: Stereotactic evacuation of intracerebral hematomas. *Appl Neurophysiol* 45:443–498, 1982
10. Cahill DW, Ducker TB: Spontaneous intracerebral hemorrhage. *Clin Neurosurg* 29:722–779, 1982
11. Chen BH, Hou DL: Surgical treatment of hypertensive intracerebral hemorrhage. *Chin Med J* [Engl] 94:723–728, 1981
12. Colombo F, Benedetti A, Alexandre A: Stereotactic exploration of deepseated or surgically unamenable intracranial space occupying lesions. *J Neurosurg Sci* 24:173–177, 1980
13. Drury I, Whisnant JP, Garraway WM: Primary intracerebral hemorrhage: Impact of CT on incidence. *Neurology* 34:653–657, 1984
14. Duff TA, Ayeni S, Levin AB, et al: Nonsurgical management of spontaneous intracerebral hematoma. *Neurosurgery* 9:387–393, 1981
15. Garde A, Bohmer G, Selden B, et al: 100 cases of spontaneous intracerebral hematoma: Diagnosis, treatment and prognosis. *Eur Neurol* 22:161–172, 1983
16. Helweg-Larsen S, Sommer W, Strange P, et al: Prognosis for patients treated conservatively for spontaneous intracerebral hematomas. *Stroke* 15:1045–1048, 1984
17. Higgins AC, Nashold BS Jr: Modification of instrument for stereotactic evacuation of intracerebral hematoma: Technical note. *Neurosurgery* 7:604–605, 1980
18. Higgins AC, Nashold BS Jr: Stereotactic evacuation of large intracerebral hematoma. *Appl Neurophysiol* 43:96–103, 1980
19. Higgins AC, Nashold BS, Cosman E: Stereotactic evacuation of primary intracerebral hematomas: New instrumentation. *Appl Neurophysiol* 45:438–442, 1982
20. Hinton DR, Dolan E, Sima AA: The value of histopathological examination of surgically removed blood clot in determining the etiology of spontaneous intracerebral hemorrhage. *Stroke* 15:517–520, 1984
21. Hondo H: CT-guided stereotactic evacuation of hypertensive intracerebral hematomas: A new operative approach. *Tokushima J Exp Med* 30:25–39, 1983
22. Hungerbuhler MD, Regli MD, Van Melle PD, et al: Spontaneous intracerebral hemorrhages (SICHs). Clinical and CT features: Immediate evaluation of prognosis. *Schweiz Arch Neurol Neurochir Psychiatr* 132:13–27, 1983
23. Kandel EI, Peresedov VV: Stereotaxic evacuation of spontaneous intracerebral hematomas. *J Neurosurg* 62:206–213, 1985
24. Kaneko M, Tanaka K, Shimada T, et al: Long-term evaluation of ultra-early operation for hypertensive intracerebral hemorrhage in 100 cases. *J Neurosurg* 58:838–842, 1983
25. Kanno T, Sano H, Shinomiya Y, et al: Role of surgery in hypertensive intracerebral hematoma: A comparative study of 305 nonsurgical and 154 surgical cases. *J Neurosurg* 61:1091–1100, 1984
26. Kase CS, Williams JP, Wyatt DA, et al: Lobar intracerebral hematomas: Clinical and CT

analysis of 22 cases. *Neurology* 32:1146–1150, 1982

27. Lunsford LD: Innovations in stereotactic technique coupled with computerized tomography. *Contemp Neurosurg* 15:1–6, 1982
28. Masdeu JC, Rubino FA: Management of lobar intracerebral hemorrhage: Medical or surgical. *Neurology* 34:381–383, 1984
29. Matsumoto K, Hondo H: CT-guided stereotaxic evacuation of hypertensive intracerebral hematomas. *J Neurosurg* 61:440–448, 1984
30. Mayr U, Bauer P, Fischer J: Nontraumatic intracerebral hemorrhage: Prognostic implications of neurological and computer-tomographical findings in 100 consecutive patients. *Neurochirurgia* (Stuttg) 26:36–41, 1983
31. Nath FP, Nicholls D, Fraser RJ: Prognosis in intracerebral hemorrhage. *Acta Neurochir* (Wien) 67:29–35, 1983
32. Schisano G, Franco A: Primary nontraumatic intracranial hemorrhage: 139 consecutive cases treated at an emergency regional hospital. *J Neurosurg Sci* 26:199–204, 1982
33. Schurmann K, Dei Anang K: Indication and contraindication for surgery of spontaneous intracerebral hematomas: Therapy and results. *Neurosurg Rev* 3:17–22, 1980
34. Scott WR, Miller BR: Intracerebral hemorrhage with rapid recovery. *Arch Neurol* 42:133–136, 1985
35. Volpin L, Cerevellini P, Colombo F, et al: Spontaneous intracerebral hematomas: A new proposal about the usefulness and limits of surgical treatment. *Neurosurgery* 15:663–666, 1984
36. Wozney P, Yonas H, Latchaw R, et al: Central herniation revealed by focal decrease in blood flow without elevation of intracranial pressure: Case report. *Neurosurgery* 17:641–644, 1985
37. Zuccarello M, Andrioli GG, Trincia G, et al: Spontaneous intracerebellar hematomas: Aspects of treatment. *Zentralbl Neurochir* 44:209–213, 1983

17. INTRACAVITARY IRRADIATION OF CYSTIC CRANIOPHARYNGIOMAS

Volker Sturm
Bernd Wowra
John Clorius
Hansjörg Sinn
Andreas Gamroth
Ulrich Steude
Stephan Kunze
Walter J. Lorenz

Craniopharyngiomas comprise 2.5% of adult and 7% of childhood intracranial neoplasms. They arise from remnants of squamous epithelium in Rathke's pouch, usually within the tuber cinereum and pituitary infundibulum [18], and extend into the sellar-suprasellar region. Rarely, these tumors extend into the frontal (2%–5%), posterior (1%–4%), or middle cranial fossae (2%) [15]. Approximately 60% of craniopharyngiomas are exclusively cystic; 9% are predominantly cystic with a smaller solid part; 15% are equally cystic and solid; and 16% are solid [17]. Because of papillary extensions and reactive gliosis, both cystic and solid craniopharyngiomas adhere closely to the surrounding brain tissue [7, 23]. This feature makes radical operative removal hazardous or even impossible, especially in larger tumors (those with diameters exceeding 3 cm) [20].

When conventional radiotherapy is given after partial surgical removal, the tumor "recurrence" rate is reduced by 70% [1]. However, even this combination therapy is not satisfactory: in addition to frequent tumor regrowth, considerable mortality and morbidity persist [1].

Because cystic craniopharyngiomas are less likely than solid craniopharyngiomas to be resected completely [10], and because the majority of clinical symptoms reflect cyst expansion, a safe method was sought to treat cystic craniopharyngioma and to solve many problems presented by patients with craniopharyngiomas. Several authors advocated repeated aspiration of cystic fluid through implanted indwelling catheters. Although this procedure may be helpful for extended periods [5, 8, 14], it is only palliative, even in exclusively cystic tumors. Some have endorsed contact irradiation of the cyst wall using colloidal suspensions of beta-ray-emitting radioisotopes, which are injected directly into the cyst fluid [3, 13, 16, 22]. In 1953, Leksell and Lidén first reported the treatment of a cystic craniopharyngioma with ^{32}Na PO_4 in an attempt to shrink the cysts permanently [11]. In this chapter, we report our experience with intracavitary contact irradiation of cystic craniopharyngiomas after

L.D. Lunsford (ed.) *MODERN STEREOTACTIC NEUROSURGERY*.

TABLE 17–1. Results of Intracavitary Beta Irradiation of cystic Craniopharyngiomas in 51 Patients*

	Intracavitary Isotope		
Effect	Yttrium-90 (N = 45)	Rhenium-186 (N = 6)	Phosphorus-32 (N = 1)
Cyst volume reduced	37 (81.8%)	1 (16.7%)	1
Cyst volume unchanged	4 (9.1%)	0	0
Cyst volume increased	4 (9.1%)	5 (83.3%)	0

* Mean follow-up duration is 3.5 years, range 1–7.5 years.

stereotactic injection of either yttrium-90 (^{90}Y), rhenium-186 (^{186}Re), or phosphorus-32 (^{32}P).

Methods and Materials

Fifty-seven patients with 72 predominantly cystic craniopharyngiomas were treated with intracystic beta irradiation between May 1979 and December 1985. Twenty-nine patients were younger than 20 years of age; 28 were 20 years or older. Patients who were treated after December 1985 and who had a follow-up time of less than one year were excluded from the study. The patients were hospitalized for various lengths of time, up to four half-lives of the isotope, depending upon which isotope was used.

Available as a colloidal silicate, ^{90}Y is a pure beta-ray emitter with mean beta energy of 0.93 MeV, a half-life of 64.1 hours, and a half-value penetrance in soft tissue of 1.1 mm. ^{186}Re sulfide emits both beta and gamma rays and has a mean beta energy of 0.36 MeV, a half-life of 90.6 hours, and a half-value penetrance in soft tissue of 0.4 mm. ^{32}P chromate is a pure beta-ray emitter with a mean beta energy of 0.69 MeV, a half-life of 14.2 days, and a half-value penetrance in soft tissue of 0.8 mm.

Stereotactic injection of the radionuclide was performed using a Riechert-Mundinger device, which we modified for use within the computed tomography (CT) scanner [21]. The technique of Leksell [11] and Backlund [2–4] was followed. The selected therapeutic beta-ray dose to the inner surface of the cyst wall was 200 Gy for both ^{90}Y and ^{186}Re and 250 Gy for ^{32}P. The dose was calculated according to the technique of Loevinger and co-workers [12]. The volume of the cysts was assessed by both CT and by radiodilution-technique, volume-dependent attenuation of the gamma-radiation of technetium-99 [2, 3, 6]. The radionuclide was implanted using intraoperative gamma-camera imaging. Additional gamma-camera investigations were performed 2 hours after operation and subsequently each day until one to two half-lives of the therapeutic agent was passed. The effect of the treatment was assessed by regular periodic clinical and CT examinations.

Results

In 72 craniopharyngioma cysts of the 57 total patients, ^{90}Y was used in 50 patients, ^{32}P in one, and ^{186}Re in six. The cyst volumes ranged from 1.5–330 ml. One patient with a giant cyst of 330 ml deserves special comment. This patient was treated successfully with ^{32}P. The cyst shrank substantially; two and one-half years after therapy the residual cyst volume was stable at 50 ml. Although minimal amounts of ^{32}P escaped from the cyst, no adverse effects were observed.

The results of the intracystic beta irradiation in 51 patients are summarized in table 17–1. Six of our patients were not evaluated by follow-up CT examinations.

^{90}Y was effective in 90.9% of the patients treated; that is, no further cyst growth occurred. In 37 patients (81.8%) treated with ^{90}Y, cysts were reduced in size or disappeared completely. Cyst shrinkage was accompanied by improved clinical symptoms in 35 of these patients. In four patients (9.1%), the cysts expanded despite ^{90}Y therapy. An example of the effect of ^{90}Y treatment is shown in figure 17–1.

Treatment with ^{186}Re was effective in only one of six patients; in this patient, an exclusively cystic craniopharyngioma completely disappeared after treatment. In five patients, further cyst growth occurred. We subsequently treated with ^{90}Y, three patients in whom ^{186}Re treatment failed. This additional treatment was successful in only one patient.

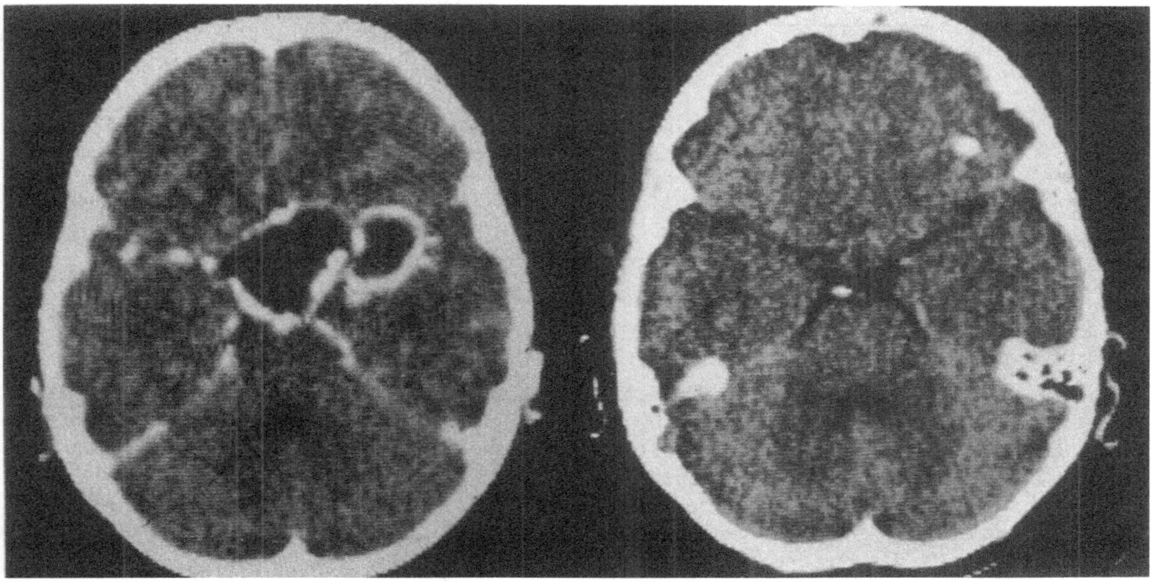

FIGURE 17–1. Axial CT section through a craniopharyngioma consisting of two communicating cysts. (This was a tumor that recurred two years after microsurgical removal in an eight-year-old boy.) Left: before therapy; right: five years after.

Complications

Sixteen of 50 patients (32%) treated with ^{90}Y eventually died, including three from causes not related to the tumor or the treatment, and one who died ten months after implantation from radiation injury to the hypothalamus. The remaining 12 deaths occurred because of progression of the solid tumor and/or from new cysts. Treatment-related clinical deterioration was observed in two patients. Despite disappearance of their cysts, one patient became blind, and an oculomotor palsy developed in another. No side effects were seen in the six patients treated with ^{186}Re, but four of these patients died because of further cyst expansion.

Escape of radioactive fluid is a potential complication of intracavitary therapy. In four of 50 patients (64 cysts) treated with ^{90}Y, small amounts of radioactivity leaked into cerebrospinal fluid (CSF) pathways. No clinical side effects were noted. Small, clinically insignificant amounts of ^{32}P were detected in the blood and CSF of the only patient treated with this isotope. In all six patients (seven cysts) treated with ^{186}Re, we detected the escape of larger amounts of radioactivity into both blood and CSF. The mortality and morbidity of intracavitary craniopharyngioma treatment are shown in table 17–2.

Discussion

Our results, after intracavitary irradiation of cystic craniopharyngiomas with ^{90}Y are similar to those reported by Backlund (personal communication, 1985). Treatment-related adverse side effects, including one death, occurred in 6% of the patients. Our data supports the high efficacy and relative safety of this therapy.

The escape of small amounts of ^{90}Y from the cyst to blood and/or CSF (observed in 8% of the cases) proved clinically insignificant.

The possibility of radiation-induced side effects with ^{90}Y prompted us to use ^{186}Re in six patients because of the lower beta-ray energy of rhenium. Szikla and co-workers successfully used this isotope to treat both cystic gliomas and craniopharyngiomas [22]. In our series, cyst leakage, causing escape of varying amounts of ^{186}Re, was observed in every patient treated with rhenium. The treatment failed in five of six cases. Three of the "nonres-

TABLE 17–2. Mortality after Intracavitary Irradiation of Cystic Craniopharyngiomas (56 patients)

	Cause of Death			
Isotope	Progression of Solid Tumor or New Cyst Formation	Radiation Damage	Other[a]	Total No. of Deaths (%)
Yttrium-90 (N = 50)	12	1	3	16 (32)
Rhenium-186 (N = 6)	4[b]	0	0	4 (66.7)

[a] Unrelated to tumor treatment.
[b] Cyst regrowth.

ponders" to ^{186}Re required additional treatment with ^{90}Y, but only one responded favorably. This poor response rate might be a result of accidental clustering of "nonresponders" in the small rhenium series or perhaps because of the induction of radioresistance after ineffective initial irradiation [19]. A more likely explanation is the short range of the beta irradiation of ^{186}Re. The tendency of ^{186}Re to leak into blood or CSF is probably related to the chemical composition. ^{186}Re is a sulfide and tends to convert to water-soluble perrhenate, whereas ^{90}Y is a stable silicate. We believe that ^{186}Re should not be used for treatment of cystic craniopharyngiomas.

Favorable results with ^{32}P have been reported by Lunsford and colleagues [13]. At present, insufficient data exist to determine whether ^{90}Y or ^{32}P is the preferred isotope for intracavitary irradiation.

In our series, 16 of 50 patients (32%) treated with ^{90}Y ultimately died, the majority despite permanent shrinkage of the treated cysts. Because ^{90}Y does not affect the solid parts of the tumor, its use is only palliative in some cases. The effectiveness of additional treatment of the solid tumor parts using stereotactic percutaneous single-dose photon irradiation [9] or the gamma knife, as described by Backlund [4], currently is being investigated. The preliminary results (four patients) are encouraging.

References

1. Amacher AL: Craniopharyngioma: The controversy regarding radiotherapy. *Childs Brain* 6:57–64, 1980
2. Backlund EO: Studies on craniopharyngiomas. III. Stereotaxic treatment with intracystic yttrium-90 *Acta Chir Scand* 139:237–247, 1973
3. Backlund EO: Studies on craniopharyngiomas. IV. Stereotaxic treatment with radiosurgery. *Acta Chir Scand* 139:344–351, 1973
4. Backlund EO, Johansson L, Sarby B: Studies on craniopharyngiomas. II. Treatment by stereotaxis and radiosurgery. *Acta Chir Scand* 138:749–759, 1972
5. Fox JL: Intermittent drainage of intracranial cyst via the subcutaneous Ommaya reservoir: Technical note. *J Neurosurg* 27:272–273, 1967
6. Georgi P, Strauss L, Sturm V, et al: Prä-und intraoperative Volumenbestimmung bei Craniopharyngiomcysten. *Nuklearmedizin* 14:187–190, 1980
7. Ghatak NR, Hirano A, Zimmermann HM: Ultrastructure of a craniopharyngioma. *Cancer* 27:1465–1475, 1971
8. Gutin PH, Klemme WM, Lagger RL, et al: Management of the unresectable cystic craniopharyngioma by aspiration through an Ommaya reservoir drainage system. *J Neurosurg* 52:36–40, 1980
9. Hartmann GH, Schlegel W, Sturm V, et al: Cerebral radiation surgery using moving field irradiation at a linear accelerator facility. *Int J Radiat Oncol Biol Phys* 11:1185–1192, 1985
10. Katz EL: Late results of radical excision of craniopharyngiomas in children. *J Neurosurg* 42:86–90, 1975
11. Leksell L, Lidén K: A therapeutic trail with radioactive isotopes in cystic brain tumor. In *Radioisotope Techniques: Medical and Physical Applications*, Vol 1. London: Her Majesty's Office, 1953, p 76
12. Loevinger R, Japha EM, Brownell GC: In Hine GJ, Brownell GL eds: *Radiation Dosimetry*. New York: Academic Press, 1956, RM 849, H662
13. Lunsford LD, Gumerman L, Levine G: Stereotactic intracavitary irradiation of cystic neoplasms of the brain. *Appl Neurophysiol* 48:146–150, 1985
14. Mann KS, Yue CP, Ong GB: Percutaneous sump drainage: A palliation for oft-recurring

intracranial cystic lesions. *Surg Neurol* 19:86–90, 1983

15. Nagasawa S, Handa H, Yamashita J, et al: Dense cystic craniopharyngioma with unusual extensions. *Surg Neurol* 19:299–301, 1983
16. Netzeband G, Sturm V, Georgi P, et al: Results of stereotactic intracavitary irradiation of cystic craniopharyngiomas: Comparison of the effects of yttrium-90 and rhenium-186. *Acta Neurochir* [*Suppl*] (Wien) 33:341–344, 1984
17. Petito CK, De Girolani U, Earle KM: Craniopharyngiomas: A clinical and pathological review. *Cancer* 37:1944–1952, 1976
18. Russell DS, Rubinstein LJ: Congenital tumors. In *Pathology of the Central Nervous System*. Baltimore: Williams & Wilkins: 1977, pp 24–64
19. Schmitt HP: Physikalische Schäden des ZNS und seiner Hullen. In Doerr W, Seifert G, Uehlinger E (eds): *Spezielle Pathologische Anatomie*, Vol 13. Berlin, Heidelberg, New York: Springer, 1983, p 777
20. Shapiro K, Till K, Grant DN: Craniopharyngiomas in childhood: A rational approach to treatment. *J Neurosurg* 50:617–623, 1979
21. Sturm V, Pastyr O, Schlegel W, et al: Stereotactic computer tomography with a modified Riechert-Mundinger device as the basis for integrated stereotactic neuroradiological investigations. *Acta Neurochir* (Wien) 68:11–17, 1983
22. Szikla G, Musolino A, Schaub C, et al: Colloidal rhenium-186 endocavitary beta irradiation of cystic craniopharyngiomas and active glioma cysts: Long-term results, side effects, and radiobiological data. *Acta Neurochir* [*Suppl*] 33:331–340, 1984
23. Zülch KJ: Die Pathologie und Biologie der Tumoren des dritten Ventrikels. *Acta Neurochir* (Wien) 9:277–296, 1961

18. INTERSTITIAL BRACHYTHERAPY FOR MALIGNANT BRAIN TUMORS: TECHNIQUE AND RESULTS

Nicholas M. Barbaro
Steven A. Leibel
Philip H. Gutin

Most malignant brain tumors are localized lesions and rarely metastasize outside the central nervous system [1, 7, 18]. Conventional external-beam radiation therapy is the most effective adjuvant treatment for malignant brain tumors, and survival increases directly with successive increases in the dose of radiation delivered up to a maximum tolerable dose, typically, 5,500 cGy [39, 40, 47, 48]. Higher, potentially curative doses of radiation that relatively spare normal brain can be delivered from radioactive sources implanted directly into localized tumors (brachytherapy) [2]. This approach offers the potential for administering a second radiation dose to recurrent tumors or of "boosting" the focal dose to a tumor immediately after conventional teletherapy is completed.

History of Brain Tumor Brachytherapy

Early in this century, interstitial irradiation was used to treat brain tumors. In 1912, Hirsch treated residual tumors by inserting radium-loaded probes into the sella by a transnasal route [17]; over the next four decades, he refined this approach for the treatment of pituitary adenomas and craniopharyngiomas. In 1914, Frazier combined external beam irradiation with the implantation of radium sources for the treatment of parenchymal tumors[9]. By 1922, he had treated 32 patients with good results. Over the next few years, several series were reported in which patients underwent either direct implantation of radioactive sources in brain tumors or instillation of radioactive fluids directly into cystic lesions [2].

The availability of stereotactic systems has made it possible to implant radioactive sources into brain tumors with relative ease [24]. Mundinger in Freiburg and Talairach in Paris used stereotactic techniques to implant encapsulated sources into deep, inoperable tumors, and their experience with thousands of patients harboring tumors of many types and in many different locations has not been equaled [30–32, 45, 46]. Both found that lower grade gliomas responded better than the more malignant, higher grade gliomas. Szikla extended Talairach's early work and implanted a number of patients who had supratentorial gliomas with removable iridium-192 (^{192}Ir) wires; brachytherapy was the initial treatment for all patients [41–44]. A multicenter study is underway in France to evaluate the combined use of external-beam irradiation and interstitial brachytherapy.

In recent years, computed tomography (CT)-directed stereotactic techniques have become available [16, 24, 28, 34]. These systems have revolutionized brain tumor brachytherapy by providing the surgeon with the ability to implant radioactive sources precisely within

This work was supported in part by NIH Program Project Grant CA-13525. We thank Pamela Silver for help with the survival data and Neil Buckley for editing the manuscript.

L.D. Lunsford (ed.) *MODERN STEREOTACTIC NEUROSURGERY*.

brain tumors. In addition, computerized treatment planning allows the choice of stereotactic targets based on precise predictions of dose distribution [38]. CT also provides an important source of follow-up data on the efficacy of brachytherapy [25].

Advantages of Interstitial Brachytherapy

Doses in conventional teletherapy, with radiation from a linear accelerator or cobalt source, are delivered at a rate of 2 Gy/minute as daily fractions, the total therapeutic dose accruing over weeks or months [14, 39]. The rate of irradiation from an implanted source is much slower, on the order of 1 cGy/minute, but it is delivered continuously. Because this lower dose rate improves the therapeutic ratio, the total dose can be delivered over a few days rather than over months.

The improvement in therapeutic ratio with brachytherapy is the result of the radiobiology of low-dose-rate irradiation and the physics of intratumoral placement of the isotope [2, 4, 10]. As the dose rate is lowered, the biological effect of radiation is reduced, principally because tissue exposed to the low-dose-rate radiation can repair sublethal damage during the time of exposure. There is evidence that normal tissues repair sublethal damage more efficiently than tumor tissue does, which may explain the efficacy of brachytherapy against a variety of tumors and the relative sparing of exposed surrounding normal tissue.

The radiophysical advantages of brachytherapy are obvious. An implanted isotope delivers a maximum radiation dose to the tumor, while the dose to surrounding tissue is reduced or essentially eliminated. This is the result of attenuation of the radiation by interposed tissues and by the constraints of the inverse square law, which states that the intensity of radiation from any point source is inversely proportional to the square of the distance from the source [2].

Based on these factors, in 1977 we began an experimental study of iodine-125 (^{125}I) brachytherapy for the treatment of malignant gliomas [19]. We have refined our technique and have treated a relatively large number of patients. A discussion of our findings follows.

Patient Selection

In our initial studies, the only candidates chosen for brachytherapy were those with focally recurrent malignant gliomas [15]. After a 68% response rate was obtained in 37 patients, we initiated an experimental protocol to deliver an interstitial "boost" dose to newly diagnosed malignant brain tumors immediately after conventional teletherapy was completed.

Solitary recurrent malignant gliomas were treated if they were well-circumscribed on CT images. This protocol was not used for diffusely infiltrative tumors, tumors with subependymal spread, or multifocal tumors. Because of the limited biological reserve of previously irradiated posterior fossa structures, tumors in the brain stem and cerebellum were not implanted.

Choice of Isotope

After the early experience with radium implantation for treatment of gliomas, gold-198 and ^{192}Ir were the isotopes most commonly used for the interstitial irradiation of brain tumors [2, 33]. ^{192}Ir is still receiving considerable attention for this purpose, but ^{125}I seems to be a better isotope because the characteristic x-rays it emits have a far lower energy (27–35 KeV) than the gamma rays emitted by iridium (300–610 KeV) [2, 21, 23]. The lower energy of photons emitted ^{125}I simplifies the problem inherent in protecting medical personnel [26]. ^{125}I is provided as a standard low activity source (0.5 mCi) that has proven useful for permanent implantation into lower grade gliomas. The large number of these low-activity sources necessary to treat faster growing, more malignant gliomas, however, makes low-activity sources less practical. Higher-activity ^{125}I sources (30–50 mCi) are available by special order (Medical Product Division, 3M Company, St. Paul, MN); implantation with a few sources provides higher, more suitable dose rates. High-activity sources cannot remain implanted permanently because of the unacceptably high dose that would result. For this reason, high-activity ^{125}I sources are implanted in catheters that can be removed after the appropriate dose has been delivered. A number of centers now have experience with removable high-activity implants for malignant brain tumors.

Implantation Technique

With a CT-stereotactic system, targets for implantation can be selected based on the tumor geometry seen on CT images, and sources can be implanted precisely within the tumor with stereotactic guidance. When the stereotactic system is integrated with a brachytherapy-treatment-planning computer program (a description follows), stereotactic targets can be determined after various source arrays and the corresponding radiation isodose lines are simulated and displayed on the computer screen. A three-dimensional appreciation of the tumor is more important in interstitial brachytherapy than in tumor biopsy procedures. Reformatting in sagittal and coronal planes provides information necessary to perform the implantation.

Any stereotactic frame can be used for brain tumor brachytherapy. Although our initial experience was obtained with the Leksell stereotactic frame [28] (AB Elekta, Decatur, GA), we now use the Brown-Roberts-Wells (BRW) stereotactic system [16] (Trentwells Inc., Southgate, CA) for implantation of ^{125}I sources.

Adults are given local anesthesia to undergo the entire procedure; children receive general anesthesia [13]. The patient is scanned with the localizing system fixed to the skull. We take 3-mm images that begin well below and end well after the lesion. A stable preoperative dose of dexamethasone must be maintained to provide the best estimate of tumor size. The computer tape from the CT scanner is taken to the department of radiation oncology and read into the planning computer.

Our treatment-planning computer program includes a VAX computer-based package that has evolved through extensive modifications of software provided by Drs. Sturm and Schlegel of the German Cancer Research Center in Heidelberg [38]. Hardware includes a VAX-11/780 computer, and FPS array processor, and a Lexidate 3700 color display system. The CT data tape is read directly by the computer. The program enables us to plan catheter arrays (number of catheters, catheter location, number of sources, source strengths, source spacing) prospectively on CT images projected onto the computer display; thus, we can visualize the isodose curves created by the arrays on axial or reformatted images (figure 18–1). Source strengths and distribution are chosen to deliver a minimum tumor dose rate of 40–60 cGy/hour to a distance 0.5 cm beyond the periphery of the tumor. When the lesion is seen to be well-covered by the appropriate isodose curves of one of the simulated arrays, the stereotactic coordinates of the catheter targets are generated quickly and trajectories planned based on skull entry points that are selected from the display screen. Either of two approaches can be used. The azimuth and declination can be specified initially, or a target within the tumor and entry point can be chosen. These correspond to the BRW and BRWT programs in the traditional BRW stereotactic system. The integration of the necessary calculations of the BRW stereotactic system into our treatment planning software has expedited this process.

One important difference between stereotactic implantation of radioactive sources and stereotactic biopsy is that the implantation array must be properly oriented within the lesion. Thus, trajectory is a major determination of dosimetry, particularly for ^{125}I sources that have an anisotropic dosage. The entry point on the skull is extremely important and must be chosen carefully. If more than one catheter is used to implant the source array, the catheters must be positioned in parallel to provide accurate dosage calculations.

Another important difference between stereotactic techniques of brachytherapy and biopsy is that the stereotactic target for implantation is the center of the array for that catheter rather than the catheter tip. Therefore, before the stereotactic target can be determined, it is necessary to calculate the overall length of the array, including the number of radioactive sources and the spacing between them. The target then is adjusted appropriately.

A coaxial, afterloaded, silicone catheter system, consisting of an outer catheter placed initially and an inner catheter that contains sources, is used to hold the radioactive sources within the often soft, necrotic tumor center and to allow removal of the sources after the desired dose has been delivered [12]. After the number of sources to be used has been determined, they are loaded into the inner catheter, and the entire assembly is autoclaved.

With stereotactic guidance, the outer catheter is inserted into the tumor with the aid of a

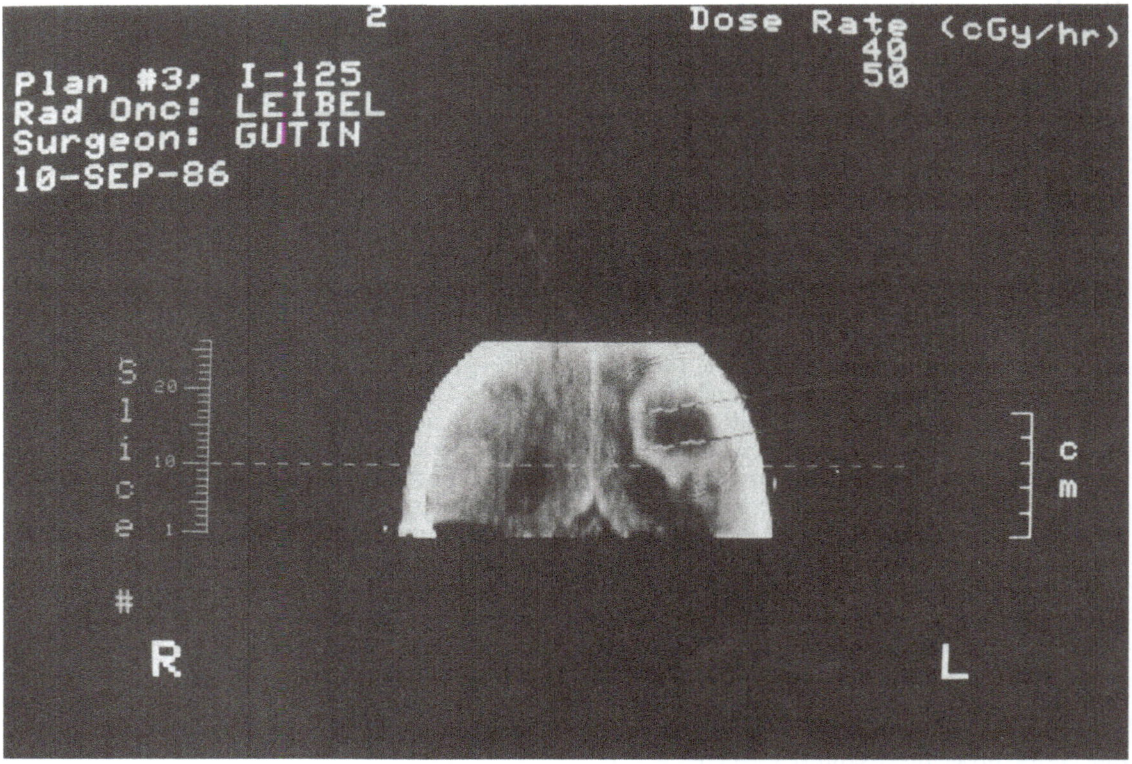

FIGURE 18–1. Treatment-planning computer simulation for a four-catheter implantation into a left parietal glioblastoma. Two catheters are visible on this slice. Isodose curves are for 50 rad/hr (inner) and 40 rad/hr (outer).

removable metal stylet introduced through either burr or twist-drill holes. The choice between the burr hole and the twist-drill technique depends on the possible presence of major vascular structures beneath the site of implantation. Burr holes are recommended for implantation over the temporal lobe near the sylvian fissure and the parasagittal region, where large bridging veins are present, and twist-drill holes may be used at other sites. The outer catheters are implanted before radioactive sources are loaded. Catheters are cut to the appropriate length and glued to a Silastic® ring, which is either cemented to the skull if a burr hole is used or sutured to the skin if a twist-drill technique is used. After all outer catheters are fixed in position, the inner catheters holding the radioactive source are placed carefully and cemented to the outer catheter (figure 18–2). Care must be taken to ensure that the inner catheter slides to the bottom of the outer catheter. Any stricture in the outer catheter that may be created by bone or dura will prevent the inner catheter from being properly positioned, which will adversely affect delivery of the intended dose.

After implantation, plain radiographs and CT scans are obtained to confirm that the sources are placed properly and to allow calculation of the correct dose (figure 18–3). The patient is isolated in a private room that is surveyed by a radiation physicist who determines the exposure time that will be safe to nurses and visitors. A helmet lined with lead foil is worn by the patient when visitors or medical personnel enter the room. Anticonvulsant medications must be monitored carefully because manipulation of the tumor during implantation can lead to increased seizures in the early postoperative period.

The dose delivered is a function of the time that the catheters are left implanted. Typically, sources are implanted for five or six days. After the calculated dose has been delivered,

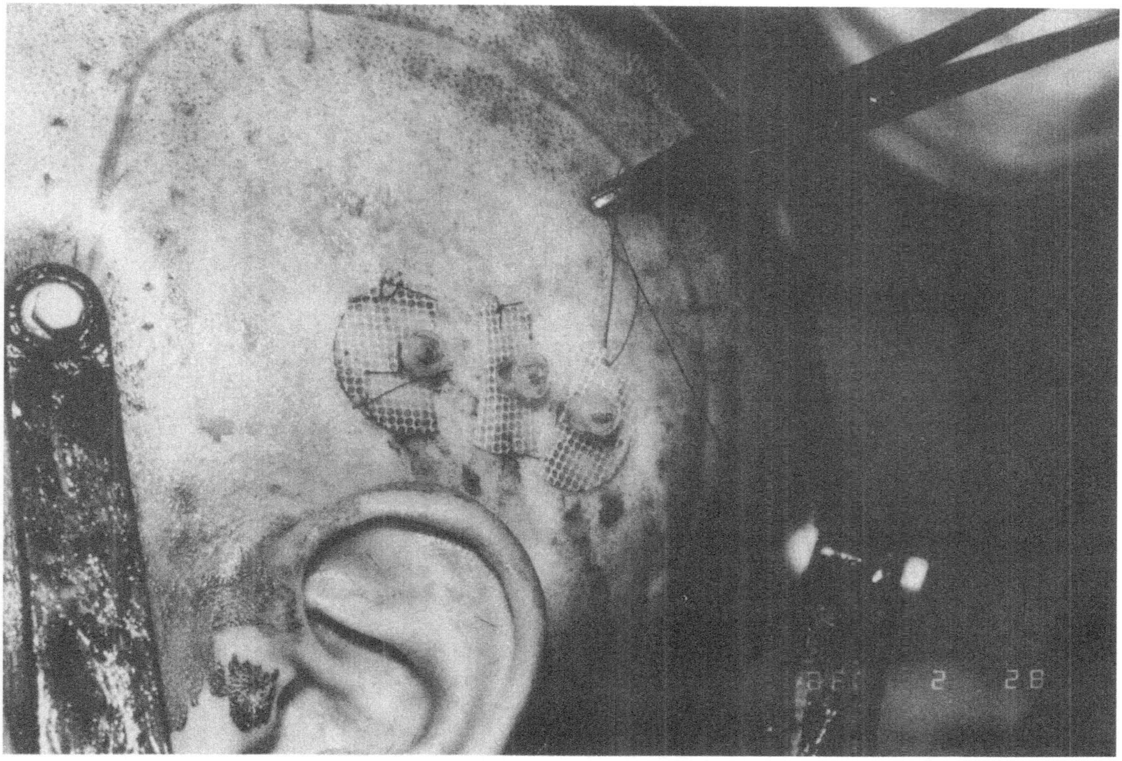

FIGURE 18-2. Intraoperative photograph shows three catheters implanted in the left parietal region via the twist-drill technique. The fixation ring is sutured to the scalp and is cemented to the outer catheter. Inner catheters have been afterloaded and cut to fit the outer catheter. Catheters can be removed in the patient's hospital room under local anesthesia.

catheters are removed, either in the operating room if a burr hole was used or in the patient's room if a twist-drill technique was used. Patients usually can be discharged the day after catheters are removed.

The follow-up examination at eight-week intervals includes a neurological examination, a CT scan, and determination of corticosteroid requirements [25]. Results of the tests are scored (−2 to +2, denoting severe deterioration to significant improvement, respectively); significant changes in the scores (two or more points) are a useful indication of the patient's condition. Patients were considered "evaluable" if they were alive and available for the first eight-week evaluation.

Results

We have reported survival data for the first 37 patients with recurrent malignant gliomas or metastatic brain tumors treated with brachytherapy (1979–1982) [15]. The overall response rate was 68% in the 34 patients who were evaluated. The survival periods of a more recent group of 41 patients with recurrent malignant gliomas are summarized in figure 18-4. Eighteen patients with glioblastomas had a median survival period after brachytherapy for recurrence of 35 weeks, two remaining alive for more than five years. For the 23 patients treated with brachytherapy for anaplastic astrocytomas, the median survival time after brachytherapy for recurrence was 153 weeks; 10 patients remained alive more than three years after brachytherapy for recurrence and four remained alive for more than four years. Both groups had significantly better outcomes ($p < 0.01$) than did groups of patients with the same diagnoses and similar general characteristics who were treated at recurrence with chemotherapy alone.

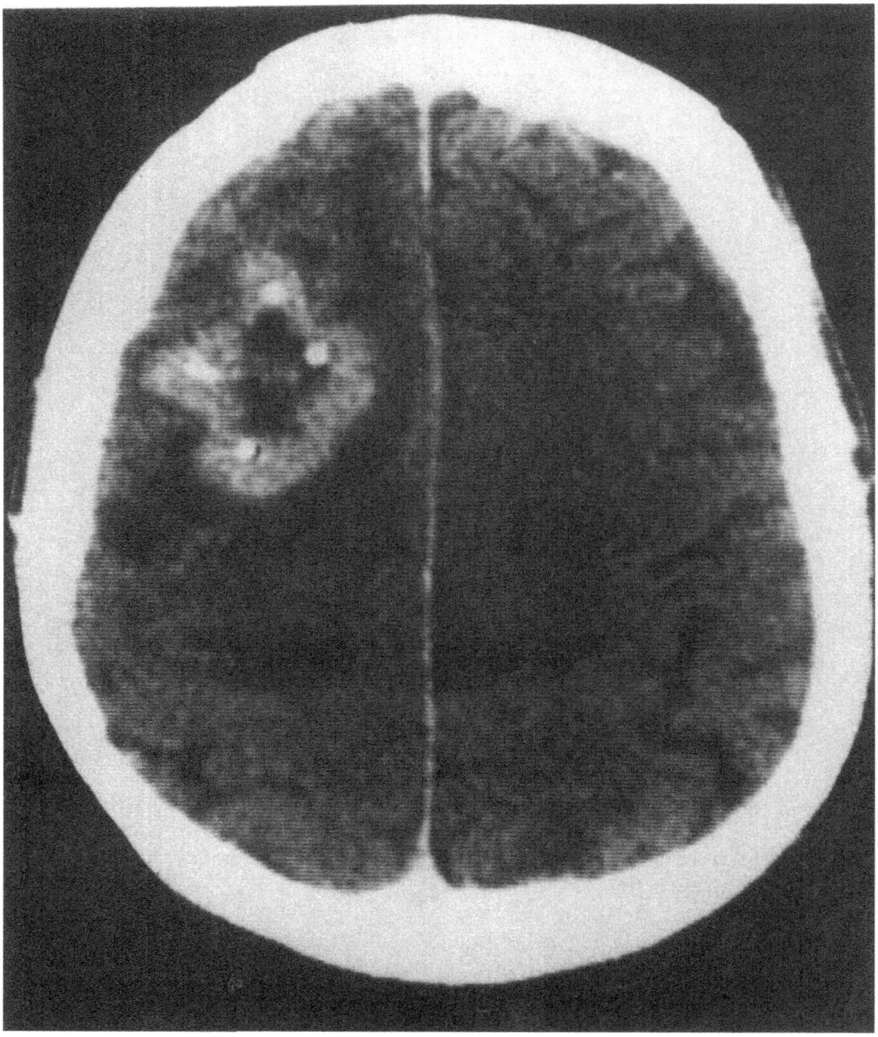

FIGURE 18–3. Postoperative CT scan shows four radioactive sources within a right frontal lesion.

Preliminary data are available on our first 77 patients with recurrent malignant gliomas treated with temporarily implanted ^{125}I sources. Forty-two patients had an histologic diagnosis of anaplastic astrocytoma, and 35 patients had a diagnosis of glioblastoma multiforme. At the time of analysis, 45% of patients with anaplastic astrocytoma and 34% of those with glioblastoma multiforme were alive (median follow-up period of 13 and 9 months, respectively). The median survival after brachytherapy for recurrence was 22 months for patients with anaplastic astrocytoma and 14.5 months for patients with glioblastoma multiforme.

Twenty-seven (35%) of 77 patients required reoperation after brachytherapy because their neurological condition had deteriorated and because there was evidence on CT images of an increase in the size of their lesions consistent with either focal radiation necrosis or tumor progression. Reoperation was performed nine to 80 weeks after brachytherapy (median, 34 weeks). At reoperation, lesions were generally firm and avascular. Patients usually improved after reoperation. In most instances, histopathologic evaluation of resected tissue showed a combination of radiation-induced necrotic tissue and recurrent tumor. There was no cor-

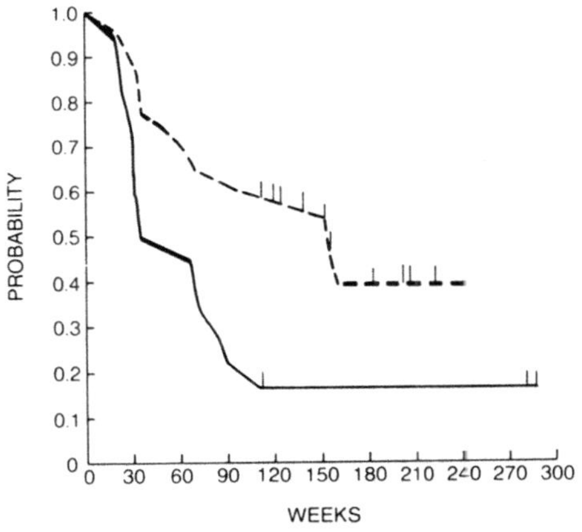

FIGURE 18–4. Kaplan-Meier survival curve for 18 patients with recurrent glioblastoma multiforme (*solid line*) and 23 patients with recurrent anaplastic astrocytoma (*broken line*). Median survival (probability = 0.5) is 153 weeks for patients with anaplastic astrocytoma and 35 weeks for patients with glioblastoma multiforme measured after brachytherapy for recurrence. Cross-hatching indicates censored patients.

relation between the histopathology of resected material and outcome, however. Compared with patients harboring the same tumor type who did not have subsequent surgery, patients who had reoperation generally had significantly improved survival rates. In addition, despite the presence in most patients of apparently viable tumor in resected specimens, tumor cells from these specimens often did not grow in culture [37]. This suggests that, although radiation did not kill these cells, many of them apparently lost the growth characteristics that lead to rapid tumor recurrence.

Complications in 77 patients treated with brachytherapy included infection in six patients, wound breakdown in two, acute cerebral edema in two, and intracranial hemorrhage in one. Preliminary evidence suggests that the incidence of infection can be reduced by the routine perioperative administration of antibiotics.

Based on the promising results of our treatment of recurrent gliomas with removable ^{125}I sources, we have begun a study through the Northern California Oncology Group in which aggressive brachytherapy is used near the beginning of treatment rather than at the time of recurrence. Patients are irradiated via conventional teletherapy with 60 Gy of radiation to the tumor volume, administered concomitantly with hydroxyurea as a radiosensitizer. Within two weeks this is followed by brachytherapy to deliver an additional minimum tumor dose of 6,000 cGy. A 12-month course of cyclical chemotherapy with procarbazine, CCNU, and vincristine then is administered. This study is based on our previous best-treatment protocol, which combines external irradiation, hydroxyurea, and the cyclical chemotherapy regimen [14].

The risk of focal radiation necrosis in patients receiving the aggressive treatment just described is unknown, as is the extent of neurological deficits that might be induced or exacerbated by such treatment. Unfortunately, the usual criteria for evaluating patients for tumor recurrence do not distinguish between recurrent disease and focal radiation necrosis [5, 8, 11, 20, 22, 35]. Preliminary evidence suggests that positron emission tomography may help distinguish between these two lesions [36]. Our experience indicates that surgery will be helpful in ameliorating these complications [6].

More than 80 patients have been placed on this protocol, but the length of follow-up is insufficient for analysis at this time. When analysis is possible, it must show brachytherapy to be dramatically superior in patients with well-circumscribed tumors, or the risk of increased deficit and the expense of this treatment will not be considered worthwhile.

Conclusions

CT-guided stereotactic surgery permits radioactive sources to be accurately placed directly into malignant gliomas. Our preliminary results with recurrent malignant gliomas are quite promising for patients with anaplastic astrocytomas, but results for patients with glioblastoma multiforme are only slightly better than results obtained with conventional chemotherapy. Better imaging of the margins of these lesions may lead to better local control; it is not clear that newer imaging modalities such as magnetic resonance imaging (MRI) will improve our ability to define the margins of these diffusely infiltrative lesions. If MRI proves to have an advantage for this purpose, then MRI-based stereotaxy might be useful in improving the results of brachytherapy. A number of issues remain to be determined including the best isotope to use, the overall number of sources that are needed, and the optimum activity of sources used.

Focal radiation necrosis is the most serious obstacle to successful brachytherapy of brain tumors. A better understanding of the mechanisms of induction of radiation necrosis might provide clues that will allow the use of higher, potentially curative radiation doses. Alternatively, combination protocols, including the use of hyperthermia and radiosensitizers, might allow an increase of the therapeutic index and thereby lower the total radiation dose needed [3, 27, 29]. Until these problems are solved, focal radiation necrosis should be anticipated in a large number of patients treated with brachytherapy. It is clear that resection of necrotic tissue is frequently of benefit in symptomatic patients.

Stereotactic implantation of radioactive sources offers great promise for the treatment of malignant brain tumors with a size and geometry suitable for implantation. Brachytherapy must be considered to be one of many experimental approaches to the treatment of these lesions until the issues described are addressed and solved. Because of the inherently experimental nature of the treatment, it is best performed in a university setting, where strict adherence to protocols and careful documentation of results can be ensured.

References

1. Alvord EC Jr: Why do gliomas not metastasize? *Arch Neurol* 33:73–75, 1976
2. Bernstein M, Gutin PH: Interstitial irradiation of brain tumors: A review. *Neurosurgery* 9:741–750, 1981
3. Coughlin JCT, Douple EB, Strohbehn JW, et al: Interstitial hyperthermia in conjunction with brachytherapy. *Radiology* 148:285–288, 1983
4. DaSilva V, Gutin PH, Deen DF, et al: Relative biological effectiveness of ^{125}I sources in a murine brachytherapy model. *Int J Radiat Oncol Biol Phys* 10:2109–2111, 1984
5. Daumas-Duport C, Blond S, Vedrenne CL, et al: Radiolesion versus recurrence: Bioptic data in 39 gliomas after interstitial, or combined interstitial and external radiation treatment. *Acta Neurochir [Suppl]* (Wien) 33:291–299, 1984
6. Edwards MS, Wilson CB: Treatment of radiation necrosis. In Gilbert HA, Kagen AR (eds): *Radiation Damage to the Nervous System: A Delayed Therapeutic Hazard.* New York: Raven Press, 1980, pp 129–143
7. Erlich SS, Davis RL: Spinal subarachnoid metastasis from primary intracranial glioblastoma multiforme. *Cancer* 42:2854–2864, 1978
8. Fike JR, Cann CE, Phillips TL, et al: Radiation brain damage induced by interstitial ^{125}I sources: A canine model evaluated by quantitative computed tomography. *Neurosurgery* 16:530–537, 1985
9. Frazier CH: The effects of radium emanations upon brain tumors. *Surg Gynecol Obstet* 31:236–239, 1920
10. Freeman ML, Goldhagen P, Sierra E, et al: Studies with encapsulated ^{125}I sources. II. Determination of the relative biological effectiveness using cultured mammalian cells. *Int J Radiat Oncol Biol Phys* 8:1355–1361, 1982
11. Graeb DA, Steinbok P, Robertson WD: Transient early computed tomographic changes mimicking tumor progression after brain tumor irradiation. *Radiology* 144:813–817, 1982
12. Gutin PH, Dormandy RH Jr: A coaxial catheter system for afterloading radioactive sources for the interstitial irradiation of brain tumors: Technical note. *J Neurosurg* 56:734–735, 1982
13. Gutin PH, Edwards MSB, Wara WM, et al: Preliminary experience with ^{125}I-brachytherapy of pediatric brain tumors. *Concepts Pediatr Neurosurg* 5:187–206, 1985
14. Gutin PH, Levin VA: Surgery, radiation, and chemotherapy in the treatment of malignant brain tumors. In Thompson RA, Green JR (eds): *Controversies in Neurology.* New York: Raven Press, 1983, pp 67–86
15. Gutin PH, Phillips TL, Wara WM, et al: Brachytherapy of recurrent malignant brain tumors with removable high-activity iodine-125 sources. *J Neurosurg* 60:61–68, 1984
16. Heilbrun MP, Roberts TS, Apuzzo MLJ, et al: Preliminary experience with the Brown-Roberts-Wells (BRW) computerized tomographic stereotaxic guidance system. *J Neurosurg* 59:217–222, 1983
17. Hirsch O: Die operative behandlung von hypophysistumoren. *Archiv Larengologie Rhiinologie* 26:529–696, 1912
18. Hochberg FH, Pruitt A: Assumptions in the radiotherapy of glioblastoma. *Neurology* 30:907–911, 1980
19. Hosobuchi Y, Phillips TL, Stupar TA, et al: Interstitial brachytherapy of primary brain tumors: Preliminary report. *J Neurosurg* 53:613–617, 1980
20. Kiessling M, Kleihues P, Gessaga E, et al: Morphology of intracranial tumors and adjacent brain following interstitial iodine-125 radiotherapy. *Acta Neurochir [Suppl]* (Wien) 33:281–289, 1984
21. Kim JH, Hilaris BJ: Iodine-125 source in interstitial tumor therapy. *AJR* 123:163–169, 1975
22. Kingsley DP, Kendall BE: CT of the adverse

effects of therapeutic radiation of the central nervous system. *AJNR* 2:453–460, 1981
23. Krishnaswamy V: Dose distributions around a ^{125}I seed source in tissue. *Radiology* 126:489–491, 1978
24. Leksell L: The stereotaxic method and radiosurgery of the brain. *Acta Chir Scand* 102:316–319, 1951
25. Levin VA, Crafts DC, Norman DM, et al: Criteria for evaluating patients undergoing chemotherapy for malignant brain tumors. *J Neurosurg* 47:329–335, 1977
26. Liu J, Edwards FM: Radiation exposure to medical personnel during iodine-125 seed implantation of the prostate. *Radiology* 132:748–749, 1979
27. Lyons BE, Britt RH, Strohbehn JW: Localized hyperthermia in the treatment of malignant brain tumors using an interstitial microwave antenna array. *IEEE Trans Biomed Eng* 31:53–62, 1984
28. MacKay AR, Gutin PH, Hosobuchi Y, et al: Computed tomography–directed stereotaxy for biopsy and interstitial irradiation of brain tumors: Technical note. *Neurosurgery* 11:38–42, 1982
29. Manning MR, Cetas TC, Miller RC, et al: Clinical hyperthermia: Results of a phase I trial employing hyperthermia alone or in combination with external beam or interstitial radiotherapy. *Cancer* 49:205–216, 1982
30. Mundinger F: The treatment of brain tumors with radioisotopes. *Prog Neurol Surg* 1:202–257, 1966
31. Mundinger F, Birg W, Ostertag CB: Treatment of small cerebral gliomas with CT-aided stereotaxic curietherapy. *Neuroradiology* 16:564–567, 1978
32. Mundinger F, Weigel K: Long-term results of stereotactic interstitial curietherapy. *Acta Neurochir [Suppl]* (Wien) 33:367–371, 1984
33. Ostertag CB, Groothius D, Kleihues P: Experimental data on early and late morphologic effects of permanently implanted gamma and beta sources (iridium-192, iodine-125, and yttrium-90) in the brain. *Acta Neurochir [Suppl]* (Wien) 33:271–280, 1984
34. Ostertag CHB, Mennel HD, Kiessling M: Stereotactic biopsy of brain tumors. *Surg Neurol* 14:275–283, 1980
35. Ostertag CB, Weigel K, Birg W: CT-changes after long-term interstitial iridum-192 irradiation of cerebral gliomas. In Szikla G (ed): *Stereotactic Cerebral Irradiation*. Amsterdam: Elsevier/North-Holland, 1979, pp 149–155
36. Patronas NJ, De Chiro GD, Brooks RA, et al: Work in progress: ^{18}F-fluorodeoxyglucose and positron emission tomography in the evaluation of radiation necrosis of the brain. *Radiology* 144:885–889, 1982
37. Rosenblum ML, Vasquez DA, Hoshino T, et al: Development of a clonogenic cell assay for human brain tumors. *Cancer* 41:2305–2314, 1978
38. Schlegel W, Scharfenberg H, Doll J, et al: CT images as the basis of operation planning in stereotactical neurosurgery. In Proceedings of the 1st International Symposium on Medical Imaging and Image Interpretation, Berlin, October 1982, ISMII 82. New York: *IEEE Trans Biomed Eng* 1982, pp 172–177
39. Sheline GE: Normal tissue tolerance and radiation therapy of gliomas of the adult brain. In *Series on Recent Results in Cancer Research* (In press)
40. Sheline GE, Wara WM, Smith V: Therapeutic irradiation and brain injury. *Int J Radiat Oncol Biol Phys* 6:1215–1228, 1980
41. Szikla G, Blond S, Daumas-Duport C, et al: Stereotaxis in the management of brain tumors: Three-dimensional angiography, sampling biopsies, and focal irradiation using the Talairach stereotactic system. *Ital J Neurol Sci [Suppl]* 2:83–96, 1983
42. Szikla G, Peragut JC: Irradiation interstitielle des gliomes. *Neurochirurgie* 21 (Suppl 2):187–228, 1975
43. Szikla G, Schilenger M, Betti O, et al: Combined interstitial and external irradiation of gliomas: A progress report. In Szikla G (ed): *Stereotactic Cerebral Irradiation*. New York: Elsevier/North Holland, 1979, pp 329–338
44. Szikla G, Schlienger M, Blond S, et al: Interstitial and combined interstitial and external irradiation of supratentorial gliomas: Results in 61 cases treated 1973–1981. *Acta Neurochir [Suppl]* (Wien) 33:355–362, 1984
45. Talairach J, Bonis A, Szikla G, et al: Stereotaxic implantation of radioactive isotopes in functional pituitary surgery: Technique and results. In Wang Y, Paoletti P (eds): *Radionuclide Applications of Neurology and Neurosurgery*. Springfield, IL: Thomas, 1970, pp 267–299
46. Talairach J, Ruggiero G, Aboulker J, et al: A new method of treatment of inoperable brain tumors by stereotaxic implantation of radioactive gold—a preliminary report. Br J Radiol 28:62–74, 1955
47. Walker MD, Alexander E Jr, Hunt WE, et al: Evaluation of BCNU and/or radiotherapy in the treatment of anaplastic gliomas: A cooperative clinical trial. *J Neurosurg* 49:333–343, 1978
48. Walker MD, Strike TA, Sheline GE: An analysis of dose-effect relationship in the radiotherapy of malignant gliomas. *Int J Radiat Oncol Biol Phys* 5:1725–1731, 1979

19. CONSIDERATIONS IN THE USAGE AND RESULTS OF CURIETHERAPY

Fritz Mundinger
K. Weigel

In the last few years, interstitial and intracavitary radiation therapies of nonresectable and/or recurrent intracranial tumors have experienced a renaissance. High expectations had followed the development of modern and increasingly sophisticated external radiation therapy techniques, but, until recently, they could not be fulfilled. Even today, problems remain, particularly with midline tumors, despite the beneficial results possible with higher depth dosage, better compatibility, and the exemption from radiation of cutaneous, osseous, and cerebral tissue within the irradiated area.

Interstitial or local radiation therapy can yield satisfactory to good results in cases of recurrent tumors that have undergone previous external radiation therapy. It also can be used for tumors remaining after surgery or prior external irradiation [12, 14, 76, 87, 99]. An additional advantage of interstitial and intracavitary therapy is that it can be repeated if the doses that will be absorbed by the midline of the brain are not excessive [14–19, 26–30]. Interstitial and intracavitary radioisotope treatment are bound necessarily to the stereotactic localization and implantation method [1–3, 14, 18, 23–25, 31, 32, 37].

Since the early 1950s, Mundinger has worked to advance the development of interstitial Curietherapy techniques. These efforts are described in numerous publications (dating back to 1953) on the stereotactic target device he developed with Riechert [85, 86], on his work (with Birg) on computer stereotaxy [6–10, 39, 55, 59–61], and on stereotaxy incorporating computed tomography (CT) and magnetic resonance imaging (MRI). The implantation of radioactive material directly into tumors initially was performed intraoperatively after tumor resection. Later, radionuclide seeds were implanted in the tumor postoperatively with the aid of simple auxiliary devices similar to stereotactic apparatus [37, 41, 46].

The stereotactic method has been used routinely since 1951 at the University-Hospital in Freiburg, West Germany. Intracranial implantation of various radioactive elements is used as both primary and secondary therapy. Table 19–1 summarizes the succession of radioisotopes used in the past by Mundinger and his co-workers [57]. By 1969, Mundinger had reported 534 cases [57], including 304 brain tumors and 206 pituitary adenomas or craniopharyngiomas. Through decades of persistent radiobiological and radiophysical investigation of the various radionuclides and comparison of statistically evaluable series, we were able to define the indications at an early stage. The results were published in detail in three reports [44, 57, 58].

It soon became evident that stereotactic implantation of radionuclides such as phosphorus-32, yttrium-90, and palladium-106 had to be limited to small-volume tumors. In cysts, these radionuclides also could be instilled as colloids or suspensions to irradiate the cyst wall [44, 57, 58, 77, 90, 96]. We observed that strong gamma-emitting isotopes, in particular cobalt-60, combined with external radiation, led to very impressive results [12, 38, 42, 44, 45, 47, 48, 57, 58].

When remaining tumor was suspected, the intraoperative implantation of radionuclides could not be used because radiation exposure

L.D. Lunsford (ed.) *MODERN STEREOTACTIC NEUROSURGERY*.

TABLE 19–1. Usage of Interstitial Radiation with Radioisotopes in Intracranial Tumors[a]

Radioisotopes	Date Usage Began	Total No. Patients Treated by 1969
Phosphorus-32	6/25/52	32
Gold-198	3/4/54	123
Yttrium-90	1/24/63	21
Cobalt-60	6/7/55	166
Tantalum-182	5/14/57	21
Iridium-192	3/15/60	87
Iridium-192-GammaMed®	6/24/64	84
Total		534

[a] Modified from Mundinger et al. [57]; patients treated in Freiberg, W. Germany.

was excessive. Furthermore, small hemorrhages caused flushing or dislocation of the radioactive material within the tissue or sometimes outside the operation area. Freehand creation of a radiation grid to guide a sufficiently high dose to the remaining tumor provided a cumbersome solution, yet only in this way could intraoperative implantation be combined effectively with tumor resection [57, 93]. For these reasons, we abandoned this method very early on. More recent attempts to implant radionuclides intraoperatively, such as those being undertaken with iodine-125 (^{125}I) seeds [74], probably will suffer a similar fate.

Alternatively, direct irradiation of the tumor resection cavity was tried, using a gamma ray-emitting element such as cobalt-60 or cesium-137 implanted by the afterloading technique, immediately after tumor resection. We initially preferred this method [57, 58]. However, when the tumor could not be totally resected either macroscopically or microscopically and the remaining tumor on the edge of the resection cavity was of varying thickness, we encountered considerable dosimetry problems. A major problem was that radiation necrosis of the healthy perifocal tissue could not be kept within acceptable limits. Therefore, we abandoned this method, too.

Our attention turned to postoperative stereotactic implantation techniques. We were aided by nuclide scintiscanning, which produced a positive-contrast image of the approximate remaining tumor volume and tumor location. Scintiscans were especially helpful in assessing deep-seated tumors, which could be shown by staining or vascular displacement from angiography or by displacement of ventricular structures from pneumoencephalography during biopsy. At present, the best radionuclides for interstitial irradiation are iridium-192 (^{192}Ir) and ^{125}I. Apart from their favorable physical characters, these radionuclides meet the requirements of radiation safety laws in most countries.

Early in our investigations, we attempted histological evaluation of mass lesions of the brain using either CT or MRI. Prior to this, we suspect that many patients erroneously underwent empirical radiation therapy. Histological verification of an intracranial mass lesion is mandatory before specific therapy is undertaken [22, 33, 34]. In deep-seated tumors located near the midline and in functionally important regions, stereotactic technique has proved to be a successful method of obtaining tissue samples for histological verification without damaging the surrounding tissue [8, 39, 51, 55, 60, 61, 63, 67, 78, 79, 83].

The introduction of improved imaging techniques such as CT and MRI has increased greatly the recognition of deep-seated brain tumors. Midline tumors still are considered nonresectable, despite the use of microsurgery, because of the major psychological and neurological impairment an operation can cause.

The biopsy needle trajectory for the verification of tumor grading and classification preceding every operation is determined by the software of modern CT and MRI scanners. If it is shown to be indicated on the basis of the biopsy diagnosis (which is obtained intraoperatively in 95% of our cases), interstitial radiotherapy can be performed immediately [4–11,

33, 34, 40, 43, 49–53, 59–61, 80–82, 89]. After biopsy in some cases, external irradiation is indicated, and, in others, the histology or tumor extent renders irradiation unnecessary.

Tumor location and volume, implantation sites (which are dependent on tumor geometry), and the optimal approach also can be determined using CT or MRI. Thus, we now are able to confine devitalization to the tumor tissue itself and largely spare the surrounding tissue.

Contrast-enhanced CT and MRI (table 19–2), preceded by the indispensable cerebral angiography and electroencephalography (table 19–3), enable the optimal trajectory and appropriate dosimetry to be selected, thus exempting large vessels from excessive radiation and preventing subsequent thrombosis and cyst formation. These imaging techniques also facilitate highly precise biopsies with very little risk to functionally important regions of the cortex (central, dominant, temporal) or in the area of the diencephalon, midbrain, and brain stem. Subsequent interstitial irradiation can be planned precisely [35, 39, 40, 45, 51, 62–74, 91, 94–97, 99–103]. The authors' CT and MRI stereotactic techniques for obtaining biopsies and for radionuclide implantation are described in detailed reports [43, 44, 53, 56–58] and other publications [40, 49, 51, 56, 59–75, 101–103].

Material and Methods

From 1951 through 1985, 1,665 patients with intracranial tumors underwent stereotactic implantation of radionuclides in Freiburg. The following pertains only to patients who were stereotactically treated between 1965 and 1985, some of whom also underwent interstitial radiotherapy. In 1981, CT was integrated into our stereotactic system [5–9, 51, 59–61]; in 1984, MRI was added [10, 75]. For the remaining patients in this series, another form of therapy was indicated. Earlier series and the results obtained after interstitial radioisotope therapy are reported elsewhere [37–75, 101, 102].

TABLE 19–2. CT Characteristics of 1,438 Intracranial Lesions

Characteristic	No. of Patients
Hypodense	420
Hyperdense	1,006
Displacement	588
Edema	1,341
Ring formation	343
Cyst formation	207

Once the intracranial target point and skull trephination site are determined, a tissue forceps is introduced into the lesion. The forceps has a diameter of 0.8 mm; the volume of the sample is 1–3 mm^3. In each puncture tract, several samples are taken at 1 to 5-mm intervals, proximal to, within, and distal to the tumor. Half of these samples are prepared immediately as smears, stained with methylene blue, and examined intraoperatively. Other samples are embedded in paraffin and analyzed with appropriate staining methods. This procedure has been described in detail in several publications [33, 34, 39, 40, 43].

If interstitial radiotherapy is indicated by the intraoperative diagnosis of the smear, radioactive sources are implanted during the same operation. In a spherical tumor, implantation is carried out through a cannula inserted into the center of the tumor. Dosimetry and determination of the radius (or radii) to be implanted and nuclide radioactivity depend on both the size and configuration of the tumor indicated on the CT or MRI images and on the histological results of the various tissue samples.

At present, ^{192}Ir in a platinum alloy and ^{125}I in seed form are the most common isotopes used in treatment of intracranial tumors. Mun-

TABLE 19–3. Electroenphalographic and Angiographic Findings in Intracranial Lesions

	Findings	No. of Patients
Electroencephalography	Pathological	1,145
	Focal	697
Angiography	Displacement of vessels	1,203
	Pathological vessels	494

TABLE 19–4. Stereotactic Biopsy and Curietherapy of Benign and Malignant Gliomas

Tumor Type	Grade	Biopsy Only	Curietherapy $^{125}I^{a}$	Curietherapy $^{192}Ir^{b}$	Total Cases
Astrocytoma	I	80	67	59	206
Astrocytoma	II	203	106	91	400
Astrocytoma	III	156	44	23	223
Astrocytoma	IV	144	20	14	178
Oligodendroglioma	II	21	11	21	53
Oligodendroglioma	III	7	2	8	17
Totals		611	250	216	1,077

[a] 1979–1985.
[b] 1965–1985.

TABLE 19–5. Stereotactic Biopsy and Curietherapy of Other Central Nervous System Tumors

	Biopsy Only	Curietherapy $^{125}I^{a}$	Curietherapy $^{192}Ir^{b}$	Total Cases
Ependymoma	6	12	6	24
Primitive neuroectodermal tumor	18	9	4	31
Germinoma	19	10	7	36
Teratoma	9	1	3	13
Metastasis	78	14	3	95
Unclassified tumor	7	1	3	11
Totals	137	47	26	210

[a] 1979–1985.
[b] 1965–1985.

dinger introduced these two elements into long-term irradiation therapy for intracranial tumors, ^{192}Ir in 1959 and ^{125}I in 1979 [46, 48, 50]. According to Hilaris [27, 28] ^{125}I is available as a 4.5 × 0.8-mm titanium seed. The seeds contain a silver rod to which the ^{125}I is bound. We use ^{192}Ir in the form of wires with a diameter of 0.3 mm; we gauge the length of the wire according to the specific activity. Both the iodine seeds and iridium wires in low doses are designed for permanent implantation (Curietherapy).

In brachy-Curietherapy, on the other hand, highly active ^{125}I seeds are inserted into a catheter and, by afterloading technique, implanted into the tumor for a specific length of time. A similar afterloading short-term irradiation technique is performed with ^{192}Ir. In 1963, Mundinger and Sauerwein developed the ^{192}Ir contact irradiation device GammaMed® for intraoperative irradiation. For a clinical accumulation dose, the radioactivity is calculated in the tumor periphery (peripheral tumor dose) at 10,000 cGy for ^{125}I and 12,000 cGy for ^{192}Ir. ^{125}I has a half-life similar to ^{192}I (64 days and 74 days, respectively) but a considerably "softer" gamma radiation (28.5 KeV for ^{125}I compared to 350 KeV for ^{192}Ir). Thus, radiation protection measures at higher levels of ^{125}I activity are eased significantly. For discussions of dosimetric problems, see [11, 50, 57].

Results

In a series of 1,551 tumor biopsies (1965–1985), stereotactic interstitial irradiation was indicated in 541 patients (tables 19–4 and 19–5). Pilocytic and fibrillary astrocytomas were frequent (42.5%) (see table 19–4). A small number of patients had other tumors, which were very unhomogeneous.

Grade I (pilocytic) astrocytomas were found

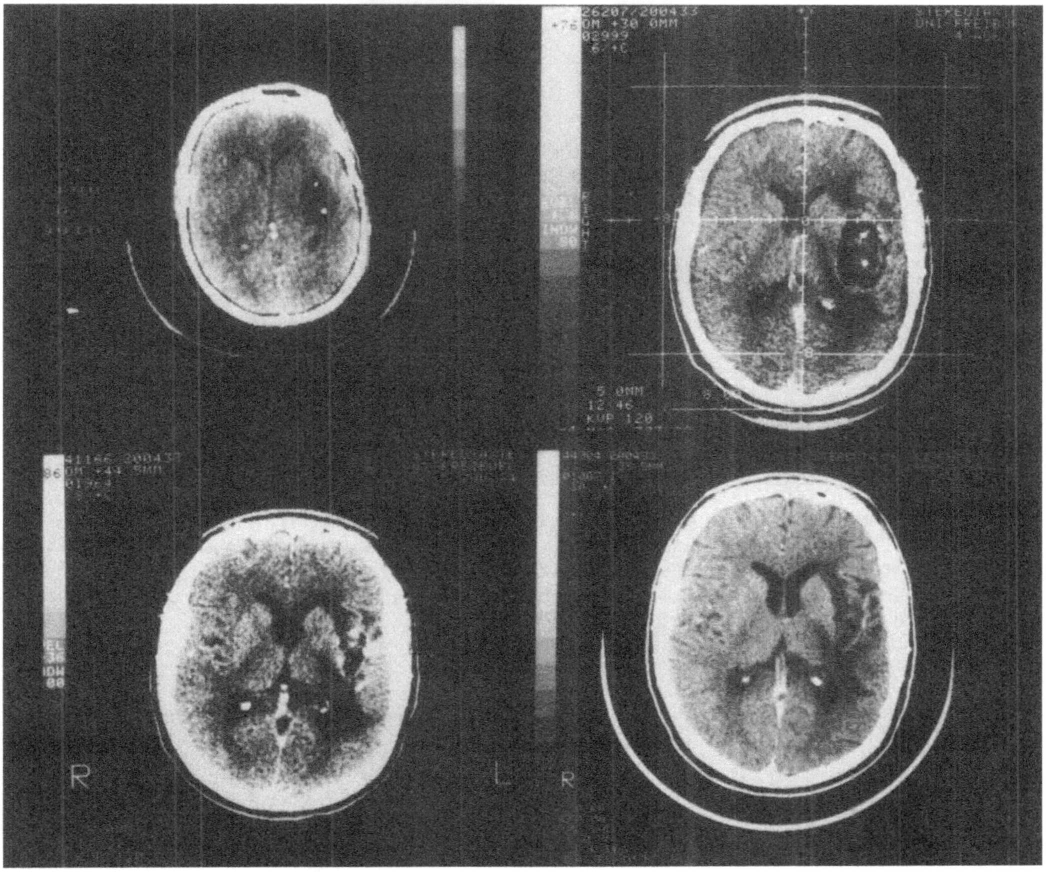

FIGURE 19–1. Stereotactic CT–confirmed grade II fibrillary astroctyoma in a 32-year-old patient. Clinical course following ^{125}I Curietherapy:
(*Top left*) CT scan defined a sharply demarcated hypodense mass immediately after ^{125}I implantation. Mass effect with compression of the ventricular system and significant perifocal edema was noted. (*Top right*) Seventeen months after ^{125}I Curietherapy, CT showed formation of a "halo" after contrast enhancement. The sources were distributed in the tumor without any change. A perifocal reaction (edema and gliosis) was noted in the parieto-occipital and mediofrontal brain.
(*Bottom left*) CT scan performed 3¾ years after ^{125}I Curietherapy showed that the ventricular system had shifted back and expanded symmetrically. The tumor mass itself had shrunk significantly and showed only a slight reaction in the surrounding tissue as well as recession of the hypodense areas (possible gliosis). There was no evidence of recurrence. (*Bottom right*) CT scan obtained five years after ^{125}I Curietherapy showed further shrinkage. The ventricular system had returned to normal. The patient was fully capable of working as a university lecturer.

chiefly in the central gray matter; the majority of these patients were under age 30. Grade II astrocytomas were identified mainly in the hemispheres (figures 19–1, 19–2), but some also occurred in the basal ganglia. The peak age for patients with grade II astrocytomas was 40–50 years (figure 19–3). Grades III and IV astrocytomas (oligodendrogliomas and glioblastomas) usually were located in the hemispheres. Interstitial implantation was carried out only if the tumors were in functionally important areas, such as the central region, and were relatively well-defined with CT. We believe that the best results are achieved when the tumor is less than 34 mm in diameter.

The primary symptom of grade I astrocytomas was an obstruction of the cerebrospinal fluid passages, as might be expected, given their

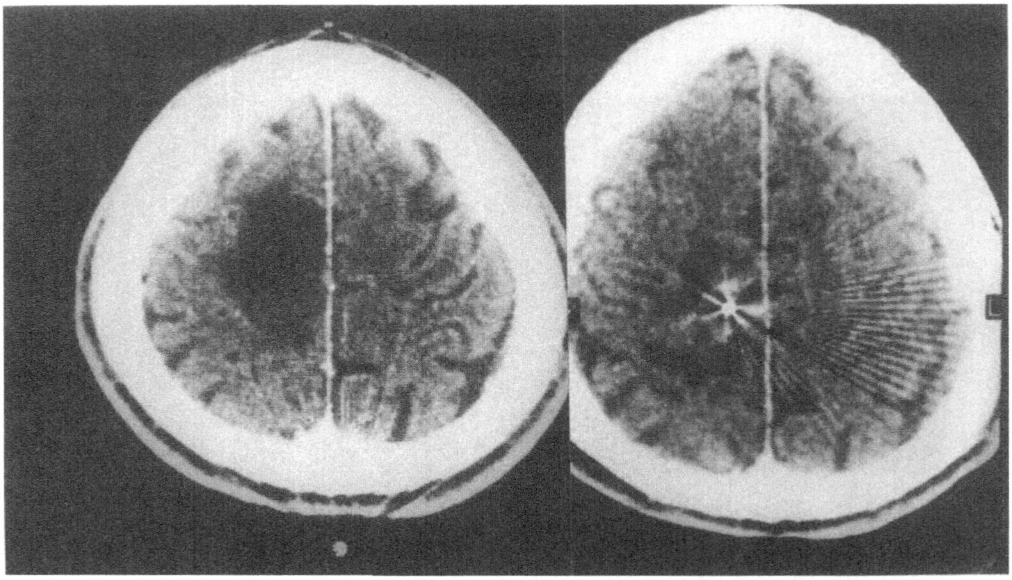

FIGURE 19–2. Stereotactic CT scan of a 21-year-old patient with a grade II fibrillary astrocytoma. (*Left*) CT revealed a relatively well-demarcated but extensive hypodense mass extending from the precentral to parietal area. (*Right*) CT performed three years after ^{125}I Curietherapy. The artifacts produced by the ^{125}I seeds can still be recognized. The central white matter still shows a hypodense area, but the sulci are enlarged. We detected no evidence of recurrent astrocytoma.

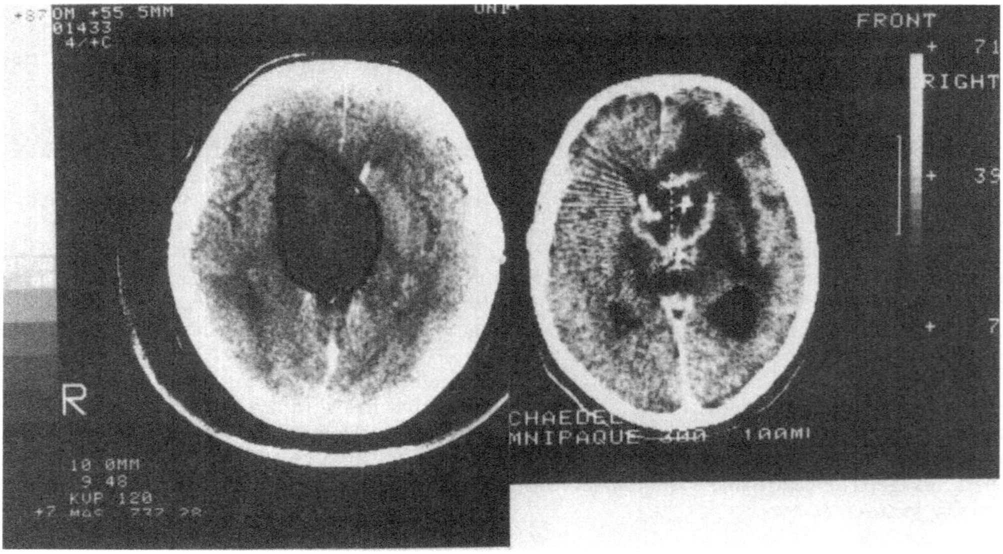

FIGURE 19–3. Extensive grade II fibrillary astrocytoma in a 33-year-old patient. The tumor bilaterally involves the diencephalon and infiltrates the right posterior frontal lobe and corpus callosum. (*Left*) CT scan defines tumor extent and mainly shows a hypodense mass (hatching) prior to Curietherapy. (*Right*) CT image 1¾ years after ^{125}I Curietherapy. The tumor has regressed significantly. The ^{125}I seeds can be seen in the center. A thin hyperdense "halo" is noted with contrast enhancement, and the center is hypodense (necrotic). Hypodense focal reactions (gliosis?) are seen mainly in the right frontal and mediotemporal regions. A dramatic improvement in the clinical findings occurred. The patient was essentially neurologically asymptomatic and capable of working.

most common site (table 19–6). The first sign of tumors located on the periphery was most frequently a convulsive disorder. Neurological deficits varied, depending on the location of the tumor. Of special interest were those midbrain tumors that usually resulted in disorders of ocular motility (table 19–7).

Certain primary symptoms or tumor locations required that general neurosurgical measures precede stereotactic puncture (table 19–8). To obtain optimal radiation effects, shunt operations and partial tumor resections frequently were performed to lower intracranial pressure. External radiation was administered to 163 patients. In 98 of these, tumor histology had not been determined; radiotherapy was indicated as a result of CT or angiographic findings alone. Table 19–9 shows the correlation between the mean implantation radii of the irradiated tumors and histology.

TABLE 19–6. Location of Intracranial Lesions that Underwent Stereotactic Biopsies[a]

Site	No. of Cases
Basal ganglia	309
Diencephalon	185
Midbrain-pons	262
Cerebral hemisphere	
Frontal lobe	318
Temporal lobe	236
Parietal lobe	191
Occipital lobe	3
Multifocal	42
Intraorbital	5
Total	1,551

[a] Freiburg, West Germany, 1965–1985.

Interstitial radiotherapy usually is a palliative measure and in rare cases a cure. Follow-up examinations took place at regular intervals. One year after local interstitial radiation, neurological deficits had improved in 40% of our patients; no changes were seen in 25%, and clinical symptoms deteriorated in 35%.

In accordance with these clinical courses,

TABLE 19–7. Preoperative Symptoms of 1,551 Intracranial Lesions

Symptom	No. of Cases
Increased intracranial pressure	807
Organic mental syndrome	756
Paresis	650
Ataxia	293
Oculomotor paresis	264
Aphasia	244
Visual impairment	183
Visual field defect	151
Other diseases	103
Extrapyramidal disorders	49
Hearing deficit	23

TABLE 19–8. Procedures Preceding Curietherapy in 571 Intracranial Lesions

Procedure	No. of Cases
Shunt	335
Partial resection	196
External irradiation	163
Without histology	98
Open biopsy	63

TABLE 19–9. Mean Implantation Radius in Interstitially Irradiated Cerebral Gliomas

		Iodine-125			Iridium-192		
Tumor	Grade	No. of Cases	Mean Implantation Radius	SE (mm)	No. of Cases	Mean Implantation Radius	SE (mm)
Astrocytoma	I	67	13.2	0.45	59	14.6	0.7
Astrocytoma	II	106	13.5	0.40	91	15.2	0.5
Astrocytoma	III	44	15.6	0.53	23	18.4	0.8
Oligodendroglioma	II	11	15.0	1.60	21	15.3	0.96
Glioblastoma		20	16.1	0.85	15	19.7	1.0

SE = standard error.

TABLE 19–10. Life Expectancy of Patients with Low-Grade Gliomas Who Underwent Interstitial Irradiation Compared with Those Who Had Biopsies Only[a]

	Tumor Type	Grade	No. of Cases	Percentage of Cases Surviving at 1 Year	3 Years	5 Years	10 Years
Iodine-125	Astrocytoma	I	67	95	70	55	
Iridium-192	Astrocytoma	I	59	94	86	78	61
Biopsy only	Astrocytoma	I	79	73	49	45	21
Iodine-125	Astrocytoma	II	106	87	31	28	
Iridium-192	Astrocytoma	II	91	86	45	31	26
Biopsy only	Astrocytoma	II	196	86	17	6	0

[a] As of June 1985.

TABLE 19–11. Complications After Stereotactic Biopsies of 1,551 Tumors[a]

Complication	Transient: No. of Cases	Transient: Percentage	Persistent: No. of Cases	Persistent: Percentage
Hemorrhage	21	1.3	15	1.0
Paresis	17	1.1	11	0.7
Aphasia	9	0.6	7	0.5
Seizure	32	2.1	8	0.5

[a] Through June 1985.

postoperative CT scans revealed a significant reduction in tumor volume in approximately half of the patients. Tumor configuration was unchanged in 16%; further tumor growth was seen in nearly 30%.

The survival probability of patients with grades I and II astrocytomas who were treated with interstitial radionuclide therapy was compared with those who underwent biopsy only (table 19–10). Fifty-five percent of patients with grade I astrocytomas were alive five years after implantation of ^{125}I seeds. For those treated with ^{192}Ir, the figure was 78%. On the other hand, the survival probability of patients with grade I astrocytomas who had biopsies alone was only 45%. The difference between groups of patients with grade II fibrillary astrocytomas were even more evident. In the group treated with ^{125}I, the probability of surviving for five years was 28%; in the group treated with ^{192}Ir, 31%. For patients who underwent biopsy alone, the rate did not exceed 6%.

Complications (table 19–11) were categorized as either a direct result of surgical intervention (i.e., the taking of tissue) or caused by radiation. Temporary neurological deterioration resulting from surgery was observed in approximately 5% of the patients; small intracerebral hemorrhage was the most frequent cause. Twenty patients (1.3%) died within seven days of surgery.

Discussion

Not all deep-seated and otherwise inoperable brain tumors located in functionally important areas are suitable for interstitial radiotherapy. As a general principle, operable extra-axial tumors, such as epidermoid cysts or meningiomas, should have open surgery. Well-defined intra-axial tumors with a radius not exceeding 40 mm can benefit from interstitial irradiation. For low-dose Curietherapy, that is, permanent implantation of ^{125}I or ^{192}Ir sources, histological findings should suggest slow tumor growth; radiosensitivity to external irradiation should be considered low to moderate. High-dose afterloaded brachy-Curietherapy, defined

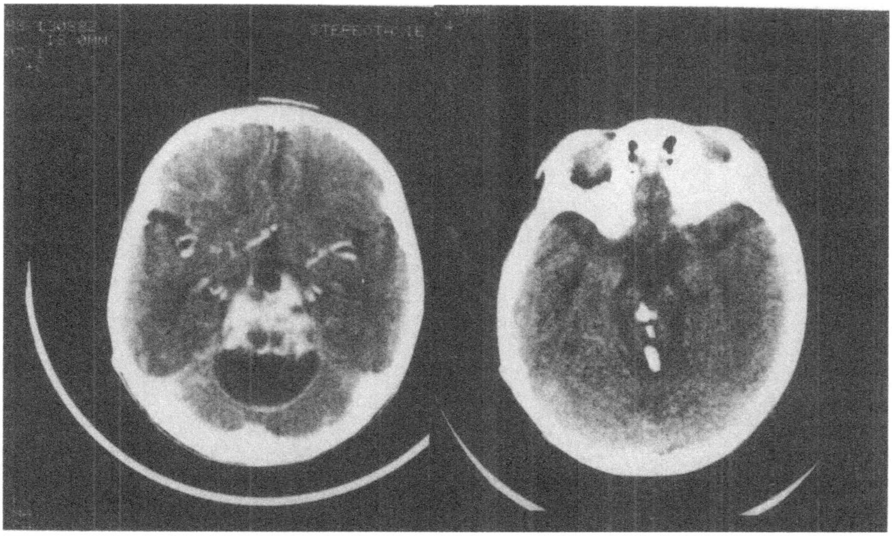

FIGURE 19–4. This 3½-year-old patient had a grade I pilocytic astrocytoma with a large cyst, which occupied the cerebellar vermis. (*Left*) A CT scan before Curietherapy demonstrated a 4-cm superior brain-stem tumor with intense contrast enhancement. (*Right*) A CT scan was performed 11 months after ^{125}I Curietherapy and stereotactic cyst implantation with a catheter and reservoir. Three consecutive cyst aspirations were performed. The ^{125}I sources are seen in the center of the tumor. The basal cisterns have reopened and cerebellar sulci can be recognized. The tumor no longer is evident. These findings were associated with dramatic clinical improvement and good physical development.

as temporary implantation of radionuclides, should be used for malignant or recurrent tumors.

For grade I or II astrocytomas, permanent radionuclide implantation is indicated. For high-grade tumors, such as anaplastic astrocytomas, permanent interstitial implantation should be performed only if the tumor is localized, small, and solid. In these instances, additional external beam irradiation must accompany permanent implantation (Curietherapy); in the case of a tumor resection, it must be combined with brachy-Curietherapy); if germinomas or primitive neuroectodermal tumors are identified histologically, external beam irradiation of the neuroaxis is indicated. In the case of a recurrent tumor, low-dose Curietherapy is indicated. The results and clinical indications of malignant tumors treated with brachy-Curietherapy are reported elsewhere [43, 51, 54, 56, 62, 69]. Radiotherapeutical measures, external or internal, should not be undertaken without decisive histological findings. As early as 1932, Cushing strongly endorsed this viewpoint when he spoke of taking "a therapeutic shot in the dark so long as the tumor's precise histological type is unknown" [13]. Reports in world-wide scientific literature reveal that until recently only about 35% of externally irradiated tumors have been histologically determined on the basis of an exploratory craniotomy [20, 36, 88, 98]. The literature also shows that total or partial resection of deep-seated tumors results in a 25% mortality rate [21, 84]. When compared to our mortality rate in this series of stereotactic operations, 0.9%, we consider exploratory craniotomy to be a method of limited appropriateness.

The favorable effects of interstitial Curietherapy on low-grade tumors are particularly evident in patients with pilocytic astrocytomas (figure 19–4). Fifty-five percent of patients with astrocytomas who received ^{125}I implantations and 78% of those treated with ^{192}Ir survived for five years after therapy, whereas only 45% who did not undergo therapy survived the fifth year. In cases of fibrillary astrocytomas, probability of survival is lower: 28% of patients implanted with ^{125}I and 31% of those treated with ^{192}Ir lived another five years (figure 19–5). Only 5% of patients not irradiated reached the five-year mark.

In addition to this distinct increase in the probability of five-year survival, Curietherapy

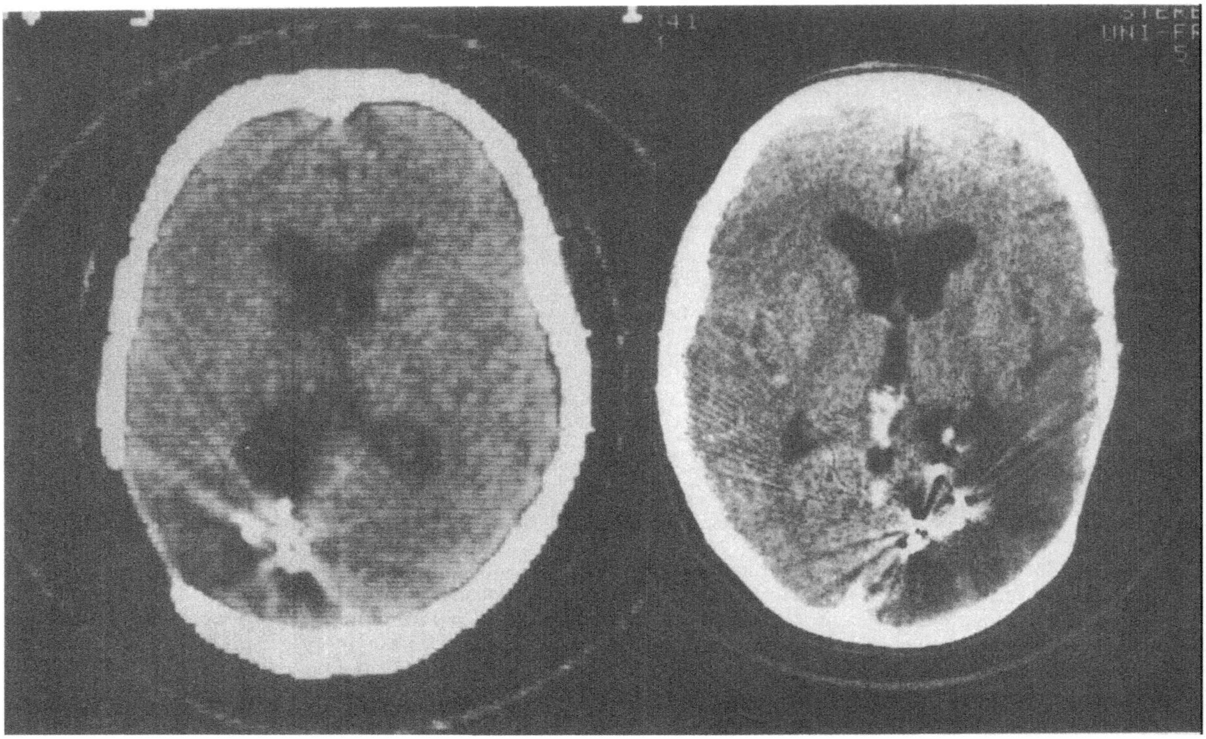

FIGURE 19–5. CT scans of a 43-year-old woman with a grade-II protoplasmic astrocytoma. She had open resection of a cystic tumor in 1963 and intraoperative implantation of tantalum-182. A recurrence prompted permanent implantation of ^{192}Ir in November 1978 and insertion of a catheter for possible drainage. (*Left*) CT image immediately after ^{192}Ir implant. (*Right*) CT image six years after ^{192}Ir implantation, 21 years following combined operative resection and interstitial Curietherapy. On the left is a parieto-occipital hypodense display of glial changes, presumably a result of irradiation. Occipitally near the posterior horn are numerous metallic artifacts caused by the radioactive implants. The ventricular system is symmetrical; the lateral fissure on the left is somewhat wider than on the right (shrinkage). With the exception of a homonymous hemianopia, the patient has no neurological symptoms. She was since given birth to a healthy child.

also often leads to improvement of neurological deficits, accompanied by CT-defined shrinking of the tumor. The tumor volume at the time of stereotactic surgery or commencement of irradiation is clearly significant: tumors with a radius not exceeding 30 mm have the best results.

We believe that our long-term results have shown the effectiveness of interstitial Curietherapy and justified its continued use.

References

1. Apuzzo MLJ, Sabshin JK: Computed tomographic guidance sterotaxis in the managment of intracranial mass lesions. *Neurosurgery* 12:277–284, 1983
2. Backlund EO: Studies on craniopharyngiomas. III. Stereotaxic treatment with intracystic yttrium-90. *Acta Chir Scand* 139:237–247, 1973
3. Bergstroem M, Greitz T, Steiner I: An approach to stereotaxic radiography. *Acta Neurochir* (Wien) 54:157–165, 1980
4. Bernstein M, Gutin PH: Interstitial irradiation of brain tumors: A review. *Neurosurgery* 9:741–750, 1981
5. Birg W, Krebber L, Mundinger F: Ein einfaches Verfahren für die Über tragung von Tomographie-Scan-Schichten auf das Röntgenbild, insbesondere für die funktionelle Neurochirurgie. *Fortschr Neurol Psychiatr* 47:637–640, 1979
6. Birg W, Mundinger F, Klar M: Computer assistance for stereotactic brain operations. *Adv Neurosurg* 4:287–291, 1977
7. Birg W, Mundinger F: Computer calculations

of target parameters for a stereotactic apparatus. *Acta Neurochir* (Wien) 29:123–129, 1973
8. Birg W, Mundinger F: CT-guided stereotaxy with the Riechert/Mundinger apparatus for biopsy and interstitial Curietherapy of intracranial processes. *J Neurooncol* 2:272–280, 1984
9. Birg W, Mundinger F: Direct target point determination for stereotactic brain operations from CT data and the calculation of setting parameters for polar-coordinate stereotactic devices. *Appl Neurophysiol* 45:387–395, 1982
10. Birg W, Mundinger F, Mohadjer M, et al: X-ray and magnetic resonance stereotaxy for functional and nonfunctional neurosurgery. *Appl Neurophysiol* 48:22–29, 1985
11. Birg W, Schneider J, Bauer S, et al: An interactive program system for the stereotactic interstitial implantation of radionuclides in brain tumors. In Szlika G (ed): *Stereotactic Cerebral Irradiation.* Amsterdam: Elsevier/North-Holland Biomedical Press, 1979, pp 77–80
12. Bond WH, Richards D, Turner E: Experiences with radioactive gold in the treatment of craniopharyngioma. *J Neurol Neurosurg Psychiatry* 28:30–38, 1965
13. Cushing H: Intracranial tumors: Notes upon a series of two thousand verified cases with surgical mortality percentages pertaining thereto. Springfield, IL: Thomas, 1932, pp 63–64
14. Danlos H: Quelques considerationes sur le traitement des dermatoses par le radium. *J Physiotherapie* (Paris) 3:98–106, 1905
15. Davis RL, Barger Gr, Gutin PH, et al: Response of human malignant gliomas and CNS tissue to ^{125}I brachytherapy: A study of seven autopsy cases. *Acta Neurochir [Suppl]* (Wien) 33:301–305, 1984
16. Davis RL, Gutin PH, DaSilva V, et al: The effect of ^{125}I brachytherapy on the radionuclide and CT scans in malignant gliomas with pathologic correlations. *J Neurooncology* 2:284–287, 1984
17. Dutreix A, Marinello G, Wambersie A: Dosimétrie en Curiethérapie. Paris: Masson, 1982
18. Dyck P: Stereotactic biopsy and brachytherapy of brain tumors. Baltimore: University Park Press, 1983
19. Frazier CH: The effects of radium emanations upon brain tumors. *Surg Gynecol Obstet* 31:236–239, 1920
20. Greenberger JS, Cassady JR, Levene MB: Radiation therapy of thalamic, midbrain and brain stem gliomas. *Radiology* 122:463–468, 1977
21. Greenwood J Jr: Radical surgery of tumors of the thalamus, hypothalamus, and third ventricle area. *Surg Neurol* 1:29–33, 1973
22. Gruskin P, Saeger KL, Carberry JN: Neuropathology of stereotactic biopsies. In Dyck P (ed): *Stereotactic Biopsy and Brachytherapy on Brain Tumors.* Baltimore: University Park Press, 1983, pp 63–78
23. Gutin PH, Bernstein M: Stereotactic interstitial brachytherapy for malignant brain tumors. *Prog Exp Tumor Res* 28:166–182, 1984
24. Gutin Ph, Phillips TL, Hosobuchy Y, et al: Permanent and removable implants for the brachytherapy of brain tumors. *Int J Radiat Oncol Biol Phys* 7:1371–1381, 1981
25. Gutin PH, Philips TL, Wara WM, et al: Brachytherapy with removable iodine-125 sources for the treatment of recurrent malignant brain tumors. *Acta Neurochir [Suppl]* (Wien) 33:363–366, 1984
26. Hall EJ, Lam YM: The renaissance in low dose-rate interstitial implants. *Front Radiat Ther Oncol* 12:21–34, 1978
27. Hilaris BS (ed): *Handbook of Interstitial Brachytherapy.* Acton, MA: Publishing Sciences Group, I 1975
28. Hilaris BS: Techniques for interstitial and intracavitary radiation. *Cancer* 22:745–751, 1968
29. Hilaris BS, Kim JA, Tokita N: Low energy radionuclides for permanent interstitial implantation. *AJR* 126:171–178, 1976
30. Jellinger K, Volc D, Pocreka I, et al: Ergebnisse der Kombinationsbehandlung maligner Gliome. *Nervenarzt* 52:41–50, 1981
31. Kelly PJ, Kall BA, Goerss SG: Computer assisted stereotactic biopsies utilizing CT digitized arteriographic data. *Acta Neurochir [Suppl]* (Wien) 33:233–235, 1984
32. Kelly PJ, Olson MH, Wright AG: Stereotactic implantation of iridium-192 into CNS neoplasms. *Surg Neurol* 10:349–354, 1978
33. Kiessling M, Kleihues P, Gessaga E, et al: Morphology of intracranial tumors and adjacent brain structures following interstitial iodine-125 radiotherapy. *Acta Neurochir [Suppl]* (Wien) 33:281–289, 1984
34. Kleihues P, Volk B, Anagnostopoulos J, et al: Morphologic evaluation of stereotactic brain tumour biopsies. *Acta Neurochir [Suppl]* (Wien) 33:171–181, 1984
35. Laitinen LV, Liliequist B, Fagerlund M, et al: An adapter for computed tomography-guided stereotaxis. *Surg Neurol* 23:559–566, 1985
36. Lee F: Radiation of intratentorial and supratentorial brain-stem tumors. *J Neurosurg* 43:65–68, 1975
37. Mundinger F: Beitrag zur Dosimetrie and Applikation von Radio-Tantal (^{182}Ta) zur Langzeitbestrahlung von Hirngeschwülsten. *Fortschr Röntgenstr* 89:86–91, 1958
38. Mundinger F: Combined treatment of experimental DS-tumors and infiltrating cerebral gliomas with interstitial Curietherapy and radiosensitizing drugs. In *Proceedings of the Fourth European Congress of Neurosurgery:*

Present Limits of Neurosurgery. Avicenum: Prag, 1972, p 77
39. Mundinger F: CT-stereotactic biopsy of brain tumors. In Voth D, Gutjahr P (eds): Langmaid C,: *Tumours of the Central Nervous System in Infancy and Childhood*. Berlin: Springer, 1982, pp 234–246
40. Mundinger F: CT stereotactic biopsy for optimizing the therapy of intracranial processes. *Acta Neurochir [Suppl]* (Wien) 35:70–74, 1985
41. Mundinger F: Eine einfache Methode der lokalisierten Bestrahlung von Großhirngeschwulsten mit radioaktivem Gold. *Münch Med Wschr* 98:23–25, 1956
42. Mundinger F: Erfahrungen mit der stereotaktischen interstitiellen Brachytherapie mit ^{192}Ir "GammaMed" bei infiltrierenden Hirntumoren. *Fortschr Röntgenstr* 110:254–261, 1969
43. Mundinger F: Implantation of radioisotopes (Curietherapy), in Schaltenbrand G, Walker AE (eds): *Textbook of Stereotaxy of the Human Brain*. Stuttgart: Thieme, 1982, pp 410–435
44. Mundinger F: Interstitial Curietherapy in the treatment of pituitary adenomas and for hypophysectomy. *Prog Neurol Surg* 6:326–379, 1975
45. Mundinger F: Interstitial radioisotope therapy of intractable diencephalic tumors by the stereotaxic permanent implantation of iridium-192, including bioptic control. *Confin Neurol* 32:195–203, 1970
46. Mundinger F: Die interstitielle Radio-IsotopenBestrahlung von Hirntumoren mit vergleichenden Langzeitergebnissen zur Röntgentiefentherapie. *Acta Neurochir* (Wien) 9:89–109, 1963
47. Mundinger F: Intraselläre iridium-192: Permanent implantation bei Hypophysenadenomen. In Busche KA (ed): Fortschritte auf dem Gebiet der Neurochirurgie. Stuttgart: Hippokrates, 1970, pp 83–87
48. Mundinger F: Die intraselläre protrahierte Langzeitbestrahlung von Hypophysenadenomen mittels stereotaktischer Implantation von Iridium-192. *Acta Radiol* (Scand) 8:55–62, 1969
49. Mundinger F: Langzeitbestrahlung nicht resezierbarer intracranieller Hirntumoren. Die CT-stereotaktische interstitielle Curie-Therapie mit Iodine-125 seeds. *MMW* 126:1176–1179, 1984
50. Mundinger F: Rationale and methods for interstitial iridium-192 brachy-Curie-therapy and iridium-192 or iodine-125 protracted long-term irradiation. In Szikla G (ed): *Stereotactic Cerebral Irradiation*. Amsterdam: Elsevier/North-Holland Biomedical Press, 1979, pp 101–116
51. Mundinger F: Stereotactic biopsy and technique of implantation (instillation) of radionuclei. In Jellinger K (ed): *Therapy of Malignant Brain Tumors*. Vienna, New York: Springer-Verlag, 1987, pp 139–194.
52. Mundinger F: Stereotactic interstitial therapy of non-resectable intracranial tumours with iridium-192 and iodine-125. In Karcher KH, et al (eds): *Progress in Radio-Oncology II*. New York: Raven Press, 1982, pp 371–380
53. Mundinger F: Die stereotaktische interstitielle Therapie nicht resezierbarer intracranieller Tumoren mit ^{192}Ir und ^{125}I. In Wannenmacher M, Schreiber HW, Gauwerky F (eds): *Kombinierte chirurgische und radiologische Behandlung maligner Tumoren*. Munich: Urban & Schwarzenberg, 1981, pp 90–112
54. Mundinger F: Stereotaktische intrakranielle Bestrahlung von Tumoren mit Radioisotopen (Curie-Therapie). In Dietz H, Umbach W, Wüllenweber R (eds): *Klinische Neurochirurgie*, Vol 2. Stuttgart, New York: Georg Thieme Verlag, 1984, Vol 2, pp 519–565
55. Mundinger F: *Stereotaktische Operationen am Gehirn Grundlagen-Indikationen-Resultate*. Stuttgart: Hippokrates-Verlag, 1975
56. Mundinger F: Technik und Ergebnisse der interstitiellen Hirntumorbestrahlung. In Heilmann HP (ed): *Handbuch der Medizinischen Radiologie*. Berlin: Springer Verlag, 1985, pp 179–214
57. Mundinger F: The treatment of brain tumors with interstitially applied radioactive isotopes. In Wang Y, Paoletti P (eds): *Radionuclide Applications in Neurology and Neurosurgery*. Springfield, IL: Thomas, 1970, pp 199–265
58. Mundinger F: Treatment of brain tumors with radioisotopes. In Krayenbühl H, Maspes M, Sweet W (eds): *Progress of Neurological Surgery*. Basel: Karger, 1966, pp 202–257
59. Mundinger F, Birg W: CT-aided stereotaxy for functional neurosurgery and deep brain implants. *Acta Neurochir* (Wien) 56:245, 1981
60. Mundinger F, Birg W: CT-stereotaxy in the clinical routine. *Neurosurg Rev* 7:219–224, 1984
61. Mundinger F, Birg W: Stereotactic biopsy of intracranial processes. *Acta Neurochir [Suppl]* (Wien) 33:219–224, 1984
62. Mundinger F, Busam B, Birg W, et al: Results of interstitial iridium-192 brachy-Curietherapy and iridium-192 protracted long-term irradiation. In Szikla G (ed): *Stereotactic Cerebral Irradiation*. Amsterdam: Elsevier/North Holland Biomedical Press, 1979, pp 303–320
63. Mundinger F, Hoefer T: Protracted long-term irradiation of inoperable midbrain tumors by stereotactic Curietherapy using iridium-192. *Acta Neurochir [Suppl]* (Wien) 21:93–100, 1974

64. Mundinger F, Jobski C, Vogt P, et al: The interstitial Curietherapy (GammaMed) after radiosensibilizing using bromdesoxyuridine/bromdesoxycytidine and antimetabolites on DS-carcinosarcoma of rats (preliminary report). *Atomkernenergie (ATKE)* 15:157, 1970
65. Mundinger F, Metzel E: Interstitial radioisotope therapy of intractable diencephalic tumors by the stereotaxic permanent implantation of iridium-192, including bioptic control. *Confin Neurol* 32:195–202, 1970
66. Mundinger F, Noetzel H, Riechert T: Erfahrungen mit der lokalisierten Bestrahlung von malignen Hirngeschwülsten mit Radio-Isotopen. *Acta Neurochir [Suppl]* (Wien) 6:171–182, 1959
67. Mundinger F, Ostertag C, Birg W, et al: Stereotactic treatment of brain lesions: biopsy, interstitial radiotherapy (iridium-192 and iodine-125) and drainage procedures. In Gildenberg PL (ed): Proceedings of the Meeting of the American Society for Stereotactic and Functional Neurosurgery. *Appl Neurophysiol* 43:198–204, 1980
68. Mundinger F, Riechert T: Hypophysentumoren, Hypophysektomie. Klinik, Therapie, Ergebnisse. Stuttgart: Thieme, 1967
69. Mundinger F, Sauerwein K: "GammaMed," ein neues Gerät zur interstitiellen, nur einige Minuten dauernden Bestrahlung von Hirngeschwülsten mit Radioisotopen, auch intraoperativ anwendbar. *Acta Radiol* (Stockh) 5:48–52, 1966
70. Mundinger F, Vogt P, Jobski C, et al: Klinische und experimentelle Ergebnisse der interstitiellen Brachy-Curietherapie in Kombination mit Radiosensibilisatoren bei infiltrieren den Hirntumoren. *Strahlentherapie* 143:318–328, 1972
71. Mundinger F, Weigel K: CT-stereotactic interstitial irradiation therapy of nonresectable and recurrent intracranial tumors in children and adolescents. In Voth D, Krauseneck P (eds): *Chemotherapy of Gliomas: Basic Research, Experiences and Results.* Berlin, New York: Walter de Gruyter, 1985, pp 241–259
72. Mundinger F, Weigel K: Indication and results of stereotactic Curietherapy with iridium-192 and iodine-125 for non-resectable tumors of the hypothalamic region. *Acta Neurochir [Suppl]* (Wien) 33:323–330, 1984
73. Mundinger F, Weigel K: Long-term results of stereotactic interstitial Curietherapy. *Acta Neurochir [Suppl]* (Wien) 33:367–371, 1984
74. Mundinger F, Weigel K: Stereotactic Curietherapy of thalamic tumours. *J Neurooncol* 2:264–278, 1984
75. Mundinger F, Weigel K, Fürmaier R, et al: CT and MRI diagnoses of intracranial tumors compared with the results of stereotactic biopsy. In Poeck K, Freund HJ, Gänshirt H (eds): *Neurology.* Berlin, Heidelberg: Springer-Verlag, 1986, pp 469–476
76. Murray KJ, Blumberg A, Strubler K, et al: Permanent radioactive iodine seed implants following radical resection in recurrent human malignant high-grade astrocytomas. *J Neurooncol* 2:277–282, 1984
77. Musolino A, Munari C, Blond S, et al: Traitement stéréotaxique des kystes expansifs de craniopharyngiomes par irradiation endocavitaire beta (^{186}Re, ^{198}Au, ^{90}Y). *Neurochirurgie* 31: 169–178, 1985
78. Pecker J, Scarabin JM, Brucher JM, et al: *Démarche Stéréotaxique en Neurochirurgie Tumorale.* Paris: Pierre Fabre, 1979, pp 1–301
79. Perry JH, Rosenbaum AE, Lunsford LD, et al: Computed tomography–guided stereotactic surgery: Conception and development of a new stereotactic methodology. *Neurosurgery* 7:376–381, 1980
80. Pierquin B: The destiny of brachytherapy in oncology. *AJR* 127:495–499, 1976
81. Pierquin B: *Précis de Curiethérapie.* Paris: Masson et Cie, 1964
82. Pierquin B, et al: The Paris system in interstitial radiation therapy. *Acta Radiol [Oncol]* 17:33–48, 1978
83. Powell M, Olney J, Darling J, et al: Correlation of target site with histology and cell culture in CT-directed stereotactic biopsy. *J Neurooncol* 2:255–265, 1984
84. Reigel DH, Scarff TB, Woodford JE: Biopsy of pediatric brain stem tumors. *Childs Brain* 5:329–340, 1979
85. Riechert T, Mundinger F: Beschreibung und Anwendung eines Zielgerätes für stereotaktische Hirnoperationen (2. Modelll). *Acta Neurochir* (Wien) 3:308–337, 1956
86. Riechert T, Mundinger F: Stereotaktische Geräte. In Schaltenbrand G, Bailey P (eds): *Einführung in die stereotaktischen Operationen mit einem Atlas des menschlichen Gehirns.* Stuttgart: Thieme, 1959
87. Rougier A, Pigneux J, Cohadon F: Combined interstitial and external irradiation of gliomas. *Acta Neurochir [Suppl]* (Wien) 33:345–353, 1984
88. Ryoo MC, Kind GA, Chung T, et al: Irradiation of primary brainstem tumors. *Radiology* 131:503–507, 1979
89. Salcman M, Sewchand W, Amin P, et al: CT-guided stereotactic surgery and interstitial irradiation for glial tumors. *J Neurooncol* 2:279–282, 1984
90. Schaub C, Bluet-Pajot MT, Videau-Lornet C, et al: Endocavitary beta irradiation of glioma cysts with colloidal rhenium-186. In Szikla

(ed): *Stereotactic Cerebral Irradiation*. Amsterdam: Elsevier/North-Holland Biomedical Press, 1979, pp 293–302
91. Scott WP: Permanent interstitial implantation technique using absorbable spacers. *Am J Roentgenol Radium Ther Nucl Med* 114:620–622, 1972
92. Selker R, Eddy M, Anderson L: A method of dosimetry planning and implantation of interstitial irradiation in glioma patients utilizing iodine-125. *J Neurooncol* 2:274–281, 1984
93. Sommermeyer K, Mittermaier L: Untersuchungen uber die Dosisverteilung in der Umgebung reiner Gammapräparate mit dem Fluoreszendosimeter. *Strahlentherapie* 102:78–87, 1957
94. Szikla G, Betti O, Szenthe L, et al: L'expérience actuelle des irradiations stéréotaxiques dans le traitement des gliomes hémisphériques. *Neurochirurgie* 27:295–298, 1981
95. Szikla G, Musolino A, Miyahara S, et al: Colloidal rhenium-186 in endocavitary beta irradiation of cystic craniopharyngiomas and active glioma cysts: Long-term results, side effects and clinical dosimetry. *Acta Neurochir* [*Suppl*] (Wien) 33:331–339, 1984
96. Szikla G, Peragut JC: Irradiation interstitielle des gliomes. *Neurochirurgie* 21:(Suppl 2) 187–228, 1975
97. Szikla G, Schlienger M, Blond S, et al: Interstitial and combined interstitial and external irradiation of supratentorial gliomas: Results in 61 cases treated 1973–1981. *Acta Neurochir* [*Suppl*] (Wien) 33:355–362, 1984
98. Villani R, Gaini SM, Tomei G: Follow-up study of brain stem tumors in children. *Childs Brain* 1:126–135, 1975
99. Walker MD: Chemotherapy: Adjuvant to surgery and radiation therapy. *Semin Oncol* 2:69–72, 1975
100. Wara WM, Gutin PH, Leibel S, et al: Treatment of malignant brain tumors with high-activity iodine-125. *J Neurooncol* 2:284–288, 1984
101. Weigel K, Mohadjer M, Mundinger F: CT-stereotaxy for differential diagnosis and radiotherapy of intracranial metastases. In Piotrowski W, Brock M, Klinger M (eds): *CNS Metastases. Neurosurgery in the Aged. Advances in Neurosurgery*, Vol 12. Berlin, Heidelberg, New York: Springer, 1984, 87–93
102. Weigel K, Ostertag C, Mundinger F: Interstitial long-term irradiation of tumors in the pineal region. In Szikla G (ed): *Stereotactic Cerebral Irradiation*. Amsterdam: Elsevier/North-Holland Biomedical Press, 1979, pp 283–292
103. Wycis HT, Robbins R, Spiegel-Adolf M, et al: Studies in stereoencephalotomy III. Treatment of a cystic craniopharyngioma by injection of radioactive ^{32}P. *Confin Neurol* 14:193–202, 1954

20. A ROBOTIC SYSTEM FOR STEREOTACTIC NEUROSURGERY

Ronald F. Young

The primary goal of stereotactic surgery is to reach a designated target within the brain safely and accurately, without directly visualizing the intended target [30]. To accomplish this, stereotactic systems have employed a frame, externally applied to the skull, which incorporates one of several coordinate systems (e.g., Cartesian, polar, spherical) to guide a probe within the brain. In addition, a reference system has been used to correlate brain anatomy and stereotactic frame settings. The original Horsley-Clarke apparatus incorporated a Cartesian coordinate system correlated with skull landmarks, (i.e., the midsagittal plane, the external auditory meatus and the orbital meatal plane) [14]. Variation in the relationship between skull landmarks and brain anatomy prevented the Horsley-Clarke apparatus from being used in humans.

Spiegel and Wycis suggested that brain targets could be localized by reference to the anatomy of the third ventricle, which was demonstrated by contrast ventriculography [25–27]. A number of atlases were then developed which related brain anatomy to certain reference points about the third ventricle, notably the anterior and posterior commissures and the foramen of Monro [1, 22, 28, 29]. Developments between 1950 and the mid-1970s provided stereotactic frames of increasing sophistication and precision, but all relied on the relationship between external frame settings and third-ventricular anatomy, demonstrated by conventional contrast ventriculography. Such techniques were reasonably accurate for attaining anatomical targets within normal brains. However, localizing pathological lesions was difficult and depended on identifying the indirect effect of the lesion on the ventricular anatomy.

A major step in improving stereotactic surgery was the advent of computed tomographic (CT) scanning. A number of stereotactic systems have been devised that correlate CT scan–identified targets to a stereotactic frame [4–7, 10, 12, 13, 17–24]. Such systems are excellent for stereotactic localization of pathological lesions but are less useful for identification of normal brain targets for several reasons. Most CT scanners do not provide sufficient resolution to identify normal brain targets (e.g., thalamic nuclei) with the precision required for functional stereotactic surgery. To use CT scanning and standard stereotactic brain atlases, CT scan images in the anterior commissure (AC)–posterior commissure (PC) plane must be reoriented. Computer reconstruction of CT images in axial, coronal, and sagittal planes is then necessary, risking further reductions in resolution. Most currently available CT stereotactic systems also require preoperative CT scanning and target calculation outside of the operating room; thus, intraoperative CT confirmation of the intended target is impossible. Consequently, if an intended target is not reached, whether for lesion biopsy or functional localization, stereotactic frame coordinates must be corrected empirically. Finally, manual transfer of CT-generated frame coordinates to the stereotactic apparatus can be cumbersome and is a potential source of

I gratefully acknowledge the contribution of Dr. Roger A. Slater to the development of the robotic system described, and Mr. Sven Olsen and the Research Foundation of Memorial Medical Center, Long Beach, CA, for financial support of the system's development. I also thank Drs. William Wild, William Hyman, and Barry Ceverah for their support.

L.D. Lunsford (ed.) *MODERN STEREOTACTIC NEUROSURGERY*. Copyright © 1988.

error. At least one commercially available CT stereotactic system utilizes a simulator to confirm the accuracy of CT frame settings prior to probe insertion.

An ideal CT-stereotactic system would permit intraoperative, real-time confirmation of the probe trajectory and final location [3]; rapid and accurate identification of the intended target; rapid calculation of CT coordinates and error-free transfer to the frame; computer display of the simulated probe trajectory in axial, coronal, and sagittal planes; and accurate attainment of the calculated target.

A new stereotactic system, designed and built by Y. S. Kwoh and colleagues [16], provides many of these features by combining three components: a dedicated CT-stereotactic operating suite with a permanently mounted CT scanner, custom-designed computer software, and a robotic system to replace the standard stereotactic frame.

Because the CT scanner is permanently mounted in the operating suite, all CT scanning for target localization, confirmation of probe trajectory, and final probe location can be performed there. The operating suite is connected to both the general operating theater and the radiology department. In a connected room, a cathrode ray tube (CRT) displaying CT scan data can be seen directly from the operating suite via two-way glass. Thus, the patient and the CT scan data can be observed simultaneously.

Custom-designed computer software digests the CT scan data and the intended target location, which is identified by a cursor on the CRT, and generates robotic coordinates to indicate the target. These coordinates, in the form of arc angles, are transmitted directly to the robotic system.

General Description of Robotics

Before considering the robotic system we have used, a brief general description of the science of robotics may be useful. The English-language term *robot* is derived from the Czechoslovakian word *robota*, which translates simply to *worker*, but implies drudgery, servitude, or forced labor [9, 11]. The term apparently was used first by Karel Capek in 1920 in a science-fiction play entitled *R. U. R. (Rossum's Universal Robots)* [8]. In the play, an artificial substitute for human beings was designed, which eliminated human failings and incorporated maximum efficiency.

A clear definition of robot is difficult. *Webster's Dictionary* defines it as "(1) a machine in the form of a human being but lacking sensitivity, (2) an automatic apparatus or device that performs functions ordinarily ascribed to human beings or operates with what appears to be almost human intelligence, (3) a mechanism guided by automatic controls." The Robotics Institute of America defines a robot as "a reprogrammable, multifunctional manipulator designed to move material, parts, tools, or specialized devices through variable programmed motions for the performance of a variety of tasks."

The author Isaac Asimov offered "The Three Laws of Robotics," which are now well accepted [2]: (1) A robot may not injure a human being, or, through inaction, allow a human being to come to harm. (2) A robot must obey the orders given to it by human beings except when such orders would conflict with the First Law. (3) A robot must protect its own existence as long as such protection does not conflict with the First or Second Law. Although these laws of robotics were constructed in a milieu of science fiction, they are clearly applicable to the use of robotics in stereotactic surgery. Most robotics applications have been in the industrial setting to perform repetitious activity, such as automobile assembly, or to function in settings that might be hazardous to human beings, such as handling radioactive materials or dangerous chemicals.

Selection of a Robot for Stereotactic Surgery

In selecting a robot for a stereotactic application, a variety of general characteristics were considered. Ideally, a stereotactic system should allow access to all areas of the head for maximum freedom of trajectories to a desired target, and it should have a reach that allows it to support the probe without obstructing the surgeon's access to the patient. The robot must be solid enough to provide a stable probe trajectory, and it should incorporate sufficient safety features to prevent damage from malfunction. The robotic system should be reliably failure-free during surgical procedures and should be relatively small and portable.

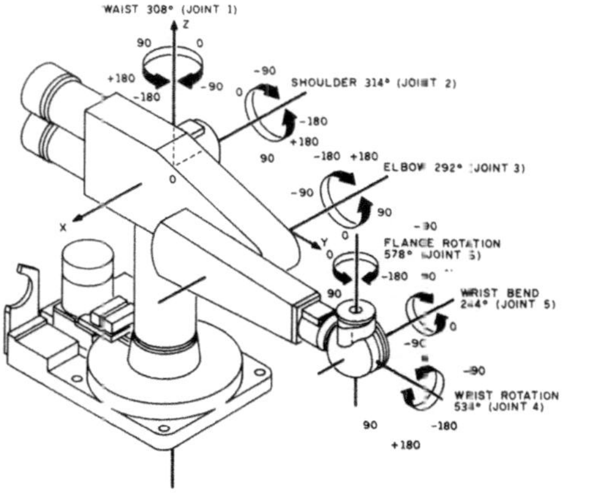

FIGURE 20-1. Diagram of robot used in stereotactic neurosurgery. (Reprinted by permission from *Robotics Age*, June 1985, copyright © 1985 Robotics Age, Inc., 174 Concord St., Peterborough, NH 03458.)

The robotic system we used initially was the Unimate Puma Mark II 200, which has been updated with the Unimate Puma 260 robot (Unimation Inc., Danbury, CT). This system, designed by Y. S. Kwoh and colleagues [16], incorporates a six-jointed, permanent-magnet, servocontrolled, motorized robotic arm (figure 20-1). In each joint, a revolute coordinate system with a wide range of angular movements allows maximum flexibility and smooth movements (figure 20-2). All servomotors contain optical incremental encoders, which provide position and velocity feedback to the robotic servosystem. The first three joints (waist, shoulder, and elbow joints, respectively) have electromagnetic brakes. The robot is mounted on an external support that allows it to be positioned in multiple locations in relation to the patient. To provide a constant relationship between the patient and the robot base, the base mount is attached to a head ring fixed to the head by skeletal fixation pins. The head ring currently used is plastic, modified from a base ring used on a previously designed prototype CT stereotactic frame. A custom-designed probe holder attached to joint six of the robotic arm allows for fine adjustment of the probe position via a screw vernier central bushing (figure 20-3). Robotic positioning is controlled by an attached Data General Eclipse

PUMA Robot	
Robot Arm	
Axes	Six revolute axes
Clearance Required	Spherical volume with shoulder at center: 0.47 m (18.5 in.) radius to hand mount flange.
Weight	129 N (29 lb)
Drive	Electric DC servomotor
Maximum Inertia Load (including Gripper)	Wrist rotation (J4) NOT exceed 1.0 in-oz-sec² Wrist Bend (J5) NOT exceed 1.8 in-oz-sec² Flange Rotation (J6) NOT exceed 0.5 in-oz-sec²
Position Repeatability	±0.05mm (±0.002 in.) within primary work envelope
Tool Velocity	1.0 m/s (3.3 fps) maximum (with maximum load within primary work envelope)
Software Movement Limits	
Waist—Joint 1	-184 to 124 (308 degree)
Shoulder—Joint 2	-247 to 67 (314 degree)
Elbow—Joint 3	-56 to 236 (292 degree)
Wrist—Joint 4	-223 to 355 (578 degree)
Wrist—Joint 5	-122 to 122 (244 degree)
Wrist—Joint 6	-222 to 312 (534 degree)

FIGURE 20-2. Functional capabilities of Puma 200 Robot. (Reprinted by permission from *Robotics Age*, June 1985, copyright © 1985 Robotics Age, Inc., 174 Concord St., Peterborough, NH 03458.)

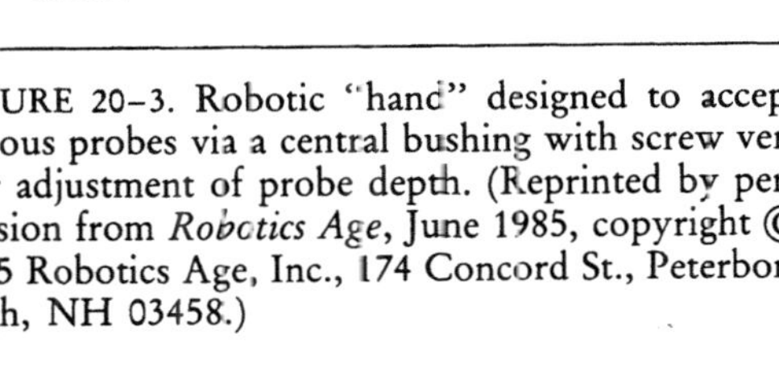

FIGURE 20-3. Robotic "hand" designed to accept various probes via a central bushing with screw vernier adjustment of probe depth. (Reprinted by permission from *Robotics Age*, June 1985, copyright © 1985 Robotics Age, Inc., 174 Concord St., Peterborough, NH 03458.)

(DEC) LSI-II minicomputer. The computer controller contains digital and analog circuits to control each robot joint and its power supply. The robot control computer is designed for robot control only and lacks the software necessary for stereotactic computation from CT-generated target identification. A host

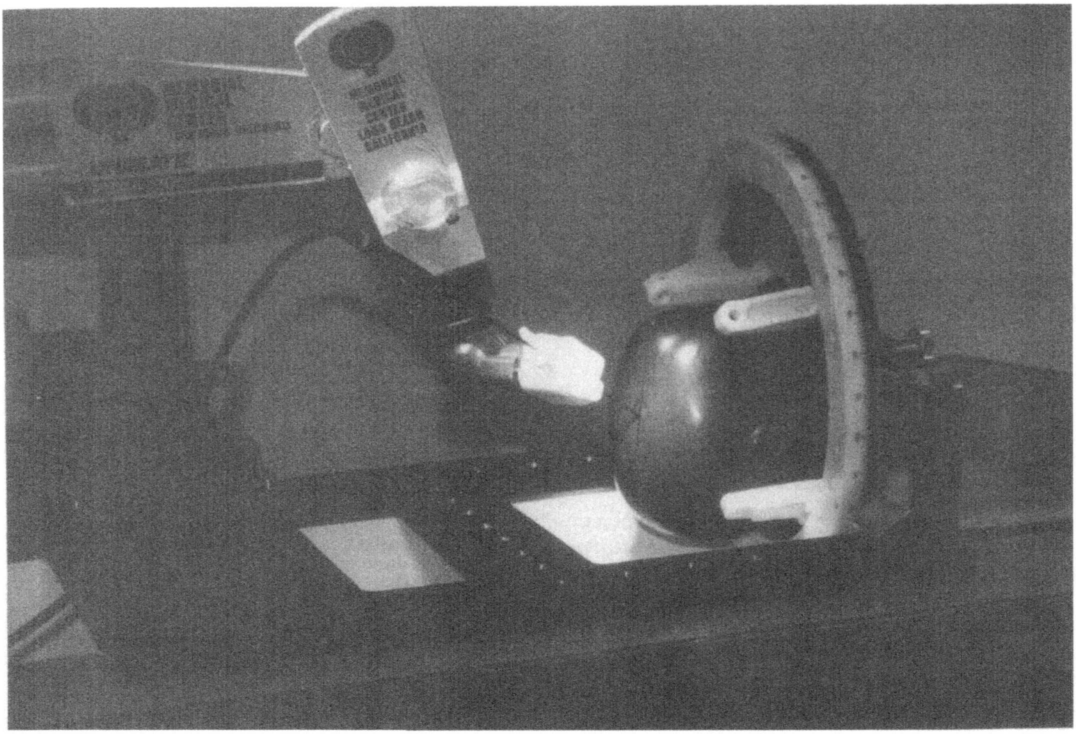

A

FIGURE 20–4. The robotic stereotactic system with simulated head. The electric drill is passed though the robotic "hand" on the predetermined trajectory toward the target, which ensures that a small cranial opening will be placed exactly (A). The robotic stereotactic system attached to a patient (B).

computer, a DEC 11/34 minicomputer, communicates with the LSI-II robot-control computer via an RS-232 link. The surgeon interacts with the host computer via the stereotactic software developed for that purpose.

The Robotic System in Operation

After local anesthetic infiltration, the patient's head is attached to the head ring with four plastic pins advanced through the scalp. Although usually positioned supine, patients may be placed in a lateral, prone, or any intermediate position (figure 20–4), depending on location of the intended target. Three plastic N-shaped locaters mounted on the head ring allow identification of the axial position (Z coordinate) of the desired target on the CT-scan images. The patient and attached head ring and N locater are advanced into the gantry of the CT scanner for preliminary imaging. The CT image demonstrating the desired target is viewed on the CRT screen, and the target is marked with a cursor. The robot is attached to the head ring in a position most convenient given the target location, intended trajectory, and position of the surgeon. The surgeon selects an approximate trajectory that will avoid functionally important regions of the brain and important vascular structures. The exact trajectory is then determined by the host computer, and appropriate commands are sent to the robotic servomotors for determination of the final position. For a lesion biopsy, a 5-mm electric drill is passed through the bushing of the probe holder to perforate the skull in the intended trajectory. A lesion biopsy is obtained with a 15-gauge biopsy needle (figure 20–5). Currently, the probe length necessary to reach the target along the intended trajectory is calculated by computer, but

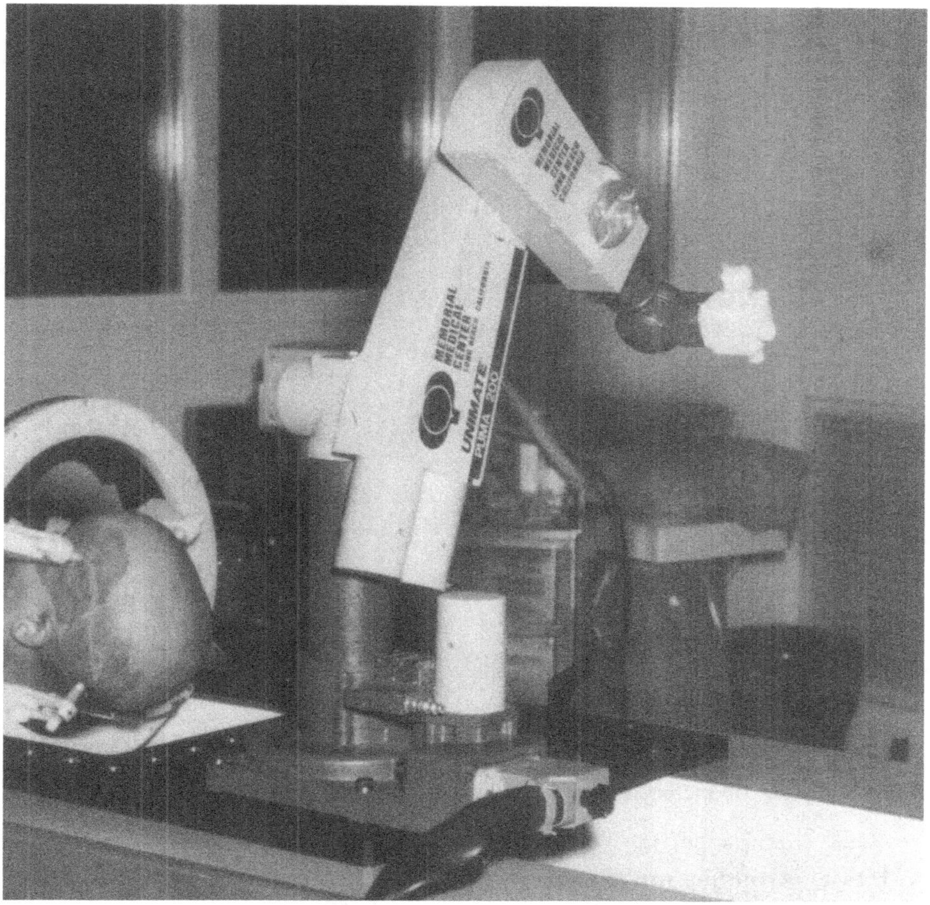

B

FIGURE 20–4. (cont.)

manually transferred to the probe by the surgeon, who then inserts the probe via the bushing in the probe holder (figure 20–6). In future development, we plan to attach the probe directly to the probe holder and accomplish insertion by robotic movement. For insertion of larger biopsy instruments, endoscopes and stimulating or recording electrodes, the twist drill is used to mark the center of the intended cranial opening, and a burr hole, trephine, or other suitable opening is created. The robotic arm is moved in and out of the surgeon's working area in seconds by the computer-controlled robotic motors, allowing unobstructed surgical manipulation. In its current form, the robotic system is capable of 0.05-mm accuracy in finding or returning to a preprogrammed target.

Advantages of Robotic Stereotactic Surgery

The robotic stereotactic system described here offers several advantages over standard CT stereotactic systems. Human errors in transferring calculations to frame settings are eliminated. Adjustments in probe trajectory can be accomplished easily by manually activated, push-button-controlled robotic movements. There are no restrictions in access or proximity to the patient's skull, which can occur when standard arc systems are used for patients with large or small skulls. The six-jointed system affords nearly unlimited access angles, so that the skull and brain can be approached easily from any direction. Finally, the robotic guide system can be moved in and out of the opera-

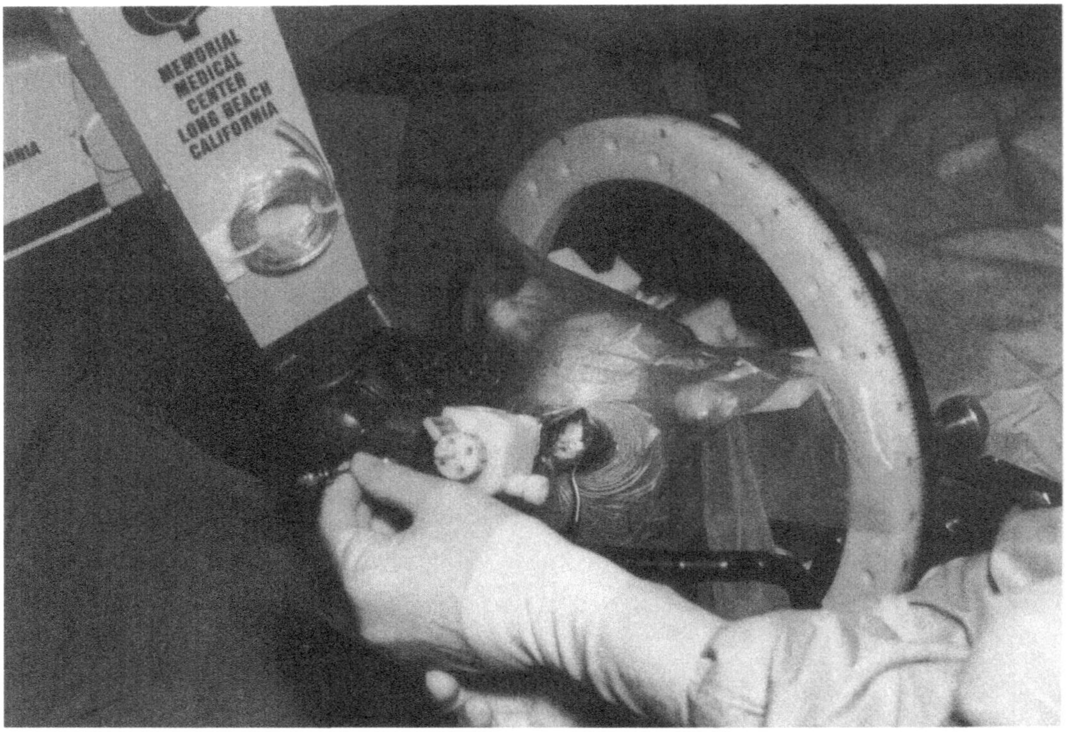

FIGURE 20-5. A biopsy probe is passed through the robotic "hand" on a trajectory predetermined by CT scan and computer-driven robotic positioning.

tive field with ease, permitting probe guidance when desired, yet always providing the surgeon unobstructed access to the patient. These advantages may be relatively minor, but potential uses of such a robotic system are exciting.

The possibility of truly "remote-controlled" stereotactic neurosurgery exists with this system. For instance, with a patient in the robotic head ring and within the CT gantry, the surgeon could observe CT images in nearly real time on the monitoring CRT screen in the adjacent room, while robotic movements were simultaneously controlled. If the robot could be combined with suitable tissue-destructive instruments (e.g., mechanical, ultrasonic, or laser devices), lesions such as tumors, abscesses, and hematomas might be removable by remote control [15]. Given the ability to monitor lesion removal at a distance by CT scan, the surgeon would avoid radiation exposure while retaining the ability to control, via robot, the movement of instruments within the brain. Such a system might allow removal of lesions in deep structures, such as the basal ganglia or brain stem, with relative safety. Hemostasis in deep structures could be a problem with such a technique, but CT observation should permit an accumulating hematoma to be observed and evacuated and the source of the hemorrhage controlled.

Concerns

Although the robotic system has some advantages over standard CT-stereotactic systems, it brings with it new problems. The robot can reach a desired target via an infinite number of trajectories. A path must be chosen for safety and convenience, and information transmitted to the robot to guide it along the selected pathway. Although it is possible to enter the necessary environmental-contour data into the computer for trajectory selection, at present such a technique is considered too time-consuming. Alternatively, all brakes and motors are inacti-

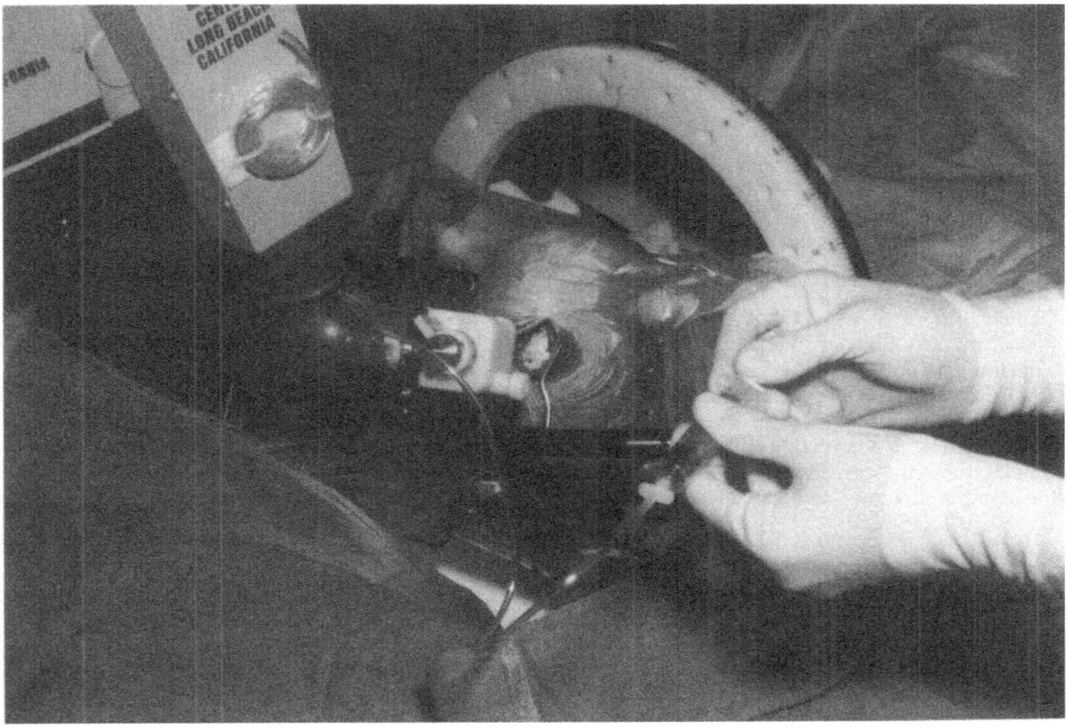

FIGURE 20-6. A biopsy specimen is obtained by aspiration. Depth of probe placement is computer-calculated but manually regulated by a movable collar.

vated, enabling the robot to move freely in all directions; the robotic arm is then directed manually toward the approximate trajectory. If computer-controlled robotic movements appear to endanger the patient or the surgeon, the robot can be stopped by a "panic button" on a manual-control unit attached to the robot.

Summary

As with other new technologies, both neurosurgeons and patients may have reservations about the safety and efficacy of a robotic system. Capek, in his play, and numerous other writers have instilled in many the fear of robot control supplanting human control. In the robotic stereotactic system described in this chapter, all aspects of system function are under human directon, as are all decisions concerning the use of the system. The robot system operates only when given directions by a human being. The robotic system was created to harness the useful features of CT scanning, computers, and the robot (i.e., rapid and accurate data collection; error-free computation; and flexible, reproducible, and extremely precise conversion of calculations into mechanical movements). The system we have described is an initial attempt to apply robotic techniques to neurosurgery. It seems likely that future developments will further refine and expand the use of robotics in neurosurgery and medicine.

References

1. Andrew J, Watkins ES: *A Stereotaxic Atlas of the Human Thalamus and Adjacent Structures: A Variability Study*. Baltimore: Williams & Wilkins, 1969
2. Asimov I: *I, Robot*. New York: Doubleday & Co, 1950
3. Bertrand G, Olivier A, Thompson CJ: Computer display of stereotaxic brain maps and probe tracts. *Acta Neurochir [Suppl]* (Wien) 21:235–243, 1974
4. Brown RA: A computerized tomography-

computer graphics approach to stereotaxic location. *J Neurosurg* 50:715–720, 1979
5. Brown RA: A stereotactic head frame for use with CT body scanners. *Invest Radiol* 14:300–304, 1979
6. Brown RA, Roberts T, Osborn AG: Simplified CT-guided stereotaxic biopsy. *AJNR* 2:181–184, 1981
7. Brown RA, Roberts TS, Osborn AG: Stereotactic frame and computer software for CT-directed neurosurgical localization. *Invest Radiol* 15:308–312, 1980
8. Capek K: *R. U. R. (Rossum's Universal Robots)*. New York: Doubleday, Page & Co, 1923
9. Engelberger JF: *Robotics in Practice*. New York: AMACOM (American Management Associations: 1980, p 278
10. Gildenberg PL, Kaufman HJH, Murthy KSK: Calculation of stereotactic coordinates from the computed tomographic scan. *Neurosurgery* 10:580–586, 1982
11. Heath L: *Fundamentals of robotics: Theory and Applications*. Reston, VA: Reston Publishing, 1985
12. Heibrun MP, Roberts TS: CT stereotactic guidance system. In Wilkins RH, Rengachary SS, (eds): *Neurosurgery*. New York: McGraw-Hill, 1985, pp 2481–2489
13. Heibrun MP, Roberts TS, Apuzzo ML, et al: Preliminary experience with Brown-Roberts-Wells (BRW) computerized tomography stereotaxic guidance system. *J Neurosurg* 59:217–222, 1983
14. Horsley V, Clarke RH: The structure and functions of the cerebellum examined by a new method. *Brain* 31:45–125, 1908
15. Kelly PJ, Alker GJ Jr: A method for stereotactic laser microsurgery in the treatment of deep-seated CNS neoplasms. *Appl Neurophysiol* 43:210–215, 1980
16. Kwoh YS, Reed IS, Chen JUY, et al: New computerized tomographic-aided robotic stereotaxic system. *Robotic Age* 7:17–22, 1985
17. Leksell L, Jernberg B: Stereotaxis and tomography: A technical note. *Acta Neurochir* (Wien) 52:1–7, 1980
18. Maroon JC, Bank WO, Drayer BP, et al: Intracranial biopsy assisted by computerized tomography. *J Neurosurg* 46:740–744, 1977
19. Mundinger F, Birg W, Klar M: Computer-assisted stereotactic brain operations by means including computerized axial tomography. *Appl Neurophysiol* 41:169–182, 1978
20. Ostertag CB, Mennel HD, Kiessling M: Stereotactic biopsy of brain tumors. *Surg Neurol* 14:275–283, 1980
21. Perry JH, Rosenbaum AE, Lunsford LD, et al: Computed tomography-guided stereotactic surgery: conception and development of a new stereotactic methodology. *Neurosurgery* 7:376–381, 1980
22. Schaltenbrand G, Wahren W: *Atlas for Stereotaxy of the Human Brain* (rev ed). Stuttgart: Georg Thieme Verlag, 1977
23. Shelden CH, McCann G, Jacques S, et al: Development of a computerized microstereotaxic method for localization an removal of minute CNS lesions under direct 3-D vision: Technical report. *J Neurosurg* 52:21–27, 1980
24. Slater RA, Rhodes ML, Glenn WV Jr: CT-assisted interactive stereotactic system. In Dyck P (ed): *Stereotactic Biopsy and Brachytherapy of Brain Tumors*. Baltimore: University Park Press, 1984, pp 149–171
25. Spiegel EA, Wycis HT: Pallidothalamotomy in chorea. *Arch Neurol Psychiatr* 64:295–296, 1950
26. Spiegel EA, Wycis HT: *Stereoencephalotomy (thalamotomy and related procedures) Part 1. Methods and Stereotaxic Atlas of the Human Brain*. New York: Grune & Stratton, 1952
27. Spiegel EA, Wycis HT, Marks M, et al: Stereotaxic apparatus for operations on the human brain. *Science* 106:349–350, 1947
28. Talairach J, David M, Tournoux P, et al: *Atlas d'anatomie stereotaxique*. Paris: Masson, 1957
29. Talairach J, Szikla G: Atlas d'anatomie stereotaxique du telencephale. Paris: Masson, 1957
30. Tasker R: Stereotactic surgery: principles and techniques. In Wilkins RH, Rengachary SS (eds): *Neurosurgery*. New York: McGraw-Hill, 1985, pp 2465–2481

III. FUNCTIONAL NEUROSURGERY

21. MESENCEPHALOTOMY AND THALAMOTOMY FOR CHRONIC PAIN

Lauri V. Laitinen

Soon after the introduction of human stereotactic neurosurgery by Spiegel and Wycis in 1947 [14], attempts were made to treat chronic intractable pain by making stereotactic lesions in the thalamus or mesencephalon [4, 13, 20]. At the mesencephalic level, the intent was to interrupt the quintothalamic or spinothalamic pain-conducting pathways. At the thalamic level the surgeon aimed at cutting these pathways at their entrance point into the thalamus (limitans nucleus) or in the specific sensory nuclei ventral posteromedial [VPM] or ventral posterolateral [VPL]. Alternatively, surgeons attempted to influence pain mechanisms by making lesions in the nonspecific nuclei (centromedian [CM], intralaminar, dorsomedial [DM], parafascicularis, and pulvinar). In this chapter these surgical procedures and their clinical importance among current neurosurgical techniques will be discussed.

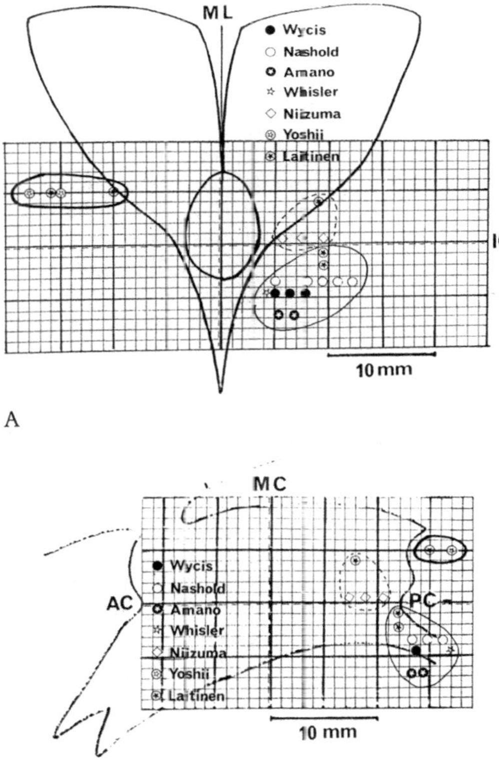

FIGURE 21-1. Anteroposterior (A) and lateral (B) demonstration of the coordinates for mesencephalotomy (*thin continuous circle*), centromedian thalamotomy (*dotted circle*) and pulvinotomy (*thick continuous circle*) of seven researchers.

Mesencephalotomy

In 1950, Wycis and co-workers reported on a patient who developed facial pain after a retrogasserian rhizotomy [20]; this patient had undergone quintothalamic mesencephalotomy in 1947 and had remained completely pain-free for more than four years. Three years later, these authors described five additional patients, all of whom had suffered from long-lasting facial neuralgias resistant to retrogasserian rhizotomies [13]. Two of these patients also had unsuccessful frontal lobotomies. The mesencephalic lesions were produced by electrocoagulation in the quintothalamic tract ventral to the posterior commissure and 5–8 mm lateral to the midline (figure 21-1). In three

L.D. Lunsford (ed.) *MODERN STEREOTACTIC NEUROSURGERY*. Copyright © 1988. Martinus Nijhoff Publishing. Boston/Dordrecht/Lancaster.

patients, additional lesions were produced in the DM nucleus. One patient with bilateral pain had undergone bilateral mesencephalotomy. Postoperatively, all patients had contralateral hemihypalgesia, hemianalgesia, and hemithermoanesthesia. One patient remained free from pain for more than nine months, and another for three years before pain returned. In a third patient, pain returned after four months. In the remaining two patients, initial pain relief was described, but the follow-up time was short. Spiegel and Wycis documented several side effects including universal postoperative drowsiness and confusion. Other side effects included a slight tactile hypesthesia, contralateral hemiparesis, tinnitus and hypoacusis, diplopia, and a loss of taste for sweet and salty substances (in a patient with bilateral lesions).

In 1969, Nashold and colleagues reported on the effects of mesencephalotomy performed in 15 patients who suffered from phantom limb pain or central dysesthesias [7]. The lesions were placed close to the target described by Wycis and associates [20], i.e., 1–5 mm caudal to the posterior commissure, 3–5 mm lateral to the midline (see figure 21–1). Two of five patients with phantom limb pain obtained complete pain relief, but three failed to improve at all. One patient with causalgia after a brachial avulsion injury had complete pain relief. The follow-up time in these patients was between 9 and 24 months. Of the nine patients with central dysesthesias, five had complete pain relief, two had partial relief, and two were not improved. The follow-up time for this group ranged between 3 and 30 months. In summary, 78% of the patients experienced complete or partial pain relief during the relatively short follow-up period reported.

Side effects were frequent: all 15 patients showed permanent loss of conjugate upward gaze, 13 had retractory nystagmus, eight had new dysesthesias, seven suffered diplopia, six had transitory loss of conjugate downward gaze, four were deeply depressed, two had hemiparesis, and one had tremor and involuntary movements in the contralateral extremities.

Amano and co-workers performed "rostral mesencephalic reticulotomy" in 15 patients who suffered from chronic intractable pain [1]. The lesion site was similar to that reported by Nashold and colleagues [7] (1–4 mm posterior to the anterior margin of the posterior commissure, 5–8 mm below the level of the intercommissural line, and 5–8 mm lateral to the midline; (see figure 21–1). A frontal approach similar to that employed by Nashold and associates [7] was used. Amano and co-workers stressed that the lesions should be very small to prevent conjugate upward-gaze pareses [1].

Whisler and Voris reported on mesencephalotomy in 40 patients with chronic pain [18]. Their target was 5 mm behind the posterior commissure, 3.5–5 mm below it and 4–5 mm lateral to the midline (see figure 21–1). Ninety-two percent of the patients were reported to be relieved of pain until their deaths. In one patient, the pain recurred nine months after surgery. Morbidity was described as low, even in far-advanced cancer cases, but few details are available. Head and neck pain responded best to these lesions, which presumably interrupted the quintothalamic tract.

To avoid the frequent ocular complications of the mesencephalotomy, we placed the lesion more rostrally in the brain stem, i.e., the limitans nucleus of the thalamus (see figure 21–1). Nineteen patients underwent surgery using this target in the early 1960s. Six patients suffered from cancer pain, five from postherpetic neuralgia, three from low back pain, two from thalamic pain, two from phantom limb pain, and one from paraplegic pain. This last patient underwent bilateral surgery. The final lesion site was determined by electrical stimulation and somatosensory evoked response (SSER) recordings. Stimulation of the quintothalamic and spinothalamic tracts or nuclei yielded a low-threshold warmth response that gradually became hot and painful as the stimulus intensity was increased. Gradually electrocoagulation resulted in dense analgesia and thermal anesthesia in the painful part of the body. The lesion seldom exceeded 5 mm in diameter. Five of 19 patients (26%) had long-lasting pain relief during the follow-up period of three years. Ten patients (53%) had side effects, including dysesthesias (eight patients), proprioceptive deficits (three), diplopia (two), a loss of conjugate upward gaze (two), hemihyperhidrosis (one), loss of taste (one), and arthralgia (one).

We believe that mesencephalotomy of the limitans nucleus area is potentially beneficial only in the treatment of patients with cancer pain.

Thalamotomy

Stereotactic thalamotomy was performed extensively in the early years of human stereotaxis. Lesion sites included the specific sensory relay nuclei (VPM, VPL) and the nonspecific nuclei that were believed to involve the paleospinothalamic pain pathways or thought to modify the emotional response to pain. These targets included the CM, the intralaminar nuclei, the parafascicular nuclei, the pulvinar, the DM nucleus, and the anterior thalamic nuclei.

Hécaen and colleagues were the first to use thalamotomy in the treatment of intractable pain [4]. In 1949, these authors reported on six patients: three had lesions in the CM and the anterior part of the VPM, two had combined lesions in the CM and the DM nucleus, and one had a CM lesion only. Five patients suffered from central pain syndrome and one from a postherpetic neuralgia. One patient died two weeks after surgery, but five were relieved of their pain for more than two months. The extent of pain perception lost varied considerably, but no side effects were reported.

White and Sweet described in detail 38 patients who underwent thalamotomy within the VPM, VPL, the nucleus parafascicularis, the DM, the ventral anterior nucleus, the CM nucleus, or the pulvinar [19]. Lesions in the specific nuclei VPM-VPL resulted in good or fair pain relief in 19 of 22 patients (86%). Seven of eight patients who had parafascicular lesions showed good or fair relief. Two of three patients with DM lesions obtained good pain relief. Two patients died soon after surgery; few side effects were observed (three patients had speech deficits, mild thalamic syndrome, or confusion).

CENTROMEDIAN THALAMOTOMY

At the Second International Symposium on Stereoencephalotomy in Vienna in 1965 Fairman discussed 30 cancer patients with intractable pain, all of whom had lesions performed in the CM and intralaminar nuclei [3]. The target coordinates were not reported. Fairman hypothesized that the lesions interrupted "the unmyelinated fibers of the nonspecific polysynaptic system of pain conduction, that is, the older fibers of the multisynaptic ascending system (MAS)." Satisfactory pain relief lasting for the rest of life (three weeks to one year) was achieved in 90% of the patients, whereas in 10% the pain returned soon after surgery. No sensory deficits were observed postoperatively. No side effects were reported.

An open transventricular approach was used to divide the intralaminar thalamic nuclei in a patient described by Sano and colleagues [11]. The posterior half of the internal medullary lamina was cut and coagulated; the depth of the incision was approximately 15–20 mm. Because the beneficial effects of this open surgery lasted for at least 2½ years, these surgeons performed stereotactic lesions of the intralaminar nuclei on ten patients, including seven who had bilateral surgery. Eight patients had good pain relief during follow-up periods ranging from one to 30 months. Aside from a transient stupor, no other side effects were reported.

In 1966 Watkins described the results of CM thalamotomy in 25 patients who had chronic pain [17]. Unilateral surgery was performed in 19 patients and bilateral surgery in six. Complete pain relief was reported in 16 and partial relief in six. Thus 88% of the patients had significant benefit. No serious complications were observed.

In the early 1960s, Laitinen performed CM thalamotomy in six patients, four of whom suffered from trigeminal deafferentation neuralgia and two of whom had central pain after strokes. Small lesions in the central area of the CM nucleus resulted in clinical improvement in four cases from six to 24 months. However, two patients had incomplete pain relief, and one had transient hemihypesthesia and loss of conjugate upward gaze, a feature that indicates posterior extension of the lesion.

Niizuma and associates carried out CM thalamatomy on 18 patients with central pain of cerebrovascular origin [8]. Their target was 7.5–11 mm posterior to the midcommissural point, 2 mm above to 1 mm below the intercommissural line, and 5.5–10 mm lateral to the midline (see figure 21–1). Fifteen patients had unilateral lesions, and three had bilateral lesions. The postoperative follow-up ranged from nine to 72 months. During that period, four patients died from recurrent strokes. In this study a good clinical result was obtained in only 56% of the patients. Because the pain often recurred within six months, these authors were pessimistic about the value of CM thalamotomy. The size of the lesions was not specified.

More recently, CM thalamotomy has been

performed in five patients suffering from intractable pain at our center. Three had central pain of cerebrovascular origin, and two had trigeminal deafferentation pain. The target was 8 mm behind the midcommissural point, 4 mm above the intercommissural line, and 9 mm from the midline (see figure 21–1). The size and the site of the lesions were confirmed with a postoperative computed tomography (CT) scan. The electrocoagulation lesions ranged from 6–8 mm in diameter (figure 21–2). Electrical stimulation of the CM nucleus prior to coagulation elicited a high-threshold response consisting of a subjective sensation of vibration in the contralateral arm. In all five patients, electrocoagulation resulted in immediate abolition of pain and no side effects were observed. The postoperative follow-up ranged from 8–18 months, and no pain recurred.

We believe that CM thalamotomy remains an effective method to treat chronic pain of both benign and malignant origin, although the lesion must be large enough to destroy most of the nucleus. Side effects are very rare.

PULVINOTOMY

Both Richardson [9, 10] and Yoshii and coworkers [21] have reported that lesions of the anterior pulvinar nucleus are effective in the treatment of chronic pain. The immediate effect of surgery generally was good, but pain tended to return so that two and one-half years later, only 25% of the patients continued to be pain-free.

In an earlier personal series (reported in 1977), 31 of 41 patients (76%) who had lesions in the anterior pulvinar were initially pain-free or improved [6]. The best results were achieved in patients with cancer pain and postherpetic neuralgia. Side effects were observed in six patients who had large medial and lateral pulvinotomies. An elderly man with phantom limb pain was confused for three days after surgery. Another patient had a feeling of numbness and heaviness in the contralateral thigh associated with hyperactive deep tendon reflexes. The cutaneous and the joint position senses were normal. Two additional patients had proprioceptive deficits. In one patient with a peripheral neuralgia following severe brain contusion and multiple injuries, diplopia was observed postoperatively. The sixth patient developed dysphasia after a large lesion in the left pulvinar. She had previously had a cancer metastasis in the left parieto-occipital lobe.

The follow-up time ranged from two to 52 months (mean 29 months). Two cancer patients died after pulvinotomy (one two months later, the other after 13 months), but both remained pain-free until death. Twenty-one patients (54%) remained pain-free, whereas 46% reported that pain returned to the preoperative level or was minimally improved. Fifty percent of the patients had medial anterior pulvinotomy (10.5 mm lateral to the midline), and the rest had an additional lateral lesion (16 mm lateral to the midline). The other pulvinar coordinates were 3 mm behind the anterior margin of the posterior commissure and 5 mm above the level of the intercommissural line (see figure 21–1).

In 1980, Yoshii and associates described 42 patients who underwent lateral pulvinotomy [22]. The target site was 15–18 mm lateral to the midline, 5 mm behind the posterior commissure, and 4 mm above the level of the intercommissural line (see figure 21–1). The lesions were much smaller than those of Laitinen (2–4 mm in diameter). Approximately 66% of their patients were pain-free or clearly improved one year after surgery.

Recently, we performed medial pulvinotomy in six cases. Two patients suffered from a brachial avulsion neuralgia and the others from pain associated with tabetic crises, facial deafferentation, thoracic zoster, or paraplegia. The target was defined by CT, which showed that the posterior margin of the pulvinar varied greatly among patients. In the first case, we found that the posterior commissure was at the same anteroposterior level as the most posterior part of the pulvinar; if the target had been determined using ventriculography, the electrode would have been in the cerebrospinal fluid (CSF) (figure 21–3). According to the atlas of Talairach and colleagues [15], the length of the pulvinar varies from 8–14 mm. Brierley and Beck studied the relation of radiological landmarks, e.g., the posterior commissure and the intercommissural line to the thalamic nuclei, but could not find any constant relationship in either the anteroposterior or vertical plane [2]. These data confirm Laitinen's preliminary CT studies, which indicate that ventriculography cannot be used reliably to determine pulvinar coordinates. In fact,

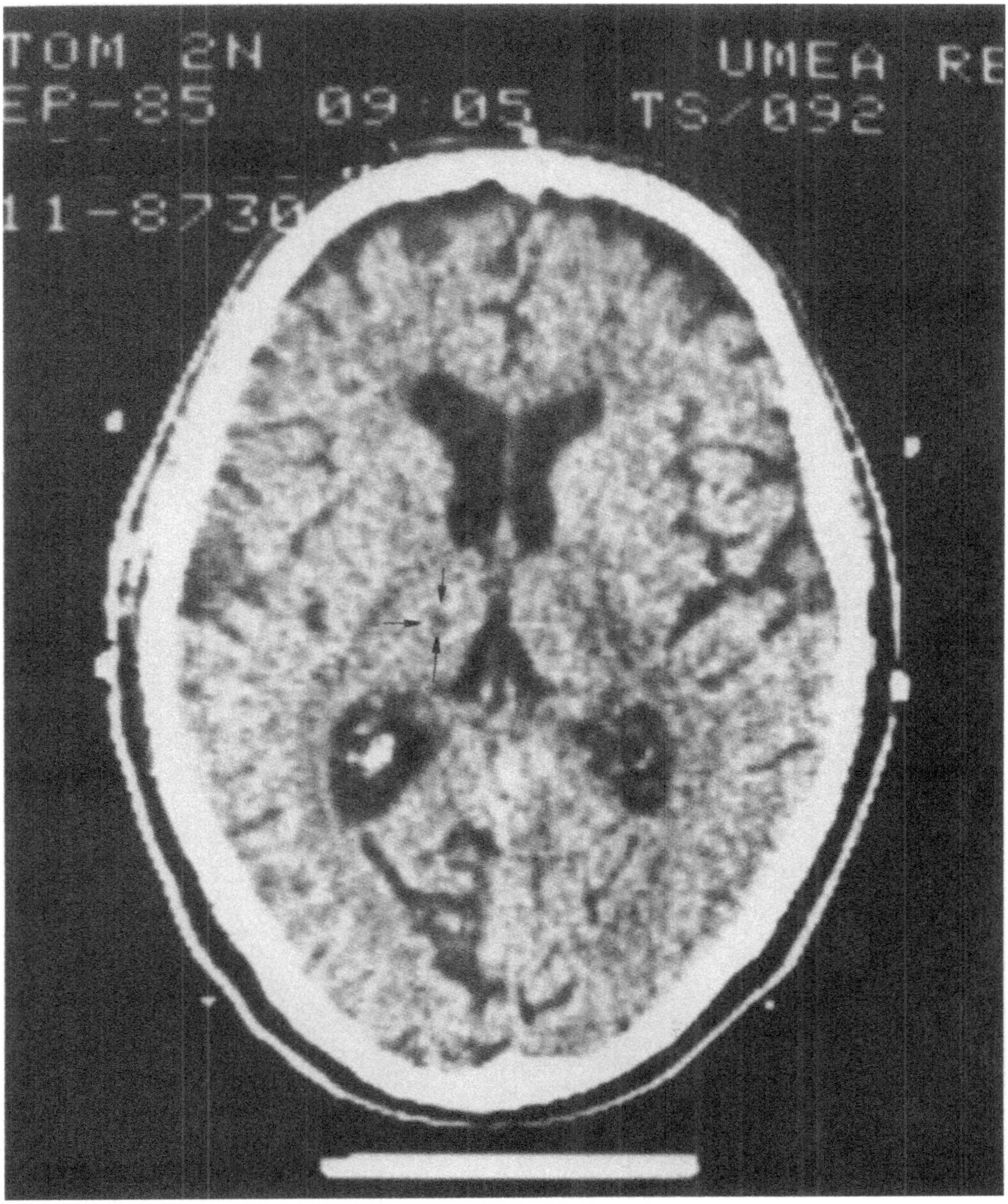

FIGURE 21–2. Arrows point to a spherical lesion with a diameter of 6 mm in the right centromedian nucelus of a 68-year-old man with trigeminal deafferentation pain. The center of the lesion is 8 mm behind the midcommissural point, 4 mm above the intercommissural line, and 10 mm from the midline of the third ventricle. The patient remained pain-free seven months after surgery, and no side effects were observed.

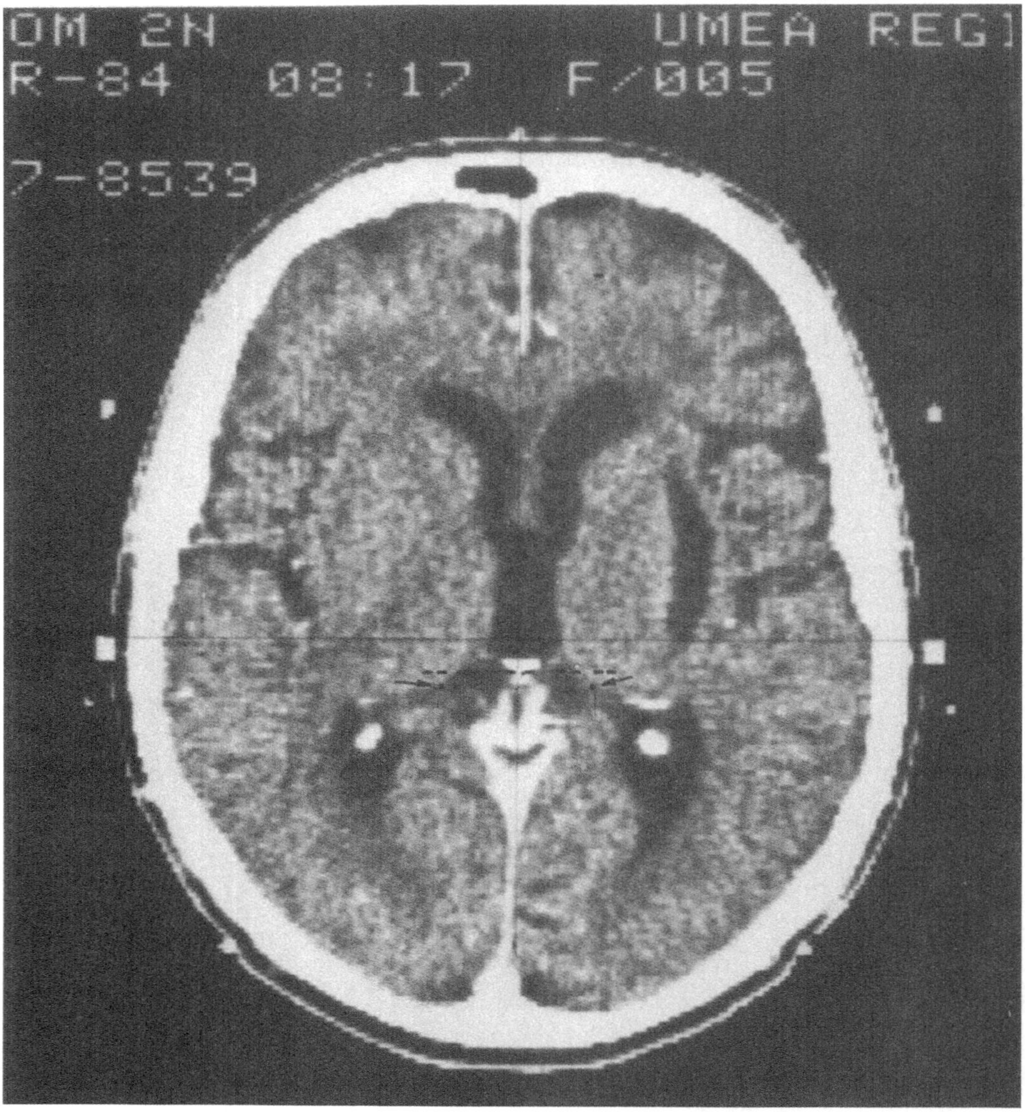

FIGURE 21–3. Dotted line indicates the vertical plane, perpendicular to the intercommissural line and passing through the anterior margin of the posterior commissure. A planned pulvinar lesion (4 mm behind the anterior margin of the posterior commissure, 4 mm above the intercommissural line, and 15 mm lateral to the midline) instead would have been placed in the cisterna ambiens (*arrows*).

it seems likely that some of the lesions performed earlier missed the pulvinar entirely and were instead in the cisterna ambiens. This may explain why some patients benefited from surgery and others did not.

Four of our six most recent patients with deafferentation pain had good early results; one patient with tabetic crises and another with facial deafferentation pain did not improve. The latter patient first had a small lesion with no improvement, after which the lesion was enlarged in a medial direction (figure 21–4). Even then, his pain did not diminish.

Pulvinotomy is often a very effective target for the stereotactic treatment of chronic pain. It may be as good as CM thalamotomy. The

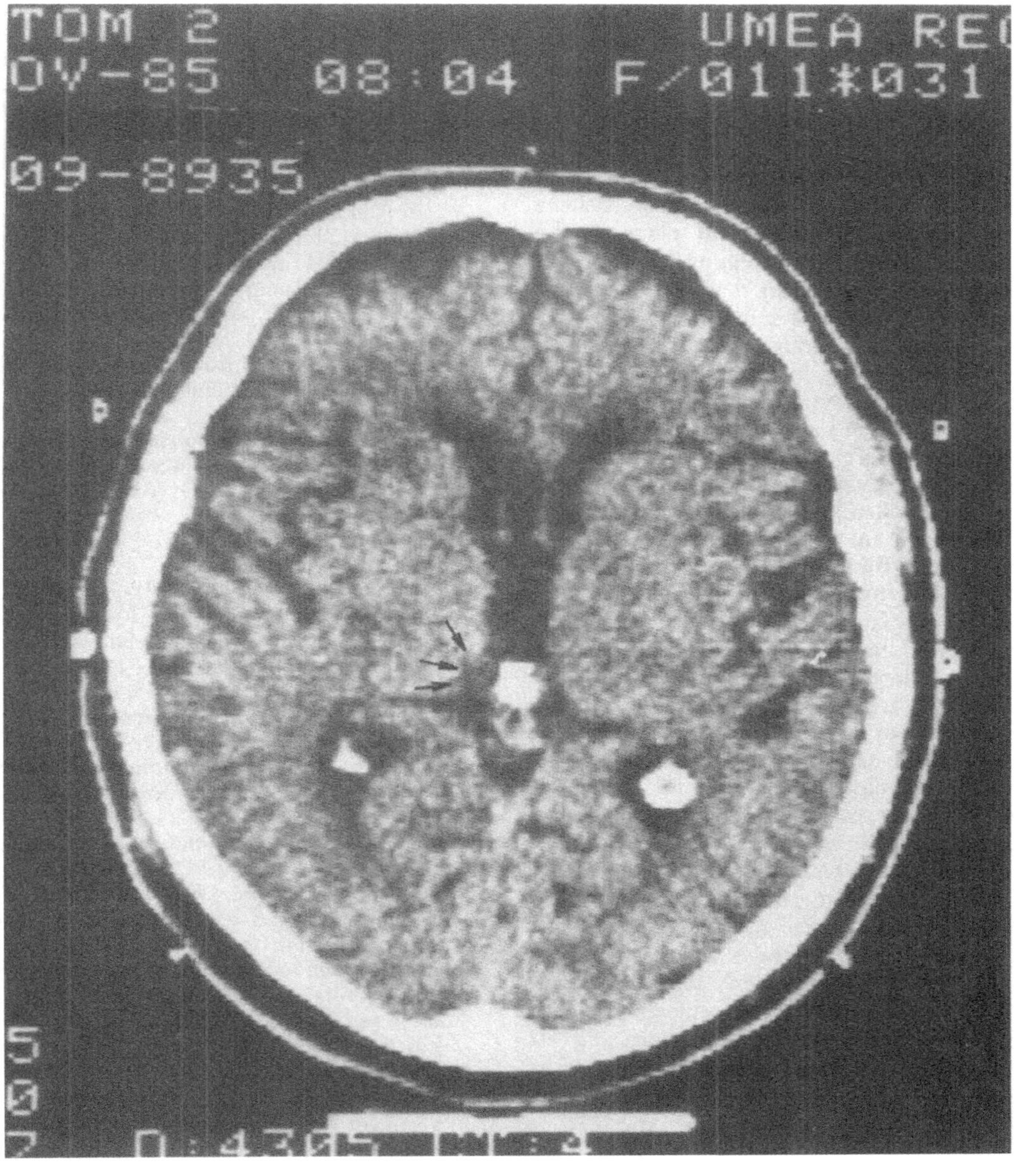

FIGURE 21–4. Electrocoagulation lesion in the medial pulvinar of a 66-year-old man with trigeminal deafferentation pain. The most lateral part of a lesion made to destroy the medial pulvinar is 12 mm from the midline and extends from 2–7 mm above the intercommissural line. Unfortunately, the pain returned two months after surgery.

recent use of CT scans or magnetic resonance imaging (MRI) to determine the pulvinar targets ensures that the lesions are placed correctly.

Assessment of Results

Based on the studies discussed here, we believe that mesencephalotomy has no place in the treatment of chronic pain. The efficacy of this approach is no better than that of nonspecific thalamotomies, but side effects are more frequent and more serious. In contrast, nonspecific thalamotomy in the CM-intralaminar nuclei is highly effective for chronic pain of both a malignant and a benign nature. The side effects are very rare. The lesions must be large enough to destroy most of the nucleus and a part of the intralaminar nuclei.

Pulvinotomy may be as effective as CM thalamotomy. Because earlier ventriculography-based determination of the target may have been inaccurate, CT-MRI-guided localization should be used instead. Postoperative CT/MRI studies and careful analysis of the clinical results are necessary before the value of pulvinotomy can be assessed [16].

A few years ago, it seemed that electrical stimulation would replace ablative thalamotomies in the treatment of chronic pain. Some neurosurgeons who have extensive personal experience with both techniques still believe this [12]. We believe that both methods must be kept in mind. Both have their advantages and short-comings, but we prefer chronic stimulation for young patients with deafferentation pain and ablative lesions for elderly patients with deafferentation and central pain and all patients with malignant pain. Many elderly patients, particularly those with cerebrovascular strokes, are unable to manage stimulators properly.

Hitchcock has pointed out that, thus far, the literature does not reveal which of the two alternatives is superior [5]. He has also discussed the expense of the stimulators, which makes their use prohibitive in many countries. We believe that ablative lesions remain a good alternative with persistent clinical value.

References

1. Amano K, Iseki H, Notani M, et al: Rostral mesencephalic reticulotomy for pain relief: Report of 15 cases. *Acta Neurochir [Suppl]* (Wien) 30:391–394, 1980
2. Brierley JB, Beck E: The significance in human stereotactic brain surgery of individual variation in the diencephalon and globus pallidus. *J Neurol Neurosurg Psychiatry* 22:287–298, 1959
3. Fairman D: Evaluation of results of stereotactic thalamotomy for the treatment of intractable pain. *Confin Neurol* 27:67–70, 1966
4. Hécaen H, Talairach J, David M, et al: Coagulations limitées du thalamus dans les algies du syndrome thalamique: Résultats thérapeutiques et physiologiques. *Rev Neurol* (Paris) 81:917–931, 1949
5. Hitchcock E: A comparison of analgesic ablative and stimulation techniques. *Zentralbl Neurochir* 42:189–202, 1981
6. Laitinen LV: Anterior pulvinotomy in the treatment of intractable pain in Sweet WH, Obrador S, Martín-Rodríguez JG (eds): *Neurosurgical Treatment in Psychiatry, Pain, and Epilepsy.* Baltimore, London, Tokyo: University Park Press, 1977, pp 669–672
7. Nashold BS, Jr, Wilson WP, Slaughter DG: Stereotaxic midbrain lesions for central dysesthesia and phantom pain: Preliminary report. *J Neurosurg* 30:116–126, 1969
8. Niizuma H, Kwak R, Ikeda S, et al: Follow-up results of centromedian thalamotomy for central pain. *Appl Neurophysiol* 45:324–325, 1982
9. Richardson DE: Thalamotomy for control of chronic pain. *Acta Neurochir [Suppl]* (Wien) 21:77–88, 1974
10. Richardson DE: Thalamotomy for intractable pain. *Confin Neurol* 29:139–145, 1967
11. Sano K, Yoshioka M, Ogashiwa M, et al: Thalamolaminotomy: A new operation for relief of intractable pain. *Confin Neurol* 27:63–66, 1966
12. Siegfried J, Hood T: Current status of functional neurosurgery In Krayenbuhl H (ed): *Advances and Technical Standards in Neurosurgery*, Vol 10. Wien, New York: Springer-Verlag, 1983, pp 19–79
13. Spiegel EA, Wycis HT: Mesencephalotomy in treatment of "intractable" facial pain. *Arch Neurol Psychiatr* (Chicago) 69:1–13, 1953
14. Spiegel EA, Wycis HT, Marks M, et al: Stereotaxic apparatus for operations on the human brain. *Science* 106:349–350, 1947
15. Talairach J, David M, Tournoux P, et al: *Atlas d'Anatomie Stéréotaxique*. Paris: Masson & Cie, 1957
16. Vilkki J: Effects of pulvinotomy and ventrolateral thalamotomy on some cognitive functions. In Sweet WH, Obrador S, Martín-Rodríguez JG (eds): *Neurosurgical Treatment in Psychiatry, Pain, and Epilepsy*. Baltimore, London, Tokyo: University Park Press, 1977, pp 673–677

17. Watkins ES: Stereotaxic thalamotomy for intractable pain. Presented at meeting of the Harvey Cushing Society, St. Louis, MO, April 19, 1966
18. Whisler WW, Voris HC: Mesencephalotomy for intractable pain due to malignant disease. *Appl Neurophysiol* 41:52–56, 1978
19. White JC, Sweet WH: *Pain and the Neurosurgeon*. Springfield, IL: Thomas, 1969
20. Wycis HT, Soloff L, Spiegel EA: Facial pain persisting after retrogasserian rhizotomy relieved by mesencephalo-thalamotomy. *Surgery* 27:115–122, 1950
21. Yoshii N, Kudo T, Shimizu S: Clinical and experimental studies of thalamic pulvinotomy. In *Abstracts of the Sixth Symposium of the International Society for Research in Stereoencephalotomy*, Oct 12–13, 1973, Tokyo
22. Yoshii N, Mizukami T, Ushikubo T, et al: Long-term follow-up study after pulvinotomy for intractable pain. *Appl Neurophysiol* 43:128–132, 1980

22. SPINAL AND PONTINE TRACTOTOMIES AND NUCLEOTOMIES

Edward Hitchcock

In stereotactic spinal surgery, a percutaneous electrode is directed to a cervical cord target via a stereotactic instrument fixed to the skull; the neck is in full flexion. It should not be confused with percutaneous cordotomies, which use simple aiming techniques, with or without micromanipulation, but which lack stereotactic precision.

Woroschiloff described a device for making intraspinal lesions in 1874 [60], and Clarke made a spinal stereotactic apparatus, which he described in 1921 [9]. Both instruments required open exposure of the cord. Nadvornik and co-workers constructed a similar device for making lesions in the lumbosacral cord [41]. Unfortunately, target identification by anatomical landmarks and evoked potentials is less reliable than identification by stimulation in the conscious patient. Rand and colleagues [47] used a stereotactic technique to place a cryoprobe via first cervical-second cervical (C1-2) interlaminar space against the anterior quadrant. Independently, Crue [11] (1967) and Hitchcock [25] (1968) performed stereotactic radiofrequency cordotomies by a posterior route. Crue used the C_{1-2} approach with the Todd-Wells apparatus; Hitchcock penetrated the atlanto-occipital space using a specially designed spinal stereotactic instrument. Crue selected a lateral coordinate 3–4 mm from the midline and penetrated the cord until the electrode struck the bone of the anterior canal.

Cadaveric experiments and surgical observations have demonstrated the relative immobility of the medulla and the first two cervical segments if the neck is fully flexed. Both lower cranial nerves and the large first dentate ligament contribute to this relative fixity. Additionally, the cord diameter varies in different positions. In extension, it is compressed axially with transverse surface folds; in flexion, the cord's smooth outline is restored, the transverse diameter remains unchanged, but the anteroposterior (AP) diameter is reduced by 20%. In conventional percutaneous cordotomies, the spine is usually extended or semiflexed, and the consequent distortion and increased mobility of the cord introduce additional errors. For these reasons, stable conditions are best achieved by fully flexing the neck and maintaining this position by fixing the stereotactic instrument to the operating table. Although fixation is not perfect (a major problem is cord distortion produced by rotation of the head on the odontoid), in practice, fixation is very satisfactory.

A clear coronal cord outline is difficult to achieve, even when open-mouth views and water-soluble contrast medium are used, but the odontoid can be used confidently as the midline landmark. The lateral target is chosen in relation to the "equatorial line" on the sagittal cord outline or relative to the anterior or posterior cord borders if the targets (arm-area spinothalamic tract or trigeminal tract) are more closely related to one of them. Some distortion is almost inevitable because of the difficulty in penetrating the tough pia, even with very sharp electrodes. Posterior-anterior electrode penetration produces less distortion than the lateral approach, although adhesion

I am grateful to Veronica Turner and to the Department of Photography, Sandwell District General Hospital, Birmingham, England, for aid in preparation of this manuscript.

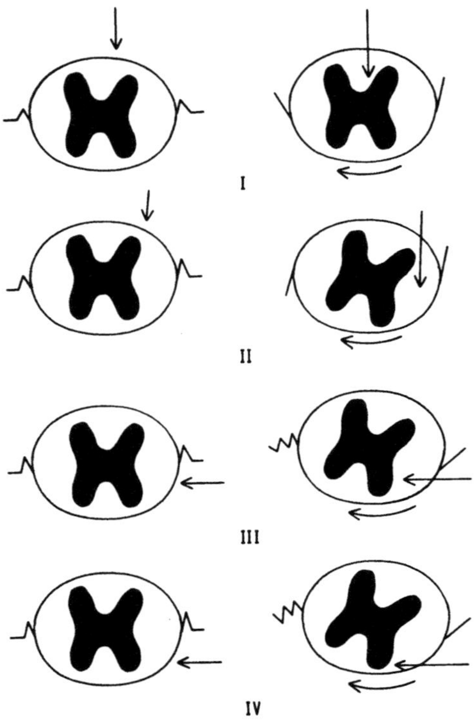

FIGURE 22–1. Diagram illustrates electrode penetration of the cervical cord by various approaches. I. Paramedial penetration with the cord stabilized by stretched dentate ligament and minimal torsion. II. Lateral penetration with more torsion but cord stability accomplished by dentate stretch. III. Lateral equatorial penetration. Large torsion and poor fixation. IV. Lateral anterior penetration. Note large torsion and poor fixation.

between the pia and the electrode can deflect the cord anteriorly, causing the original chosen target point to appear some millimeters short of a correct position. However, when a lateral lesion is desired, the posteroanterior approach can induce even greater distortion than results from the lateral approach (figure 22–1).

The rapid, functional changes of fiber systems within very short distances demand that the electrode holder be capable of fine adjustment (tenths of a millimeter) to permit recognition of the electrode track. With the posterior approach, laterality is accurate within one millimeter. The depth may deviate up to 5 mm (average 2 mm), however, indicating cord distortion and the need for electrophysiological recognition before placing a lesion. Because a particular response can result from stimulation of any of several different sites, repeated testing at various depths is essential for accurate recognition.

In the brain, it is possible to identify the electrode track and the target with a fine recording electrode, which is then replaced with a lesion-making probe. In the cord, however, because of the infinitely greater difficulties of electrode penetration and passage, this technique is unacceptable. The smaller confines of the cord require electrodes of smaller diameter than those used in the brain. Originally, fine tungsten-wire electrodes were used, which permitted the recording of evoked potentials. The temperature-monitoring electrode generally used today allows greater control during lesion production. The adhesion between the pia and the electrode can be partially overcome by rapid, almost complete, penetration of the cord followed by withdrawal of the electrode to the target point. In placing lateral cord lesions, the posterior approach may produce greater torsion than the lateral, but for lesions in the anteromedial part of the cord (to produce upper-body analgesia), the posteroanterior approach is most suitable. The lateral approach should be reserved for lower-body analgesia.

A major problem with this technique is that the exact positions of spinal cord tracts are ill-defined. Taren and co-workers [56] furnished gross measurements, and Nadvornik and associates [42] presented models for experimental lumbosacral spinal cord stereotaxy. Zlatos and Cierny [61, 62] provided more detailed maps, but the exact location of the fiber tracts that make up the bulk of the cord is often disputed because of considerable variability among patients. As the results accumulate for lesion production after stimulation studies, the traditional concept of the spinothalamic fibers as simple laminated dermatomal layers is being replaced by a concept of more complex patterns. The general pattern of lower-body fibers lying posteriorly and upper-body fibers anteriorly has been confirmed many times. It is also evident that a relatively large proportion of these fibers supply functionally important areas, such as the hand. A "spinothalamic homunculus" and "posterior column homunculus" (figure 22–2)

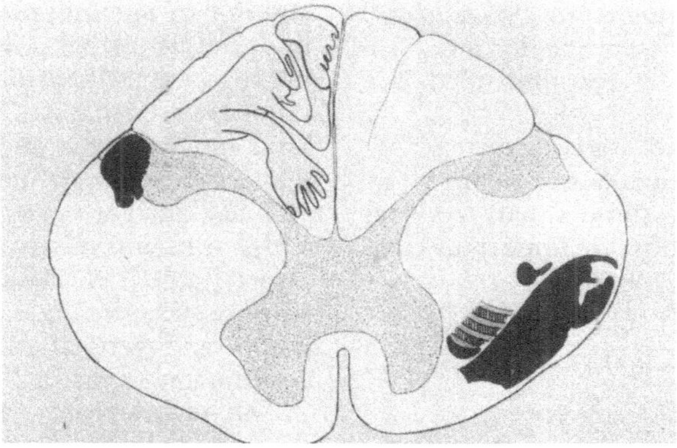

FIGURE 22–2. Spinal cord homunculi. The autonomic fibers controlling respiration and micturition are close to associated spinothalamic fibers.

were described [19, 24], and these concepts were supported by others [33, 50, 57]. A simple functional map of the high cervical cord helps in the recognition of electrode position and trajectory. Experience with the effect of open cordotomies indicates that the spinal pathways of respiration and micturition bear a somatotopic relationship to the spinothalamic tract. The respiratory fibers are closely related to the cervicothoracic fibers [26], and micturition fibers lie close to the sacral fibers [27].

Stimulation remains the most useful method of determining electrode position, because the patient's reaction depends on the electrode track [19, 31]. When the cord is traversed by an electrode aiming for the spinothalamic tract, the patient commonly experiences a shock-like sensation in the ipsilateral arm or face as the fasciculus cuneatus or trigeminal tract is penetrated. Increased penetration and low-frequency stimulation produce movement in the ipsilateral arm or leg as the corticospinal tract is traversed with the electrode advanced further; spinothalamic tract stimulation at 50 Hz produces an unpleasant or warm sensation in the contralateral arm or leg. A more medial approach elicits tingling, movement, or shock-like sensations in either leg as the electrode penetrates the fasciculus gracilis; if the electrode is close to the midline, increasing the voltage produces sensations in both legs. With deeper penetration, sensations are often experienced in the more distal portions of the leg and often in either arm, suggesting that the posterior columns are organized somatotopically with the distal extremity fibers located centrally. In the central portion of the cord, stimulation at low frequencies may provoke coughing or apnea, and at higher frequencies, nausea or truncal burning sensations. Central stimulation often causes an indescribable, but characteristic, unpleasant sensation that is widespread. The change from ipsilateral sensory responses to contralateral responses is usually very distinct.

An incremental radiofrequency lesion is made until acceptable anesthesia is achieved. Sensation and motor power are tested frequently to ensure that analgesia is adequate and that no paresis or incoordination occurs. Given a local anesthetic without premedication, patients tolerate these procedures extremely well, but diazepam administered intravenously is useful in the apprehensive patient. Impedance measurements, initially good guides to cord contact, become unreliable because cerebrospinal fluid (CSF) enters the needle track, lowering the impedance. The absolute values of impedance vary with the electrode size, but invariably we and others have found increases when passing from CSF to cord contact and a greater increase upon cord penetration.

The major advantage of stereotactic spinal percutaneous procedures is the ability to make selective lesions with considerable accuracy. This is especially important in young patients for whom sensory disabilities in an uninvolved limb or autonomic disorders are serious risks. Stereotactic cordotomies result in fewer respiratory or micturition tract injuries than do other percutaneous procedures. In patients with respiratory inadequacy, neither type of procedure should be attempted. Stereotactic pontine tractotomy, mesencephalotomy, or some other procedure is recommended for these patients.

Both percutaneous and stereotactic cordotomies require cooperative and oriented patients. Invasive cervical tumors and cervical spine deformity or infection are important contraindications.

Stereotactic Spinothalamic Tractotomy

The technique for spinothalamic tractotomy is a modification of that used for all spinal stereotactic procedures. The patient is placed on the operating table in the sitting position. Three-point fixation is selected: the central anterior pin should be placed about 2 cm above the nasion; the two posterior pins, about 3 cm above and behind the ear. It is unnecessary to shave the patient's head for fixation, but small circles of skin should be shaved at the fixation points, which then are infiltrated with a local anesthetic. Facing the patient, the neurosurgeon applies the frame and pushes the anterior pin through the skin and onto the frontal bone in the midline. The frame is held parallel to the interpupillary line while the posterior screws are fixed. The patient's neck then is put in full flexion, and the fixation pieces are secured to the operating table to maintain this position. It is important to ensure that the patient is seated squarely on the table and that the neck, trunk, and head are not rotated. Next, the whole operating table is tilted so that the stereotactic square is parallel to the floor, and the operative area is draped. A small area of skin at the nape of the neck is shaved.

The L-grid is applied in the odontoid plane, which lies at the mastoid tip. An x-ray cassette is inserted in the posteriorly fixed cassette holder, and an open-mouth roentgenogram is taken at 3–4.5 mm. The odontoid is identified, and a line bisecting it is projected at right angles to the horizontal ruler, thus defining the lateral offset (figure 22–3). The L-grid then is applied posteriorly at that offset, which is now the odontoid midline. A cisternal puncture is made, a water-soluble contrast agent (2–3 ml) is injected, and a lateral radiograph is obtained.

The target is chosen according to the analgesic level required. Thus, the target will be anterior to the midpoint of the cord (equatorial line) and its medial or lateral extent will depend upon whether upper or lower body analgesia is required. Coordinates for upper body analgesia are 3 mm from the midline and 3–4 mm anterior to the equatorial line. Coordinates for lower body analgesia are 5 mm from the midline and 1 mm anterior to the equatorial line. The target point is marked on the roentgenogram, and lines are drawn at right angles to the horizontal and vertical rulers to obtain X and Y coordinates (figure 22–4).

The quadrant arc is fixed at the chosen coordinates, and the cistern is penetrated by the "split needle technique." This permits fixation of the distal needle in the apparatus and the free passage of the electrode within it. Because of the difficulty in penetrating the skin, a small entry incision should be made with the point of a scalpel. The split needle is advanced steadily through the soft tissue of the neck until the cistern is penetrated. Removing the stylet allows the escape of CSF and confirms penetration. Even within the rigid apparatus, penetration of the cistern is detected as a sudden loss of resistance. When penetration is completed, the distal portion of the split needle is fixed in the extension piece, and the inner needle and proximal part of the split needle are removed. The electrode is fixed in the electrode holder once it has been confirmed that the electrode tip reaches the center of the arc. It is then carefully inserted into the distal split needle and steadily advanced with the micromanipulator until the impedance suddenly increases. This is usually associated with a sensation in the ipsilateral leg (medial tract) or in the face or the arm (lateral tract). The electrode then is withdrawn a few millimeters and then quickly advanced to penetrate the pia and a few millimeters of the cord (figure 22–5). The patient usually complains of a sensation in the ipsilateral arm when the fasciculus cuneatus is penetrated. Stimulation is delivered at 2 Hz to elicit motor responses and at 50 Hz for sensory responses. All of these responses are obtained with less than 1 V, although 2–3 V occasionally are necessary to produce a response. As the corticospinal tract is stimulated, the ipsilateral arm or leg contracts, and, with further penetration, the patient complains of either a warm or unpleasant sensation in the contralateral limbs or trunk. When the target point is reached, a confirming roentgenogram should be obtained.

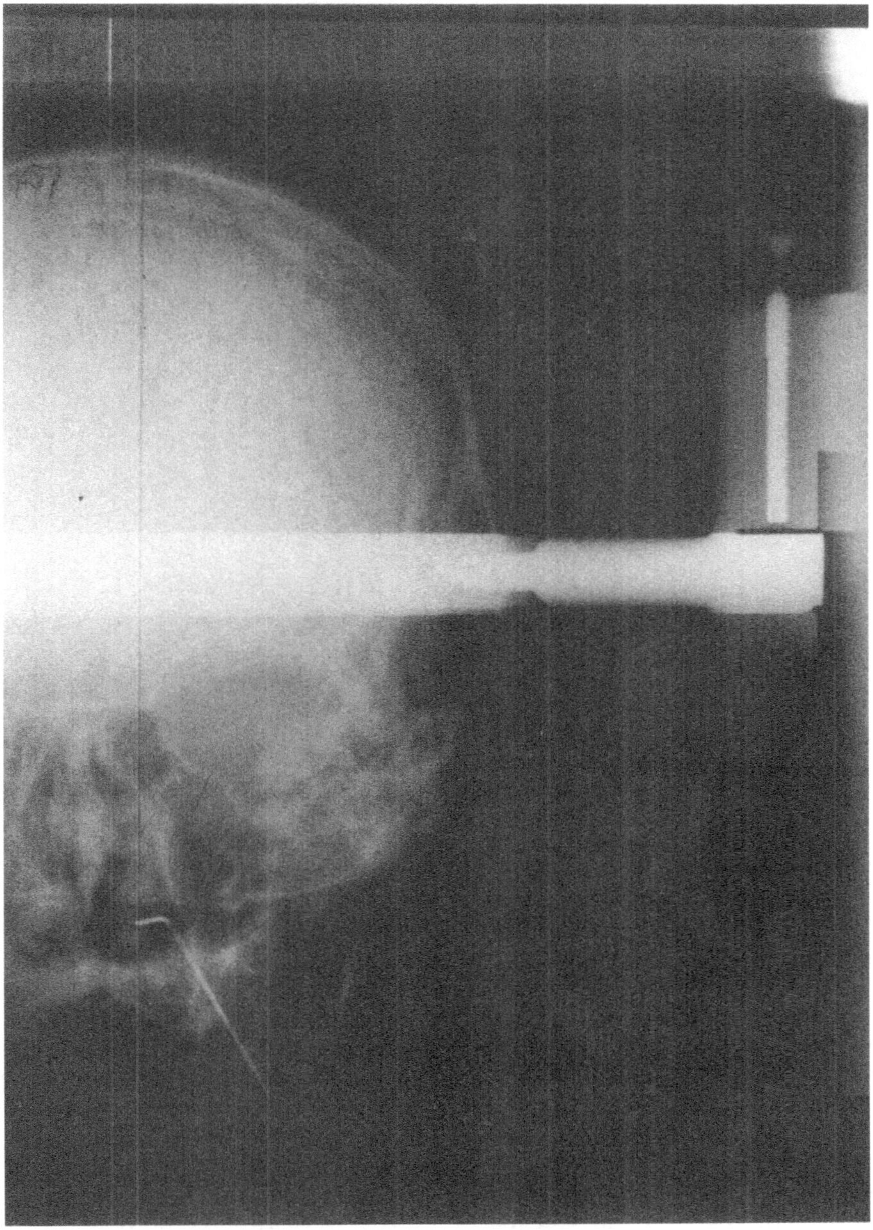

FIGURE 22-3. AP radiograph showing perpendicular projection through odontoid to horizontal ruler.

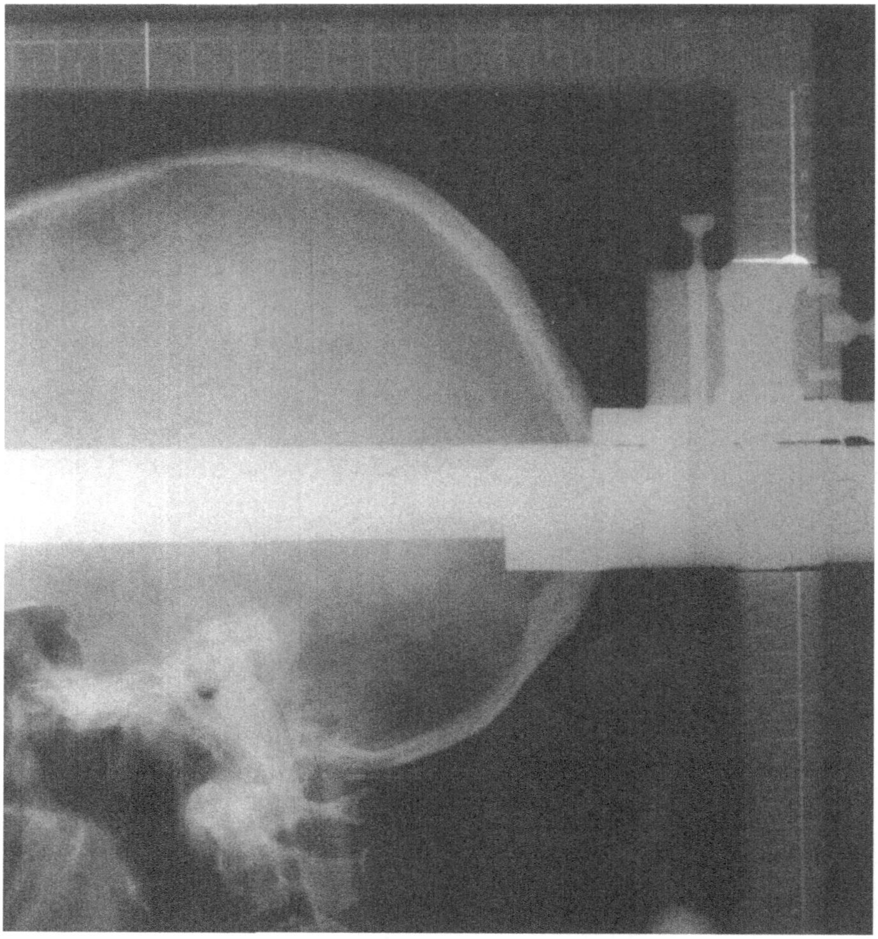

FIGURE 22–4. Horizontal and vertical projections from C_1 cord target.

Then the electrode is advanced or retracted according to the response to stimulation. A spinal atlas should be consulted regarding responses to stimulation so that the structures traversed can be plotted.

When a satisfactory response is obtained, a radiofrequency lesion is made incrementally while power, coordination, and sensory loss are monitored carefully. The patient's response at the time of initial cord penetration is important, as this entry point defines the trajectory. With this technique, it is sometimes clear that the cord has rotated and that the needle trajectory is directed away from the target. When that happens, the electrode should be removed, and the angle of insertion changed to take the rotation into account. A second insertion is quite permissible and often required, but, in general, it is wise to limit the number of insertions to three, as further improvement by repositioning is unlikely.

SPECIAL CONSIDERATIONS

Bilateral cervical cordotomies are dangerous and should be avoided, even with stereotactic technique. In fact, severe respiratory impairment can occur after unilateral cordotomies, particularly with the high cervical lesions that are usually necessary for the arm or chest pain produced by such diseases as lung cancer [5]. In producing a contralateral spinothalamic lesion, the adjacent respiratory fibers can be damaged as they pass to the ipsilateral intact respiratory apparatus. Although unaffected, the

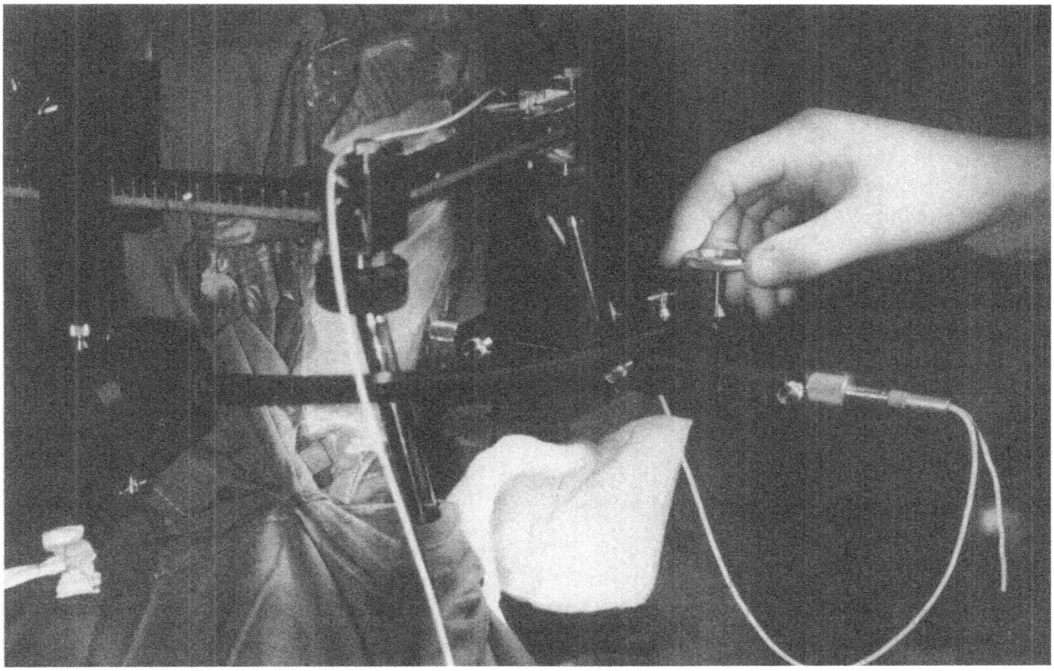

FIGURE 22–5. The electrode is advanced through the distal split needle held in the extension collet.

contralateral descending respiratory pathway may descend to an ineffective respiratory apparatus. In any case, a significant reduction of respiratory capacity is inevitable; and high cervical cordotomies should not be performed for any patient with a forced expiratory volume at one second of less than 1.5 l. Partial injury to these descending respiratory fibers will produce sleep apnea even in patients with normal bilateral respiratory function. Because the descending corticospinal voluntary pathways are used, the patient can breathe with some difficulty when awake, but when drowsy or sleepy, the patient becomes apneic as a result of the damage to the automatic reticular spinal respiratory pathway (Ondine's curse).

A similar situation exists for patients with pain from unilateral pelvic disease involving the bladder. Patients with adequate but abnormal micturition can develop retention or incontinence following a unilateral lesion involving the lumbosacral spinothalamic tract if there is injury to the adjacent micturition pathway.

RESULTS

Both percutaneous and stereotactic cordotomies [50] initially relieve pain effectively in a high percentage of patients. All reports in the literature include a large number of terminal patients; therefore, in a one-year follow-up, duration of pain relief is assessed on a progressively decreasing number of survivors. In a series by the author [22], of the 90% who obtained good to excellent pain relief initially, 88% maintained that level of relief six months later, which fell to 80% at nine months; this rate remained static at one year and beyond.

These figures indicate that although pain relief may be long lasting, a more realistic assessment is based on the duration of pain relief relative to life span. Sixty-four percent of the patients in our series had good to excellent relief until death or until their last follow-up, which was more than two years after surgery in 8%. Eighteen percent had moderate pain recurrence in the few weeks before death, and another 18% had major pain recurrence. Paresis occurs transiently in both percutaneous (average 13%) and stereotactic (average 10%) procedures. Paresis lasted more than a few days in only 3% of our patients. Rosomoff [48] reported transient bladder disorder in 10% of patients who underwent a percutaneous cordotomy, whereas equally brief bladder disorders have been reported in only 5% of stereotactic cordotomies. Despite this low incidence, cystometrogram changes can be demonstrated even in asymptomatic patients [27]. In patients with preexisting bladder disorders, the risk of postoperative incontinence or retention is relatively high. Similarly, some respiratory dysfunction was common with both procedures in symptomatic and asymptomatic patients. Using a spinal stereotactic technique and a modified Hitchcock instrument, Schvarcz was able to obtain high levels of analgesia without any respiratory disorders and suggested that the stereotactic procedure had fewer contraindications than percutaneous cordotomy [50].

Stereotactic Trigeminal Tractotomy and Nucleotomy

In 1937, Sjoquist [53] sectioned the spinal tract of the trigeminal nerve 8–10 mm above the obex by incising the posterolateral aspect of the medulla. The procedure was generally regarded as high-risk, yielding an appreciable rate of mortality and morbidity, and was rarely performed [15, 17]. Later Kunc perfected a simpler procedure at the cervical level and was able to section the tract selectively using local anesthesia [35]. Hosobuchi and Rutkin refined Sjoquist's procedure, using the microscope and a radiofrequency electrode after careful electrophysiological monitoring [32]. Although Bricolo [7] commends this procedure for pain from malignancy, it is a major undertaking, and, because it must be performed under general anesthesia, the ability to observe a patient's response to stimulation is lost.

Trigeminal tractotomy was developed independently by Crue and co-workers [12] in 1967 and Hitchcock [23, 25], in 1968. Both groups used the cisternal route. Crue had th patient prone and used coordinates 6.5 mm from the midline and 4 mm anterior to the posterior part of the brain stem. It is easier, however, to have the patient sitting with the neck fully flexed, because the cord is less mobile than when the head is in the neutral position. Flexion is much easier to achieve and safer in the sitting position than in the prone; monitoring also is facilitated. Coordinates 6 mm from the midline and 3 mm anterior to the posterior aspect of the cord at the first cervical segment places the electrode in the "caudal trigeminal dermatome." Targets that are further lateral, anterior, and rostral produce more central face analgesia. The intermedius, glossopharyngeal, and vagal components of the tract lie more posteriorly and medially. These are approximate measurements, based on a study of brain-stem and cord sections, and they make no allowance for cord displacement. As previously mentioned, even in the relatively fixed, fully flexed cord, some anterior displacement is inevitable.

The usual pattern of sensory loss after C_1 trigeminal tractotomy demonstrates central facial sparing, because the rostral trigeminal dermatomes are closer to the medulla. Although these areas often can be reached by angling the electrode up towards the lower medulla, it is difficult and sometimes impossible. When central facial analgesia is essential, pontine trigeminal tractotomy may be a preferable procedure.

The Radionics (Radionics, Inc., Burlington, MA) temperature-monitoring electrode is suitable for impedance stimulation and lesion production. The technique is similar to that previously described for spinothalamic tractotomy, with an the approach through the atlanto-occipital membrane. Placement of the tip within the trigeminal tract invariably is followed by the complaint of ipsilateral facial pain, whereupon the electrode tip is advanced or retracted according to the patient's responses. When appropriate responses are obtained, a radiofrequency lesion is made in incremental steps; analgesia, power, and coordination are tested at each step. It usually is not necessary to move the electrode once an ipsilateral facial sensory response is obtained. Analgesia extends and deepens as radiofrequency current is increased. If central facial or mucosal analgesia cannot be achieved, it usually is better to withdraw the electrode and reinsert it at a higher level rather than attempt adjustments at the initial insertion. Widespread analgesia in both head and neck dermatomes demonstrates the extensive overlap of sensory fibers within the caudal part of the trigeminal spinal nucleus (figure 22–6). This method has considerable advantages over conventional open medullary tractotomy. The extent of the lesion and the patient's reactions can be monitored, and the operation is relatively minor and undoubtedly the easiest of all the stereotactic spinal procedures.

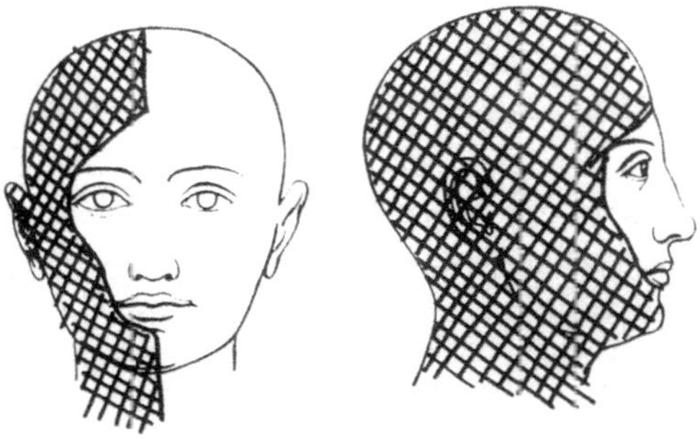

FIGURE 22-6. Cross-hatching represents the extensive analgesia produced by trigeminal nucleotomy and tractotomy.

CASE REPORTS

The following case reports illustrate the type of patient suitable for the procedure and the results likely with each.

Alveolar Carcinoma (Trigeminal Pain). A 64-year-old man had carcinoma of the left alveolus, resulting in a pathological fracture of the mandible. He suffered severe intractable pain, and a left stereotactic trigeminal tractotomy was chosen. Upon placement of the electrode, he developed complete analgesia of the left face and head, extending from the circumoral region to about the C_2 dermatome. This faded within a few minutes, and a radiofrequency lesion then was placed. The resultant analgesia involved the whole head, sparing the central face from mid-eyebrow to mid-mandible. The electrode was advanced 2 mm, and another radiofrequency lesion placed. The analgesia then spread to the midline and inferiorly as far as C_2. The patient was relieved of pain completely; his pathological fracture could be manipulated without pain. He remained pain-free on the left side of the face but developed pain in the right tongue from extension of the growth. He remained free of pain in his left jaw until his death.

Malignant Ulcer of the Tonsillar Fauces and Soft Palate (Glossopharyngeal Pain). A 62-year-old man had a faucial/soft palate ulcer following radiotherapy for a lymphoepithelioma of the right tonsil. He was in severe pain that prevented his eating or drinking adequately, and a trigeminal tractotomy was chosen. Insertion of the electrode to the target point caused him to complain of pain in the right jaw and neck. A radiofrequency lesion was performed, producing a wide area of analgesia involving the peripheral portion of the face and the C_2 region with sparing of the central face. Immediately thereafter, it was possible to palpate the ulcer without pain. He continued to be free of pain with well-maintained analgesia for more than two years.

Carcinoma of the Ear (Trigeminal, Nervus Intermedius, Glossopharyngeal, Vagal, and Cervical Pain). A 63-year-old woman suffered from very severe pain in the right temporal, facial, ear, and neck regions resulting from an ulcerating squamous cell carcinoma of the right ear. She felt extreme pain during dressing of the large ulcer cavity, and she required large doses of analgesics and hypnotics to control her constant pain. A stereotactic trigeminal tractotomy was performed. A radiofrequency lesion was placed at a site where ear pain was produced on stimulation. Postoperatively, she no longer complained of pain, and all analgesics were stopped. No definite analgesia could be demonstrated, but she continued to be painfree until death, in particular, tolerating dressings of the ulcer cavity without the administration of hypnotics or analgesics.

RESULTS

In an early series of 21 patients who underwent stereotactic trigeminal tractotomies, there was no operative mortality, but transient mild paresis or ataxia occurred in 40%. One patient had severe although transient ataxia, attributed to loss of electrode insulation that resulted in a lesion larger than intended. One patient had a diminished corneal reflex, and one had severe dysesthesias for several weeks. Pain relief was good to excellent until death in 47%, but 40% developed minor recurrent pain. The best results were obtained in patients with pain from malignancy: 66% achieved good to excellent relief until death, and only 22% experienced major recurrence. This procedure has continued to be used for selected patients with malignant face or head pain with similar results.

The possibility of destroying the nucleus as well as the tract encouraged the use of stereotactic trigeminal tractotomy in patients with postherpetic trigeminal neuralgia with some success [28]. Following herpes, facial pain is second in frequency only to truncal pain and almost invariable involves the ophthalmic division. Most medical and surgical treatments have been unsuccessful. Because some of this pain may be a deafferentation phenomenon, the results of brain stimulation have been encouraging.

Open trigeminal tractotomy appears to be only slightly more successful than other forms of treatment. This may be because of the interconnections between the nuclear masses, the polysynaptic ascending intranuclear pathway described by Stewart and co-workers [55], and the fact that there is considerable overlap between the cervical and facial segments of the nucleus. The inflammatory lesions of herpes zoster and the sensory ganglia, root entry zone, and posterior horn cells [13, 38] are especially prominent in segments related to the cutaneous eruption. Deafferentation pain may be caused by hyperexcitable neuronal pools within the substantia gelatinosa or its homologue, the trigeminal nucleus. Thus, radiofrequency destruction of this nucleus destroys these pools, removing both hypoesthesia and deep background pain. The relatively high percentage of success in the first three patients was encouraging, and the method has continued to be used. Schvarcz reported that seven of eight patients with postherpetic neuralgia achieved either reduction or elimination of burning pain [49].

Stereotactic trigeminal tractotomy and nucleotomy have been used for many types of facial pain, including pain from malignancy, postherpetic neuralgia, anesthesia dolorosa as well as atypical facial pain and trigeminal neuralgia. Schvarcz [55] reported 104 stereotactic neucleotomies: relief was obtained in 57% of patients with anesthesia dolorosa and in 72% of patients with "dysesthesia." He reported an enviably high success rate of 87% for postherpetic neuralgia and nearly the same rate of relief for pain due to malignancy. In general, however, the procedure should be limited to patients with oropharyngeal head malignancy and selected cases of atypical facial pain or facial deafferentation pain. It is important to note that if the lesions are too far medial and placed within an already-crossed lateral spinothalamic tract and ventral secondary trigeminal accending tract, contralateral anesthesia of the body and face may result. However, such sensory losses occur only with a lesion in the low medulla.

Myelotomy (Central Cord Lesion)

This 60-year-old procedure currently is enjoying a resurgence of interest, partially because it has proved effective for a variety of pain syndromes, but largely because the sensory changes produced can be explained only by new concepts of pain mechanisms. Thoracolumbar mediolongitudinal section of the cord was reported by Armour in 1927 [2]. The aim of this procedure was to interrupt "all the pain-conducting fibers crossing at the level of the incision." For nearly 50 years, all subsequent operations and their modifications were performed on the basis of this theory, i.e., division of the decussating spinothalamic fibers produces bilateral analgesia to an extent determined by the segmental length of the incision. In advocating the operation, its originator pointed out that visceral pain from the abdominothoracic organs could not be relieved by a unilateral cordotomy, possibly because visceral sensations ascended equally in each anterolateral column. There were clearly many advantages to this procedure, in comparison with anterolateral cordotomy. First, the risk of injury to the laterally placed corticospinal tract was much reduced. Second, for relief of bilateral or central pain, a single incision sufficed instead of bilateral incisions into the anterolateral columns. Subsequently, Leriche [37] and others [18, 40, 58, 59] developed the procedure. The effects appeared unpredictable, however, and classical spinothalamic sensory losses were not always achieved [40]. Mansuy and colleagues [40] and Wertheimer and Lecuire [58] obtained objective losses of pain and temperature sensation in only 30% of patients. They attributed their success to a five- or six-segment decussation of individual pain fibers. Performing myelotomies primarily at T_{10}–T_{12} and occasionally a few segments higher or lower, Sourek obtained an analgesic girdle area but noted pain relief in lower dermatomes in which normal pain sensation was preserved. Utilizing the arousal reaction in electroencephalograms, he noted a longer latency between stimulation of areas without disorder of pain sensations than in the analgesic girdle area. This he

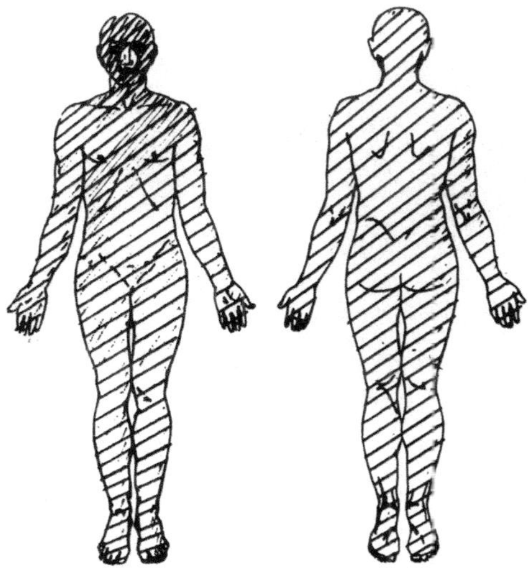

FIGURE 22–7. Extensive body-wide analgesia produced by a single C_1 central cord lesion is shown by hatching.

ascribed to a disorder of the mediodorsal system [54].

In 1934, Putnam [46] independently devised cervical myelotomy, again aiming to interrupt decussating spinothalamic fibers by splitting the commissure from C_4 to T_3 to produce analgesia from C_5 to T_9. Pain relief continued despite the return of normal sensation a week or two after surgery. Lembke [36] also performed myelotomy in the lower cervical cord and obtained similar sensory changes. The available evidence supported the view that the spinothalamic fibers decussated within a few segments of their posterior horn origin in the cervical region, but that at lower levels (pelvic dermatomes), the decussation took place over several segments. All of these procedures split the cord for at least three or more segments.

In 1968, Hitchcock [20] introduced stereotactic cervical myelotomy and noted analgesia from a single central thermocoagulation at the C_{1-2} level (figure 22–7). Even if as many as eleven segments are traversed prior to complete decussation, a solitary C_1 lesion could not produce such widespread analgesia simply by interrupting spinothalamic fibers. Furthermore, as cordotomy at the C_1 segment produced satisfactory analgesia and pain relief in the leg, the findings could be explained only on the basis of two separate modalities of pain sensation. The production of analgesia *above* the level of the lesion was even more difficult to explain. These findings since have been confirmed by others using thoracic or lumbosacral myelotomy after limited C_{1-3} commissurotomy [8, 10, 16, 34, 39, 44]. Schvartz [49, 50, 52] and Eiras and colleagues [14] have reported their experience with stereotactic cervical myelotomy and have confirmed Hitchcock's early findings and subsequent experience [21, 22].

PROCEDURE

The procedure for central cord lesion myelotomy is the same as that used for stereotactic spinothalamic tractotomy with a central cord target. Several points are chosen along the anterior and posterior margin of the cord image, and a line is drawn down the cord halfway between them. This line is assumed to demarcate the central canal. A suitable point is chosen along this line that will allow the passage of the electrode through the occipitocervical interval. In some patients, the occipitocervical interval is fused, but the C_{1-2} interval in these patients usually is sufficiently wide (with full neck flexion) to allow passage of the electrode posteriorly or, failing that, laterally (figure 22–8). The electrode is inserted in the needle by the electrode holder. During passage, impedance is recorded, and the abrupt change is noted when the posterior cord surface is reached. The electrode then is withdrawn 1 cm and sharply advanced to penetrate the cord. The patient usually will complain of an electric shock–like sensation in one or both legs if the midposition of the dorsal column is penetrated. Complaint of pain in the arm or face indicates that the electrode is off the midline and is penetrating the fasciculus cuneatus or trigeminal tract. If this occurs, the electrode should be withdrawn, and the cannula arc angle readjusted. As long as satisfactory midline responses are obtained, the electrode is advanced further. In the absence of responses to mechanical stimuli, electrical stimulation (50 Hz, 0.2 msec duration, 1.2 V) can be used. With continued fine advances of the electrode and further stimulation, sensory responses will be obtained in the legs and perineum and, subsequently, both arms. It is important to realize

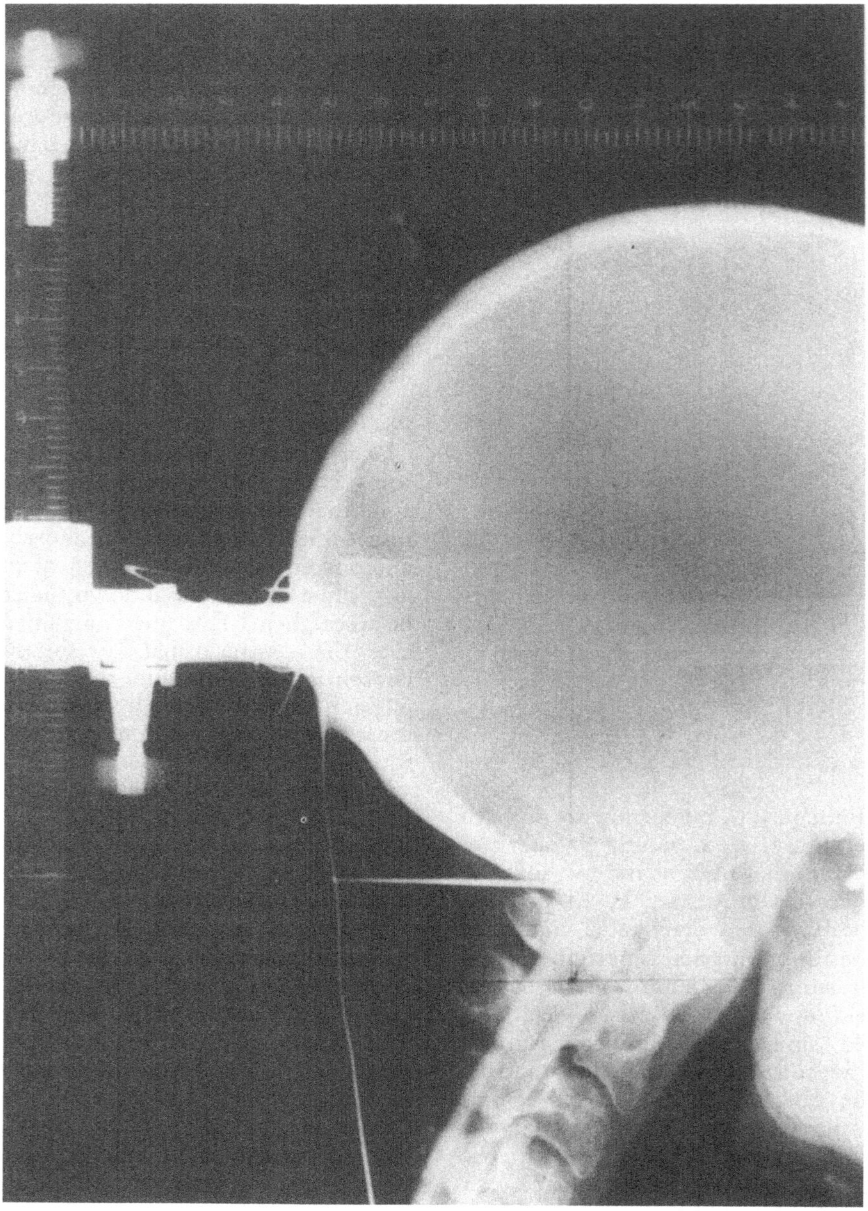

FIGURE 22-8. C_{1-2} target for lateral-entry central cord lesion.

that the target point will usually be short of the center of the cord because the cord is pushed by the electrode as much as 5 or 6 mm anteriorly. Physiological verification of position by stimulation is therefore vital. The central cord is reached approximately 2 mm after the bilateral sensations in legs or arms have ceased. Stimulation at the central cord often produces a whole-body paresthesia and, frequently, an unpleasant central-chest and abdominal sensation. At this point, radiofrequency coagulation should be performed in small temperature increments up to 75°C at 30 sec intervals. After each increment, careful sensory and motor testing should be performed. Bilateral hypalgesia usually is noted at lower temperatures, but a complete lesion should be made, providing no proprioceptive or corticospinal disorder is found.

RESULTS

The sensory changes have been debated incompletely and are at variance with established neuroanatomical knowledge. Additionally, it is difficult to explain why pain from pelvic structures innervated by sacral segments is relieved better by a myelotomy higher than that used for leg pain. A lower thoracic myelotomy seems to be more effective for leg pain than an upper thoracic myelotomy.

In general, central cord lesion myelotomy has been used for patients with bilateral pain, especially pelvic. A group of 19 patients with neoplastic pain was followed for up to four years or until death; eight remained pain-free without further procedures or analgesics, and five required only weak analgesics. In six patients who had little or no sensory loss, pain relief was poor or transient, but of the remaining 13 patients who achieved good relief, nearly 80% had well-marked analgesia [21]. Schvarcz also reported good results in 45 patients with a variety of painful conditions, 35 of whom had neoplastic pain [52]. In this group, 30 obtained good relief, and five developed recurrence of pain. Cook and Kawakami studied 25 cases of commissural myelotomy and concluded that, even without sensory loss, pain relief can be obtained [10]. These authors argued that the central cord lesion interrupts pathways entering, within, or leaving the spinothalamic complex.

Pontine Spinothalamic Tractotomy

Pontine stereotactic spinothalamic tractotomy was introduced in 1970 [24]. The procedure was said to provide major advantages: precise target localization and destruction enabled high analgesic levels to be achieved without injury to adjacent tracts. Because of the separation of autonomic and pain pathways [4, 6, 43, 45], micturition and respiratory disorders could be avoided. Subsequently, Barbera and coworkers reported their experience with this stereotactic technique in five patients, all of whom achieved pain relief without serious complications [3].

Neurophysiological studies in animals indicate that autonomic fibers, including respiratory and micturition pathways, are in the posteromedial pons, close to the medial longitudinal fasciculus. This supports the concept that pontine spinothalamic tractotomies are less likely than spinal procedures to be followed by autonomic disorder. Other important pathways and cranial nerve nuclei lie close by, and very precise stereotactic stimulation technique is required.

METHOD

The stereotactic procedure is performed with the patient in a recumbent sitting position. Local anesthesia is used, sometimes supplemented with intravenous diazepam. The stereotactic instrument is fixed to the skull, and water-soluble contrast ventriculography is performed via a frontal twist-drill hole to outline the third and fourth ventricles (figure 22–9). Using a pontine coordinate atlas, the target is marked in relation to a line drawn through the floor of the fourth ventricle, and a second line is drawn at right angles to it, passing through the fastigium (figure 22–10). The relationship of the fastigium to the fourth ventricle is inconstant, but it serves as a useful and well-defined landmark for mid-pons, and the easiest target to delineate is that within the fastigial plane.

Temperature-monitoring electrodes (1.1 mm by 7 mm) are used with a Radionics RFG-3B radiofrequency generator (Radionics Inc., Burlington, MA). During passage of the electrode through a posterior fossa burr hole, the results of stimulation are recorded at different points along the tract. In general, the angle chosen for the electrode passes through the cerebellum and inferior cerebellar peduncle before penetrating the trigeminal nucleus and fibers, facial nerve, and often the cochlear and vestibular nuclei. Occasionally, quintothalamic fibers are penetrated (figure 22–11). Stimulation is performed at various frequencies ranging from 2–100 Hz; the lower frequencies are used to explore motor responses, and the higher frequencies (most commonly 50 Hz) are used to elicit sensory responses. The pulse duration is normally 2 msec with voltages varying from 0.3–6 V. Sensory responses from stimultion of nuclei are obtained by less than 1 V, but higher voltages are sometimes necessary to produce responses from tract stimulation. In general, voltages less than 1.5 V have produced

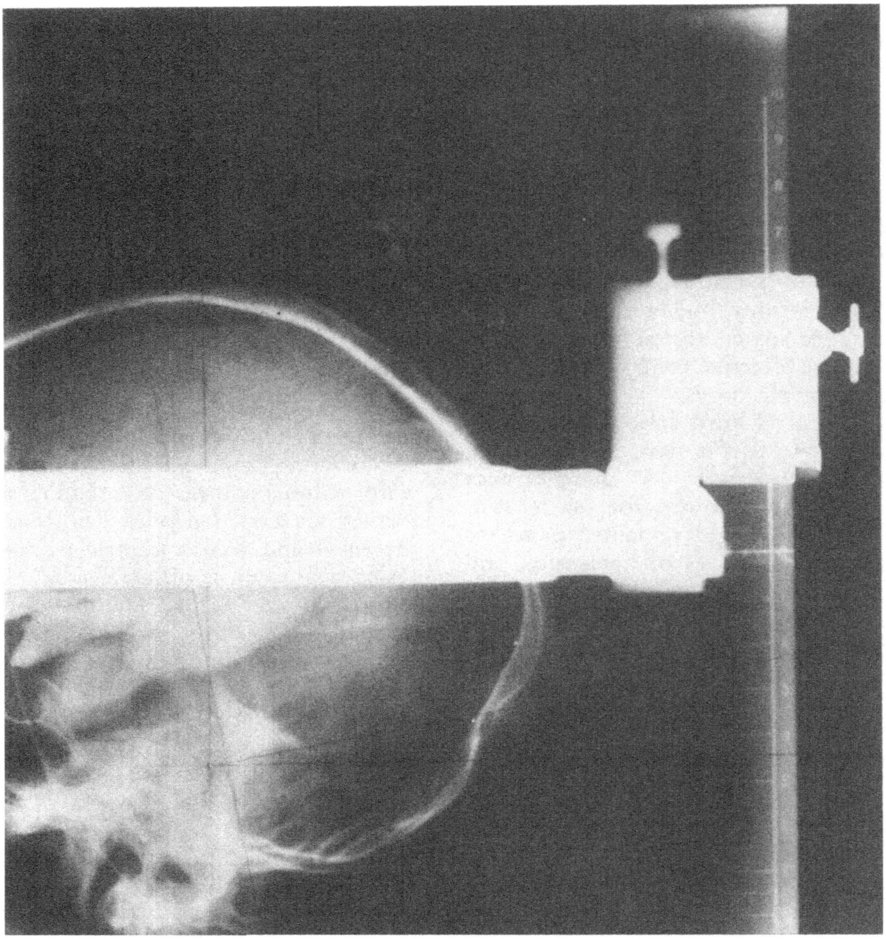

FIGURE 22–9. Pontine target delineated in relation to fourth ventricular floor and fastigial line.

responses, although voltages more than 3 V sometimes have been necessary.

During passage through cochlear and vestibular nuclei, the effects of stimulation are studied closely. Vestibular stimulation induces profound vertigo and nystagmus, and cochlear stimulation results in a clicking sound in the ipsilateral ear at the same rate as the stimulation frequency. Stimulation within the trigeminal nucleus produces ipsilateral facial pain, stimulation of the facial nerve, and ipsilateral whole-face contraction. Contralateral facial pain occurs with stimulation within the quintothalamic fibers. Further progression and stimulation evokes a warm or occasionally painful sensation in the opposite side of the body, indicating that the electrode is within or close to the spinothalamic tract.

Although radiological confirmation is needed to choose the primary target, close observations of the effects of stimulation are vital. If satisfactory responses cannot be obtained, a new trajectory should be chosen a few millimeters medial or lateral until the desired responses are obtained. Roentgenograms should be taken to confirm correct electrode position. If satisfactory responses are unobtainable, no lesion should be made, even if the electrode position seems correct using radiological criteria.

RESULTS

Our first experience involved seven patients, six of whom had pain caused by cancer [24]. Although pain relief was good, long-term follow-up was not possible, because the patients selected had terminal conditions. High analgesic levels were reached easily (figure 22–

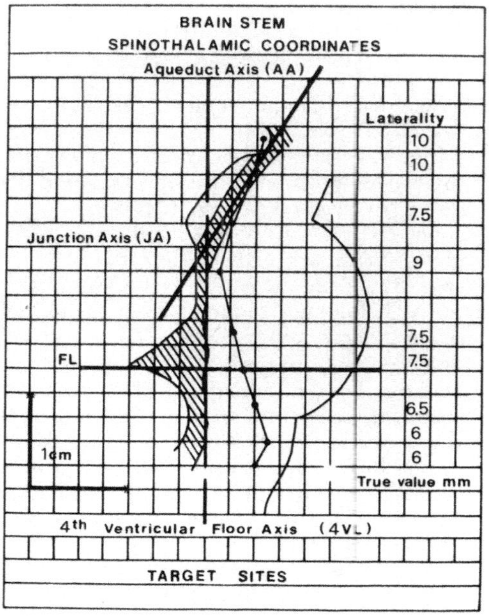

FIGURE 22–10. Pontine coordinates for spinothalamic tract.

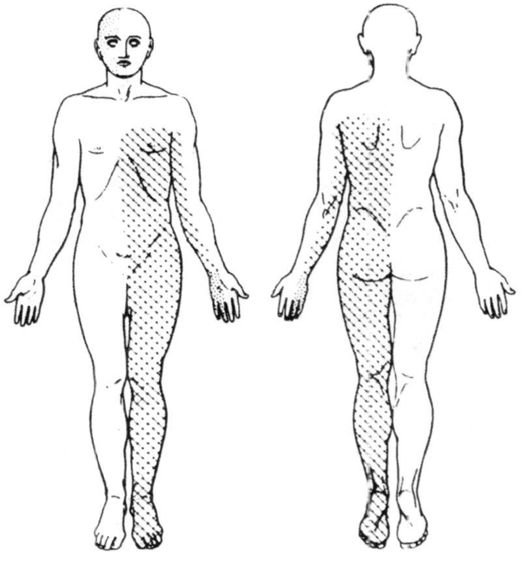

FIGURE 22–11. Right pontine lesion produces right facial analgesia and left spinothalamic loss.

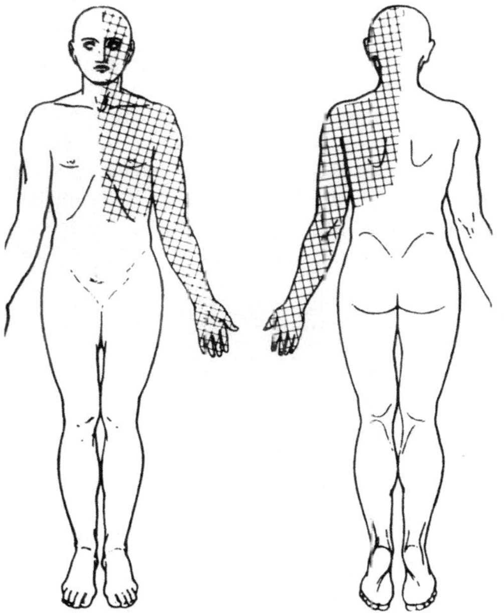

FIGURE 22–12. High right pons lesion produces deep facio-brachio-truncal analgesia.

12). Our most recent experience included eight cancer patients who had poor respiratory conditions or required high levels of analgesia [29]. One patient died a few days following surgery and demonstrated evidence of an unusually extensive lesion from a large electrode (1.8-mm tip, 3-mm diameter). Six patients achieved pain relief until death or the last follow-up. One patient had severe pain recurrence 12 weeks after the procedure. The procedure is less complex and less difficult than might appear, but it does require precise instrumentation and some knowledge of pontine anatomy. It is very dependent upon good patient cooperation and is not suitable for patients who are unable to cooperate for any reason. Our experience with the procedure is limited to 18 patients, although more patients have been accepted for this procedure in recent years. Barbera and colleagues reported good results in five patients and continue to use the method [3]. Two of their patients had deafferentation pain from brachial plexus destruction, and they obtained good relief. Schvarcz has also used the procedure with success (personal communication).

There are no reliable stereotactic coordinates for the important zone in the brain stem that extends several millimeters above and below the fastigial line. The atlas of Afshar and associates has a 10-mm gap in its representation of the spinothalamic tract around the fastigial plane [1]. A simple atlas has been described [24, 29], but this atlas must be regarded as a relatively crude guide to a most complex neuroanatomical area. The lateral coordinates probably should be 1–2 mm more medial than described.

The stereotactic approach has major advantages over an open exposure. The procedure is better tolerated by patients who are in poor general condition, as those requiring this surgery often are. It is more precise than open exposure and radiofrequency coagulation by a freehand method. The single operative death that has occurred must be weighed against the hazards of attempting other definitive analgesic procedures in a patient with an exceptionally severe respiratory inadequacy. It is possible that for such patients, the risks cannot be greatly reduced, even by pontine tractotomy. But for many others, pontine spinothalamic tractotomy offers deep, sustained high-level analgesia at less risk than many other procedures. The procedure can be compared favorably with mesencephalotomy [30].

References

1. Afshar F, Watkins ES, Yap JC: *Stereotactic Atlas of the Human Brain Stem and Cerebellar Nuclei.* New York: Raven Press, 1978, pp 80–88
2. Armour D: Lettsonian lecture on the surgery of the spinal cord and its membranes. *Lancet* 1:691–697, 1927
3. Barbera J, Juan L, Barcia-Salorio JL, et al: Stereotaxic pontine spinothalamic tractotomy. *Surg Neurol* 11:111–114, 1979
4. Beattie J, Brown GR, Long CNH: Physiological and anatomical evidence for existence of nerve tracts connecting the thalamus with spinal sympathetic centres. J Soc (Lond) Series B 106:253–275, 1930
5. Belmusto L, Brown E, Owens G: Clinical observations on respiratory and vasomotor disturbance as related to cervical cordotomy. *J Neurosurg* 20:225–232, 1963
6. Bradley WE, Conway CJ: Bladder representation in the pontine-mesencephalic reticular formation. *Exp Neurol* 16:237–249, 1966
7. Bricolo A: Medullary tractotomy for cephalic pain of malignant disease. In Bonica JJ, Ventafridda V (eds): *Advances in Pain Research and Therapy*, Vol 2. New York: Raven Press, pp 453–462
8. Broager B: Commissural myelotomy. *Surg Neurol* 2:71–74, 1974
9. Clarke RH: Investigation of the central nervous system: Methods and instruments. *Johns Hopkins Hosp Report* 1:1–159, 1921
10. Cook AW, Kawakami K: Commissural myelotomy. *J Neurosurg* 47:1–6, 1977
11. Crue BL, Todd EM, Carregal EJA: Posterior approach for high cervical percutaneous radiofrequency cordotomy. *Confin Neurol* 30:41–52, 1968
12. Crue BL, Todd EM, Carregal EJM, et al: Percutaneous trigeminal tractotomy. *Bull Los Angeles Neurol Soc* 32:86, 1967
13. Denny Brown D, Adams RD, Fitzgerald PJ: Pathologic features of herpes zoster: A note on "geniculate herpes." *Arch Neurol Psychiatry* 51:216–231, 1944
14. Eiras J, Garcia J, Gomez J, et al: First results with extralemniscal myelotomy In Advances in Stereotactic Functional Neurosurgery Part 4. *Acta Neurochir* [*Suppl*] (Wien) 30:1980
15. Falconer MA: Intramedullary trigeminal tractotomy and its place in the treatment of facial pain. *J Neurol Neurosurg Psychiatry* 12:297–311, 1949
16. Gildenberg P, Hirshberg R: Limited myelotomy for the treatment of intractable cancer pain. *J Neurol Neurosurg Psychiatry* 47:94–96, 1984
17. Guidetti B: Tractotomy for the relief of trigeminal neuralgia. *J Neurosurg* 7:499–500, 1950
18. Guillaume I, Mazars G: Valletean de mouillac: La myelotomie commisurale. *Presse Med* 53:666–667, 1945
19. Hitchcock E: Electrophysiological exploration of the cervico-medullary region. In Somjen G (ed): *Neurophysiology Studied in Man.* International Congress Series 253. Amsterdam: Excerpta Medica, 1971, pp 237–245
20. Hitchcock E: Stereotactic cervical myelotomy. *J Neurol Neurosurg Psychiatry* 33:224–230, 1970
21. Hitchcock E: Stereotactic myelotomy. *Proc Soc Med* 67:771–772, 1974
22. Hitchcock E: Stereotactic spinal surgery. In *Proceedings of the Sixth International Congress of Neurological Surgery.* Amsterdam/Oxford: Excerpta Medica, 1977, pp 271–280
23. Hitchcock E: Stereotactic trigeminal tractotomy. *Ann Clin Res* 2:131–135, 1970
24. Hitchcock E: Stereotaxic pontine spinothalamic tractotomy. *J Neurosurg* 39:746–752, 1973
25. Hitchcock E: Stereotaxic spinal surgery: A preliminary report. *J Neurosurg* 31:386–392, 1969
26. Hitchcock E, Leece B: Somatotopic representa-

tions of the respiratory pathways in the cervical cord of man. *J Neurosurg* 27:320–329, 1967
27. Hitchcock E, Newsome D, Salama M: The somatotopic representation of the micturition pathways in the cervical cord of man. *Br J Surg* 61:395–401, 1974
28. Hitchcock E, Schvarcz JT: Stereotactic trigeminal tractotomy for post-herpetic facial pain. *J Neurosurg* 37:412–417, 1972
29. Hitchcock E, Sotello MG, Kim MC: Analgesic levels and technical method in stereotactic pontine and spinothalamic tractotomy. *Acta Neurochir* (Wien) 77:29–36, 1985
30. Hitchcock E, Teixeira M: A comparison of results from center median and basal thalamotomy for pain. *Surg Neurol* 15:341–351, 1981
31. Hitchcock E, Tsukomoto Y: Physiological correlates in stereotactic spinal surgery. *Acta Neurochir [Suppl]* (Wien) 121:119, 1974
32. Hosobuchi Y, Rutkin B: Descending trigeminal tractotomy: Neurophysiological approach. *Arch Neurol* 25:115–125, 1971
33. Illingworth RD, Molina Negro P: Spontaneous and electrically evoked activity in the anterolateral column of the spinal cord in dogs. *J Neurosurg* 40:58–64, 1974
34. King RB: Anterior commissurotomy for intractable pain. *J Neurosurg* 47:7–11, 1977
35. Kunc Z: Tractus spinalis nervi trigemini. Rozprovny Ceskoslovenska, Akademic Red., 1964
36. Lembke W: Ueber die mediolongitudinale chordotomie im Halsmarkberieich. *Zentralbl Chir* 89:439–443, 1964
37. Leriche R: Traitement de la douleur dans les cancers abdomineux et pelviens inoperables ou recidives. *Gaz Hop* (Paris) 109:917–922, 1936
38. Lhermitte J: Lesions spinales du zona: La myelite zosterienne. *Rev Neurol* (Paris) 40:361–364, 1924
39. Lippert RG, Hosobuchi Y, Nielsen SL: Spinal commissurotomy. *Surg Neurol* 2:373–377, 1974
40. Mansuy L, Lecuire J, Accassat L: Techniques de la myelotomie commissurale posterieuse. *J Chir* (Paris) 60:202–213, 1944
41. Nadvornik P, Frohlish J, Jezek V, et al: New apparatus for spinal cord stereotaxis and its use in the microsurgery of lumbar enlargement. *Confin Neurol* 34:311–314, 1972
42. Nadvornik P, Nemecek S, Petr R, et al: Model maps for experimental spinal cord stereotaxis. *Confin Neurol* 30:273–279, 1968
43. Orville A, Smith JR, Clarke N: Central autonomic pathways: A study in functional neuroanatomy. *J Comp Neurol* 3:399–406, 1964
44. Papo I, Luongo A: High cervical commissural myelotomy in the treatment of pain. *J Neurol Neurosurg Psychiatry* 39:705–710, 1976
45. Plum F, Posner JB: *The Diagnosis of Stupor and Coma*, (2nd ed). Philadelphia: FA Davis, 1972, p 26
46. Putnam PH: Myelotomy of the commissure: A new method of treatment for pain in the upper extremities. *Arch Neurol Psychiatr* (Chicago) 32:1189–1193, 1934
47. Rand RW, Baner RO, Smart CR, et al: Experience with percutaneous stereotaxic cryocordotomy. *Bull Los Angeles Neurol Soc* 30:142–147, 1965
48. Rosomoff HL: Percutaneous radiofrequency cervical cordotomy for relief of intractable pain. In Bonica JJ (ed): *Advances in Neurol*, Vol 4. New York: Raven Press, 1974, pp 683–688
49. Schvarcz JR: Postherpetic craniofacial dysaesthesiae. Their management by stereotactic trigeminal nucleotomy. *Acta Neurochir* (Wien) 38:65–72, 1977
50. Schvarcz JR: Spinal cord stereotactic surgery. In Sano K, Ishii S (eds): *Recent Progress in Neurological Surgery*. Amsterdam: Excerpta Medica, 1974, pp 234–241
51. Schvarcz JR: Spinal cord stereotactic techniques re trigeminal nucleotomy and extralemniscal myelotomy. *Appl Neurophysiol* 41:99–112, 1978
52. Schvarcz JR: Stereotactic extralemniscal myelotomy. *J Neurol Neurosurg Psychiatry* 39:53–37, 1976
53. Sjoquist O: Studies on pain conduction in the trigeminal nerve. *Acta Psychiatr Neurol [Suppl]* 17, 1938
54. Sourek K: Commissural myelotomy. *J Neurosurg* 31:524–527, 1969
55. Stewart WA, Stoops WL, Pillone PR, et al: An electrophysiological study of ascending pathways from nucleus caudalis of the spinal trigeminal nuclear complex. *J Neurosurg* 21:35–48, 1964
56. Taren JA, Davis R, Crosby EC: Target physiologic corroboration in stereotaxic cervical cordotomy. *J Neurosurg* 30:569–584, 1969
57. Tasker RR: The merits of percutaneous cordotomy over the open operation. In Morley TP (ed): *Current Controversies in Neurosurgery*. Philadelphia: Saunders, 1976, pp 496–501
58. Wertheimer P, Lecuire J: La myelotomie commissurale posterieure: A propos de 107 observations. *Acta Chir Belg* 52:568–574, 1953
59. Wertheimer P, Santot J: Les resultants de la myelotomie commissurale posterieure. *Concours Medicale* 71:413–414, 1949
60. Woroschiloff C: Der verlanf der motorischen und sensiblen bahnen durch das lendenmark des kannchens. *Ber Verh Sächs Ges Wiss (Leipzig)* 26: 248–304, 1874
61. Zlatos J, Cierny G: Method of determining topometric values of some structures of the human spinal cord. *Appl Neurophysiol* 38:104–109, 1975
62. Zlatos J, Cierny G: Statistical model map of the spinal cord and its use. *Appl Neurophysiol* 38:225–239, 1975

23. THALAMOTOMY FOR PARKINSON'S DISEASE: MICROELECTRODE TECHNIQUE

Ronald R. Tasker
K. Yamashiro
F. Lenz
J. O. Dostrovsky

Surgery is the most effective means for treating disabling tremor in patients with Parkinson's disease. An appropriately placed stereotactic lesion relieves tremor permanently and eliminates or greatly reduces rigidity on the opposite side of the body. Whether bilateral surgery can arrest the progress of the disease is a controversial issue [38, 47].

Selection of Patients

Candidates for surgery are selected from that small portion, perhaps 10%, of all patients with parkinsonism in whom tremor is severe. Akinesia, which responds dramatically to therapy with L-dopa and not at all to surgery, is often less pronounced in such patients. Indeed, they often appear to have an unusually slowly progressing and "less malignant" form of the disease. Yet tremor shows a disappointing response to L-dopa, either failing to be adequately relieved by large doses, or intermittently "breaking through" during the day, or alternating with periods of dopa-induced dyskinesia, depending on the drug regimen used. In addition, many patients with severe tremor lack the proper indications for its use, especially if their tremor is not adequately controlled. The long-term use of L-dopa is expensive, fraught with complications, and may be destined to fail. It is not widely known that the surgical lesion that relieves parkinsonian tremor also prevents dopa dyskinesia on the contralateral side of the body.

Surgery should be considered only if simpler therapy has failed. In deciding whether to operate, the likely gains in relief of disability should be weighed against the risks of the operation. Also, it must be determined that tremor, and not akinesia, is the disabling feature of the disease, interfering with important manual skills, very occasionally with gait or stance. Tremor must be more than just a psychosocial embarrassment. It is essential to dispel the notion, often secretly held by the patient, that surgery will accomplish more than the control of tremor and rigidity.

Stereotactic surgery also controls rigidity, although rigidity rarely is disabling: the helpless, rigid-looking patient with parkinsonism is nearly always akinetic and may not benefit from surgery. Surgical treatment of Parkinson's disease is contraindicated in the following patients for fear their deficits will worsen: (1) those with chronic progressive or potentially fatal diseases, (2) those with bleeding diatheses, (3) those with deterioration of higher intellectual function, and (4) those with episodes of organic brain syndrome unexplained by drug toxicity (over and above the mild forgetfulness of words and names and the antisocial self-consciousness so typical of Parkinson's dis-

Supported in part by PSI Foundation of Ontario, Parkinson Foundation of Canada, and the Medical Research Council of Canada.

L.D. Lunsford (ed.) *MODERN STEREOTACTIC NEUROSURGERY*. Copyright © 1988.
Martinus Nijhoff Publishing. Boston/Dordrecht/Lancaster. All rights reserved.

ease). Patients deemed unsuitable for surgery for any of these reasons often show slow wave patterns on their electroencephalograms (EEGs). Hypertension, the incidence of which is reduced in patients with Parkinson's disease, has not been a contraindication in the authors' experience. It is possible to carry out successful thalamotomy on patients into their mid-seventies, other things being equal, although after age 70, the general risks increase.

Finally, one still sees occasionally, though increasingly less often, patients with Parkinson's disease who are relatively young, or whose disease truly is limited to one-half of the body, or who have obviously spontaneously arrested parkinsonism (in the authors' experience, always unilateral). The cause of Parkinson's disease in these patients is presumably encephalitis. If tremor is a major problem in such patients, surgery is the treatment of choice; within about a year after surgery they appear (and will remain) essentially normal.

History of Microelectrode Technique in Thalamotomy

Spiegel and Wycis introduced human stereotactic surgery by combining radiological localization with the use of the stereotactic frame; it then became possible to perform Russell Meyers' procedure of surgically removing the globus pallidus much more safely and effectively by stereotactic means. Hassler and Riechert and, at the same time, Cooper then demonstrated that a lesion in the ventrolateral nucleus of the thalamus, which receives projections from the globus pallidus, was even more effective than pallidotomy in controlling dyskinesias.

Despite the guidance of the stereotactic frame and ventriculography, the anatomy of human brains proved variable within the fabric of the brain; thus, physiological corroboration of the target site was also necessary for optimal results. At first, attempts were made to use deep EEG recordings for this purpose, but eventually most surgeons began to rely on macrostimulation. They watched for stimulation-induced conscious sensory effects in order to demarcate and to avoid the ventrobasal complex. They searched for the zone in which stimulation suppressed tremor, a target area just rostral to the ventrobasal complex. Subsequently, the use of evoked potential recordings was explored. Finally Albe-Fessard and Guiot introduced the use of microelectrode recording [1–6, 16].

During the same period, a variety of techniques was used to produce lesions: destructive chemical agent injections, small leukotomes, and cold. Eventually, most surgeons settled on radiofrequency heat lesions as the most effective means of destroying the neurons apparently responsible for tremor. The alternative of implanting a long-term stimulating electrode at the target site recently has become available for patients in whom the risks of creating lesions are best avoided [47].

The Surgical Target in Parkinsonism—Macrostimulation

It is customary to describe the target for the relief of parkinsonian tremor in terms of the anterior commissure (AC)–posterior commissure (PC) line and the sagittal plane at a site remarkably constant among different surgeons [32]. Because of anatomical variations among individuals, however, such descriptions can be considered only approximations to be verified physiologically. In our experience, the usual target for controlling the typical disabling tremor in the dominant hand of a victim of Parkinson's disease is, in nucleus ventralis intermedius (V.i.m.) 15 mm from midline, a few millimeters above the intercommissural line, and just rostral to the manual digital tacile area. Individual variation from the radiologically identified site is less than 1 mm in 40%–50% of patients, 1–2 mm in 25%–40%, and more than 2 mm in the rest [50]. The accuracy of stereotactic equipment is usually ±1 mm. Although 2–3 mm may not seem like much, the possibility of such an error in any one of three planes is a substantial obstacle in the operating room, particularly when a microelectrode is used.

The physiological identity of the V.i.m. target can only be conjectured. Though there are some convincing data, it is still uncertain whether the lesion destroys tremor pacemakers or interrupts a long loop whose pathological activity is responsible for the tremor [8–10, 13, 29, 32, 33, 35, 38, 39, 43, 44, 50, 52]. Because lesions at the same target are also effective in controlling a variety of dyskinesias besides parkinsonian tremor [50], no specific relationship can be implied between these target cells and the tremor with which they are involved. The target cells must be involved not only in tremor but also in a variety of other dyskinetic disorders, all of which are susceptible to surgical control by a lesion at the same site. They are simply part of a motor control apparatus capable of similar participation in diverse conditions.

An understanding of the function of the target area is revealed by studies of macrostimulation. For this purpose, we have used extensively a concentric bipolar stimulating electrode about 1.1 mm in diameter and 0.5 mm in pole separation. The technique includes using current-monitored threshold stimulation with 60-Hz negative square waves of 3-msec duration delivered by a Grass stimulator* [47–50]. Most significant responses occur at less than 0.5 mA; at this level, the computed spread of effective current extends to 2 mm. We found that the usual target lay just rostral to sites in which such macrostimulation-induced paresthesias referred to contralateral lips or hand. Stimulating the target area itself with parameters similar to those eliciting the paresthesias often somatotopically produced contralateral conscious sensory effects which suggested motor connotations: a sense of pulling, tightening, drawing, or pressure, and rarely of "negative" motor effects such as weakness, heaviness, or fatigue. We interpreted these responses, also seen by others, as arising from stimulation of muscle-afferent pathways. These may include the spindle-afferent pathway, which Goto and co-workers consider one of the conscious somatosensory tracts [15], and which, animal studies indicate, traverses this area [36]. Somewhat rostral to such effects, we often elicited unusual motor effects, different from the more familiar tetanization. These we construed as arising from transsynaptic activation of the corticospinal tract through stimulation of dentatothalamic fibers. Such motor responses, seen both in humans and in experimental animals, occur with the onset of a train of stimulation and do not continue during the train. Moreover, voluntary movement is not impaired once the original "on" effect subsides. Such motor "on" responses appear to arise in the rostral V.i.m. and ventral oral posterior (VOP) nuclei. On occasion, we also elicited a totally different type of response in V.i.m. with similar parameters of stimulation, though not so sharply localized—a sense of rotation of the whole body or nonspecific dizziness, faintness, or nausea—which were thought to be caused by activation of the rostral vestibulothalamic tract through the V.i.m. [26]. All these observations seemed logical; nevertheless, we were surprised that the sensory motor, motor "on," and vestibular responses were seen so much less frequently than the paresthetic responses. Although such responses are useful in localizing certain areas in the thalamus, and thereby surgical targets, some other macrostimulation-induced effects locate the surgical target more definitely. Macrostimulation nearly always alters tremor in patients with parkinsonism at sites where sensory motor, motor "on," and vestibular effects occur (rostral to the paresthetic effects in the ventrobasal complex). Tremor was arrested or suppressed at 73% of sites and driven at 27%, precisely marking the location of an effective lesion. In nonparkinsonian tremor, such stimulation effects the tremor in only 38% of patients, driving it in 67%. We have not frequently used rates other than 60 Hz for macrostimulation, but we believe that 300-Hz stimulation alters dyskinesias much more often, usually suppressing them.

History of Microelectrode Recording in Thalamotomy

Albe-Fessard and Guiot made several interesting observations while using microelectrodes [1–6, 16]: (1) They were able to identify the somatosensory cells of the ventrobasal complex by virtue of the receptive fields of the cells and the quality of their effective stimulus; (2) they discovered "tremor cells" that appeared to fire in bursts synchronous with the patient's tremor; and (3) they learned that the effective lesion should be made just rostral to ventrobasal responses for tremor of lip or manual digits. This target was approximately 14–15 mm from the midline in an area inhabited by "tremor cells" and was just rostral to the site where slow waves, recorded from their semimicroelectrodes in response to tactile stimuli, reversed polarity as the electrode was advanced from posterior to anterior. These exciting discoveries inspired several investigators to begin using microelectrode technique for guiding stereotactic operations [7, 13, 28, 35].

Bertrand, Jasper, Hardy, and their associates reported very sophisticated studies of human thalamic neurons [8–10, 17–23]. These investi-

* Grass Instrument Co., Quincy, MA

gators identified a core of tactile cells located inferiorly and caudally in the ventrobasal complex; rostral to this area were cells responding to pressure, followed by kinesthetic cells responding to tendon stretching and musculoskeletal compression. Even further rostral were voluntary cells that fired only in relationship to a specific contralateral voluntary act. Three types of tremor cells were identified: (1) those that had no particular features but were prevalent in the lateral thalamus in patients with Parkinson's disease; (2) those clearly evoked by tremor because they were kinesthetic; and (3) those that were not evoked yet were tremor-synchronous and were located in the voluntary cell zone. These last cells were considered to be autonomous "tremor cells" and possibly "tremor pacemakers." Therapeutic lesions should be designed to destroy these tremor-synchronous cells.

Narabayashi and Ohye and co-workers concluded that the target should be the kinesthetic tremor cells, which were thought to be the large cells seen histologically in the area [14, 26, 38–44], and that a carefully positioned lesion of no more than 40 cubic mm could permanently abolish parkinsonian tremor.

Although we have used microelectrode recording of thalamic neurons during stereotactic surgery for ten years, it has been a routine part of our procedures only in the last four. Two years ago, we replaced macrostimulation with microstimulation, using the microelectrode from which selected deep evoked potentials also are recorded.

Stereotaxis

The procedure is performed in two stages: radiological localization with the patient under general anesthesia, and physiological localization with the placement of lesions under local anesthesia [50].

The first stage is performed with the computed tomography (CT)-compatible Leksell frame applied to the head with four skull pins. The distance these pins project beyond the frame is measured to allow future repositioning without repeated imaging. With the patient supine, a burr hole is made at about the level of the coronal suture, ipsilateral to the target, and the same distance from the midline as the intended target, so that exploratory electrode trajectories will be parasagital and therefore more easily mapped. With lateral imaging, a brain needle is introduced into the lateral ventricle, and a small quantity of air is injected to outline the foramen of Monro. A plastic brain cannula is introduced through the foramen of Monro and monitored with a C-arm image intensifer. A drop of positive contrast medium is administered to outline the PC. X (anterior-posterior) and Y (superior-inferior) coordinates of the PC are now determined by aligning the cross wires of plastic inserts that fit into the side bars of the Leksell frame. The inserts are at identical settings on both sides of the frame, so that the images of the PC are superimposed on those of the two sets of cross wires (figure 23–1, B). The Z (left-right) coordinate is determined by superimposing the images of plastic bars (applied to the back and front of the frame) with cross-wire riders identically positioned on one another and on the midline of the posterior third ventricle. The patient now is placed in the semisitting position, and a specially designed clamp is used to fix the Leksell frame to the operating table. The patient's head is flexed somewhat; if necessary, additional contrast medium is given until the AC is outlined (figure 23–1, A). The X, Y, and Z coordinates are determined in the same way as for the PC. With access to a high-quality CT scanner, the coordinates of the AC and PC can be read directly from the CT scan (figure 23–2).

The coordinates are supplied to a computer graphics program that generates hard copies adapted from the sagittal plates of the Schaltenbrand and Bailey atlas at four times natural size [24]. The atlas brain outlines for the patient's frame position can be shrunk or stretched in the anterior-posterior direction to ensure that the intercommissural distance conforms to that of the patient (figure 23–3).

At the second stage of the procedure, the patient is supine and comfortably placed in a lounge chair position. The frame is reapplied to the skull in precisely the same position used in phase one. The burr-hole incision is infiltrated with local anesthesia but not opened. The appropriate sagittal diagram containing the target (usually 15 mm from midline for parkinsonian tremor) is chosen and the target selected, usually in the center of the inferior third of the V.i.m. and 2–4 mm above the intercommissural line. The X and Y coordinates are read from the computer-generated diagram and set on the frame. Usually, a secondary target is chosen 2 mm posterior to this in the ventrocaudal (VC) nucleus. A hollow tube with a stylet is used; it must be large enough to accept the microelectrode and have the same outer diameter as the lesion-making electrode. Both are fitted with length markers so that when passed into the brain, mounted via the arc of the Leksell frame, they will stop at the center of the sphere described by rotation of the arc. By virtue of geometry with the X, Y, and Z coordinates set, the electrode reaches the intended target. The lesion-making electrode is positioned so that the center of its 3-mm bare tip is at the target while the introductory cannula for the microelectrode is drawn back, usually 10 mm superficial to the target. This ensures that the microelectrode will traverse this distance through the brain. The microelectrode is driven by a hydraulic microdrive with calibrations that determine the position of the microelectrode tip at any time during the operation. A longer trajectory risks bending the microelectrode. The angular coordinates are read from the frame and recorded at each position, which enables the surgeon to plot the (virtually parasagittal) trajectory of approach to target. On the computer-generated brain diagram, the surgeon calculates the deviation of the electrode from the parasagittal plane over the distance along which the trajectory is explored; this deviation is 0.5 mm or less within 5 mm of the target, if the medial-lateral deviation is the usual 5° or less from perfectly parasagittal. At the same time, the trajectory is plotted on a large sheet of paper at a magnification of 50 times to facilitate hand-plotting of the microelectrode-recording data.

Microelectrode

The microelectrode consists of a platinum-iridium wire electrolytically etched to 3–4 microns, then insulated with sintered glass to an impedance of 2–4 megohms at 1,000 Hz. Occasionally, a tungsten wire is used instead. The distal 1 cm is sheared off and inserted in a 26-gauge stainless steel tube insulated with polyamide (Capton-Niemad Industries, New York). The junction between glass and polyamide is insulated with epoxylite, and the whole assembly is cut to length. The microelectrode then is put into a stainless steel carrier tube that has a set screw at the upper end to lock the electrode in place. Before being sterilized with gas for use in the operating room, the microelectrode tip is plated with platinum to reduce its impedance to 100,000 500,000 ohm and still retain its microscopic size. The microelectrode assembly is fitted to a modified hydraulic microdrive (David Kopf Instruments, CA), which incorporates a high impedance preamplifier. The microelectrode is inserted into the stereotactically positioned electrode guide and advanced with the microdrive after the set screw is released. Knowing the stereotactic location of the guide-tube tip and the microdrive reading at which the microelectrode tip extrudes from its guide tube, the surgeon can accurately follow and plot the progress of the microelectrode tip through the brain.

Data Processing

The output of the preamplifier is fed into an amplifier, displayed on an oscilloscope, and stored on tape. The signal is also relayed to the operating room by a delay-line circuit and storage oscilloscope, the output of which is also stored on tape. Either the raw or discriminated signal is fed into an audio amplifier. Up to eight channels of electromyogram (EMG) are recorded and monitored on an oscilloscope; five of these channels can be recorded on the tape along with a voice record.

The tape is studied off-line to verify observations made in the operating room. It also can be used for various investigations of tremor synchrony and latency and for studies of cross-correlation between neuronal and EMG activity. Histogram analysis of discriminated cells is performed by aligning all records to EMG onset during repetition of a voluntary movement. Baseline thalamic cell firing is calculated from the first eight bins. A significant response is defined as greater than the mean plus two standard deviations. The cumulative sum and change of slope of cumulative sum are computed to identify increased neuronal firing related to, and in advance of, the EMG in voluntary movement. Cross-correlation analyses of tremor cells and EMG activity are performed by examining neuron spike auto power at tremor frequencies and coherence function between thalamic firing and the EMG. Latency between thalamic firing and EMG activity is measured by averaging EMG activity in rela-

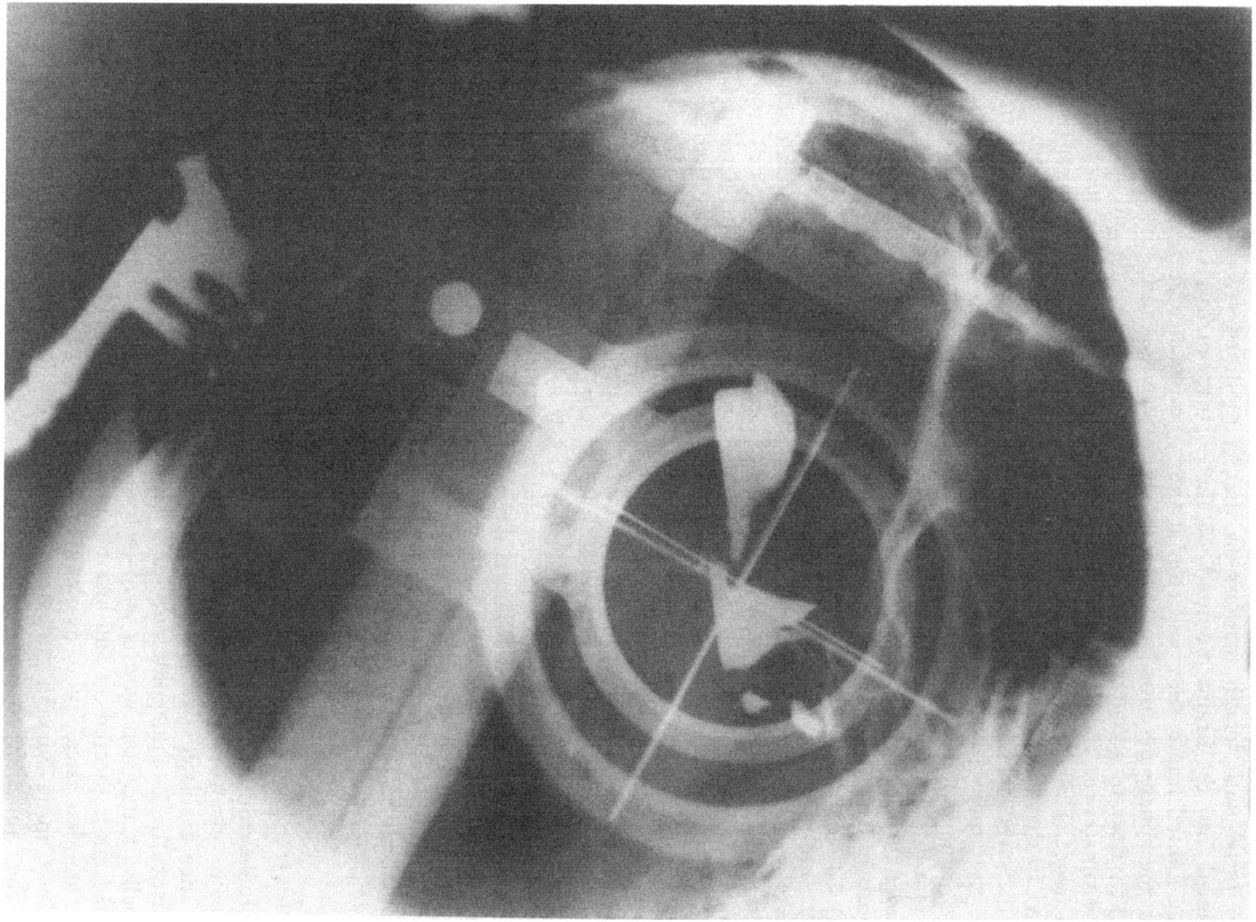

FIGURE 23–1. Positive-contrast ventriculogram outlining the posterior commissure (A) and anterior commissure (B). Superimposed are images of the cross wires of plastic inserts fitted into the Leksell frame side bars and identically positioned on both sides. The X and Y frame coordinates are read directly.

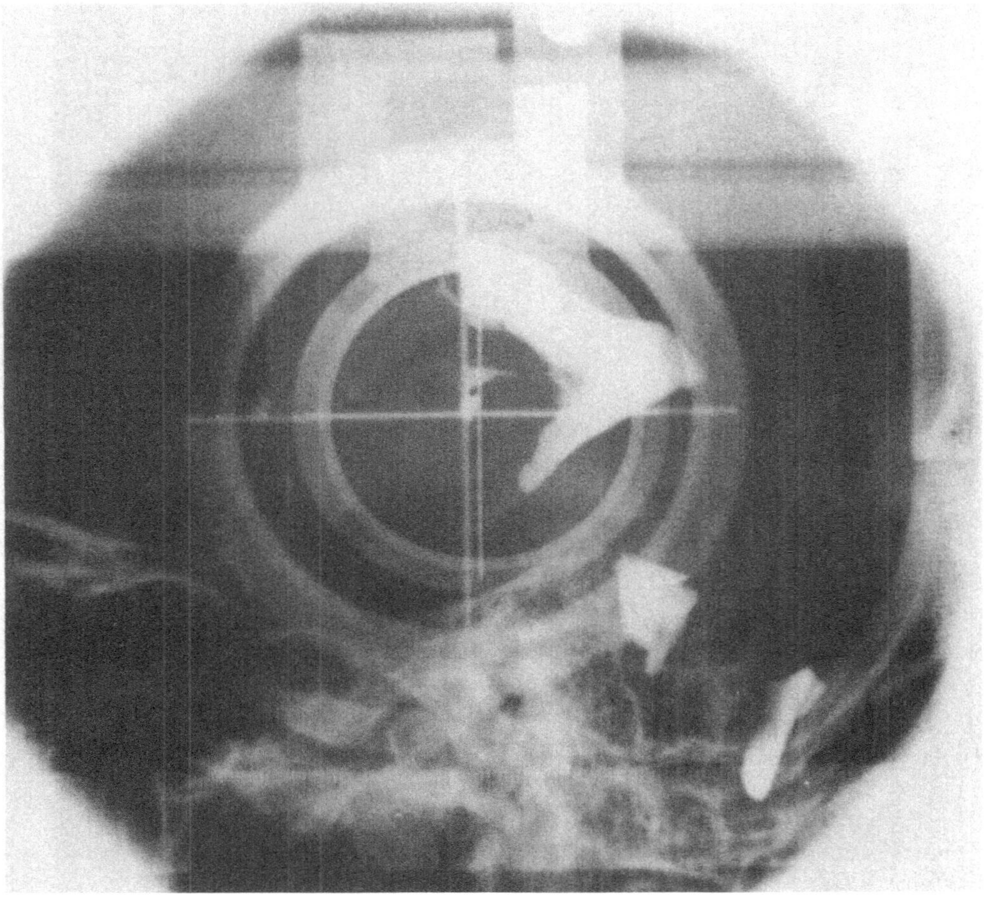

B
FIGURE 23-1. (cont.)

tion to the occurrence of thalamic action potentials [32–34].

We use only a microelectrode that can record action potentials and that is sophisticated enough to discriminate unit recordings. Ohye has demonstrated that such fine electrodes, by virtue not only of their impedance but also their tiny tip size, are less suited for assessing background activity than is a semi-microelectrode of similar or slightly smaller impedance but larger tip geometry [39]. He measured background activity with an integrating circuit connected to a "noise meter" and was able to recognize certain brain structures by their "noise signature" as the semi-microelectrode traversed them. This feature enabled Ohye to locate the "ballpark" somatosensory and tremor cells. The microelectrode we use is less effective for this purpose but better equipped to zero in on the "players" once the "ball park" is entered; it also allows rigorous physiological off-line analyses.

If anatomical variation among patients did not exist, the microelectrode directed towards the V.i.m. would always record a series of tremor, kinesthetic, and voluntary cells with the appropriate responses to microstimulation and evoked potential recording; the microelectrode proceeding to the VC nucleus would pass through a fringe of tremor and kinesthetic cells and enter a zone of tactile cells. Unfortunately, at least half of the patients do not conform to the expected pattern, and the actual sequence of observed events may differ from that expected. When this occurs, another trajectory must be selected. On the basis of the imaging

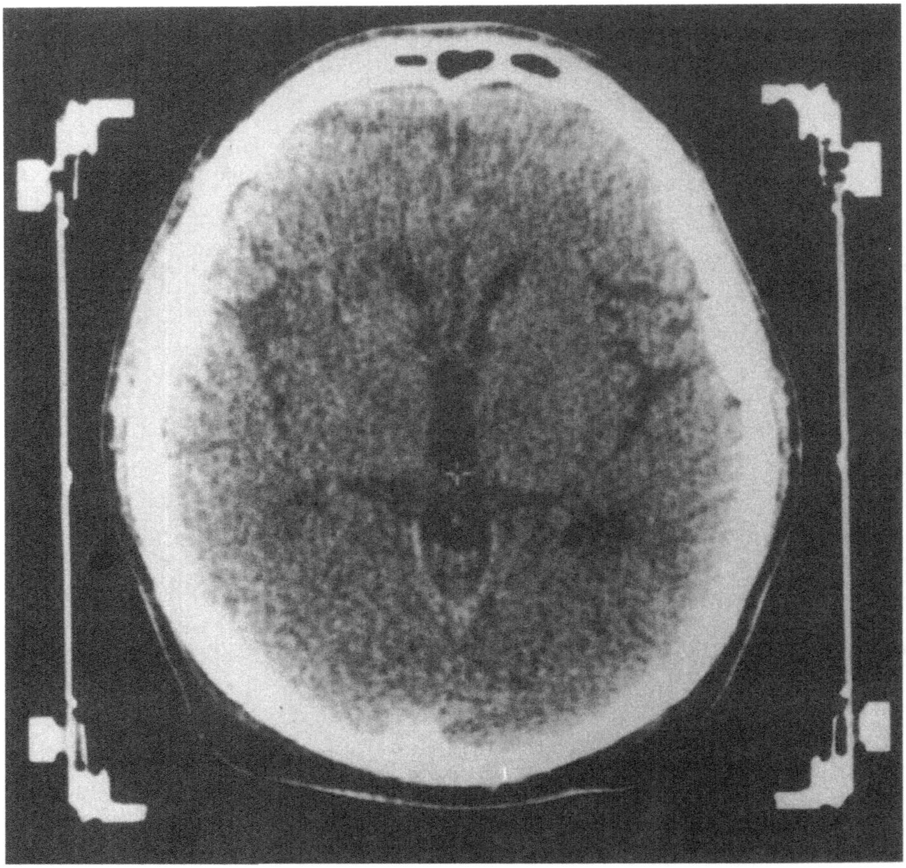

A

FIGURE 23–2. Identification of the posterior commissure (A) and anterior commissure (B) by CT using the CT-compatible Leksell frame. The locations of the commissures and of the six fiducial bars on either side of the frame allow the X, Y, and Z coordinates to be read directly from the CT images.

and the trajectories studied thus far, this trajectory will carry the microelectrode tip into either the V.i.m. or VC nucleus. When deviation in a patient is great, this can be a tedious process that is mitigated by the Ohye technique of using a "noise meter."

The microelectrode is advanced cautiously just into brain until the electrical activity of neurons is recognized, which ensures the integrity of the electrode. At the beginning of the extrusion, the microelectrode tip usually lies near the dorsum of the ventral tier of thalamic nuclei. Unitary activity is studied at 0.5-mm intervals, and microstimulation is carried out with the same electrode after recording at each particular site is completed. Microstimulation is performed with manually controlled trains of usually 300 Hz (0.1–0.2 msec duration up to 120 microamperes); manually controlled trains of negative square waves from a Grass S8 stimulator are used. After the microstimulation or, retrospectively, at the conclusion of the trajectory, evoked potentials are recorded with a four-channel Nicollet CA 1000 averager at selected sites. The same microelectrode is used, and stimulation is performed at either the contralateral median or the tibial nerve.

During microrecording, spontaneous activity is observed, particularly for bursts of neural firing at tremor frequencies. It is noted whether these bursts occur only when there is peripheral tremor or whether they appear to be

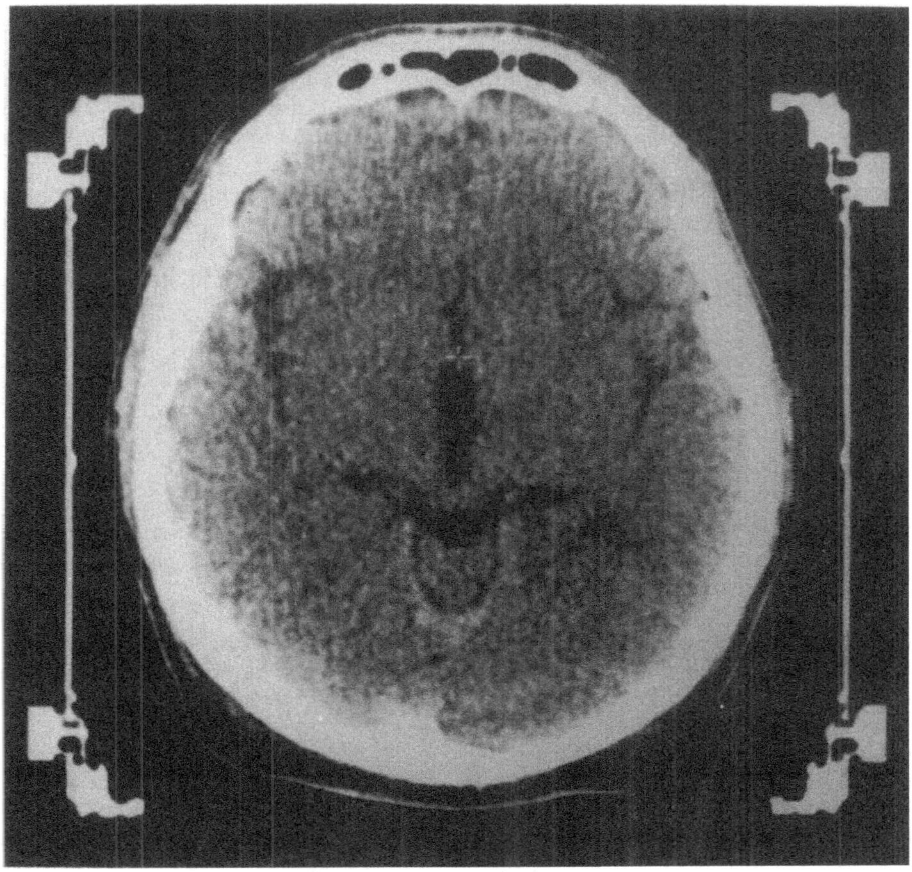

B

FIGURE 23–2. (cont.)

synchronous with such tremor. Samples of activity plus five channels of EMG are stored for later analysis.

Activity and response to superficial or deep tactile stimuli, muscle squeeze, joint stretching, or voluntary activity is elicited, and receptive fields are plotted; responses are categorized as either rapidly adapting or slowly adapting. Taped records are analyzed later to determine relationships among stimuli, EMG activity, latency, and timing with respect to voluntary EMG.

Microstimulation is carried out at threshold to detect the presence of the following perceived responses: paresthesias; a sense of muscular activity occurring without movement (monitored on the EMG); temperature-coded somatosensory effects; sound; a sense of dizziness, faintness, or rotation. The surgeon notes the effects on tremor and determines whether movement is induced, either typical tetanization or motor "on" effects. The microelectrode is advanced, and data are collected until the previously described target is defined.

Potentials evoked by median nerve stimulation in the inferior half to two-thirds of the VC show well-defined P15 and N19 waves; we found the former to be of thalamic origin [7]. This evoked-potential pattern shows rapid attenuation in all directions outside the VC nucleus.

Lesion Production

After the target site has been adjusted on the basis of the physiological studies, the lesion is made. The lesion is designed to destroy the inferior 5 mm of the V.i.m. serving the hand. The electrode has a 1.1-mm outer diameter and is insulated except for its 3-mm tip (Diros

Technology Inc., 965 Page Ave., Toronto, Canada, M4K 3V6). The lesion is made with radiofrequency current from the OWL cordotomy system (Diros Technology). For lesion production, the low, rather than the high, output mode is employed. Starting at 35 mA for 60 seconds of current flow, the lesion is enlarged cautiously. Current is gradually increased to 60–80 mA. Current should not be increased because the lesion would become too large. During lesion placement, the patient is tested continually for the onset of finger-to-nose ataxia, subjective numbness, and dysarthria. If untoward effects appear, lesion production is stopped at once. The procedure can continue if the paresthesias are reported at the onset of current flow, but soon end spontaneously while current is flowing.

If precisely positioned, the resulting single lesion (3 × 3–4 × 4 mm in diameter or 15–35 mm^3, according to warm-egg-albumin experiments) should suffice to control parkinsonian tremor and reduce rigidity. Inadequate control or premature termination of lesion placement because of side effects results from less-than-optimum siting and requires repositioning of the electrode and repetition of the lesion-making process. If tremor control in the lower extremity is required, lateral extension of the lesion may be necessary, unless the original physiological localization included "leg" cells.

At the conclusion of the procedure, the positions of the skull pins are recorded and the frame removed. The incision is sutured to prevent cerebrospinal fluid leakage. The patient is observed for six to eight hours or until stable, after which medication is resumed. Immediately after surgery, the patient is warned and protected against falling because of the contralateral hypotonia frequently induced by the lesion. Hypotonia usually subsides in a few days. In 10% of cases, tremor recurs up to two to three months postoperatively. Recurrence of tremor may necessitate enlargement of the lesion.

Table 23–1 summarizes our experience with microelectrode recording in the thalamus and compares these results with those of microstimulation using the same electrode at the same sites [32–34, 47, 48].

Tactile Cells

Tactile cells are located most posteriorly in the inferior one-half to three-quarters of the VC nucleus and presumably represent the lemniscal thalamic relay. These cells respond to either superficial pressure (light cotton wisps) or deep pressure (tapping or stroking) in (usually) discrete, contralateral small receptive fields. (Occasionally, perioral sites will produce ipsilateral responses.) Such neuronal representation is most commonly found periorally or in the digits, where receptive fields are smallest (some only a few millimeters in diameter). We believe that deep tactile cells lie rostral to superficial cells, but we have not been able to confirm this statistically. Once encountered in a parasagittal trajectory, these tactile cells show a remarkable monotony of somatotopic representation. Cells extending as far as 5 mm on a parasagittal trajectory have similar or overlapping receptive fields. However, a 1–2 mm shift of trajectory into a new sagittal plane may produce quite striking somatotopic changes. The somatotopographic arrangement, at least for the face and upper-limb digits (which are represented inferiorly in the nucleus), appears to be in the form of parasagittal books of medially to laterally arranged lamellae, which are convex laterally.

Microstimulation at sites where 200 such tactile cells were recorded (whether superficial or deep, at thresholds as low as 3–4 μA at 100–300 Hz and 0.1 msec) induced paresthetic responses in 157 cells. These sites usually referred to the same area on the body as the cells' receptive fields. The quality of induced response was described as painful by six patients, burning by three, pressure or stretching by 16, and warm or cold by four. Based on animal studies, such cells are likely to be located in the ventrobasal complex in the lemniscal relay. It is important to identify this region, which probably extends no more than 2–4 mm anteroposteriorly, 4 mm medially to laterally, and 4–5 mm dorsoventrally. A lesion to control manual tremor should be placed just rostral to the tactile finger area, but it should not invade this area because of the risk of causing sensory loss.

Kinesthetic Cells

Immediately rostral to the area containing tactile cells is a small zone of units that respond to passive joint movement and muscle belly squeezing but not to cutaneous stimulation. (The two types do not appear to be spatially separated from one another.) The response

TABLE 23–1. Results of Microrecording and Microstimulation During Stereotactic Thalamotomy

Microrecording	Microstimulation	Anatomical Site	Probable Structure
Tactile unit RA, SA, responding to light touch	Paresthesias same as RF of tactile unit	Inferior VC	Lemniscal relay
Tactile unit responding to deep stimuli RA, SA	Paresthesias same as RF of tactile unit	Inferior VC,? rostral to superficial tactile	Lemniscal relay
Kinesthetic unit responding to muscle belly squeeze or tendon, joint stretch RA or SA	Paresthesias or sense of movement	Inferior V.i.m.	Lemninscal relay, ? + spindle afferent
Kinesthetic unit with evoked tremor synchronous activity	Paresthesias or sense of movement + tremor reduction or arrest	Inferior V.i.m.	Lemniscal relay, ? + spindle afferent
Voluntary cell	Motor "on" effect	Inferior?, rostral V.i.m., VOP	? Dentatothalamic tract to Betz cells
Voluntary cell plus RF	? Motor "on" effect	Inferior?, rostral V.i.m., VOP	? Dentatothalamic tract to Betz cells
Voluntary cell with tremor synchrony	Motor "on" effect + tremor reduction or arrest	Inferior?, rostral V.i.m.	? Dentatothalamic tract to Betz cells
Bursting cell, not tremor rate or tremor synchronous	None	Throughout V.i.m.	Unknown
Tremor rate, not synchronous	None	Throughout V.i.m.	Unknown
Axons	Paresthesias, larger fields	Medial lemniscus	Medial lemniscus
Axons, ? small cells	Hot, cold, sometimes paresthetic effects to lower limb, trunk	Inferior rim of VC, ? V.i.m. adjacent to medial geniculate	? Spinothalamic tract
Auditory cells (contralateral RF)	Low-pitched sound	Medial geniculate	Primary auditory path
Not recognized	Faint, dizzy, rotatory	V.i.m.	Rostral vestibulothalamic path

RA = rapidly adapting; SA = slowly adapting; RF = receptive field; VC = ventrocaudal nucleus of thalamus; V.i.m. = ventral intermediate nucleus of thalamus; VOP = ventral oral posterior nucleus of thalamus.

may be tonic or phasic, as indeed the tactile cells may be, and is elicited from a part of the body somatotopically similar to the tactile cells that are immediately caudal. This somatotopic arrangement seems to be similar to that of tactile cells. Microstimulation was performed at 41 sites where such cells were recorded and produced the following responses: paresthesias in parts of the body similar to the receptive fields at 23 sites; a feeling of muscle movement or stretching at three; hot, cold, or burning effects at three; and motor "on" effects at four.

In patients with Parkinson's disease or other types of tremor, these kinesthetic cells are potential tremor cells, firing with evoked rhythmic patterns at rates rigorously synchronous with peripheral tremor. (In our experience, this is not true for patients without tremor.) Studies of discriminated kinesthetic neurons show a high degree of autopower at tremor frequencies and tight correlation with tremor recorded in the EMG of upper limb muscles. Tremor appears to be synchronous throughout all upper limb muscles. The evoked tremor activity of these cells stops when the tremor ceases spontaneously or in response to a voluntary movement or tactile stimulus; it then resumes with the degree of synchrony becoming more significant the longer the tremor continues. Microstimulation at the sites of kinesthetic tremor cells alters tremor. As frequency of stimulation is increased, an effect first appears at about 20–30 Hz, becoming more pronounced up to 300 Hz, at which point tremor arrest nearly always occurs. When the stimulation train is first applied, it may disrupt or accelerate the tremor pattern. The longer the current flows, the more likely the suppression of the tremor.

We believe that these kinesthetic cells, whether or not they function as tremor cells, lie in the V.i.m., but it is unclear if they are lemniscal cells or if their afferent path is via other routes, such as the spinocerebellar tract. Possibly more than one cell population is involved, some representing lemniscal-kinesthetic cells and others representing spindle-afferent cells.

Voluntary Cells

More rostral to kinesthetic cells lies a narrow zone containing "voluntary cells" that increase or occasionally decrease firing in response to a particular voluntary movement involving contralateral musculature (e.g., protruding the tongue, making a fist, or pointing the index finger). These cells do not respond to passive movement of the same or any other body part, and they appear to be less numerous than kinesthetic cells. The responsible movement involves parts of the body somatotopographically similar to the area related to the kinesthetic and tactile cells located caudal to them. They appear to lie either in the rostral portion of the V.i.m. or the caudal part of the VOP. Analyses of neuronal firing and related EMG show that these cells fire as much as 850 msec in advance of voluntary movement. Microstimulation at sites where voluntary cells are recorded may induce a motor "on" effect involving the muscles that fire them. This suggests that the effect arises from the transsynaptic firing of Betz cells and that the cells are located in the dentatothalamic tract. On other occasions, sensory effects are perceived with motor connotations.

Some voluntary cells are also tremor cells, firing synchronously with, and in advance of, peripheral tremor, which suggests that they may be tremor pacemakers. Microstimulation in areas where voluntary cells are also tremor cells can arrest tremor.

Voluntary Cells With Sensory Fields

Intermingled with voluntary cells are a few cells that have sensory receptive fields in addition to their motor characteristics. Some of these may function as tremor cells in Parkinson's disease. Examination of latencies precludes the possibility that their firing is evoked by the tremor via their sensory input. These cells fire in advance of both the voluntary movement and the EMG of tremor. Their latencies indicate that they could be firing through the corticospinal tract as tremor pacemakers. Therefore, they may have a tremor-generating role. In our experience, the effective lesion for controlling parkinsonian tremor and reducing rigidity encompasses the tremor cells in the kinesthetic and voluntary cell zone of the thalamus.

Other Tremor Cells

Two other types of tremor cells are intermixed with the kinesthetic and voluntary cells and also extend more dorsally in the V.i.m. Some of these fire at tremor frequency but demonstrate neither receptive fields nor association with voluntary movement. Some fire at rates other than tremor frequency. The functions of both groups are difficult to discern.

Other Responses

If the microelectrode trajectory traverses inferoposteriorly past the V.i.m. or the ventrobasal nuclei, additional effects can be recognized. Most neurons that fire in response to contralateral auditory stimuli are encountered in the medial geniculate, where microstimulation produces low-pitched contralateral auditory effects. Between the medial geniculate and the ventrobasal complex lies a small area where microstimulation occasionally produces contralateral feelings of tingling but usually feelings of cold, warmth, or burning. Instead of being referred to the hand or face, as the responses encountered throughout most of the trajectories through the V.i.m. and the ventrobasal nuclei, these responses are referred to the foot, leg, or trunk. Microrecording here reveals small neurons and axons, with occasional fields receptive to pinprick in the same bodily parts as those in which the stimulus-induced effects are produced. Thus, there is an abrupt discontinuity between masses of neurons throughout most of the trajectory and an area with few neurons and mostly axons. The monotonous overlapping of receptive fields involving the face or manual digits is abruptly broken, and responses shift to the lower part of the body.

The quality of response typically changes from paresthesias through the ventrobasal complex to hot, cold, or burning responses in the distal body sites that lie posteroinferiorly. We believe this area corresponds to the spinothalamic relay [50], as reported by Kniffki and Mizumura [30]. More rostrally and medially, deep to ventrobasal neurons, the electrode may enter the medial lemniscus, where neurons are replaced by axons. At this location, paresthetic responses to stimulation persist, often at very low thresholds. However, the responses refer to bodily parts that are larger than those obtained in the VC nucleus but are otherwise similar. If the electrode is advanced still further through the medial geniculate, as the electrode tip impinges on the pia of dorsal brain stem, the patient may feel deep aching that can be referred to the ipsilateral eye or forehead [50].

It is useful to explain the microelectrode technique with reference to a particular patient.

Case History

A 48-year-old woman noted tremor in her right index finger two years before surgery. The tremor steadily spread throughout her hand and, one year before surgery, to the left hand and slightly to the left lower limb. Though right-handed, she began using her left hand for tasks requiring dexterity and complained of pain in the right forearm musculature. Constant severe rest tremor was noted in the right upper extremity, especially distally, despite L-dopa therapy. She also had severe rigidity on the right side, especially in the upper extremity and ankle. Tremor and rigidity were less marked in the left upper extremity. Repetitive manual skills were severely impaired on the right, much less so on the left; handwriting was impossible with either hand. Gait and stance were well preserved, although she exhibited "petit pas" on turning. She had no spontaneous arm swing and carried the right upper extremity in a dystonic posture.

Figure 23–3 (upper panel) shows the computer-generated operative diagram described

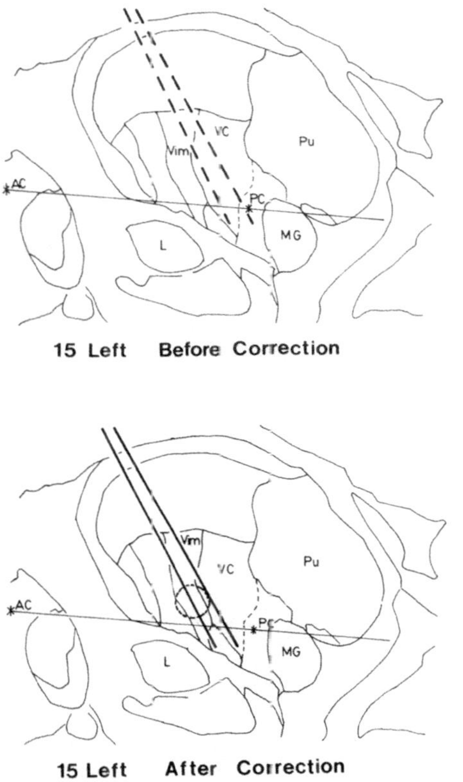

FIGURE 23–3. *Top*: Computer-generated diagram of the thalamus in 15-mm sagittal plane, prepared on the basis of radiologically located anterior and posterior commissures. Pu = pulvinar, L = corpus Luysii, MG = medial geniculate nucleus. The left (anterior) hatched line represents an electrode trajectory ending in rostral VC nucleus, as located by ventriculography, where manual tactile neurons would have been expected. Instead (see figure 23–4), responses more typical of the V.i.m. were found in this trajectory, and a second trajectory (right, more posterior hatched line) was explored, which yielded responses expected in the first.
Bottom: The two trajectories above have been replotted, each 2 mm more rostrally (to the left), so that recorded physiological responses now match anatomical structures. Thus, the lesion to control tremor (hatched circle 1.5–2.0 mm in radius) must be placed 2 mm more caudally than the site selected by radiological localization alone.

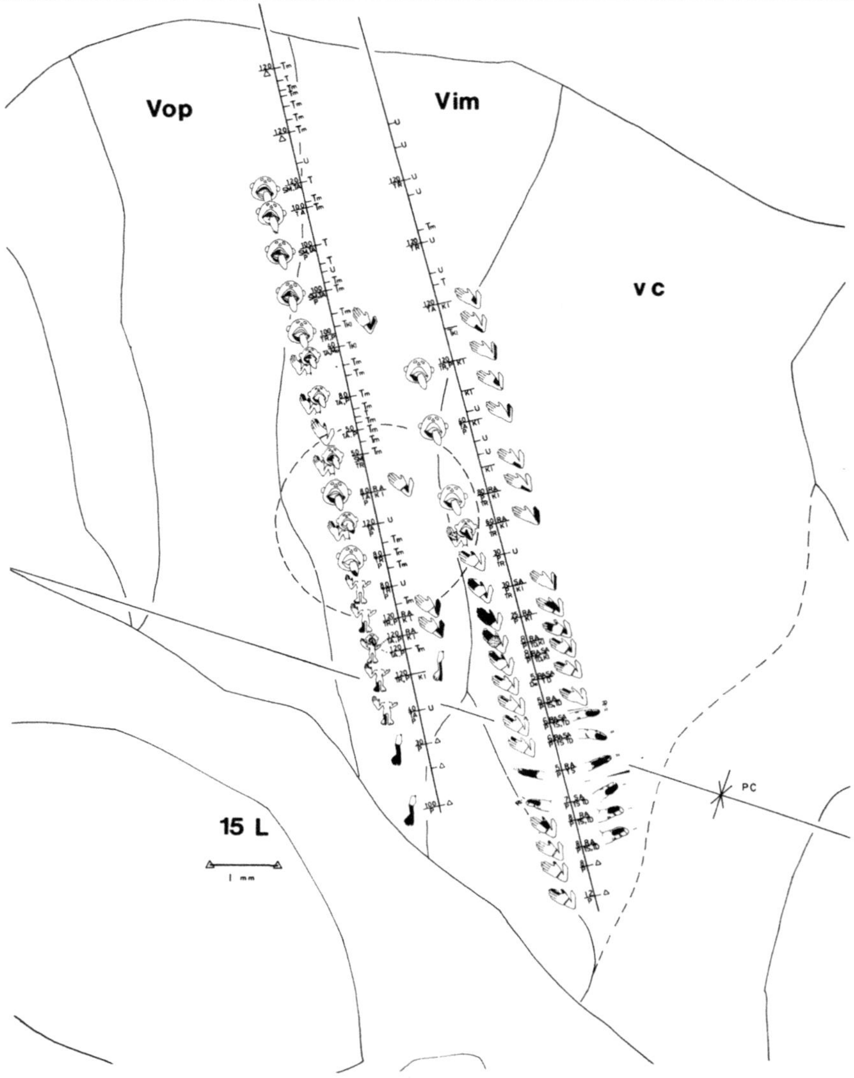

FIGURE 23–4. Physiological data collected along two trajectories (from figure 23–3, bottom) by microelectrode recording (*right*) and microstimulation (*left*), plotted 2 mm anteriorly to (to left of) actual recording sites, so that data conform to anatomical structures. Lesion site and size are indicated by hatched circle. (See scale, lower left.) In the superior portions of both trejectories (in V.i.m.) many tremor cells T = not synchronous with EMG; (Tm = synchrons with EMG) are seen; some that are located inferiorly also have receptive fields to kinesthetic stimuli (KI). At many tremor cell sites, microstimulation (threshold indicated in microamperes to the left of each trajectory) induced sensations of muscle contraction without any actual movement (SM) and also caused tremor arrest (TA) or reduction (TR). One motor "on" site affecting the thumb is seen in the left anterior trajectory in dorsal V.i.m. More inferiorly and posteriorly in the V.i.m., stimulation induced paresthesias (P) even at sites where kinesthetic (KI) cells were recorded. In the more caudal (right) trajectory, inferiorly and posteriorly, the kinesthetic and tremor cells were replaced by (first) deep (TD) then superficial (TS) tactile cells that have very discrete receptive fields; this occurred at sites where stimulation induced paresthesias at low thresholds (5–8 A) in bodily areas similar to the receptive fields. Tremor reduction was not seen here. U = unidentified neuron; RA = rapidly adapting; SA = slowly and apting.

earlier, with a target in the rostral part of the VC nucleus and the trajectory (rostral dotted line) with which it was explored. Figure 23–4 illustrates the responses obtained with microstimulation and microrecording. Figure 23–5 demonstrates the results of evoked potential recordings at this site. Expected tactile responses were not found initially, and an additional trajectory was chosen more caudally. The desired tactile effects were recorded (caudal hatched line, figure 23–3, top). These findings indicate that the anatomical target we sought was 2 mm caudal to the site selected on the basis of imaging. In figure 23–3 (bottom), the trajectories have been redrawn 2 mm more rostrally, so that they are now correctly oriented to the anatomical structure. Figure 23–4 shows that the most rostral trajectory does not contain expected tactile cells, but rather tremor and kinesthetic cells and stimulus-induced sensorimotor and tremor-suppressive effects typical of the V.i.m. The second, more caudal trajectory contains occasional tremor and kinesthetic cells typical of the V.i.m. superiorly, with tactile responses typical of the VC inferiorly, along with appropriate stimulus-induced effects. The lesion was placed 2 mm more caudally than the imaging would have suggested (see figures 23–3 and 23–4). The lesion completely and permanently arrested the patient's tremor and rigidity on the contralateral side without complications and restored her ability to perform tasks requiring manual dexterity such as handwriting.

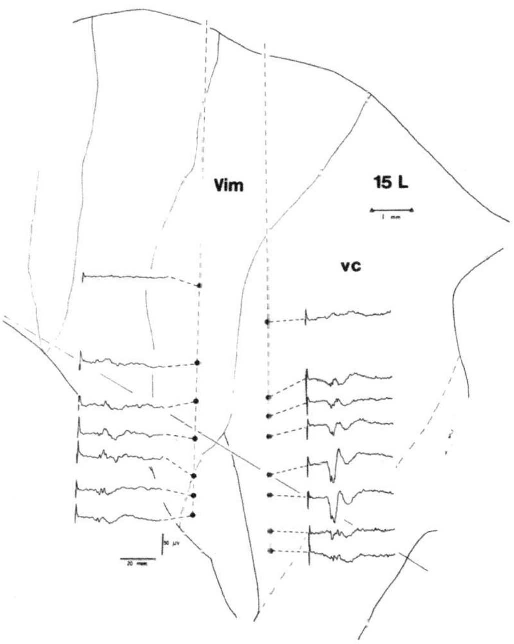

FIGURE 23–5. Same mapping as figure 23–4, showing evoked potential recordings elicited by contralateral median nerve stimulation at various thalamic sites with the same microelectrode used for unit recording and microstimulation. Voltage and time base are shown at lower left. The prominent P15 N19 complex, clearly illustrated, attenuates rapidly outside the inferior VC nucleus.

Results

The relatively recent adoption of microelectrode recording (in the late 1970s), particularly the technique of stimulating and recording evoked potentials with the same microelectrode (in the mid-1980s), has greatly improved the accuracy and reduced the morbidity of our surgical treatment of Parkinson's disease. A prospective study of 75 of 190 cases operated upon unilaterally between 1965 and 1982, chiefly using macrostimulation, revealed that no deaths occurred, and there was only one instance (in 1975) of severe morbidity [51]. This patient sustained a hemorrhage at the lesion site and lost position sense in half of the body.

Three months postoperatively, 71.6% of the patients reviewed were free of contralateral manual digital tremor; another 10.4% were nearly free of this disability. Wrist tremor was eliminated in 74.6% and almost so in 4.5%; 83.6% were free of proximal upper-limb tremor and 11.9% almost so; 92.5% were free of proximal lower-limb tremor and 4.5% nearly free; and 83.6% were relieved of ankle tremor, with 3.0% mostly relieved. During simultaneous rapid contralateral hand patting at this time, rigidity was absent from the hand in 69.9%, from the wrist in 41.3%, from the proximal upper limb in 55.5%, from the proximal lower limb in 61.9%, and from the ankle in 50.8%. Three percent suffered from increased postoperative interference of locomotion caused by dystonic posturing of the ankle. This complication usually developed several days postoperatively, and its cause was uncertain. Significant worsening of speech occurred in 1.3% of these patients. About one-quarter of the patients experienced transient or minor complications, such as subjective numbness of the contralateral corner of the mouth or fingers (12.0%), transient contralateral hypotonia (6.7%), transient neglect or ataxia of the hand (5.3%), transient foot dystonia (2.7%), transient or minor worsening of dysarthria (2.7%), and transient confusion (12.0%). Yasui and colleagues found a similar incidence of hand ataxia in patients undergoing thalamotomy and a much higher rate among patients subjected to subthalamotomy [55].

Conclusion

Thalamic lesions of 30 mm^3 stereotactically placed in the V.i.m. remain the sole reliable means of permanently controlling severe contralateral parkinsonian tremor and, to a lesser extent, rigidity [27]. The location of the lesion site must, however, be corroborated by physiological techniques. The most elegant of these techniques entails locating kinesthetic and voluntary tremor cells for (usually) the dominant hand, just rostral to tactile cells for the same body part. Physiological technique should include microelectrode recording correlated with microstimulation and evoked potential recordings performed at the same sites with the same microelectrode.

References

1. Albe-Fessard D: Electrophysiological methods for the identification of thalamic nuclei. *Z Neurol* 205:15–28, 1973
2. Albe-Fessard D, Arfel G, Derome P, et al: Electrophysiology of the human thalamus with special reference to trigeminal pain. In Hassler R, Walker AE (eds): *Trigeminal Neuralgia: Pathogenesis and Pathophysiology*. Philadelphia: Saunders, 1970, pp 134–148
3. Albe-Fessard D, Arfel G, Derome P, et al: Thalamic unit activity in man. *Electroencephatogr Neurophysiol [Suppl]* 25:132–142, 1967
4. Albe-Fessard D, Arfel G, Guiot G: Activitiés electriques caractéristique de quelques structures cérébrales chez l'homme. *Ann Chir* 17:1185–1214, 1963
5. Albe-Fessard D, Arfel G, Guiot G, et al: Electrophysiological studies of some deep cerebral structures in man. *J Neurol Sci* 13:37–51, 1966
6. Albe-Fessard D, Guiot G, Hardy J: Electrophysiological localization and identification of subcortical structures in man by recording spontaneous and evoked activities. *Electroencephalogr Clin Neurophysiol* 15:1052–1053, 1963
7. Bertrand C, Martinez SN, Hardy J, et al: Stereotactic surgery for Parkinsonism: Microelectrode recording, stimulation, and oriented sections with a leukotome. In Krayenbuhl H, Maspes PE, Sweet WH (eds): *Progress in Neurological Surgery*, Vol 5. Basel: Karger, pp 79–112
8. Bertrand G, Jasper H: Microelectrode recording of unit activity in the human thalamus. *Confin Neurol* 26:205–208, 1965
9. Bertrand G, Jasper H, Wong A: Microelectrode study of the human thalamus: organization in the ventrobasal complex. *Confin Neurol* 29:81–86, 1967
10. Bertrand G, Jasper H, Wong A, et al: Microelectrode recording during stereotactic surgery. *Clin Neurosurg* 16:328–355, 1969
11. Cordeau JP: Further studies on patterns of central unit activity in relation with tremor. *J Neurosurg* 24:213–218, 1966
12. Cordeau JP: Discussion. In Purpura DP, Yahr MD (eds): *The Thalamus*. New York: Columbia, 1966, pp 384–386
13. Crowell RM, Perret E, Siegfried J, et al: "Movement units" and "tremor phasic units" in the human thalamus. *Brain Res* 11:481–488, 1968
14. Fukamachi A, Ohye C, Narabayashi H: Delineation of the thalamic nuclei with a microelectrode in stereotaxic surgery for parkinsonism and cerebral palsy. *J Neurosurg* 39:214–225, 1973
15. Goto a, Kosaka K, Nakamura R, et al: Thalamic potentials from muscle afferents in the human. *Arch Neurol* 19:302–309, 1968
16. Guiot G, Hardy J, Albe-Fessard D: Délimitation précise des structures souscorticales et identification des noyaux thalamiques chez l'homme par l'electrophysiologie stéréotaxique. *Neurochirurgia* (Stuttg) 5:1–18, 1962
17. Hardy TL, Bertrand G, Thompson CJ: Organization and topography of sensory responses in the internal capsule and nucleus ventralis caudalis found during stereotactic surgery. *Appl Neurophysiol* 42:335–351, 1979
18. Hardy TL, Bertrand G, Thompson CJ: Position and organization of thalamic cellular activity during diencephalic recording. *Appl Neurophysiol* 43:18–27, 1980
19. Hardy TL, Bertrand G, Thompson CJ: Position and organization of thalamic cellular activity during diencephalic recording. II. Joint- and muscle-evoked activity. *Appl Neurophysiol* 43:28–36, 1980
20. Hardy TL, Bertrand G, Thompson CJ: Thalamic recordings during stereotactic surgery I. Surgery topography of evoked and nonevoked rhythmic cellular activity. *Appl Neurophysiol* 42:185–197, 1969

21. Hardy TL, Bertrand G, Thompson CJ: Thalamic recordings during stereotactic surgery. II. Location of quick-adapting touch-evoked (novelty) cellular responses. *Appl Neurophysiol* 42:198–202, 1979
22. Hardy TL, Bertrand G, Thompson CJ: Topography of "bilateral-movement-evoked" thalamic cellular activity found during diencephalic recording. *Appl Neurophysiol* 43:67–74, 1980
23. Hardy TL, Bertrand G, Thompson CJ: Touch-evoked thalamic cellular activity: The variable position of the anterior border of somesthetic S1 thalamus and somatotopography. *Appl Neurophysiol* 44:302–313, 1981
24. Hawrylyshyn PA, Rowe IH, Tasker RR, et al: A computer system for stereotactic neurosurgery. *Comput Biol Med* 6:87–95, 1976
25. Hawrylyshyn PA, Rubin AM, Tasker RR, et al: Vestibulothalamic projections in man: A sixth primary sensory pathway. *J Neurophysiol* 41:394–401, 1978
26. Hirai T, Nagaseki Y, Kawashima Y, et al: Large neurons in the thalamic ventrolateral mass in humans and monkeys. *Appl Neurophysiol* 45: 245–250, 1982
27. Hirai T, Shibazaki T, Nakajima G, et al: Minimal effective lesion in the stereotactic treatment of tumor. *Appl Neurophysiol* 42:307–308, 1979
28. Hongell A, Wallin G, Hagbarth KE: Unit activity connected with movement initiation and arousal situations recorded from the ventrolateral nucleus of the human thalamus. *Acta Neurol Scand* 49:681–698, 1973
29. Jasper HH, Bertrand G: Thalamic units involved in somatic sensation and voluntary and involuntary movements in man. In Purpura DP, Yahr MD (eds): *The Thalamus*. New York: Columbia, 1966, pp 365–390
30. Kniffki KD, Mizumura K: Responses of neurons in VPL and VPL-VL region of the cat to algestic stimulation of muscle and tendon. *J Neurophysiol* 49:649–661, 1983
31. Laitinen LV: Brain targets in surgery for Parkinson's disease. *J Neurosurg* 62:349–351, 1985
32. Lenz FA, Tasker RR, Kwan HC, et al: Cross-correlation analysis of thalamic "tremor cells" and EMG activity in patients with Parkinsonian tremor. *Appl Neurophysiol* 48:305–309, 1986
33. Lenz FA, Tasker RR, Kwan HC, et al: Functional classes of "tremor cells" in the ventral tier of lateral thalamic nuclei of patients with parkinsonian tremor. In Brock M (ed): *Modern Neurosurgery*. Springer-Verlag, 1986
34. Lenz FA, Tasker RR, Kwan HC, et al: Techniques for the analysis of spike trains in the human central nervous system. *Acta Neurochir* [Suppl] (Wien) 33:57–61, 1984
35. Li CL, Van Buren JM: Micro-electrode recordings in the brain of man with particular reference to epilepsy and dyskinesia. In Somjen GG (ed): *Neurophysiology Studied in Man*. Amsterdam: Excerpta Medica, 1972, pp 49–63
36. Maendly R, Rüegg DG, Wiesendanger M, et al: Thalamic relay for group I muscle afferents of forelimb nerves in the monkey. *J Neurophysiol* 46:901–917, 1981
37. Matsumoto K, Schichijo F, Fukami T: Long-term follow-up review of cases of Parkinson's disease after unilateral or bilateral thalamotomy. *J Neurosurg* 60:1033–1044, 1984
38. Narabayashi H: Tremor mechanisms. In Schaltenbrand G, Walker AE (eds): *Stereotaxy of the Human Brain*. Stuttgart, New York: Thieme Verlag, 1982, pp 510–514
39. Ohye C: Depth microelectrode studies. In Schaltenbrand G, Walker AE (eds): *Stereotaxy of the Human Brain*. Stuttgart, New York: Thieme Verlag, 1982, pp 372–389
40. Ohye C, Fukamachi A, Narabayashi H: Spontaneous and evoked activity of sensory neurons and their organization in the human thalamus. *Z Neurol* 203:219–234, 1972
41. Ohye C, Hirai T, Miyazaki M, et al: V.i.m. thalamotomy in the treatment of various kinds of tremor. *Appl Neurophysiol* 45:275–280, 1982
42. Ohye C, Nakamura R, Fukamachi A, et al: Recording and stimulation of the ventralis intermedius nuclei of the human thalamus. *Confin Neurol* 37:258, 1975
43. Ohye C, Narabayashi H: Physiological study of presumed ventralis intermedius neurons in the human thalamus. *J Neurosurg* 50:290–297, 1979
44. Ohye C, Saito Y, Fukamachi A, et al: An analysis of the spontaneous rhythmic and non-rhythmic burst discharges in the human thalamus. *J Neurol Sci* 22:245–259, 1974
45. Raeva SN: Unit activity of some deep nuclear structures of the human brain during voluntary movement. In Somjen GG (ed): *Neurophysiology Studied in Man*. Amsterdam: Excerpta Medica, 1972, pp 64–78
46. Scott RM, Brody JA, Cooper IS: The effect of thalamotomy on the progress of unilateral Parkinson's disease. *J Neurosurg* 32:286–288, 1970
47. Tasker RR: Effets sensitifs et moteurs de la stimulation thalamique chez l'homme. Applications cliniques. *Rev Neurol* (Paris) 142: 316–326, 1986
48. Tasker RR, Lenz FA, Dostrovsky J, et al: Thalamocortical contributions to sensory motor integration. International Symposium on Contributions to Sensory Motor Integration, Munich, April 21–24, 1986 (In press)
49. Tasker RR, Organ LW, Hawrylyshyn P: Investigation of the surgical target for alleviation of involuntary movement disorders. *Appl Neurophysiol* 45:261–274, 1982
50. Tasker RR, Organ LW, Hawrylyshyn PA: The

thalamus and midbrain of man. In Wilkins RH (ed): *A Physiological Atlas Using Electrical Stimulation*. A monograph in the Bannerstone Division of American lectures in neurosurgery. Springfield, IL: Thomas, 1982

51. Tasker RR, Siqueira J, Hawrylyshyn P, et al: What happened to V.i.m. thalamotomy for Parkinson's disease. *Appl Neurophysiol* 46:68–83, 1983
52. Tatton WG, Lee RG: Evidence for abnormal long-loop reflexes in rigid parkinsonian patients. *Brain Res* 100:671–676
53. Van Buren JM, Borke RC, Modesti LM: Sensory and nonsensory portions of the nucleus "ventralis posterior" of chimpanzee and man. *J Neurosurg* 45:37–48, 1976
54. Walker AE: Stereotaxic surgery for tremor. In Schaltenbrand G, Walker AE (eds): *Stereotaxy of the Human Brain*. Stuttgart, New York: Thieme Verlag, 1982, pp 515–521
55. Yasui N, Narabayashi H, Kondo T, et al: Slight cerebellar signs in stereotactic thalamotomy and subthalamotomy for parkinsonism. *Appl Neurophysiol* 39:315–320, 1976–77

24. SELECTIVE THALAMOTOMY FOR MOVEMENT DISORDERS: MICRORECORDING STIMULATION TECHNIQUES AND RESULTS

Chihiro Ohye

Using semi-microelectrodes adapted to the Leksell stereotactic apparatus, a technique has been developed for physiologically controlled selective thalamotomy to treat tremor, partial dystonia, choreoathetosis, and other involuntary movement disorders [22, 23, 25, 29].

This chapter describes preoperative assessment, the operative technique, and postoperative results.

Preoperative Assessment

PATIENT EVALUATION

Neurological examination remains of paramount importance in establishing both the diagnosis and the appropriate therapeutic approach. The various elements of each movement disorder should be carefully analyzed, because most movement disorders consist of mixtures of several types of tremor, chorea, athetosis, or ballism.

Two useful methods for analyzing movements are the electromyogram (EMG) and film or videotape recordings. EMG can be recorded using a multipurpose, multichannel electroencephalogram (EEG) machine and surface electrodes attached to the skin over the bellies of the appropriate muscles. Simultaneous recordings from antagonistic muscles (e.g., the flexors and extensors of the elbow) are essential. In any abnormal movement, several factors should be studied. In the case of tremor, the following characteristics are important: (1) frequency, (2) amplitude, (3) distribution of tremor in the affected limb, and (4) conditions under which the tremor appears (resting, postural, intentional). These characteristics are used to determine the size of the therapeutic lesion and its specific location within the thalamus [7].

Motion picture or videotape recording is another useful method of analyzing the features of abnormal movements. At Gunma University, 16-mm films are taken before and after each operation to document the abnormal movements and how surgery has affected these movements. Retrospective observation of the abnormal movements is thereby easily accomplished and the effects of therapy more objectively assessed.

STEREOTACTIC COMPUTED TOMOGRAPHY (CT)

Using a special recently developed craniometric method, the intercommissural (IC) line can be drawn precisely on a simple lateral skull x-ray [27]. A tentative target point on this IC line is selected and an appropriate site for electrode insertion and trajectory to the target is chosen, usually entering in the prefrontal area. A line is drawn on the x-ray from the selected entry site to the target point, usually making an angle of about 30° with the IC line. This guideline on the lateral skull x-ray can be transferred to the patient's scalp and a CT scan made in this plane on the line as well as 5 mm rostral and caudal to it (figure 24–1).

One of the CT images thus taken theoretically contains the region of the nucleus ventra-

L.D. Lunsford (ed.) *MODERN STEREOTACTIC NEUROSURGERY*.

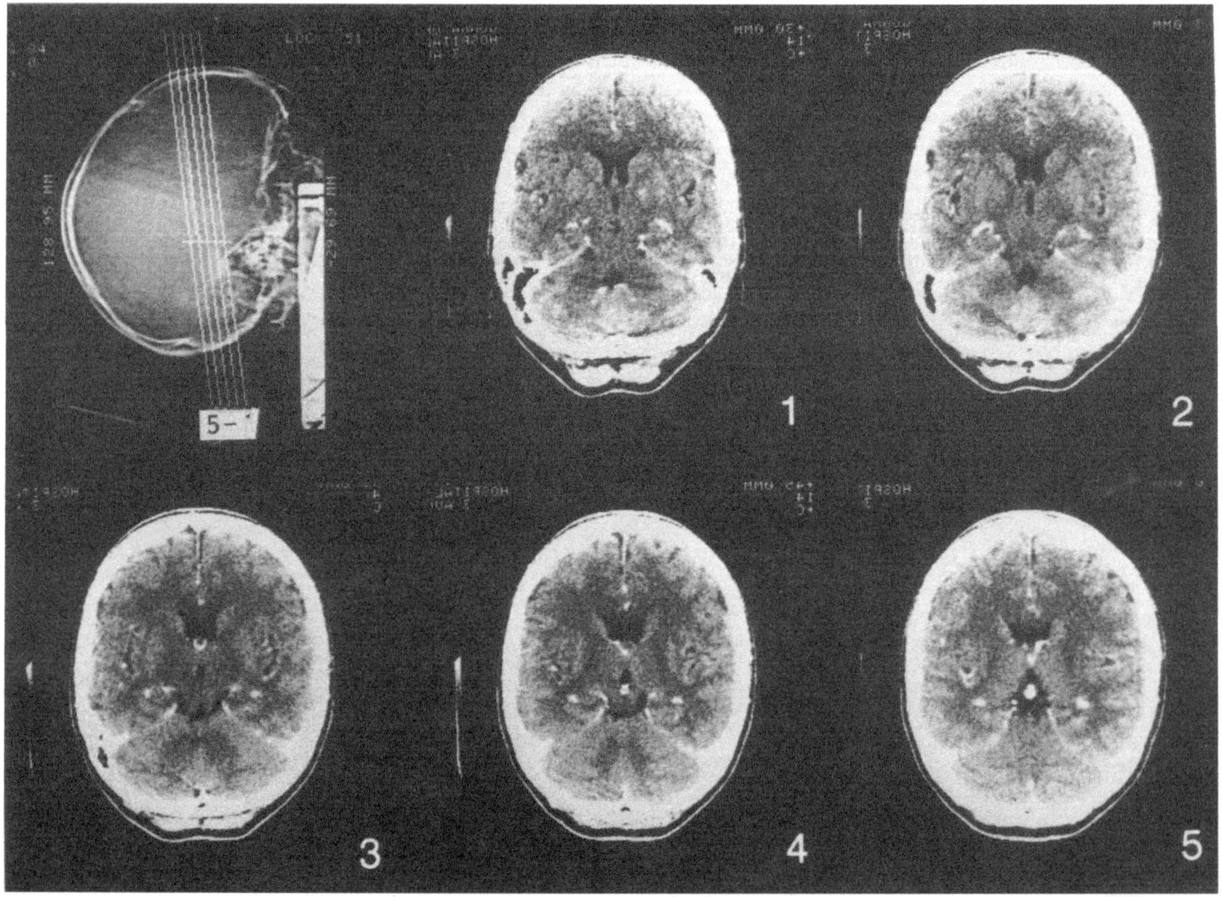

FIGURE 24–1. Five stereotactic CT images (1–5) for the direct aid of the stereotactic thalamotomy. Each image clearly shows gray and white matter, especially the caudate nucleus and thalamus. Referring to the foramen of Monro (in image 2) and the cerebral aqueduct (in image 3), image 3 was chosen as a guide plane in this case. (See also figure 24–4.) The five parallel lines in the left "scout" view correspond to the level (5–1) of each image. The angle and the tentative target point are arrived at by a craniometric method.

lis intermedius (V.i.m.) or at least the thalamic area close to it. This selected CT image will be in the plane through which the electrode would pass intraoperatively, assuming the electrode angle is adjusted as described later in this chapter. Using this stereotactic CT method, the geographical relationship of the subcortical structures to the ventricular system and any deformity that might exist can be determined before surgery. In addition, the distance can be measured from the inner table of the skull at the proposed electrode insertion site to both the target and to specific nuclei encountered en route. This method has proven to be a reliable operative strategy and can be adapted to stereotactic approaches in other regions of the brain, as well.

Operative Technique

OPERATING ROOM EQUIPMENT

Some electronic equipment is inevitably required to perform stereotactic surgery that includes depth recording and stimulation. At Gunma University, this includes (figure 24–2) the following mandatory equipment:

Semi-microelectrodes: bipolar concentric needle type (steel-steel)—outer diameter 0.6–0.3 μm; interpolar distance, 0.3–0.5 mm; tip, about 20 μm; electrical resistance, about 100 kOhm (the same electrode is used for recording and stimulation)
Oscilloscope: main and slave types
Multipurpose EEG machine
FM tape-recorder
Loud speaker
Electrical stimulator

The following equipment is optional:

Signal level meter
Micromanipulator—facilitates controlled approach to target
Digital meter—to measure automatically the distance from the target to the electrode tip
Data processor
Personal computer

PREPARATION OF THE PATIENT

The surgery may be performed with the patient in the sitting, semisitting, or supine positions. We prefer the supine position using the Leksell stereotactic apparatus. The operation is usually performed under local anesthesia in order to observe the patient's abnormal movements as the operation proceeds. As with all operations performed in the awake state, the patient's cooperation is essential during this procedure. However, in cases with severe abnormal movements, some sedation is given, and in patients under ten years of age, a general anesthetic is preferred. Premedication usually is unnecessary, but in some cases, prophylaxis or treatment of excessive oral secretions or nausea is administered. For EEG and EMG monitoring and recording, the appropriate scalp and surface electrodes are attached.

We modified the original method of Leksell [12] by performing ventriculography at the time of operation. After fixing the stereotactic frame, a burr hole (diameter 1.5 cm) is made at a point already chosen using the stereotactic CT scan. It is usually 2–3 cm rostral to bregma and about 3 cm lateral to the midline. After making a cruciate dural incision, the lateral ventricle is tapped. After withdrawing 15–20 ml cerebrospinal fluid (CSF), a small amount of radiopaque substance (metrizamide, 3–5 ml) and room air (about 10 ml) are injected. Lateral and posteroanterior skull x-rays are then taken immediately. With the patient in the supine position, the posterior commissure is made visible by the denser radiopaque substance, and the anterior commissure by the room air. The tentative target point is then selected on the IC line, 5 mm anterior to the posterior commissure and 15 mm lateral to the midline. This is the optimal standard target point, corresponding to the inferior border of the V.i.m., according to the Schaltenbrand and Wahren atlas of the human thalamus [6].

Next, the semicircular arc of the Leksell apparatus is fixed so that the midpoint between the two adjacent electrodes in the apparatus is on a direct trajectory to the target. The angle of the arc will closely approximate that of the stereotactic CT scan (figure 24–3). Thus, a central electrode will reach its target through a path shown on the stereotactic CT scan. If the burr hole is sited accurately, the difference between the angle on the stereotactic CT scan and the angle of the electrode trajectory is negligible (less than 5°) [27]. In unusual circumstances, such as when a very large underlying cortical vein is found, the burr hole may need to be enlarged.

As the Leksell frame requires two needles

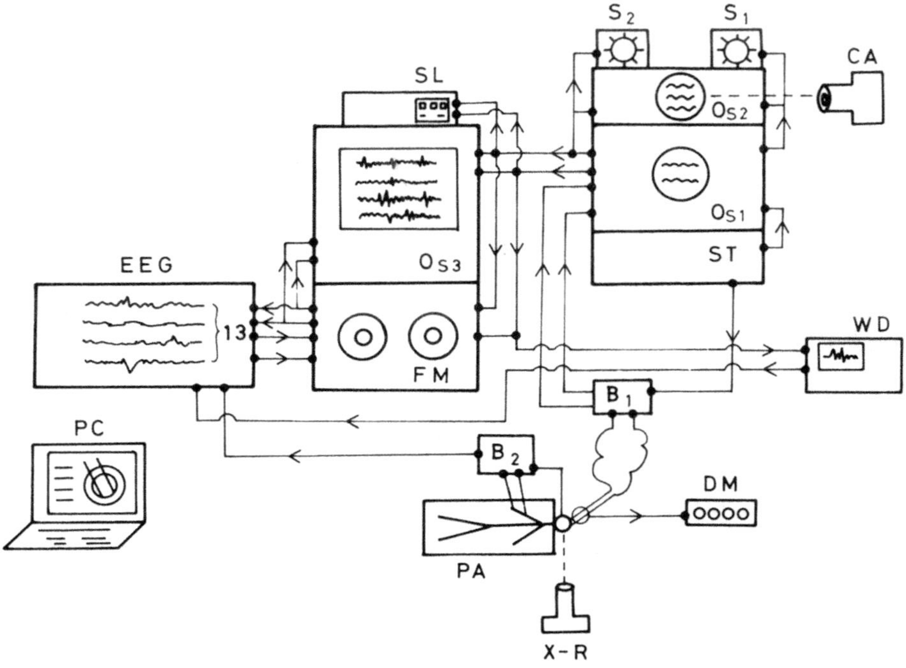

FIGURE 24–2. Arrangement of equipment in our operating room at Gunma University. B_1, input box for recording and stimulation; B_2, input box for EEG and EMG; CA, camera for filming abnormal movements; DM, digital meter; EEG, multipurpose machine; FM, magnetic tape; O_{s1-3}, oscilloscopes; S_{1-2}, speakers; SL, signal level meters; PA, patient; PC, personal computer; WD, window discriminator; X–R, x-ray tube.

for final bipolar thermocoagulation [12], a set of two semi-microelectrodes is used for recording and stimulation before placing the lesion. The semi-microelectrodes are inserted in place of the stylet, with the coagulation needle serving as a guide (see figure 24–3). To measure the distance from the target point to the tip of the electrode, a slit gear-gauge micromanipulator adapted to the electrode holder is connected to a digital meter (10-μm steps). The zero point of the micromanipulator (the target) is verified on the frame beforehand by moving the electrode tip to the center of the arc before the arc is attached to the frame. At this zero point, the digital meter is also set at zero. This ensures that the digital meter consistently displays the distance from the target point to the tip of the electrode with 10-μm precision. This distance can be confirmed by comparing it to the distance derived from the stereotactic CT scan. The second electrode can be set at any point relative to the central electrode; we usually use a 3-mm separation between tips, which are oriented parallel to the midsagittal plane. The tips may be rotated to make them parallel to the frontal or coronal planes.

INTRAOPERATIVE PHYSIOLOGICAL STUDIES

Since the beginning of stereotaxy, neurosurgeons have tried various methods to accurately reach deep-seated target sites. Most have relied on anatomical landmarks, such as the sella turcica, the calcified pineal gland, and the ventricles. After more than two decades of experience, however, physiological identification of targets using subcortical recordings of electrical activity is generally accepted as one of the most reliable and direct methods to reach clinical targets safely and accurately [1, 11, 17]. Therefore, this technique is described in some detail.

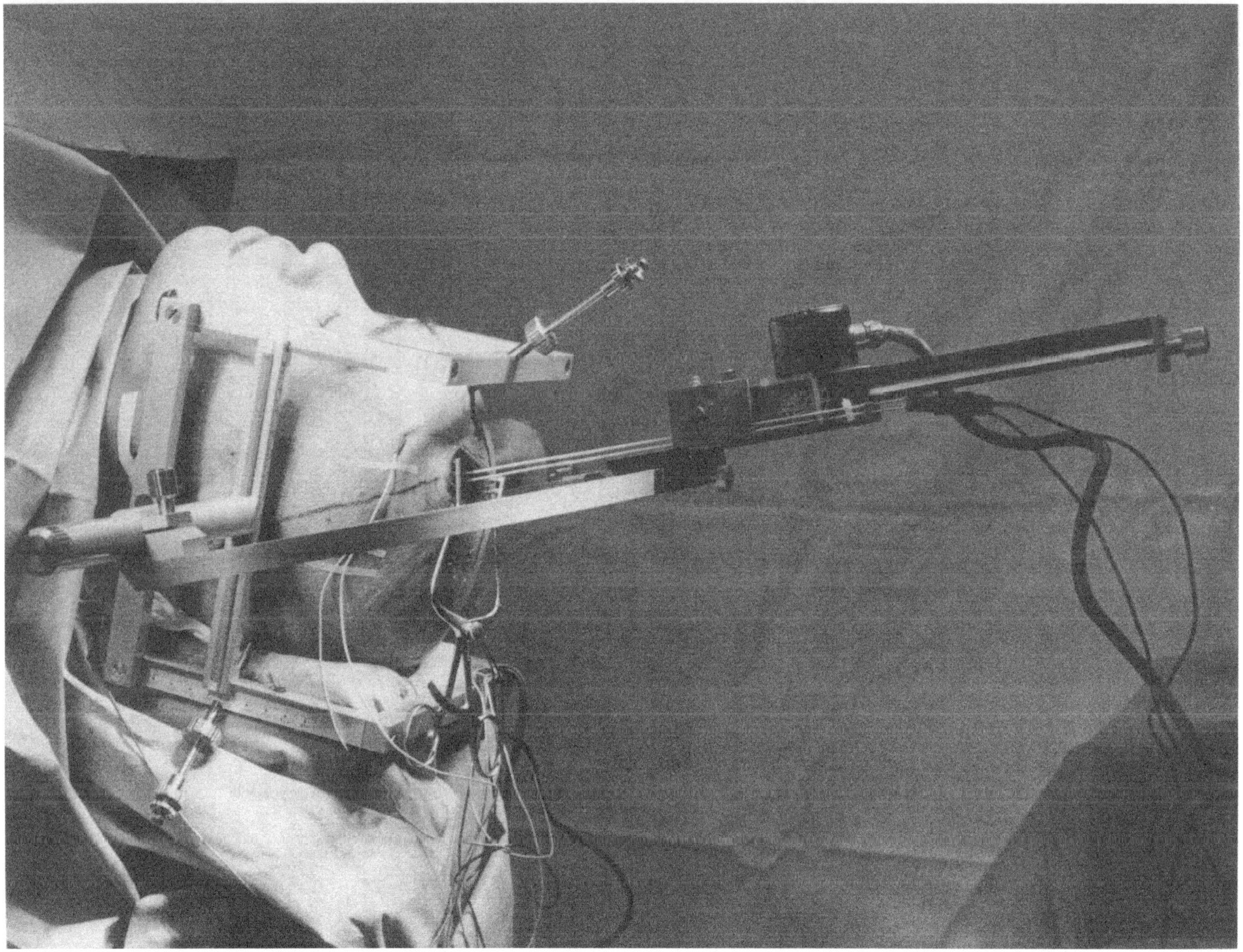

FIGURE 24–3. Stereotactic instrument fixed on a patient's skull. The semicircular arc is set at the same angle as that of the stereotactic CT scan (indicated by a line on the scalp). Note that a burr hole is opened on this line. A pair of recording electrodes will be introduced into the brain with the aid of a micromanipulator.

Recording. Using the micromanipulator, recording begins from the cortical surface. The surface contact point is about 60–70 mm from the target (zero) point, and this distance can again be verified by the stereotactic CT. On the way to the target, the electrodes pass through cortical gray matter, white matter, the caudate nucleus, and another small strip of white matter, until they finally enter the thalamus. The sequential penetration of these subcortical structures is clearly indicated by the characteristic electrical activity recorded for each (figure 24–4). Cortical gray matter exhibits high-amplitude rapid oscillation with superimposed large spikes. This pattern appears for a distance of about 15–20 mm, followed by a sudden decrease in electrical activity marked by only small positive spikes, indicating that the tip of the electrode has penetrated white matter. At about 30 mm from the target point, the electrical activity increases again, shown by irregular oscillations of about 30 Hz and superimposed sporadic spike discharges of moderate amplitude and long duration (2–3 m sec). This pattern continues for some 10 mm and corresponds to the caudate nucleus, as confirmed by standard stereotactic atlases and the stereotactic CT image. If the electrode approach is more lateral, one observes only small positive spikes on a low level of background activity, denoting white matter; whereas, if the electrode travels more medially, there is an interval without electrical activity, because the lateral ventricle has been entered. Thus, before penetrating the thalamus, caudate activity confirms the trajectory of the electrode, as predicted by the stereotactic CT image. Caudate activity thus can be used as a "pilot structure."

Just beneath the caudate nucleus, the electrical activity usually decreases again, indicating a short zone of white matter between it and the thalamus. Approximately 15–20 mm from the target, the electrical activity again increases, signifying that the tip of the electrode has entered the roof of the thalamus. Because the roof of the thalamus is curved, the tips of the electrode pair penetrate it at slightly different distances from the target. One can thereby estimate the curvature or shape of this portion of the thalamus [4, 14].

Within the thalamus, the electrical activity also exhibits characteristic patterns that allow nuclear localization. Differences in spontaneous activity between dorsal and ventral and between rostral and caudal regions are particularly dramatic, the ventral and caudal portions being more active. This may be due to the disparate cellular compositions of the various thalamic subnuclei [5]. Here, the angle of the electrode approach in relation to the configuration of the thalamic subnuclei is very important. If the electrodes approach the thalamic ventrolateral mass at an acute angle, penetration of the V.i.m. is more likely (figure 24–5). However, if the electrode path is more vertical, there is a greater risk of missing the V.i.m. nucleus, because it is a narrow structure in its anterior-posterior dimension. Using a sagittally oriented pair of electrodes 3 mm apart, we have found that one or both electrodes may reach the V.i.m. though the posterior electrode usually arrives first. The electrical activity of the V.i.m. is distinctly different from that of the surrounding structures. In nine out of ten cases, the posterior electrode, which penetrates the V.i.m., exhibits very high background activity and slight oscillation of 25–30 Hz superimposed on a high-amplitude spike discharge. Meanwhile, the anterior electrode is usually in the ventrolateral (VL) nucleus, where only small spikes over relatively low background activity are found. Typically, this difference is so marked that the anterior border of the V.i.m. is easily recognized. The clear separation of the electrical background activity between VL and V.i.m. can be attributed to differences in cytoarchitechture [8, 9]. The majority of the neurons in the VL nucleus are small (about 300 μm^2) and densely packed, whereas neurons in the V.i.m. are large (about 500 μm2) and sparsely distributed.

In the high-background activity zone, distinguishable single- or multiple-unit spike discharges can be separated with the help of the micromanipulator. Among these, rhythmic discharges time-locked to the contralateral tremor can be found readily, particularly in patients with spontaneous tremor (figure 24–6). A loudspeaker is quite helpful in recognizing these rhythmic bursts. Frequently, when advancing the electrodes, the rhythmic activity of tremor-synchronous neurons can be heard above the background noise, even if the spikes are not individually distinct. Further careful descent of the electrode via the micromanipulator often separates the rhythmic grouped spikes from the background noise.

After reaching and identifying this electrical

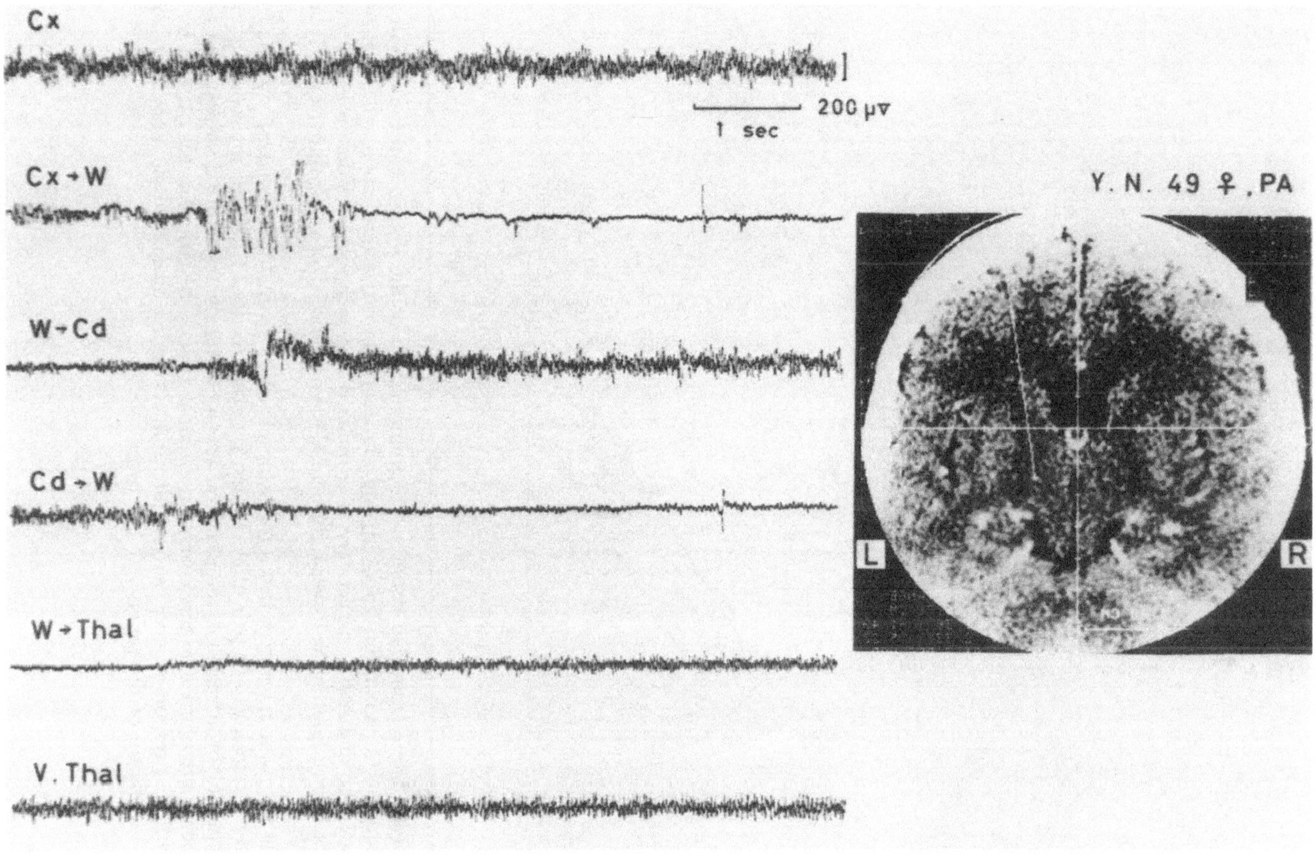

FIGURE 24–4. Examples of characteristic electrical activities in the cortical and deep subcortical structures are shown along the trajectory toward the tentative target point. The expected direction of the trajectory is drawn (*white line*) on the stereotactic CT image on the right.

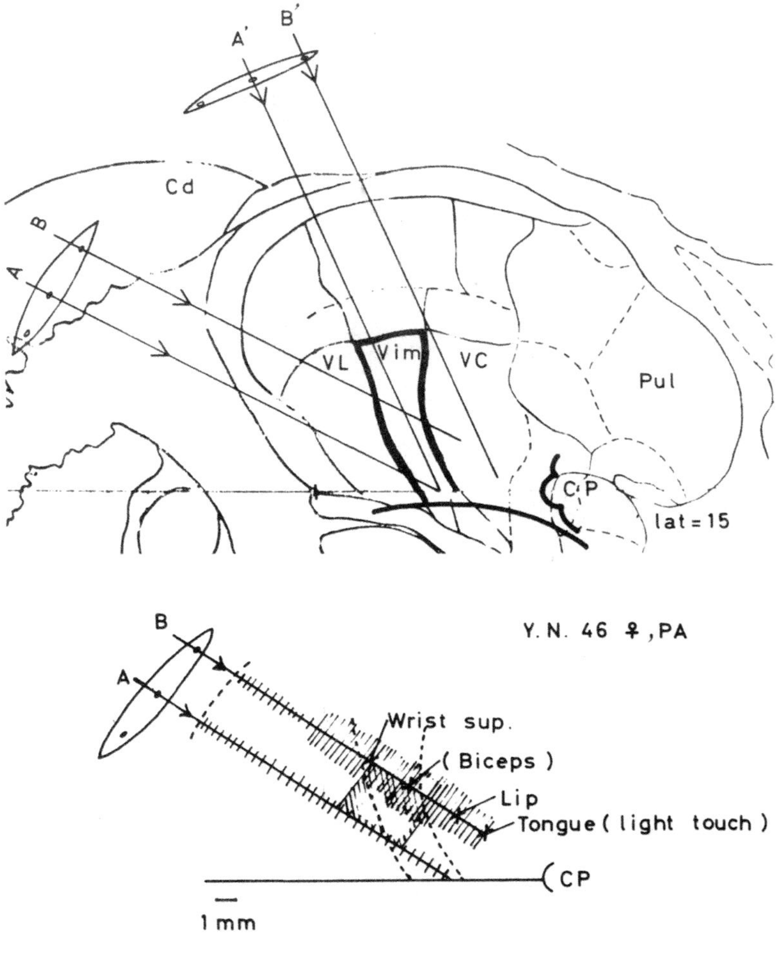

FIGURE 24–5. *Top:* The relationship between the configuration of the V.i.m. and the angle of the pair of recording electrodes. The maximum (inclined) and minimum (more vertical) approaches that we have used are shown by lines AB and A′B′, respectively. The inclined approach increases the probability of traversing the V.i.m. Thick curved lines in the lower right denote the posterior part of the third ventricle and posterior commissure (CP).
Bottom: Example of an intraoperative data processing chart. A profile of the thalamic V.i.m. zone (within dotted lines) and the trackings of a pair of electrodes, referring to the CP and the intercommissural line. The approximate amplitude of the background electrical activity along the trajectory is shown, and several points of thalamic response are plotted on this chart. An essential zone to be coagulated is marked by the hatched area. The four different responses were: wrist supination, stretching biceps muscle (not clear), tap on the lip, and light touch on the tip of the tongue.

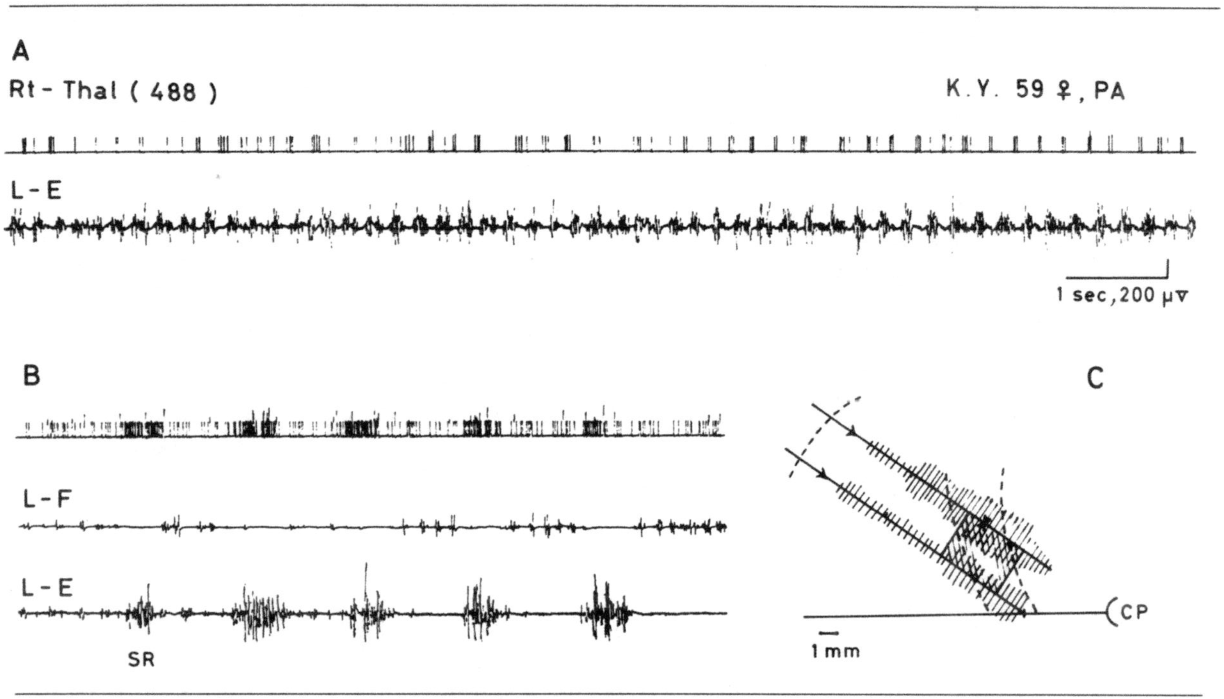

FIGURE 24–6. (A) Rhythmic burst discharge in the thalamus (right V.i.m., 488 × 10 μm from the target marked by X in drawing C) time-locked with the contralateral grouped discharge of tremor in EMG (*lower trace*). The original spike discharge was converted to a pulse and recorded on a thermopen-writing EEG machine. (B) The same thalamic discharge responds to stretching forearm extensor muscle (L-E). (C) A simple data processing chart, similar to that seen in figure 24–5, analyzing the data noted (A) and (B).

activity, we determine whether a variety of passive or active contralateral limb movements can modify this rhythmic bursting. About 20% of neurons in the V.i.m. respond to limb motions and often exhibit tremor-synchronous firing. These units are very modality-specific in their response; their firing is not affected by other sensory stimulation, such as a light touch. They are therefore called "kinesthetic units" [31]. It should be noted that they do not always show tremor-related firing and in fact may be found in patients without tremor. They should not be confused with units showing rhythmic or irregular bursting without kinesthetic or other sensory responses. The latter may be found close to the kinesthetic units but tend to be in the more dorsal portion of the V.i.m. [24, 32].

These kinesthetic units have been found in at least 90% of cases, usually on the first or second electrode tracking. They tend to cluster in the last 10 mm of the tracking, and in our anterolateral-to-posteromedial trajectory, they are invariably the first sensory neurons identified in the thalamus, and in turn theoretically correspond very nicely to the V.i.m. The micromanipulator has helped enormously in recognizing these units.

These kinesthetic neurons show a topographical organization within the V.i.m. In general, neurons responding to stimulation of the face and the upper and lower limbs are found in the most medial, ventromedial, and dorsolateral parts of the V.i.m., respectively [23]. Therefore, upon reaching the high-activity V.i.m. zone, the kinesthetic response is most likely found by examining the lower limbs, but at the end of tracking, attention should be focused on the upper limb or face area.

Identifying at least one unequivocal kinesthetic response is the most essential part of selective thalamotomy. Its location is a crucial factor in deciding on the location and size of the therapeutic lesion(s).

After a stable kinesthetic neuron and its peripheral receptive field are found, the corresponding peripheral nerve is electrically stimulated percutaneously, using a stimulus weaker than the motor (and usually the sensory) threshold. (A very weak paresthesia may occur.) The kinesthetic units invariably respond with latencies of approximately 11–12 m sec for the upper limb area [31]. Because there is always a fixed latency in a given unit, it is probable that the ascending pathway from the peripheral nerve to the contralateral V.i.m. neurons is direct and possibly mono- or oligosynaptic. This pathway may well be the spinothalamic tract [19, 34, 35].

Stimulation. Sensation and/or modulation of movement provoked by thalamic stimulation are other important methods to confirm that the tip of the electrode is in the V.i.m. We stimulate the point in the thalamus where the kinesthetic unit is recorded, using the same electrodes as for recording 60–100 Hz, 0.3–0.6 mA, 0.5 ms, about 1 s) [31]. It is interesting to note that at threshold stimulus intensities, the majority of patients describe electric-like sensations in the contralateral body part corresponding to the peripheral receptive field. Some describe a feeling of numbness in the same area. Thalamic stimulation modifies spontaneous tremor in (mainly) the corresponding area of the receptive field (figure 24–7) and may either augment or suppress the tremor.

In a series of stereotactic operations performed in the 1960s, we used the thalamocortical potentials evoked by low-frequency (about 6 Hz) thalamic stimulation as a major physiological tool to identify thalamic nuclei [28, 38]. However, with the advent of thalamic recording, we have relied much more on physiological information directly obtained from the thalamus. The thalamocortical evoked potentials are now used only as supplementary procedures.

Recording and stimulation around the V.i.m. nucleus. As previously noted, physiological findings outside the V.i.m. nucleus differ substantially from those inside. Anteriorly in VL nucleus, the background activity is low and without large spike discharges, and kinesthetic neurons are not found. Several investigators have observed VL neurons discharging with voluntary movement of the contralateral limbs [2, 11]. However, we found no such voluntary units in this area. Certainly, some of the kinesthetic neurons in the V.i.m. discharge with voluntary as well as passive movements. Analysis of the time relationship between these thalamic discharges and corresponding EMG discharges has been difficult, and it has not been possible to ascertain with certainty which came first. Furthermore, we

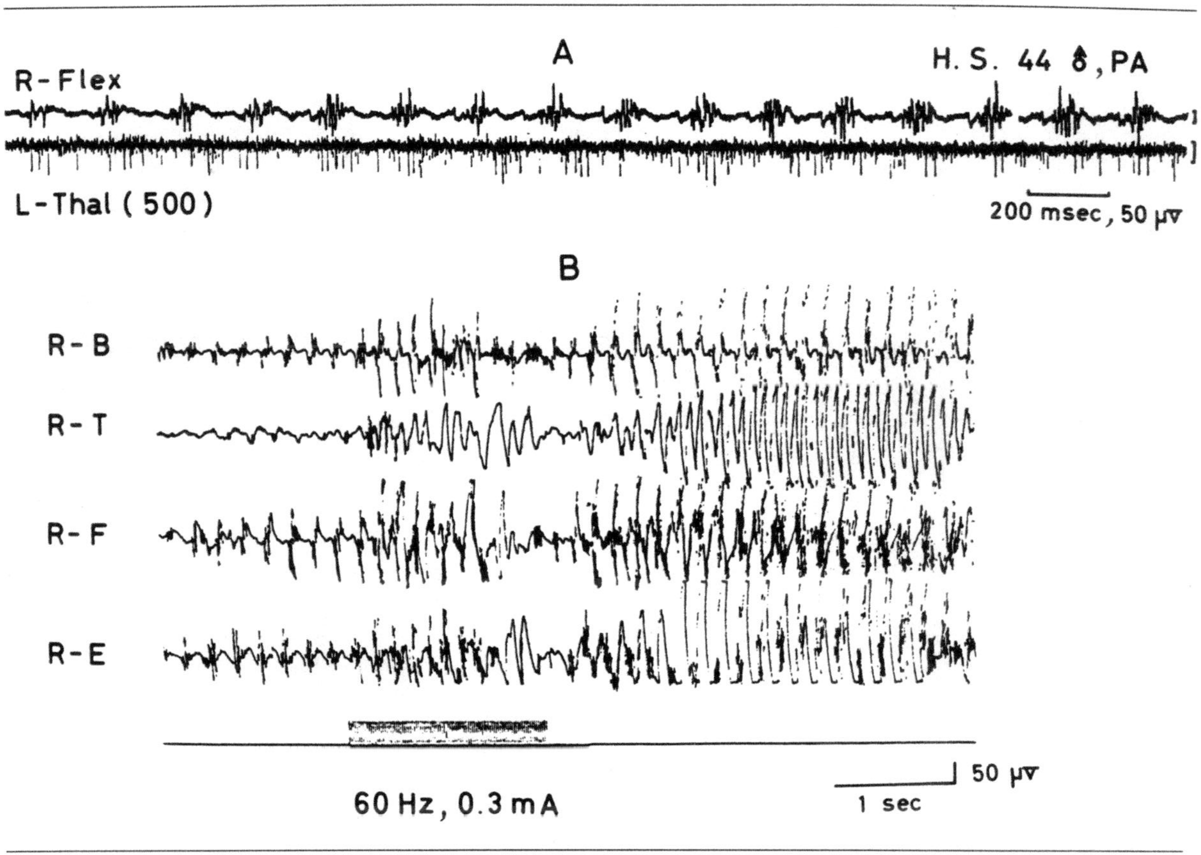

FIGURE 24–7. Effect of electrical stimulation on the thalamic point where tremor synchronous activity was recorded. (A) Rhythmic discharge recorded from the left thalamus (L-Thal, 500 × 10 μm from the target point), synchronous to the peripheral tremor. Upper trace: EMG from the right forearm flexor (R-Flex). (B) Electrical stimulation (60 Hz, 0.3 mA, for 1.5 sec) of this point produced augmentation of the tremor (amplitude and frequency) on the contralateral limbs. Note that the effect was strongest in the forearm flexor muscle, which corresponded to the peripheral receptive field of the thalamic unit shown in (A). R-B, right biceps; T, triceps; F, forearm flexor; E, forearm extensor.

have found that electrical stimulation in the VL produces a general increase in stretch reflex discharge in the contralateral extremities as well as a marked thalamocortical evoked potential in the cortical motor area [28].

Posterior to the V.i.m. is the ventrocaudal (VC) nucleus. Here, the background activity is also high, and large-amplitude spikes are found. Thus, it is difficult to differentiate VC from V.i.m. simply by spontaneous activity. However, the VC neurons respond to light touch on the contralateral extremity. Usually their receptive field is very small, often being only a circumscribed area several mm in length [17]. As there is no functional overlap between the V.i.m. (kinesthetic) and VC (tactile) neurons, the difference in modality is the most reliable way to distinguish these regions. Finally, electrical stimulation of the VC nucleus produces paresthesia or numbness [37]. The threshold seems to be less than that for V.i.m. activation.

Just lateral to the V.i.m. is the internal capsule, which consists only of nerve fibers. Because their electrical activity is extremely low and there is no response to sensory stimulation, the internal capsule is easily avoided. When the internal capsule is stimulated directly, jerky flexion is often produced in the contralateral limb.

When physiological studies are complete, a final x-ray is taken to check the electrode position.

Therapeutic Lesion Technique

TREMOR

The location and size of the therapeutic lesion(s) are determined after assessing the characteristics of the tremor and the results of physiological testing. Intraoperative data processing has proven very helpful in integrating these findings and in preventing any misinterpretations of the geographical relationships indicated by the physiological testing and the complex three-dimensional configuration of the V.i.m. The necessary programs for processing these factors quasi on-line with the aid of a personal computer were recently developed. If a computer is not available, a simple hand drawing as shown in figure 24–5 is a great aid.

The Leksell stereotactic apparatus utilizes two electrodes for placing bipolar lesions. In this way, the size of the lesion can be more precisely controlled and estimated (figure 24–8). The location of lesions should include the point where a tremor-synchronous unit is recorded, or, if this is not possible, the point where a kinesthetic neuron is recorded. Lesions must be larger than these areas to have a sustained therapeutic effect. However, a lesion of any size should include portions of these areas to have a significant tremor-reducing result.

The recording electrodes are replaced by the thermocouple stylets, and a pair of coagulation needles (used previously as guide needles for recording) is set in the correct position on the initial target point. An initial lesion here often dramatically reduces the tremor, which may already have been reduced by the concussive effect of the passing electrodes.

Once the initial lesion is made, subsequent lesion placement also depends on physiological findings. For example, if tremor-synchronous units have been identified, another lesion placed 1–2 mm higher in the electrode trajectory than the first, thereby overlapping it, is usually sufficient to produce effective and sustained results (figure 24–9). If the tremor involves both upper and lower limbs, a third lesion is made, as well.

When kinesthetic units associated with the arm are discovered, lesions should be placed there and then the electrodes should be rotated so that further coagulation can be performed in more lateral parts of the V.i.m., covering leg-related areas as well. If leg-related kinesthetic units were found, the reverse would of course apply. This takes full advantage of the topographical representation of body parts in the V.i.m.

The specific number and volume of lesions required have been studied in some detail. In Parkinson's disease and essential tremor patients, two to three lesions of about 40–60 mm^3 (in one quadrant of a 3-mm radius cylinder) are enough to arrest the tremor in the contralateral extremities [7, 26]. In contrast, tremor developing after trauma or cerebrovascular accidents has somewhat different clinical and therapeutic features [10]. First, the tremor frequency tends to be slower (about 3 Hz), while its amplitude is higher, and it is quite coarse. It more often involves the proximal trunk muscles. It remains a mystery why a V.i.m. area related to trunk muscles has **not** yet been identified in humans. Second, the electrical activity in the thalamus, especially in the ventrolateral mass (including the V.i.m.) is often different from that in Parkinson's disease.

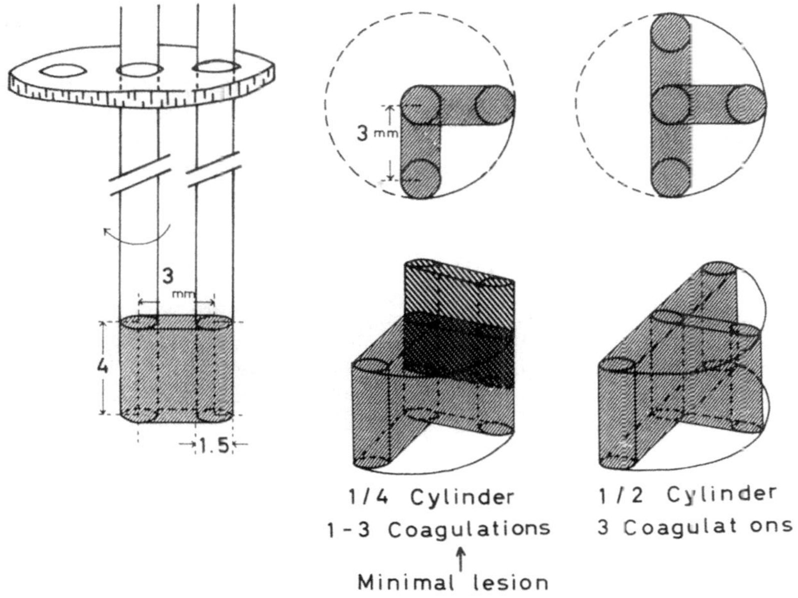

FIGURE 24-8. Schematic drawing of the tip of coagulating needles shows our standard coagulative lesion. Far left: a unit lesion (*shaded area*) with the possibility of adding the second lesion within an imaginary cylinder of a 3-mm radius around a center electrode. Overview and oblique, respectively, view of our minimal lesion (*center, top and bottom*) and an additional larger lesion (*right, top and bottom*).

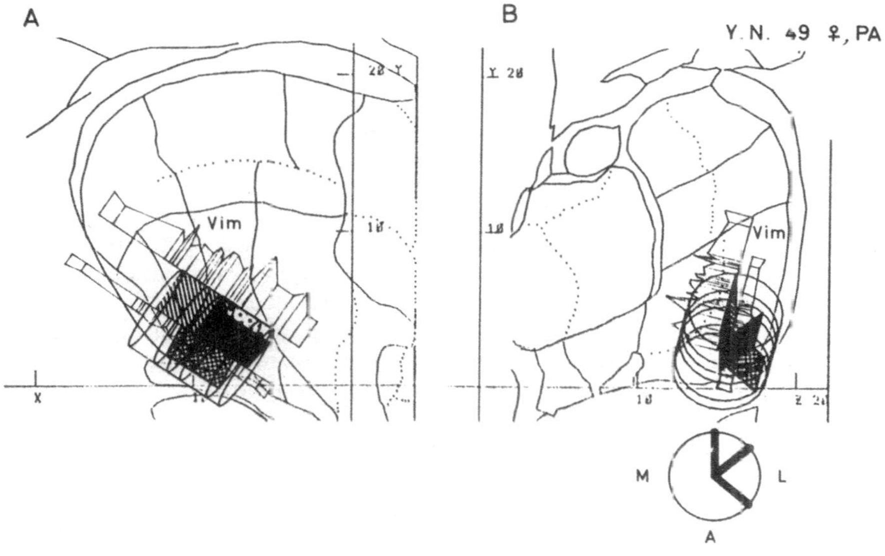

FIGURE 24-9. Computer graphics demonstrate the actual coagulation lesion in a Parkinson's disease patient with tremor and rigidity. Background atlas of the thalamus is from Hassler's standard atlas, displayed in an appropriate enlargement determined by the physiological findings in this case. (A) Lateral view. (B) Frontal view. In this case, four lesions (shown by different patterns) were made, some of them overlapped, within a quarter and a half cylinder. Overview is shown at bottom right.

Background activity is generally reduced (at times dramatically so) either diffusely or in patches, with kinesthetic neurons being difficult to find in either case. This is likely due to the effect of the underlying insults on the thalamus. In such cases, every effort should be made to find even a "fragment" of V.i.m. activity, which would greatly increase the probability of successfully placing a therapeutic lesion in these difficult patients. Such "fragments" are often to be found anteriorly in the VL or posteriorly in VC nuclei, apparently "displaced" by the insults [33]. Because of altered thalamic organization, therapeutic lesions in these patients usually need to be larger (some more than 200 mm^3) and to cover wider areas than those for Parkinson's disease [7, 26]. Without the benefit of physiological studies, the lesions might need to be larger still, entailing greater risks of undesirable side effects.

RIGIDITY

For the treatment of rigidity (defined as exaggerated tonic stretch reflex) [36] and partial dystonia, the lesion is placed not in the V.i.m. but its anterior part, bordering on the VL nucleus. Based on our experience with selective thalamotomy, we assume that the VL nucleus is associated more with rigidity than with tremor [18]. The VL nucleus exhibits no particular physiological characteristics to enable positive identification; its background activity is low, and the small spikes that do occur do not respond to sensory or motor stimuli. Therefore, the VL nucleus is defined secondarily, after identification of the V.i.m., on the basis of their geographical relationship.

In cases of Parkinson's disease with both tremor and rigidity, the V.i.m. is identified first and coagulated to relieve tremor. Then its rostral part is coagulated to ameliorate rigidity. The latter procedure is accomplished by turning one of the coagulation electrodes to the anterior position of the frame's guide cylinder (see figures 24–8 and 24–9). By coagulating first V.i.m. and then the VL, effects on tremor and then rigidity, respectively, can be seen clearly.

OTHER MOVEMENT DISORDERS

The principles of selective thalamotomy have been applied to partial dystonia associated with cerebral palsy or other causes, choreoathetotic movements, and other movement disorders [3, 30]. These principles have been most effectively used with patients suffering primarily from tremor and rigidity. The extent of lesions in these cases has likewise been determined principally by the physiological character of the abnormal movement. In most of the cases, combined VL and V.i.m. thalamotomy is recommended, though the extent of either lesion may be adjusted to suit the particular patient.

Results

Experience with well over 200 cases has shown the results of physiologically controlled selective thalamotomy to be very satisfactory. In cases in which the V.i.m. could be physiologically identified, there has been an immediate and dramatic therapeutic effect following coagulation. This effect has been sustained for the entire five- to ten-year follow-up period [13]. If tremor has recurred, it generally has been manifest within two to three weeks of operation. In such cases, an additional lesion(s) usually is made, again utilizing physiological control.

In cases in which tremor-synchronous units have been identified in the thalamus and used as a guide to placing lesions, the tremor has never recurred in the corresponding extremity. This further highlights what we believe to be a critical relationship between the thalamic "tremor units" and contralateral peripheral tremor. It can be said with little exaggeration that parkinsonian tremor and essential tremor can now be almost completely controlled, if not cured (figure 24–10). Even in suboptimal cases in which some tremor remains, it is invariably much improved and usually not troublesome enough to affect activities of daily living. Unfortunately, such dramatic effects cannot always be expected after stroke or head injury, even with the physiologically controlled method. Coarse tremors may persist partially, but even if abolished, the paresis often present may continue to be the most troublesome problem. In these cases, therefore, the surgeon must assess the degree to which the tremor or rigidity contributes to the underlying disability. Conversely, even a mild improvement may mean a great deal to this group of patients.

In general, untoward side effects of selective thalamotomy have been rare and minimal [13]. Most patients complain of an unusual feeling of weakness in the contralateral extremities im-

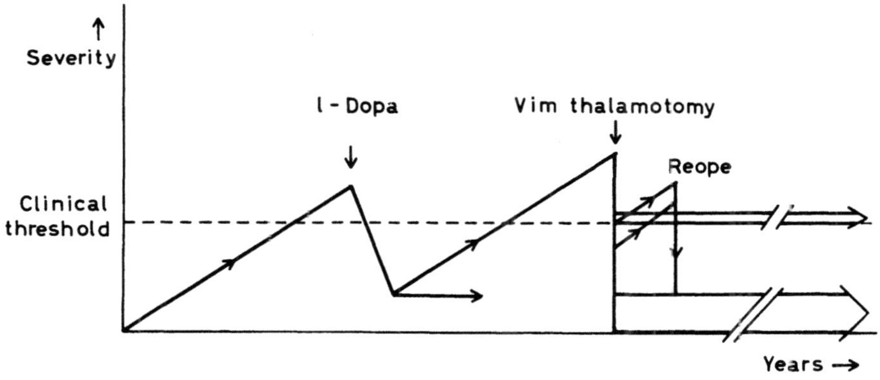

FIGURE 24–10. Schematic drawing illustrates possible course of Parkinson's disease (especially with tremor) in relation to L-dopa therapy and thalamic surgery. V.i.m.-thalamotomy is effective and sustained in the majority of cases; in less than 10% of cases, recurrence of tremor necessitates reoperation.

mediately after the surgery. Detailed examination shows that, in most cases, this feeling is not associated with objective weakness or upper motor neuron signs and therefore cannot be attributed to impingement on the internal capsule. This feeling may be better described as "lightness" in the limb, in contrast to the "heaviness" described by patients with genuine pareses. Usually, this sensation subsides within ten to 14 days, but in rare cases it has persisted for several months. In almost every case, it has not interfered with activities of daily living.

Paresthesia of the tip of the thumb or index finger, the lip, or the tongue has occurred in about 10% of cases immediately after the operation. This is presumably because the lesions have been placed close to the VC nucleus, where they may induce secondary, invariably temporary changes. Fortunately, persistent paresthesias are rare, occurring in 1%–2% of cases. Most of the time this phenomenon subsides within a month.

Language disturbance is another problem, related especially to bilateral thalamotomy. In our series, two patients exhibited significant dysarthria following surgery performed one year after a previous thalamotomy on the opposite side. Both occurred early in our series, when the lesions were made slightly larger than at present. In a recent minimal lesion series, although no persistent speech disturbance has occurred, temporary symptoms have been noted, surprisingly even after unilateral lesions on either the right or left side. These sequelae pose important challenges for future improvement.

Summary and Conclusion

The continuous refinement of stereotactic techniques, which has led to the current approach, has traditionally sought to produce the minimum lesion with the maximum effect [16, 20]. It seems reasonable that precise localization is a prerequisite for this goal. The current technique offers the following advantages in line with historical stereotactic principles:

1. It allows use of the smallest lesions currently thought feasible for relief of tremor, with success rates as high or higher than other techniques.
2. It allows lesions to be placed where the thalamic targets actually exist in each individual patient, rather than where standard atlases indicate they should be. That the V.i.m. is not always where it should be is evident in the cases of thalamic reorganization after trauma or stroke. Furthermore, functional localization allows in vivo confirmation of the target site, whereas stereotactic atlases invariably depend on postmortem anatomy. A physiological technique overcomes these biological variations.
3. It has identified groups of neurons with very specific behaviors that very likely underlie the tremor in all patients. We believe that V.i.m. neurons play a primary role

in tremor mechanisms. At present, we assume that they are involved in the tremor-mediating system, if not in the tremor genesis [15, 21].
4. It can give some measure of prediction of a sustained therapeutic effect, based on the types of units identified in the thalamus.
5. It can, theoretically, improve the complication rates by using the smallest possible lesions.

In conclusion, we believe that only selective, well-defined stereotactic lesions will contribute to our understanding of the neural mechanisms underlying involuntary movement disorders such as tremor.

References

1. Albe-Fessard D, Arfel G, Guiot G: Activités éléctriques caractéristiques de quelques structures cérébrales chez l'homme. *Ann Chir* 17:1185–1214, 1963
2. Bertrand G, Jasper H, Wong A, et al: Microelectrode recording during stereotactic surgery. *Clin Neurosurg* 16:328–355, 1969
3. Fukamachi A, Ohye C, Narabayashi H: Delineation of the thalamic nucleus with a microelectrode in the stereotaxic surgery for parkinsonism and cerebral palsy. *J Neurosurg* 39:214–225, 1973
4. Fukamachi A, Ohye C, Saito Y, et al: Estimation of the neural noise within the human thalamus. *Acta Neurochir [Suppl]* (Wien) 24:121–136, 1977
5. Grover FS, Buchwald JS: Correlation of cell size with amplitude of background fast activity in specific brain nuclei. *J Neurophysiol* 33:160–171, 1970
6. Hassler R: Architectonic organization of the thalamic nuclei. In Schaltenbrand G, Wahren W (eds): *Atlas for Sterotaxy of the Human Brain*, (2nd ed). Stuttgart: G Thieme, 1977
7. Hirai T, Miyazaki M, Nakajima H, et al: The correlation between tremor characteristics and predicted volume of effective lesions in stereotaxic Vim-thalamotomy. *Brain* 106:1001–1018, 1983
8. Hirai T, Nagaseki K, Kawashima Y, et al: Large neurons in the thalamic ventrolateral mass in humans and in monkeys: Their special references to Vim-thalamotomy. *Appl Neurophysiol* 415:245–250, 1982
9. Hirai T, Wada H, Nagaseki K, et al: Cell sparse zone in the ventrolateral thalamic mass in humans, monkeys and cats. *Appl Neurophysiol* (in press)
10. Isobe I, Nojiri K, Tsukahara Y, et al: Correlation between the neural noise in the thalamus after cerebrovascular disease and computerized tomography. *Appl Neurophysiol* 39:212–215, 1976/1977
11. Jasper HH, Bertrand G: Thalamic unit involved in somatic sensation and voluntary and involuntary movements in man. In Purpura DP, Yahr MD (eds): *The Thalamus.* New York: Columbia University Press, 1966, pp 365–390
12. Leksell L: *Stereotaxis and Radiosurgery: An Operative System.* Springfield, IL: Thomas, 1977
13. Nagaseki Y, Shibazaki T, Hirai T, et al: Long-term follow-up after selective Vim-thalamotomy. *J Neurosurg* 65:296–302, 1986
14. Nakajima H, Fukamachi A, Isobe I, et al: Estimation of neural noise—Functional anatomy of the human thalamus. *Appl Neurophysiol* 41:193–201, 1978
15. Ohye C: Anatomy and physiology of the thalamic nucleus ventralis intermedius. In Ito M (ed): *Integrative Control Functions of the Brain*, Vol 1. Tokyo: Kodansha, 1978, pp 152–163
16. Ohye C: Changing feature of stereotactic surgery. *Neurol Surg* 12:227–236, 1984 (Jpn)
17. Ohye C: Depth microelectrode studies. In Schaltenbrand G, Walker AE (eds): *Stereotaxy of the Human Brain.* Stuttgart, New York: G Thieme. 1982, pp 372–389
18. Ohye C: Role des noyaux thalamiques dans l'hypertonie et le tremblement de la maladie Parkinson. *Rev Neurol* (Paris) 142:362–369, 1986
19. Ohye C: Experimental tremor in monkey. In Sasaki K, Hongo T (eds): *Handbook of Physiology*, (2nd ed). Tokyo: Igaku-Shoin. (in press)
20. Ohye C: Idea of stereotactic surgery. *Brain and Nerve* 29:481–488, 1977 (Jpn)
21. Ohye C: Neurons of the thalamic ventralis intermedius nucleus. Their special reference to tremor. *Adv Neurosci* 29:224–231 (Jpn)
22. Ohye C: Stereotactic selective thalamotomy for tremor. *Neurol Surg* 13:707–716, 1985 (Jpn)
23. Ohye C: Stereotactic surgery for parkinsonism-selective thalamotomy. In Hirayama K (ed): *Parkinson's Disease and Parkinsonism.* Tokyo: Kimposha, 1984, pp 95–103
24. Ohye C, Albe-Fessard D: Rhythmic discharges related to tremor in humans and monkeys. In Chalazonitis N (ed): *Abnormal Neuronal Discharges.* New York: Raven Press, 1978, pp 37–48
25. Ohye C, Fukamachi A, Miyazaki M, et al: Physiologically controlled selective thalamotomy for the treatment of abnormal movement by Leksell's open system. *Acta Neurochir* (Wien) 37:93–104, 1977
26. Ohye C, Hirai T, Miyazaki M, et al: Vim thalamotomy for the treatment of various kinds of tremor. *Appl Neurophysiol* 45:275–280, 1982
7. Ohye C, Kawashima Y, Hirato M, et al:

Stereotactic CT scan for the direct aid of stereotactic thalamotomy and biopsy. *Acta Neurochir* (Wien) 71:55–68, 1984
28. Ohye C, Kubota K, Hongo T: Ventrolateral and subventrolateral thalamic stimulation: Motor effects. *Arch Neurol* 11:423–434, 1964
29. Ohye C, Miyazaki M, Hirai T, et al: Primary writing tremor treated by stereotactic selective thalamotomy. *J Neurol Neurosurg Psychiatry* 45:988–997, 1982
30. Ohye C, Miyazaki M, Hirai T, et al: Stereotactic selective thalamotomy for the treatment of tremor type cerebral palsy in adolescence. *Childs Brain* 10:156–167, 1983
31. Ohye C, Narabayashi H: Physiological studies of presumed ventralis intermedius neurons in the human thalamus. *J Neurosurg* 50:290–297, 1979
32. Ohye C, Saito Y, Fukamachi A, et al: An analysis of the spontaneous rhythmic and non-rhythmic burst discharges in the human thalamus. *J Neurol Sci* 22:245–259, 1974
33. Ohye C, Shibazaki T, Hirai T, et al: Plastic change of the thalamic organization in the cases with tremor after stroke. *Appl Neurophysiol* 48: 288–292, 1985
34. Ohye C, Shibazaki T, Hirai T, et al: Possible neural circuit mediating experimental tremor in monkeys (Abstract). *J Physiol Soc Jpn* 46:381, 1984
35. Shibazaki T, Hirai T, Nagaseki Y, et al: Ascending pathways to kinesthetic neurons in the monkey thalamus. *Neurosci Lett* [*Suppl*] 17:154, 1984
36. Shimazu H, Hongo T, Kubota K, et al: Rigidity and spasticity in man. *Arch Neurol* 6:10–17, 1962
37. Tasker RR, Organ LW, Hawrylyshyn PA: The thalamus and midbrain of man. Springfield, IL: Thomas, 1982
38. Yoshida M, Yanagisawa N, Shimazu H, et al: Physiological identification of the thalamic nucleus. *Arch Neurol* 11:435–443, 1964

25. THALAMOTOMY FOR PARKINSON'S DISEASE

Jean Siegfried
G. L. Rea

Despite the significant impact of dopamine replacement and other adjuvant medical therapies on the lives of patients with Parkinson's disease, the role of surgery in this disorder has gained renewed interest [32, 57]. To evaluate the position surgical therapy should hold in the treatment of Parkinson's disease symptoms, it is necessary to understand the incidence, etiology, pathology, and natural history, of the disorder and to weigh the benefits and complications of both medical and surgical therapies. This chapter reviews the literature and examines the long-term results in patients with Parkinson's disease who have been treated at the University of Zurich. The indications for surgical therapy are reviewed and reconsidered in light of these current findings.

Incidence and Etiology

Parkinson's disease is a significant health problem, affecting approximately 500,000 persons in the United States alone; 36,000 new cases are diagnosed each year [18, 19]. The incidence among Caucasians is reported to be 106–187 cases per 100,000 persons. Parkinson's disease may affect up to 1% of the population over age 60 and 2.5% over age 75 [18, 19, 30]. Although Orientals appear to have a lower incidence, the occurrence of Parkinson's disease among American blacks is not significantly different from that of Caucasians when age-adjusted prevalence ratios are considered [19, 41, 53] Recent studies also have shown that despite the lack of new cases related to von Economo's encephalitis, the incidence of Parkinson's disease has remained relatively constant during the past 20 years, which suggests that the number of cases related to that encephalitis epidemic were far fewer than originally thought [48].

The cause of primary Parkinson's disease remains elusive. It has been suggested that research into its cause has been slowed by the initial spectacular success of L-dopa therapy [39]. Although genetic factors have been considered important by some researchers, current studies indicate minimal hereditary influence [38, 69]. The relationship of Parkinson's disease to atherosclerosis, premature aging, metabolic defects, and infection all have been studied, but no consistently significant correlations have been found [6, 40, 41]. Recently, the possibility of a toxic cause has gained some credibility because of the discovery in heroin addicts of a syndrome resembling Parkinson's disease [1, 33]. A toxic substance, MPTP (N-methyl-4-phenyl-1,2,3,6-tetrahydropyridine), has produced a parkinsonian syndrome in nonhuman primates that is pathologically quite similar to Parkinson's disease in humans; some researchers are concerned that chronic exposure to even small quantities, coupled with the effect of aging, could be important in the development of the disorder [9, 12].

Pathology

In contrast to the lack of research into its cause, many investigations have been undertaken into the histological and biochemical pathology of Parkinson's disease. Histological findings commonly include cell drop-out, primarily in the zona compacta of the substantia nigra and also in the sympathetic ganglia [16, 67]. In virtually 100% of the cases, these areas

L.D. Lunsford (ed.) *MODERN STEREOTACTIC NEUROSURGERY*.

also contain Lewy bodies [17]. In addition, cell loss in the substantia innominata, locus ceruleus, the cortex, striatum, pallidum, and ventral tegmental area is described consistently [46, 67, 68].

The underlying biochemical pathology in Parkinson's disease is thought to be a deficiency of dopamine in the basal ganglia; the degree of this deficiency has been shown to correlate with melanin-containing neuronal loss in the pars compacta of the substantia nigra [16, 37]. Areas outside the nigrostriatal system that show decreased dopamine include the frontal cortex, the nucleus accumbens, and the olfactory tubercle [23, 27, 52]. Several authors have attempted to correlate these pathological and biochemical findings with the heterogenous clinical incidence of Parkinson's disease. Price and colleagues found that bradykinesia is associated with low dopamine levels in the accumbens-caudate pathway, whereas mental and affective changes were linked with low levels in the parolfactory gyrus–putamen connections [47]. Bernheimer and co-workers [5] reported similar findings: the decrease of dopamine and homovanillic acid in the caudate corresponded most directly with akinesia, but tremor correlated with the decrease of homovanillic acid in the pallidum. Uhl and associates postulated that the loss of pigmented cells in the ventral tegmental area could lead to the akinesia and cognitive problems of Parkinson's disease patients because this structure has wide connections with the mesolimbic and prefrontal cortex [68]. The dementia in some patients has also been related to the lack of dopamine in the cerebral cortex [24, 52].

Natural History

Until the widespread use of L-dopa in the late 1960s, the disease described by James Parkinson in 1817 was essentially unaltered by the many medical therapies proposed for its treatment. In 1967, Hoehn and Yahr reviewed the natural history of Parkinson's disease in more than 800 patients. They proposed a classification system for disease severity, considered the possibility that disease progression varied among individuals, and noted the important clinical characteristics of this pre-L-dopa population [22]. Of the 802 patients evaluated, 672 had a diagnosis of primary Parkinson's disease. The mean age of onset was 55.3 years. Tremor was the initial complaint in 71%, gait disturbance in 12%, and stiffness or slowness in 20%. The disability scale of Hoehn and Yahr ranged from I–V:

I. Unilateral involvement only; minimal or no functional impairment
II. Bilateral or midline involvement, no balance difficulty
III. Evidence of impaired righting reflex; unstable turning by patient may be demonstrated when patient is pushed from standing equilibrium position; disability mild to moderate
IV. Fully developed; severe disability; able to stand and walk unassisted, but markedly incapacitated
V. Confined to bed or wheelchair unless significant aid is available

Patients with primary Parkinson's disease were found to have a yearly mortality rate three times that of age and sex-matched control groups; their average age of death was 67.0 years. Although statistics were bleak for the patient population as a whole, Hoehn and Yahr believed that disease progression was quite slow in a subset of patients whose righting reflexes and balance were preserved during 10 years of illness and who had only minimal disability for 20 years. Of those patients who had Parkinson's disease for more than 10 years, 34% remained in a grade I status. Unfortunately, the only clinical clue to the identity of these patients was a suggestion that during the first 10 years of illness, disease progression was slower when tremor was the initial symptom.

This possibility that Parkinson's disease might have different courses has been supported more recently by neuropsychological [43] genetic [3], and clinical studies showing the syndrome to have both benign and malignant forms [8, 51]. Zetusky and associates [71] studied 334 patients and found that the subgroup of patients with tremor as their primary problem appeared to have a more favorable prognosis than did patients with rigidity, bradykinesia, or postural instability. This tremor subgroup was associated with a relative preservation of mental status, earlier age of disease onset, and a family history of parkinsonism. The realization that disease progression may vary has significant implications in evaluating reports of therapeutic efficacy and in planning treatment regimens for newly diagnosed patients.

Medical Therapy of Parkinson's Disease

Dopamine replacement therapy has been important, not only in improving the quality of life of patients with Parkinson's disease, but also in providing the first opportunity to treat a chronic degenerative disease of the central nervous system [2, 6, 35, 59]. L-dopa (used instead of dopamine, which does not cross the blood-brain barrier) has been found to improve the symptoms of bradykinesia and rigidity and, to a lesser extent, tremor [6]. Approximately 75% of patients responded to L-dopa; unfortunately, the doses required were quite high because 95% of it is peripherally decarboxylated and thus peripherally inactivated. The high doses caused significant nausea and vomiting problems, which were alleviated by the addition of a peripheral decarboxylase inhibitor. This inhibitor reduced the necessary L-dopa dosage by about 75%; it also lessened the side effects and the time necessary to reach optimum dosage and resulted in a greater number of patients improving [6, 11, 62, 70]. This replacement therapy has been shown to increase the longevity of patients and to lengthen the time spent in each clinical grade [20, 21, 26]. After three to five years of therapy, however, a significant number of patients begin to develop abnormal involuntary movements related to peak dosage, and sometimes the medications become ineffective in maintaining the patient's functional status [3, 7, 20, 65]. Although the actual number of patients who experience iatrogenic involuntary movements is unknown, Bergmann and colleagues [4] reported it to be as high as 93%. It also appears that 7%–30% of patients have abnormal involuntary movements that are dose-limiting [7, 20]. Because of these features of L-dopa therapy, other medications have been developed. The apomorphines, such as N-prophylnoraprophine, are dopamine agonists and have been examined as adjuvant therapy in Parkinson's disease [6, 14]. The ergoline class of compounds has also been used to produce the dopamine agonists bromocriptine, lisuride, pergolide, and mesulergine [6, 25, 31]. These medications have been somewhat successful in prolonging the effectiveness of therapy and decreasing the severity of "on-off" effects. However, they also cause some notable side effects that can limit their usefulness [6, 25, 31]. Other drugs that can increase the effectiveness of L-dopa are the monoamine oxidase (MAO)-B inhibitors. Compounds such as deprenyl act to inhibit MAO-B that degrades dopamine in the central nervous system and appears to aid in therapy for a while [6, 15].

Other medications such as amantadine, which is thought to cause the release of dopamine from terminals, and the anticholinergics, which aid in restoring the acetylcholine-dopamine imbalance in Parkinson's disease, may be mildly effective for a short time. However, they have been replaced largely by the use of L-dopa and the dopa decarboxylase inhibitors.

History of Surgical Therapy

Although before the mid-1950s, more than 20 different surgical procedures were advocated for the treatment of Parkinson's disease, since 1955 the procedure of choice has been a stereotactic interruption of the pallido-thalamo-cortical pathway [13, 32, 36, 57]. The stereotactic methods and frames used for this interruption are many, but they are all based on the same principle of combining radiography, atlas measurements, and physiological techniques to aid in localizing the target point [58]. The lesion is produced mechanically, chemically, or electrically.

The sites used most often to interrupt the pallido-thalamo-cortical system include the medial pallidum; the ventrolateral thalamic nuclei, ventro-oralis-anterior (VOA), ventro-oralis-posterior (VOP), and ventrointermedius (V.i.m.); or the subthalamic area, with its concentrations of pallido-fugal fibers [29, 32, 44, 45, 61, 66, 70]. Each of the various stereotactic frames, lesioning methods, and target sites has its advocates, and each has enjoyed some success in treating Parkinson's disease.

There have been many reports concerning the effectiveness of surgery in Parkinson's disease. Three relatively representative studies are those of Riechert in 1973 [49] Kelly and Gillingham in 1980 [28], and Matsumoto and coworkers in 1984 [42]. Riechert reviewed his surgical results in 2,000 cases of tremor [49]. He found that stereotactic procedures resulted in long-term tremor control, that is, tremor was never seen or was seen only with emotional stress in 81.4% of unilateral or bilateral cases. With pallidotomy or thalamotomy, rigidity was improved immediately in 86.5%, and long-term symptom control was obtained in 50.9%. In evaluating patients' total function, he used a point scale that included rigidity, tremor, akinesia, and secondary symptoms [50]. According to this evaluation system, symptoms substantially improved in 90% immediately after a unilateral procedure; improvement decreased to 82% with longer follow-up. In bilateral operations, improvement decreased from 84% initially to 59% with follow-up. The surgical morbidity included an incidence of intracranial bleeding (0.43%), transient dysphasia (0.57%), persisting paresis (0.14%), pneumonia (0.36%), and embolism (0.36%). Although there were some postoperative deaths early in the series, after Riechert began to use a temperature-regulated electrode, 1,000 patients underwent surgery with no mortality.

Kelly and Gillingham reported the results of thalamotomy in 60 patients who were followed for ten years, with evaluations every two years [28]. In 57 patients with preoperative tremor, the success rate after two years was 90%, after four years 73%, and after ten year 57%. The results in patients with rigidity was similar. In 42 patients treated with L-dopa, these researchers found the success rate of tremor treatment at two years was 25%, at four year 29% (some had had a thalamotomy), and at six year 16%. Sixty-nine percent of the L-dopa patients had significant rigidity at six years. They reported no mortality with surgery and noted the decreased incidence of L-dopa-induced dyskinetic movements on the side contralateral to the thalamotomy.

Matsumoto and associates evaluated 86 of 103 patients receiving ventral lateral thalamotomy, either bilateral or unilateral, between 1964 and 1969, prior to L-dopa therapy [42]. Although they did not evaluate the specific effect of surgery on tremor or rigidity, they did examine the effects of thalamotomy on clinical grade ten years after surgery. They found that 31% of 64 patients receiving unilateral thalamotomy had no progression after ten years. They also found that, ten years after the second surgery in bilateral cases, 14 of 22 had no clinical grade deterioration. No perioperative mortality was noted, but 10% of the patients experienced transient confusion, and 8% had some hemifacial weakness. The confusion and weakness cleared during hospitalization. They again noted that L-dopa dyskinesias were virtually absent on the side operated on.

Stereotactic Surgery at the University of Zurich

At the University of Zurich, the Riechert-Mundinger frame [50], stereotactic ventriculography, and intracerebral stimulation techniques are used to localize the VOP and V.i.m. nuclei of the thalamus and the subthalamic region. High-frequency electrocoagulation is used to produce the lesion. During placement of the frame and subsequent surgery, only local anesthesia is used. Patients with multiple sclerosis receive corticosteroids one day before surgery, but no other antibiotics or premedications are given routinely. This decreases the chance of an adverse drug reaction and allows the patient to be wide awake and fully cooperative during the procedure.

While the patient is in a supine position and the frame is in place, a lateral roentgenogram is obtained. A line is drawn on the film from bregma to the dorsum sellae, and the length of the line is measured and then multiplied by a constant factor of 0.6874. The resulting figure becomes a distance that is measured along the reference line on the roentgenogram, beginning at bregma. The target for the ventricular catheter is a point 3–5 mm posterior to this point along the bregma-dorsum line [60]. This method of localizing the foramen of Monro is successful in 92% of cases. Using a 2.5-mm drill, a burr hole is made without an incision in a small area of shaved scalp at a point approximately 5 mm anterior to the coronal suture and 3 cm from the midline. After coagulation of the dura, the cannula is inserted, 10 cm^3 of cerebrospinal fluid is removed, and 15–20 cm^3 of air is injected. The use of the bregma-dorsum sellae line to locate the foramen of Monro allows precise placement of the cannula tip so that sufficient filling of the third ventricle and, usually, the aqueduct and fourth ventricle are obtained. The position of the target for tremor, VOP/V.i.m., is located along the foramen of Monro–posterior commissure reference line. When this line measures 23.5 mm, the target point is 12.5 mm posterior to the foramen of Monro and 11 mm lateral to the third ventricle border. After these calculations are determined, an identical second burr hole is made, and an electrode is introduced. We use an electrode made in our department; it is 2 mm in diameter and has a 2-mm exposed tip. It also contains a second (0.7-mm) electrode, which has the capability of lateral extension and is controlled by a micromanipulator.

The anatomical placement of the electrode is confirmed by 50–100 Hz stimulation using biphasic wave forms of 1–2 msec duration. Such stimulation enables us to identify the internal capsule as well as points at which the tremor is arrested, initiated, or facilitated. For surgical procedures on the dominant side, it also allows us to observe the effects of stimulation on speech. Next, a lesion is made, while the patient is observed for evidence of weakness or other untoward effects. The size of the lesion is increased until the tremor is absent even with facilitating measures, unless, of course, weakness or dysphasia occurs. If the lesion must be made outside the axis of the electrode pass, extension of the string electrode laterally with the micromanipulator is invaluable, for it obviates the need for another electrode pass. Using computer-calculated target points, we are able to perform the entire operation in one stage in no more than 75 minutes. The patient is transferred back to the room fully alert and is usually discharged in fewer than six days.

This method has been used in more than 1,500 patients since 1958. We have found it to be successful in 85% of the cases in which it was performed for unilateral tremor and have had similar results with rigidity. Transient postoperative contralateral facial paresis, lateropulsion, and foot-dragging were seen in 30% of closely monitored patients, but these side effects lasted only a few days to a few weeks. In 10% of patients who had surgery in the dominant hemisphere, dysphasia appeared and was usually longer lasting.

When patients were observed closely for learning and memory changes following thalamotomy, we found that the left-sided lesions affected mainly verbal memory and that right-sided lesions affected nonverbal memory. These alterations, however, were limited in content and duration, and did not affect attention span or short-term memory [29]. In our series, the peroperative mortality rate was 0.2%. Although the success rates reported earlier in unilateral cases were similar for bilateral procedures, speech, balance, and swallowing difficulties developed in 20%–30% of patients after a lesion was placed in the second side. For this reason, bilateral procedures are performed only in exceptional cases and only after an interval of at least one year.

These results have also been examined in patients over 70 years of age. The results were the same, and the incidence of complications was no higher. The only significant difference is that the elderly patients were hospitalized longer, for both social and rehabilitative reasons [63].

Discussion

After considering the incidence and natural history of Parkinson's disease, the results of medical therapy, and current reports of surgical therapy, some guidelines can be constructed for selecting patients most likely to benefit from a surgical procedure.

Incidence and prevalence studies show that Parkinson's disease affects a large number of elderly persons; as the average life span increases, the total number of these patients will increase. The greater number of patients will demand more of society's resources; therefore, all forms of therapy should be evaluated in terms of lifetime cost, efficacy, and ability to free the patient from the health care system. Parkinson's disease has a wide range of effects; some patients experience tremor alone for many years, while others suffer rapidly progressing rigidity, bradykinesia, and dementia. Although it is difficult to separate these patient groups clearly, we believe that patients with tremor only should have stereotactic surgery, which offers the potential for an efficient, complete cure of the tremor. In cases of tremor, surgery is much more effective than medical therapy for both the short and long term.

Medical therapy of Parkinson's disease initially alleviates the most physically debilitating symptom of bradykinesia but does not adequately treat the socially debilitating symptom of tremor. Furthermore, in a significant number of patients, continuous use of medications in doses required to treat bradykinesia effectively often leads to severe abnormal involuntary movements. To be capable of even minimal movement, the patient must tolerate severe involuntary movements. Abnormal involuntary movements repeatedly have been shown to be prevented or stopped by stereotactic thalamotomy [28, 32, 61, 64]. In the long run, surgical control of tremor is significantly better than medical control [28, 32, 42, 61]. As noted previously, major studies also indicated the very important fact that iatrogenic dyskinesias can be controlled by stereotactic procedures [28, 42, 44, 54, 55, 58, 59]. This functionally widens the therapeutic range of the medications and improves the patient's status. The morbidity and mortality in unilateral procedures is quite small, and with careful monitoring and patient selection, is acceptable [61, 63].

The literature suggests that those patients who are young, those with a family history of Parkinson's disease, and those with unilateral tremor, have a prolonged and more benign course of their disease. In this group, surgery should be considered as initial therapy. Patients with significant unilateral tremor that is not controlled with medications also should be considered for surgery. In addition, patients with severe unilateral abnormal involuntary movements are important surgical candidates, because surgery aided by medication results in a longer period of functional activity.

It is important to understand that, although stereotactic ablative procedures can improve the symptoms of Parkinson's disease in these patients, it is not the final tool at the disposal of the functional neurosurgeon. Other surgical alternatives, such as thalamic stimulation, cell transplantation, and intraventricular infusion techniques, may offer future benefits for patients with Parkinson's disease.

References

1. Ballard PA, Tetrud JW, Langston JW: Permanent human parkinsonism due to MPTP: Seven Cases. *Neurology* 35:949–956, 1985
2. Barbeau A: L-dopa therapy in Parkinson's disease: A critical review of nine years' experience. *Can Med Assoc J* 101:791–800, 1969
3. Barbeau A, Pourcher E: New data on the genetics of Parkinson's disease. *Can J Neurol Sci* 9:53–66, 1982
4. Bergmann KJ, Mendoza MR, Yahr MD: Parkinson's disease and long-term levodopa therapy. Presented at the VIIIth International Symposium on Parkinson's Disease, June 9–12, 1985, New York, NY
5. Bernheimer H, Birkmayer W, Hornykiewicz O, et al: Brain dopamine and the syndromes of parkinsonism and Huntington: Clinical, morphological and neurochemical correlation. *J Neurol Sci* 20:415–455, 1973
6. Bienchne JR: Drugs for Parkinson's disease, spasticity, and acute muscle spasms. In Gilman AG, Goodman LS, Rall TW, et al (eds): *The Pharmacological Basis of Therapeutics.* New York: Macmillan, 1985, pp 473–490
7. Birkmayer W, Danielczyk W, Riederer P: Symptoms and side effects in the course of Parkinson's disease. *J Neural Transm [Suppl]* 19:185–199, 1983
8. Birkmayer W, Reiderer P, Youdin JBH: Distinction between benign and malignant types of Parkinson's disease. *Clin Neurol Neurosurg* 81:158–164, 1979
9. Blume E: Street drugs yield Parkinson's model. *JAMA* 250:13–14, 1983
10. Burns RS, Chiuch CC, Markey SP, et al: A primate model of parkinsonism: Selective destruction of dopaminergic neurons in the pars compacta of the substantia nigra by MPTP. *Nat Acad Sci USA* 80:4546–4550, 1983
11. Calne DB: Progress in Parkinson's disease. *N Engl J Med* 310:523–524, 1984
12. Calne DB, Langston JW: Aetiology of Parkinson's disease. *Lancet* 2:1457–1459, 1984
13. Cooper IS: Neurosurgical treatment of dyskinesias. *Clin Neurosurg* 24:367–390, 1977
14. Cotzias GS, Papavasiliou PS, Tolosa ES, et al: Treatment of parkinsonism with apomorphines: Possible role of growth hormone. *N Engl J Med* 294:567–572, 1976
15. Da Prada M, Keller HH, Pieri L, et al: The pharmacology of Parkinson's disease: Basic aspects and recent advances. *Experientia* 40:1165–1172, 1984
16. Ehringer H, Hornykiewicz O: Verteilung von noradrenalin und dopamin im gehirn des menschen und ihr verhalten bei erkrankungen des extrapyramidalen systems. *Klin Wochenschr* 38:1236–1239, 1960
17. Forno LS: The Lewy body in Parkinson's disease. Presented at the VIIIth International Symposium on Parkinson's Disease, June 9–12, 1985, New York, NY
18. Gilroy J, Meyer JS: *Medical Neurolgy* (2nd ed). New York: Macmillan, 1975
19. Harada H, Nishikawa S, Takahashi K: Epidemiology of Parkinson's disease in a Japanese city. *Arch Neurol* 40:151–154, 1983
20. Hoehn M: Parkinsonism treated with levodopa: Progression and mortality. *J Neural Transm [Suppl]* 19:253–264, 1983
21. Hoehn M: Parkinson's disease: progression and mortality. Presented at the VIIIth International Symposium on Parkinson's Disease, June 9–12, 1985, New York, NY
22. Hoehn MM, Yahr MD: Parkinsonism: Onset,

progression and mortality. *Neurology* 17:427–442, 1967

23. Hornykiewicz O: Biochemical abnormalities in some extrastriatal neuronal systems in Parkinson's disease. In Rinne UK, Klingler M, Stamm G (eds): *Parkinson's Disease: Current Progress, Problems and Management.* Amsterdam: Elsevier, Biomedical Press, 1980, pp 109–119
24. Hornykiewicz O: Current concepts and controversies in Parkinson's disease. (Symposium) *Can J Neurol Sci* 11 (Suppl 1):89–240, 1984
25. Jankovic J: Long-term study of pergolide in Parkinson's disease. *Neurology* 35:296–299, 1985
26. Joseph C, Chassan JB, Koch ML: Levodopa in Parkinson's disease. *Ann Neurol* 227:75–88, 1982
27. Jovoy-Agid F, Agid Y: Is the mesocortical dopaminergic system involved in Parkinson's disease? *Neurology* 30:1326–1330, 1980
28. Kelly PJ, Gillingham FJ: The long-term results of stereotaxic surgery and L-dopa therapy in patients with Parkinson's disease. *J Neurosurg* 53:332–337, 1980
29. Kocher U, Siegfried J, Perret E: Verbal and nonverbal learning ability of Parkinson patients before and after unilateral ventrolateral thalamotomy. *Appl Neurophysiol* 45:311–316, 1982
30. Kurland LT, Kurtzke JF, Goldberg ID: Epidemiology of neurologic and sense organ disorders. Cambridge, MA: Harvard University Press, 1973, pp 41–63
31. Kurland R, Miller C, Lewy R, et al: Long-term experience with pergolide therapy of advanced parkinsonism. *Neurology* 35:738–742, 1985
32. Laitinen LV: Brain targets in surgery for Parkinson's disease. *J Neurosurg* 62:349–351, 1985
33. Langston JW, Ballard PA, Tetrud JW: Chronic parkinsonism in humans due to nine products of meperidine-analog synthesis. *Science* 219:979–980, 1983
34. Langston JW, Forno LS, Robert CS, et al: Selective nigral toxicity after systemic administration of MPTP in the squirrel monkey. *Brain Res* 292:390–394, 1984
35. Lesser RP, Fahn S, Snider SR, et al: Analysis of the clinical problems in parkinsonism and the complications of long-term levodopa therapy. *Neurology* 29:1253–1260, 1979
36. Manen J, Speelman JD, Tans KJJ: Indications for surgical treatment of Parkinson's disease after levodopa therapy. *Clin Neurol Neurosurg* 86:207–212, 1984
37. Mann DMA, Yates PD: Possible role of neuromelanin in the pathogenesis of Parkinson's disease. *Mech Ageing Dev* 21:193–203, 1983
38. Martin WE, Young WI, Anderson VE: Parkinson's disease: A genetic study. *Brain* 96:495–506, 1973
39. Marttila RJ: Etiology of Parkinson's disease. In Rinne UK, Klingler M, Stamm G (eds): *Parkinson's Disease: Current Progress, Problems, and Management.* Amsterdam: Elsevier, Biomedical Press, 1980, pp 3–16
40. Marttila RJ, Rinne UK: Arteriosclerosis, heredity, and some previous infections in the etiology of Parkinson's disease: A case control study. *Clin Neurol Neurosurg* 79:45–56, 1976
41. Marttila RJ, Rinne UK: Epidemiology of Parkinson's disease: An overview. *J Neural Transm* 51:135–148, 1981
42. Matsumoto K, Shichijo F, Fukami T: Long-term follow-up review of cases of Parkinson's disease after unilateral or bilateral thalamotomy. *J Neurosurg* 60:1033–1044, 1984
43. Mortimer JA, Pirozzola FJ, Hansch EC, et al: Relationship of motor symptoms to intellectual defects in Parkinson's disease. *Neurology* 32:133–137, 1982
44. Narabayashi H, Yokochi F, Nakajima Y: Levodopa-induced dyskinesia and thalamotomy. *J Neurol Neurosurg Psychiatry* 47:831–839, 1984
45. Ohye C, Hirai T, Miyazaki M, et al: V.i.m. thalamotomy for the treatment of various kinds of tremor. *Appl Neurophysiol* 45:275–280, 1982
46. Oppenheimer DR: Diseases of the basal ganglia, cerebellum and motor neurons. In *Greenfield's Pathology* (3rd ed). New York: Wiley, 1976, pp 608–651
47. Price KS, Farley IJ, Hornykiewicz O: Neurochemistry of Parkinson's disease: relation between striatal and limbic dopamine. In Roberts PJ, Woodruff GM, Iversen LL (eds): *Advances in Biomedical Psychopharmacology*, Vol 19. New York: Raven Press, 1978, pp 293–300
48. Rajput AG, Offord KP, Beard CM, et al: Epidemiology of parkinsonism: Incidence, classification, and mortality. *Ann Neurol* 16:278–282, 1984
49. Riechert T: Stereotaxic surgery for treatment of Parkinson's syndrome. *Prog Neurol Surg* 5:1–78, 1973
50. Riechert T, Mundinger F: Beschreibung und anwendung eines Zielgeraetes for stereotaktische hirnoperationen (II. Model). *Acta Neurochir [Suppl]* (Wien) 308:337, 1955
51. Rinne UK, Sonninen V, Siirtola T, et al: Long-term responses of Parkinson's disease to levodopa therapy. *J Neural Transm [Suppl]* 16:149–156, 1980
52. Scatton B, Ronguier L, Jovoy-Agid F, et al: Dopamine deficiency in the cerebral cortex in Parkinson's disease. *Neurology* 32:1039–1040, 1982
53. Schoenberg BS, Anderson DW, Haerer AF: Prevalence of Parkinson's disease in the biracial population of Copiah County, Mississippi. *Neurology* 35:841–845, 1985

54. Selby G: The influence of previous stereotactic thalamotomy on L-dopa therapy in Parkinson's disease. *Proc Aust Assn Neurol* 13:55–60, 1976
55. Siegfried J: Deux and d'experience avec la L-dopa associeé a un inhibiteur de la decarboxylase. *Rev Neurol* (Paris) 122:243–248, 1970
56. Siegfried J: Is the neurosurgical treatment of Parkinson's disease still indicated? *J Neural Transm [Suppl]* 16:195–198, 1980
57. Siegfried J: Neurosurgical treatment of Parkinson's disease. Present indications and value. In Rinne UK, Klingler M, Stamm G (eds): *Parkinson's Disease: Current Progress, Problems and Management*, North Holland: Elsevier, Biomedical Press, 1980, pp 369–376
58. Siegfried J: *Die Parkinsonsche Krankheit und ihre Behandlung*, Vol 1. Wien, New York: Springer Verlag, 1968, p 262
59. Siegfried J: The place of L-dopa in the treatment of Parkinson's disease. *Progr Neurol Surg* 5:387–405, 1973
60. Siegfried J, Brandli-Graber S: Repérage radiologique simple du trou de Monro sur les radiographies crâniennes à vide. *Neurochirurgie* 26:387–389, 1980
61. Siegfried J, Hood T: Current status of functional neurosurgery. In Krayenbuhl H (ed): *Advances and Technical Standards in Neurosurgery*, Vol 10. New York: Springer-Verlag, 1983, pp 19–79
62. Siegfried J, Klaiber R, Perret E, et al: Treatment of Parkinson's disease with L-dopa and a decarboxylase inhibitor. *German Medical Monthly* 15:315–318, 1970
63. Siegfried J, Zumstein H: Thalamotomies stereotaxiques pour troubles fonctionnels chez les personnes agees. *Neurochirurgie* 22:536–539, 1976
64. Svennilson E, Torvik A, Lower R, et al: Treatment of parkinsonism by stereotactic thermolesions in the pallidal region: A clinical evaluation of 81 cases. *Acta Psychiatr Neurol Scand* 35:358–377, 1960
65. Sweet RD, McDowell FH: Five years' treatment of Parkinson's disease with levodopa: Therapeutic results and survival of 100 patients. *Ann Intern Med* 83:456–486, 1975
66. Tasker RR, Organ LW, Hawrylyshyn P: Investigation of the surgical target for alleviation of involuntary movement disorders. *Appl Neurophysiol* 45:261–274, 1982
67. Turner B: Pathology of paralysis agitans. In Vinken PJ, Bruyn GW (eds): *Diseases of the Basal Ganglia. Handbook of Clinical Neurology*, Vol 6. Amsterdam-North Holland, 1968, pp 212–217
68. Uhl GR, Hedreen JC, Price DL: Parkinson's disease: Loss of neurons from the ventral tegmental area contralateral to therapeutic surgical lesions. *Neurology* 35:1215–1218, 1985
69. Ward CD, Duvoisin RC, Ince SE, et al: Parkinson's disease in 65 pairs of twins and in a set of quadruplets. *Neurology* 33:815–824, 1983
70. Yahr MD: Overview of present day treatment of Parkinson's disease. *J Neural Transm* 43:227–238, 1978
71. Zetusky WJ, Jankovic J, Pirozzola FJ: The hetrogeneity of Parkinson's disease: clinical and prognostic implications. *Neurology* 35:522–526, 1985

26. POSTTRAUMATIC MOVEMENT DISORDERS

Dennis E. Bullard
Blaine S. Nashold

Practical Indications

INCIDENCE

Death and disability are major problems of closed head injuries. It has been estimated that, in the United States alone, head injury causes approximately 24 deaths/100,000 population [16]. Perhaps more troubling is the morbidity that occurs among those who survive severe head injuries: six months after their accident, 1%–5% of patients remain vegetative and 5%–18% severely disabled [17]. These disabled individuals represent a significant proportion of the population. In the United States, their number is not clearly defined. In Britain, where head injuries are somewhat less common, (9 deaths/100,000 population) the number of individuals with major handicaps persisting after head injury has been estimated at 150/100,000 persons; one in 300 British families has such a member [1, 16]. Reduced speed limits and mandatory seat belt laws are likely to increase further the population of surviving, disabled patients.

Strich reviewed the relationship between head injury and subsequent neurological disease [28, 29]. Head injury has been linked tenuously with Alzheimer's disease [9, 15], Pick's disease [21], motor neuron disease, and Jakob-Creutzfeldt disease. In contrast, a clear association exists between severe head injury and the subsequent development of movement disorders (MD) [2, 7, 18, 23], although the true nature of these MD is unclear. In his extensive review of prolonged posttraumatic coma, Bricolo stated that extrapyramidal and cerebellar syndromes were among the possible neurological sequelae of severe head injury, and he described various combinations of these syndromes, including tremor and rigidity [4]. However, reports of such extrapyramidal syndromes following severe head injury are relatively rare. Grimberg, in 1934, related closed head injury to the subsequent development of Parkinson's disease [12]. Kremer and colleagues later reported nine patients who had dysarthria and ataxia after head injury [18]. Of these, three had coarse postural tremors believed to be secondary to midbrain damage. Andrew and co-workers described eight patients with involuntary MD after closed head injury. In seven of these, volitional movement aggravated the MD [2]. Niizuma and associates (1982) reported on three patients with posttraumatic MD, characterized by hemiparesis with coarse and irregular postural and kinetic tremors involving primarily the arm [23].

SYNDROME

The findings of the previous authors are similar to our findings in 14 patients with posttraumatic MD (table 26–1) [6]. Virtually all of these patients sustained severe head injuries and had prolonged comas. At the time of head injury, pupillary dysfunction, stereotypic reflex posturing, and other signs of brain-stem dysfunction were evident. As the level of consciousness improved, a severe MD developed. In most instances, this was noted as soon as purposeful movement occurred. In some patients, the MD fluctuated in intensity over the next three to six months but then stabilized and did not change substantially thereafter. These patients usually had other overt sequelae of the trauma. The most common deficit was dysarthria. Thirteen of the 14 patients in our series demonstrated

L.D. Lunsford (ed.) *MODERN STEREOTACTIC NEUROSURGERY*.

mild to moderate dysarthria. Eleven had some degree of psychomotor retardation, eight had hemiparesis, and seven had ocular motility problems. A variety of MD were observed, and more than one type was seen in 11 patients. These consisted of action or intention tremors in ten, choreoathetoid movements in four, and truncal ataxia or titubation in two. We also saw asynchronous, violent movements in 11. We first described these as hemiballismus, based upon their sudden, violent nature and severity. The dominant MD often was seen when the patient was at rest, but it worsened characteristically when a fixed posture was assumed and increased most strikingly during action. The MD was coarse and irregular and involved varying muscle groups. Often, the patient either used the contralateral limb to restrain the involved side or sat on the involved hand. This particular MD was most often the patient's disabling problem during the postinjury recovery period. The majority of patients had difficulty feeding themselves, writing, and, in certain instances, walking because the MD was so severe.

MEDICAL MANAGEMENT

Attempts at treating posttraumatic MD medically generally have failed. Andrew and colleagues reported on eight patients, one of whom believed that alcohol improved the MD [2]. In another, propranolol reduced the MD somewhat. Two patients received tetrabenazine, and one haloperidol, without benefit. In contrast, Starosta-Rubinstein and co-workers (1983) described a posttraumatic intention myoclonus [27] in a 54-year-old woman who had sustained a closed head injury at the age of four. After the injury, she was comatose. She eventually improved but was left with dysarthria and asynchronous, asymmetric jerking movements of the face, tongue, and all limbs. Taking oral clonazepam at a dose that eventually reached 1 mg twice daily, she improved, and maintained satisfactory response for four and one-half months. Chadwick and associates reported on 15 patients with myoclonus, one of whom developed the disorder following severe head injury [8]. Eight of the fifteen patients (including the patient with the posttraumatic disorder) improved with 5-hydroxytryptophan, tryptophan in combination with a monoamine oxidase inhibitor, and clonazepam. In our series, we used a wide variety of agents including haloperidol, carbidopalevopdopa, trihexyphenidyl hydrochloride, ethopropazine, benztropine mesylate, diphenhydramine amantadine phenytoin, clorazepate dipotassium, phenobarbital, diazepam, propranolol, valproic acid, carbamazepine, and clonazepam. However, medical management did not produce satisfactory clinical responses in our patients. It is difficult to determine whether the posttraumatic myoclonus is the same syndrome as posttraumatic MD. Clinically, the descriptions are similar; however, the reports of posttraumatic intention myoclonus generally have been included in larger series with postanoxic myoclonus [20]. Posttraumatic and postanoxic syndromes appear to be closely related, both clinically and pharmacologically [8, 20], but unlike posttraumatic MD, postanoxic myoclonus did not respond to thalamotomy [10]. This suggests that more than one syndrome exists.

SURGICAL INDICATIONS

The practical indications for consideration of a stereotactic thalamotomy for a posttraumatic MD are: that the disorder is significantly disabling, that it has shown no evidence of spontaneous improvement one year after the injury, and that a reasonable trial of medical management has been completed. This last criterion is the most difficult to determine. In our experience, quite extensive trials of medical management consistently failed to provide satisfactory relief. Among our patients, the median duration of symptoms before referral for surgical evaluation has been five years, with a range of 1–28 years. However, the patient population in our tertiary referral center is skewed toward those who have failed medical treatment. Thus, it is difficult to establish from our data which agents should be tried before proceeding with thalamotomy. Based upon the broad responses to drugs of other MD, propranolol and clonazepam should be tried before surgery is considered. Exhaustive trials of multiple drugs and unnecessary delays before considering surgery are not indicated, however.

PREOPERATIVE EVALUATION

Preoperatively, patients should undergo electroencephalograms (EEG), computed tomography (CT), detailed speech and memory testing (SMT) [6], and videotaping. The EEG is performed to exclude an underlying seizure focus, the CT to rule out a mass lesion, and SMT to evaluate the risks of postoperative speech and memory dysfunction. The patients at maximal risk for developing speech and memory problems are those with evidence of generalized brain atrophy or significant encephalomalacia on CT, those in whom a dominant thalamotomy is to be performed, and those with poor preoperative SMT scores. The most frequently encountered significant postoperative dysfunction, however, is dysarthria. Those most at risk for this are patients with a degree of preoperative dysarthria and, to a lesser extent, patients undergoing dominant thalamotomies. Other postoperative dysfunctions include dysphagia and contralateral weakness, usually in the leg. These dysfunctions are often transient.

TECHNIQUE

ANESTHESIA

Crucial to a successful operation is the preoperative establishment of a close rapport with the patient. The day before surgery, the procedure should be discussed in great detail with the patient and the patient's family. The coldness of the operating room, the discomfort associated with local anesthesia, and the strange sensation and pain of having one's head fixed within a frame are best dealt with in advance to minimize their impact. We stress this because we believe it is important to avoid using preoperative sedatives, which potentially can alter the MD and/or the patient's intraoperative ability to cooperate. The patient fasts overnight and undergoes the stereotactic procedure as the first case of the day, so that he or she does not have to await surgery while fasting and anxious. When sedation is absolutely required, we use a short-acting narcotic-sedative compound, such as fentanyl, before the head is shaved, washed, and anesthetized. In such anxious patients, the head is placed in the stereotactic frame before the burr hole is placed; normally, this sequence is reversed. During this time, it is crucial to maintain an atmosphere as soothing as possible to prevent the need for further sedation.

VENTRICULOGRAPHY

To prepare the head, we cut all of the hair and cleanse the head with an iodinated soap, iodine, and alcohol. A burr hole is made at the approximate level of the coronal suture and centered 2 cm from the midline, after infiltration of this area with 1% lidocaine. The patient then is placed in a Todd-Wells stereotactic frame and anteroposterior (AP) and lateral roentgenograms are obtained to evaluate the position of the head within the frame. In our operating rooms, fixed lateral and AP radiography machines provide the necessary studies with known magnification factors. Because roentgen rays travel in a radial rather than a parallel fashion, parallax and magnification occur. To compensate for this, the stereotactic frame must be centered within the roentgen-ray beam and its position confirmed before each case. Also, the degree of magnification must be known. This can be determined by taking a roentgenogram of a radiopaque ruler or other object of known length and then measuring its length on the film. The discrepancy between this measurement and the object's length indicates the magnification factors. This must be done for both AP and lateral films unless the roentgen-ray tubes are the same distance from the center of the frame.

In positioning the patient, it is crucial that no tilt or rotational misalignment occur before the stereotactic procedure is performed. We position the head so that a point 2 cm above the dorsum sellae, corresponding to the approximate position of the foramen of Monro, is centered within the frame.

Next, a ventriculogram is obtained. Originally, we used a water-insoluble positive-contrast medium, which was introduced into the ventricular system through a silicone elastomer cannula. More recently, we have used metrizamide, a water-soluble contrast agent, (1–3 ml, 250 mg of iodine per ml). If the structures are not adequately visible, this dose may be repeated once. While this conceivably could cause a seizure because of the epileptogenic potential of metrizamide, we had no untoward problems using this regimen for all intraoperative ventriculograms. Others have use metrizamide for ventriculography in more than 500 patients, reporting only one major adverse reaction, a seizure [26]. Investigators who recorded EEG before, during, and after injecting metrizamide and performed serial analysis of the cerebrospinal fluid found no evidence of significant changes after injecting the metrizamide [30]. We chose this regimen because it enables excellent visualization of the anterior

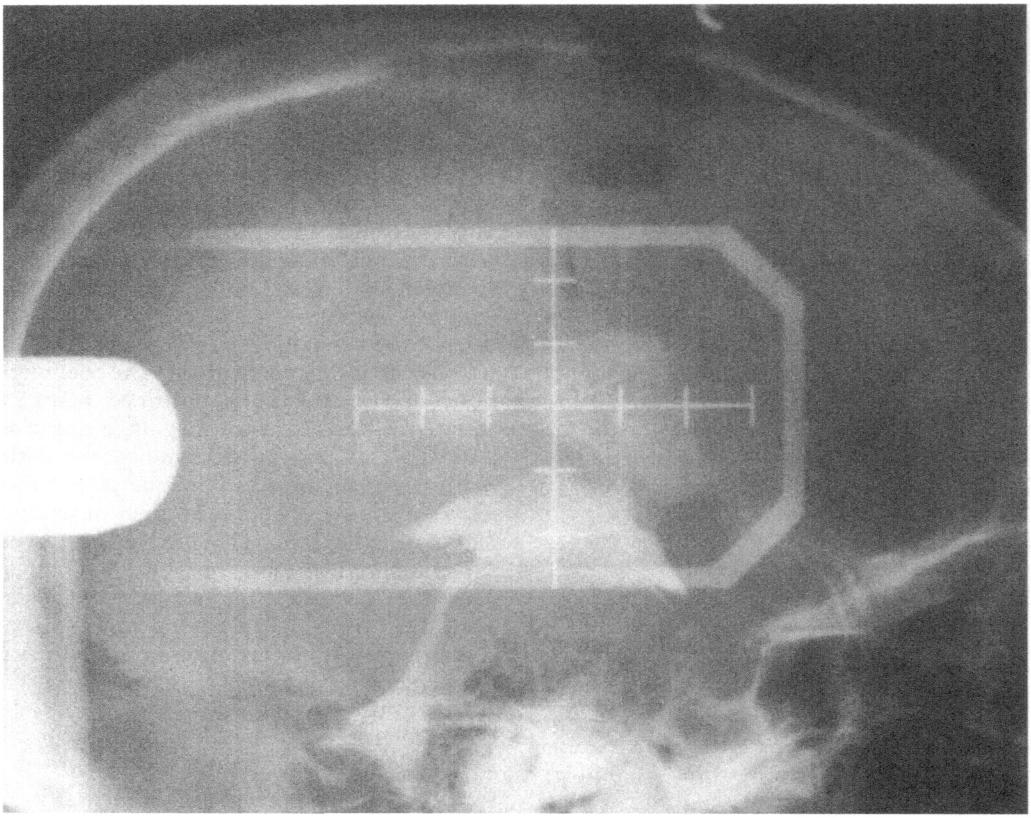

A

FIGURE 26–1. Intraoperative anteroposterior ventriculogram with metrizamide clearly shows the third ventricle (A). Intraoperative lateral ventriculogram performed in sequence clearly delineates the anterior and posterior commissures (B). The AC–PC line is superimposed.

commissure (AC) and posterior commissure (PC) and because the water-soluble dye is excreted (figure 26–1, left). The metrizamide is injected through a ventricular catheter, premeasured to extend no deeper than 5 cm below the cortex. The catheter is inserted more medially and anteriorly than is usual for a ventriculostomy. For general landmarks, we use the medial canthus of the eye and a point just anterior to the central cross hairs of the Todd-Wells frame. This corresponds intracranially to a point just anterior to the foramen of Monro. The majority of the contrast usually is injected into the third ventricle, rather than into the lateral ventricles, and the catheter tip does not obscure any of the third-ventricular landmarks. Immediately after injection, AP and lateral roentgenograms are obtained. The AC-PC line and the width of the third ventricle then are determined. Both of these parameters must be clearly established in order to select appropriate initial radiographic target coordinates (see figure 26–1).

SELECTION OF INITIAL TARGET

Selecting targets for treating MD is somewhat confused by a rather poor understanding of the true nature of MD and the variations both in individual anatomy and in nomenclature. An excellent review of nomenclatures was published by Gildenberg [11]. The earliest lesions for treating MD were placed in the globus pallidus for Parkinson's disease. In 1959, however, Bravo and Cooper demonstrated that a

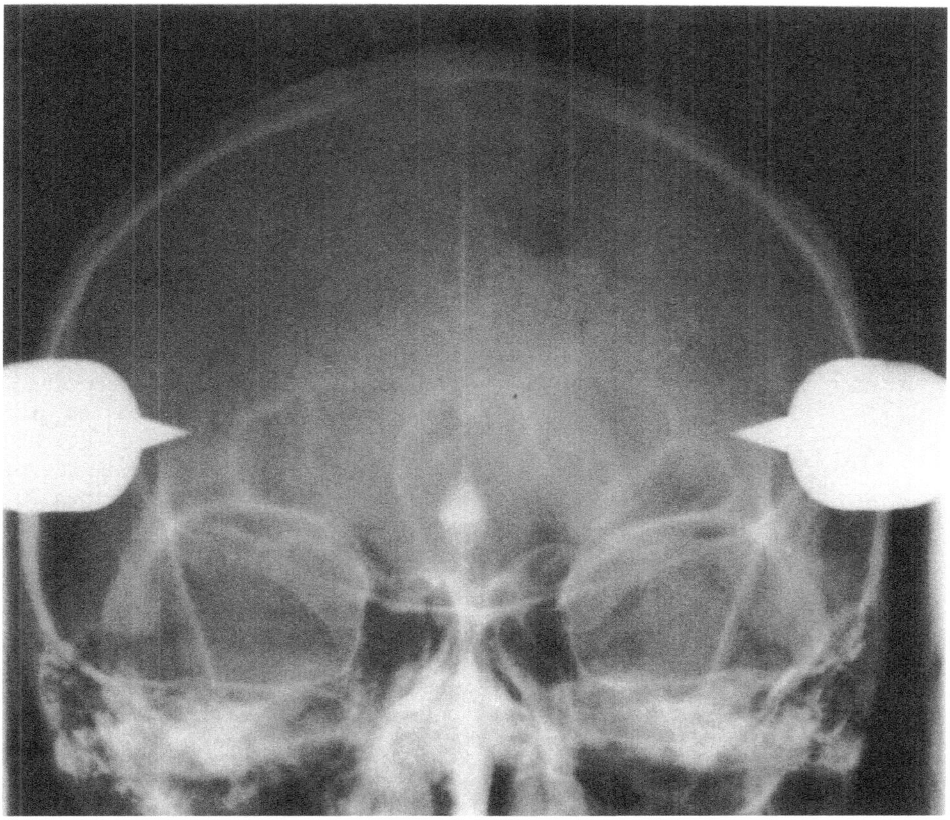

B

FIGURE 26–1. (cont.)

stereotactic lesion in the ventrolateral (VL) nucleus of the thalamus effectively reduced the tremor and rigidity of this disease. Subsequently, the VL and the interconnecting fiber tracts, the ansa lenticularis and fields of Forel became the most common targets [3]. Tasker and colleagues (1982) reviewed stereotactic targets for control of MD. Their data suggested that a common target in the inferior ventrointermedius (V.i.m.) nucleus, in the 13.5-mm sagittal plane, was effective for the control of a wide variety of dyskinesias [31]. Lesions made in this general area were capable of reducing the rigidity, dystonia, chorea, and tremor associated with many causes, including multiple sclerosis, Parkinson's disease, cerebellar degeneration, and posttraumatic or postanoxic injuries. For cerebellar tremor per se, targets ranged over the inferior ventro-oralis anterior (VOA), ventro-oralis posterior (VOP), and V.i.m. nuclei (figure 26–2). However, various MD, including the cerebellar type, have been controlled satisfactorily with lesions in other areas within the VL nucleus, varying by 6–7 mm, and in the pallidofugal fibers of the fields of Forel or the zona incerta [19].

Although some recommend that specific symptoms be matched with particular coordinates, this approach seems to be consistently effective only in Parkinson's disease, in which rostral lesions appear to have more influence on rigidity than on tremor. Many recommend either absolute coordinates for the initial target point or proportionate systems. Gildenberg recommends the following empiric coordinates: 2 mm anterior to the midpoint of the intercommissural (AC–PC) line, 9.5 mm lateral to, and 3 mm above the line for rigidity; for tremor 2 mm posterior to the mid AC–PC line, 11.5 mm lateral to, and 3 mm above, the AC–PC line. He also recommends the posterior target coordinates for tremor having other causes

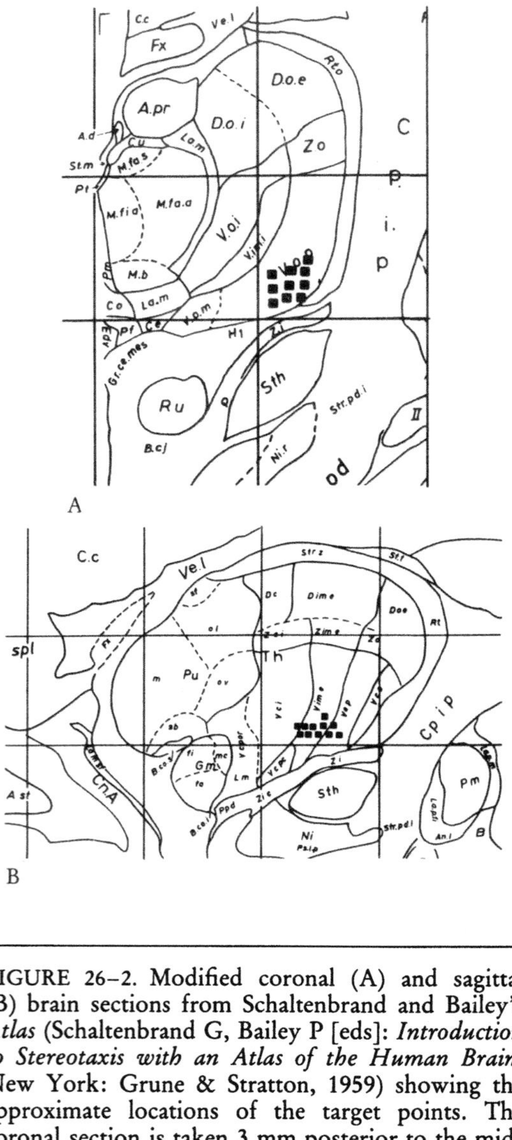

FIGURE 26–2. Modified coronal (A) and sagittal (B) brain sections from Schaltenbrand and Bailey's *Atlas* (Schaltenbrand G, Bailey P [eds]: *Introduction to Stereotaxis with an Atlas of the Human Brain.* New York: Grune & Stratton, 1959) showing the approximate locations of the target points. The coronal section is taken 3 mm posterior to the mid-AC–PC line. The sagittal section is 15 mm from the midline. Th = thalamus; Pu = pulvinar; Cpip = internal capsule, posterior limb; vci = nucleus ventrocaudalis interna (ventral-posteromedial nucleus), Vim = nucleus ventro-intermedius, Vop = nucleus ventro-oralis posterior, Voa = nucleus ventro-oralis anterior (the last three correspond to the ventrolateral nucleus in American nomenclature).

[11]. In contrast, Guiot and associates (1969) recommended a target that is 5/12ths of the intercommissural distance, 14.5 mm lateral to the midline and 3 mm above the AC–PC line [13]. Ojemann and Ward used a more superior target: 9 mm anterior to the PC along the AC–PC line, 12–15 mm lateral to the midline, and 6–12 mm above the AC–PC line [24]. Other authors have instead stressed the variations in individual anatomy and have used proportionate systems. Using a proportionate system, Molina-Negro (1979) reported cessation of tremor in more than 200 patients upon the initial passage of an electrode [22]. The only exceptions occurred when pathological hydrocephalus with an AC–PC line greater than 30 mm or craniosynostosis or microcephaly with a length of less than 20 mm was present. Their data indicate that alteration in the width of the third ventricle did not change the length of the AC–PC line. Their coordinates for tremor relief were 8/10ths of the length of the AC–PC line behind the AC, 5/10ths of the AC–PC line laterally, and at the level of the plane of the AC–PC line.

In the past, our initial target corresponded to a point 1–7 mm behind the mid AC–PC line and 10–15 mm lateral to the midline of the third ventricle at the level of the AC–PC line. This agreed generally with the target sites used by many other functional surgical centers [19]. More recently, we have selected the initial target spot based upon a proportionate system, the target being approximately 80% of the total length of the AC–PC line behind the AC, and 60% of the total length lateral to the midline. This point is centered and confirmed by repeated AP and lateral roentgenograms. Physiological localization is then performed.

PHYSIOLOGICAL LOCALIZATION

The purpose of radiographic localization techniques and/or the use of stereotactic atlases is to determine the approximate anatomic position of the electrode. Before placing a lesion, physiological localization is mandatory.

In 1959, Brierley and Beck showed that the intercommissural line and PC did not have a constant anatomic relationship to the thalamic nuclei [5]. Subsequent data reinforced the pertinence of this observation. Tasker and coworkers reviewed the literature on variations between anatomic and physiological localization and found differences of 1 mm in 15%–

56% of patients, 2 mm in 21%–52%, 3 mm in 11%–30%, and 4 mm in 2%–15% [32]. This disparity demonstrates the need for physiological localization prior to final lesion placement. Many methods have been used for this purpose. These include electrical stimulation, microelectrode recording of evoked potentials, recording of electrical impedance, transient tissue cooling or heating, infiltration with procaine hydrochloride, localized pressure, ultrasonic inactivation, and incremental lesion making [33]. In general, however, physiological localization is performed with either microelectrode recordings or electrical stimulation. Tasker and Walker both provided elegant comparisons of these two techniques [32, 33]. Microelectrode recording offers higher spatial definition, less dependence on patient cooperation, and an excellent ability to detect somatopy within certain areas. However, this method requires sophisticated electronic equipment and has limited ability to anatomically compensate if the initial trajectory does not pass through structures that are easy to identify physiologically. In contrast, stimulation is much faster and can identify a wide variety of intracranial structures, thereby allowing greater flexibility for appropriate coordinate adjustments. Currently, stimulation is the more commonly used of the two systems [32]. However, either system is reliable in experienced hands.

We prefer electrical stimulation. A thermistor electrode (Radionics, Inc., 72 Cambridge Street, Burlington, MA) is inserted to the target. We have used a monopolar electrode, which has a tip length of 5 mm and a tip diameter of 1.6 mm, and a bipolar electrode, with a tip length of 4 mm and a tip diameter of 1.1 mm. The impedance monitoring system of a Radionics (RFG-3-B) radiofrequency lesion generator is used to record impedance at intervals along the probe's trajectory from the cortex to target. The Radionics system uses a 50 kHz measuring frequency, which drives a sinewave constant current relative to the unknown impedance at the tissue-electrode interface. The resulting voltage is rectified to produce a measurable direct current signal proportional to tissue impedance. Changes in impedance measurements among white matter, gray matter, and ventricular fluid allow gross identification of anatomic boundaries such as the thalamic-ventricular interface and the thalamus-subthalamus border [25]. At the target, stimulation then is performed. For effective stimulation, the frequency, wave form, and peak-to-peak current of the stimulus are all important factors. Frequencies of 2–100 Hz, a biphasic wave form with pulses 1 msec in duration, and a constant current usually are optimal. We use frequencies of 2–100 Hz at voltages ranging from 0.1 to 10 mV with a current of 1 mA for 1 msec. The motor and sensory responses are recorded at threshold voltage. It is important that only the threshold response is taken, because excessive current can result in spread, with loss of localizing value. The motor response obtained identifies the posterior limb of the internal capsule. Therefore, stimulation posterior only to the midpoint of the AC–PC line is most often useful. The location of the internal capsule depends to some extent on the width of the third ventricle. If the ventricle is narrow (1–5 mm), the internal capsule is usually 16–20 mm lateral to the midline, whereas if the third ventricle is wider (6–14 mm), the medial fibers of the capsule may be up to 19–23 mm lateral to the midline. [14]. We found that using frequencies of 5–20 Hz (at less than 2 mV thresholds) caused contralateral synchronous motor responses when the target point was too near the internal capsule. Tonic motor responses were noted at higher frequencies at less than a 1-mV threshold. Sensory responses tend to occur when the target is too far posterior and at frequencies greater than 50 Hz. In general, target lesions are satisfactory when stimulation causes either reduction or increase in the MD. Our results largely have agreed with Walker's observation that destruction of a target point that, when stimulated, arrested a tremor, uniformly improved the MD, whereas destruction of the target that facilitated or initiated the tremor commonly, but inconsistently, improved the MD [33].

In our earlier work, we usually placed two lesions. The first was made at 75–80°C for 60 seconds and the second lesion was made at 75°C for 30 seconds after a 3–5 mm withdrawal of the electrode. More recently, we have limited our lesions to a single 60-second, 80°C lesion at the target. During this procedure, the patient is instructed to count and to hold extended the contralateral arm and leg. Early evidence of dysarthria, dysphagia, or weakness thus may be detected. Following placement of the lesion, the patient is observed for 10–15 minutes in the operating room. If the tremor returns, the procedure is repeated.

Results

PATIENT POPULATION

Our study involved 14 patients, ten men and four women (table 26–1). The median age at the time of trauma was 16 years, with a range of six to 46 years. The median duration of symptoms was five years (range, one to 28 years). The median age at surgery was 20 years (range, 10–47 years). Ten patients had action tremors, 12 had hemiballismus, three had choreoathetoid movements, three had bilateral involvement, two had truncal ataxia, and ten had multiple MD. The majority of patients had other posttraumatic sequelae: dysarthria (12 patients), psychomotor retardation (11), cranial nerve dysfunction (seven) and hemiparesis (eight).

CT scans and EEG were used for preoperative evaluation of 13 patients. On CT scans, four patients were normal, four demonstrated generalized atrophy, and five had focal and generalized tissue loss. The EEG was normal in six individuals, showed nonspecific slowing in six, and showed seizure activity in one. Seven of the patients underwent right thalamotomies, and seven left thalamotomies. One patient (Case 7) also had a lesion placed in the subthalamic nuclei. Two patients had second thalamotomies one week after the initial surgery because of early recurrence of the MD.

IMMEDIATE POSTOPERATIVE RESULTS

In all patients, some improvement in the MD was noted. Eight patients demonstrated marked improvement, four achieved moderate improvement, and two only minimal improvement that was not considered functionally significant. In two persons, initial improvement of left-sided action tremors disappeared after the first 24 hours. Following second procedures performed approximately one week later, both improved considerably.

In ten patients, the preoperative dysarthria worsened in the immediate postoperative period. Six had undergone left VL thalamotomies and four right VL thalamotomies. In four of these patients, the dysarthria was mildly aggravated for three to ten days. In two, exacerbation was moderate, and dysarthria was still present, although improved, at the time of discharge. In four individuals, the postoperative dysarthria was considered severe. In all of these patients, a relatively severe dysarthria and associated dysphagia had been present preoperatively. One patient demonstrated signs of moderately worse dysphagia postoperatively, specifically, difficulty eating and handling oral secretions. Previously, this patient had suffered severe dysarthria and had a baseline difficulty with oral secretions. Dysphagia was severely increased postoperatively in three patients, who were totally unable to eat or handle oral secretions. Significant dysphagia and dysarthria had been present preoperatively in these three. Postoperative testing revealed that they also had decreased velopharyngeal functioning and a reduction in the oral-nasal pressure differential. SMT was performed postoperatively on two of the patients with severe dysarthria and dysphagia. Their comprehension of spoken language was intact, but they showed mild-to-moderate alterations in memory and/or language dysfunction. All of the patients with dysarthria and dysphagia experienced a decreased range of tongue motion. In general, some clinical improvement in dysarthria and dysphagia occurred prior to discharge. Baseline dysarthria apparently improved postoperatively in two of those who had had right VL thalamotomies (Cases 3 and 7).

Thirteen patients manifested some facial asymmetry following surgery; this improved in all instances. A bilateral decrease in lower facial movement was noted in one patient (Case 5). In three individuals, contralateral weakness increased in the postoperative period. In two of these three, the weakness was most pronounced in the lower extremity.

LONG-TERM RESULTS

Twelve patients were available for follow-up evaluation for two months to three years after surgery (table 26–2). All 12 maintained some improvement in their MD, ranging from two months to one year. In one patient (Case 3), functional improvement that was noted at three months and at one year was no longer present at three years. At three years, this person showed a marked increase in extensor tone in the lower extremity, although the MD had not returned. Three months after surgery, another patient demonstrated a moderate increase in contralateral lower extremity tone that was not

TABLE 26–1. Patient Population

Case No.	Age, Sex	Posttrauma Interval (years)	Disorders of Cranial Nerve Function	Movement Disorders	Computer Tomography Findings
1	42, M	28	Mild dysarthria	B choreoathetoid and ballismus	Low density area R frontal region, ipsilateral frontal horn enlargement, enlargement of lateral and third ventricles
2	19, M	6	L ptosis, mild dysarthria	R action tremor, titubation	Normal
3	13, F	5	Severe dysarthria and dysphagia	L choreoathetosis, hemiballismus	Normal
4	20, M	1	Severe dysarthria and dysphagia	B action tremor, hemiballismus	Generalized brain atrophy
5	23, M	17	Moderate dysarthria	R hemiballismus	Normal
6	15, F	1	Skew deviation, bilateral intranuclear, ophthalmoplegia, L hemianopsia, pseudobulbar palsy, severe dysarthria and dysphagia	R action tremor, truncal ataxia	Generalized brain atrophy L frontal encephalomalacia
7	33, M	11	Decreased upward gaze, moderate dysarthria	B choreoathetosis, L hemiballismus	
8	16, M	1	L optic atrophy, R facial palsy, severe dysarthria and dysphagia	R action tremor, hemiballismus	Mild cerebral atrophy, caudate atrophy
9	21, M	7	L optic atrophy, L oculomotor and R facial palsies, moderate dysarthria	L action tremor, hemiballismus	Ventricular asymmetry with R hemispheric atrophy
10	17, M	7	Decreased adduction on conversion, R facial palsy, moderate dysarthria	R action tremor, hemiballismus	Mild ventriculomegaly, loss of tissue in temporal lobe
11	10, F	3	B superior oblique palsies, moderate dysarthria	R action tremor, hemiballismus	Generalized cortical atrophy and ventriculomegaly
12	21, F	5	Intact	R action tremor, hemiballismus	Generalized brain atrophy with severe brain-stem and cerebellar atrophy
13	47, M	1	Mild dysarthria	L action tremor	Generalized atrophy with tissue loss in left hemisphere
14	20, M	3	Normal	L action tremor	Normal

L = left; R = right; B = bilateral.

TABLE 26–2. Postoperative Results

Case No.	Postoperative Interval (months)	Clinical Examination
1	6	Improved tremor
2	3	Improved tremor
3	3	Improved tremor
	12	Further improvement in tremor
	36	Increased spasticity, dystonic posturing
4	3	Improved tremor, increased dysarthria and dysphagia
	9	Further improvement in tremor; improvement in dysarthria and dysphagia
6	3	Improved tremor, increased dysarthria, further improvement in tremor and dysarthria
8	6	Improved tremor and baseline speech
9	2	Improved tremor
	12	Further improvement in tremor
10	3	Improved tremor, dysarthria and dysphagia, further improvement in all areas
11	4	Improved tremor, increased dysarthria and dysphagia
	12	Further improvement in tremor, dysarthria and dysphagia
12	5	Improved tremor, mild dysarthria
13	3	Improved tremor, increased spasticity
14	1	Improved tremor
	3	Further improvement

associated with a change in functional ability nor recurrence of the MD. Five patients (Cases 3, 4, 6, 10, 11) evaluated at serial intervals continued to show significant improvement in their MD at the second examination. A sixth patient (Case 9) evaluated both two months and two years after surgery, had continued but less striking improvement in tremor at the second examination.

In nine patients, preoperative dysarthria became worse immediately after surgery. Eight of these patients had a follow-up examination. In five of the eight, speech had improved three to six months postoperatively. In the other three, no improvement was noted at three or four months. However, subsequent evaluation of those three patients (at 9, 12, and 36 months, respectively) demonstrated continued improvement in dysarthria, although a residual dysfunction still existed.

Eleven patients had CT scans within two weeks postoperatively. In three (all of whom had significant postoperative dysarthria and dysphagia), the low-attenuation lesion seen in the left thalamic region appeared to extend into the internal capsule. In the other eight patients, a low-density area was seen in the thalamus only. A generalized but mild increase in ventricular size was noted in one patient.

Summary

Posttraumatic MD occurs after severe head injury. In general, the MD is a moderate-to-severe intention tremor coinciding with variable other posttraumatic sequelae. In most cases, however, the MD is the major source of disability for the patient. Some advocate medical management, including propranolol and clonazepam. In our experience, however, none of these agents has been effective. Stereotactic thalamotomy has a high rate of clinical success, however, and should not be delayed unnecessarily. Before surgery, the minimal evaluation should include a CT scan, EEG, and speech and language evaluation to determine treatable causes for the MD and to assess the potential risks associated with surgery. Each of our 14 patients experienced postoperative improvement in their MD: eight, a marked improvement; four, moderate improvement; and two minimal improvement.

The major risks associated are contralateral weakness, increased dysarthria, and postoperative memory and language dysfunction. Patients most at risk for these last two complications include those undergoing dominant thalamotomies, those demonstrating ventriculomegaly or significant encephalomalacia on CT scan, and those with poor preoperative performance on memory and language testing. Overall, stereotactic thalamotomy provides a satisfactory response in patients with posttraumatic MD and should be considered as the recommended form of therapy.

References

1. Adams JH: Head injury. In Adams JH, Corsellis JAN, Duchen LW (eds): *Greenfield's Neuropathology* (4th ed). New York: Wiley, 1984, pp 85–124
2. Andrew J, Fowler CJ, Harrison MJG: Tremor after head injury and its treatment by stereotaxic surgery. *J Neurol Neurosurg Psychiatry* 45:815–819, 1982
3. Bravo GJ, Cooper IS: A clinical and radiological correlation of the lesions produced by chemopallidectomy and thalamotomy. *J Neurol Neurosurg Psychiatry* 22:1–10, 1959
4. Bricolo A: Prolonged post-traumatic coma. In Vinken PJ, Bruyn GW (eds): *Handbook of Clinical Neurology*, Vol 24. New York: American Elsevier, 1976, pp 699–755
5. Brierley JB, Beck E: The significance in human stereotactic brain surgery of individual variation in the diencephalon and globus pallidus. *J Neurol Neurosurg Psychiatry* 22:287–298, 1959
6. Bullard DE, Horner J, Walker J, et al: Evaluation of memory and language function pre and postthalamotomy with an attempt to define those patients at risk for postoperative dysfunction. In press, 1986
7. Bullard DE, Nashold BS: Stereotactic thalamotomy for the treatment of posttraumatic movement disorders. *J Neurosurg* 61:316–321, 1984
8. Chadwick D, Hallett M, Harris R, et al: Clinical, biochemical, and physiological features distinguishing myoclonus responsive to 5-hydroxytryptophan, tryptophan with a monoamine oxidase inhibitor, and clonazepam. *Brain* 100:455–487, 1977
9. Corsellis JAN, Brierley JB: Observations on the pathology of insidious dementia following head injury. *J Mental Sci* 105:714–720, 1959
10. Fahn S: Posthypoxic action myoclonus: Review of the literature and report of two new cases with response to valproate and estrogen. In Fahn S, Davis JN, Rowland LP (eds): *Advances in Neurology*, Vol 26. New York: Raven Press, 1979, pp 49–84
11. Gildenburg PL, Kaufman HH, Murthy KSK: Calculation of stereotactic coordinates from the computed tomographic scan. *Neurosurgery* 10:582–586, 1982
12. Grimberg L: Paralysis agitans and trauma. *J Nerv Ment Dis* 79:14–42, 1934
13. Guiot G, Derome P: The principles of stereotaxic thalamotomy. In Kahn EA, Crosby EC, Schneider RC, et al (eds): *Correlative Neurosurgery*. Springfield, IL: Thomas, 1969, pp 376–401
14. Hardy TL, Bertrand G, Thompson CJ: Position of the medial internal capsular border in relation to third-ventricular width. *Appl Neurophysiol* 42:234–247, 1979
15. Hollander D, Strich SJ: Atypical Alzheimer's disease with congophilic angiopathy presenting with dementia of acute onset. In Wolstenholme GEW, O'Connor M (eds): *Alzheimer's Disease and Related Conditions*. CIBA Foundation Symposium. London: Churchill, 1970, pp 105–124
16. Jennett B, Teasdale G: *Management of Head Injuries*. Philadelphia: FA Davis, 1981
17. Jennett B, Teasdale G, Galbraith S, et al: Severe head injuries in three countries. *J Neurol Neurosurg Psychiatry* 40:291–298, 1977
18. Kremer M, Russell WR, Smyth GE: A midbrain syndrome following head injury. *J Neurol Neurosurg Psychiatry* 10:49–60, 1947
19. Laitinen LV: Brain targets in surgery for Parkinson's disease: Results of a survey of neurosurgeons. *J Neurosurg* 62:349–351, 1985
20. Marsden CD, Hallett M, Fahn S: The nosology and pathophysiology of myoclonus. In Marsden CD, Fahn S (eds): *Neurology 2: Movement Disorders*. New York: Butterworth Scientific, 1982, pp 196–248
21. McMenemey WH, Grant HC, Behrman S: Two examples of "precinct senile dementia" (Pick's disease and Stern-Garcin syndrome) with a history of trauma. *Arch Psychiatr Nervenkr* 208:162–176, 1965
22. Molina-Negro P: Functional surgery of abnormal movements. In Rasmussen TT, Marina R (eds): *Functional Neurosurgery*. New York: Raven Press, 1979, pp 89–121
23. Niizuma H, Kwak R, Ohyama H, et al: Stereotactic thalamotomy for postapoplectic and posttraumatic involuntary movements. *Appl Neurophysiol* 45:295–298, 1982
24. Ojemann GA, Ward AA Jr: Abnormal movement disorders. In Youmans JR (ed): *Neurological Surgery*. Philadelphia: Saunders, 1973, pp 1829–1867
25. Robinson BW, Tompkins HE: Impedance method for localizing brain structures: An ex-

tension of the method. *Arch Neurol* 10:563–574, 1964

26. Sortland O, Hovind K: Ventriculography with water-soluble contrast media. *Acta Radiol [Suppl]* (Stockh) 355:223–236, 1977
27. Starosta-Rubinstein S, Bjork RJ, Snyder BD, et al: Posttraumatic intention myoclonus. *Surg Neurol* 20:131–132, 1983
28. Strich SJ: Cerebral trauma. In Blackwood W, Corsellis JAN (eds): *Greenfield's Neuropathology* (3rd ed). London: Edward Arnold, 1976, pp 327–360
29. Strich SJ: The pathology of brain damage due to blunt head injuries. In Walker AE, Caveness WF, Critchley M (eds): *The Late Effects of Head Injuries*. Springfield, IL: Thomas, 1969, pp 501–524
30. Suzuki S, Ito K, Iwabuchi T: Ventriculography with non-ionic water-soluble contrast medium, Amipaque (metrizamide). *J Neurosurg* 47:79–85, 1977
31. Tasker RR, Organ LW, Hawrylyshyn P: Investigation of the surgical target for alleviation of involuntary movement disorders. *Appl Neurophysiol* 45:261–274, 1982
32. Tasker RR, Organ LW, Hawrylyshyn PA: *The Thalamus and Midbrain of Man: A Physiological Atlas Using Electrical Stimulation*. Springfield, IL: Thomas, 1982
33. Walker AE: Stereotaxic surgery for tremor. In Schaltenbrand G, Walker AE (eds): *Stereotaxy of the Human Brain: Anatomical, Physiological, and Clinical Applications*. New York: Thieme-Stratton, 1982, pp 515–521

27. THE ROLE OF ANTERIOR INTERNAL CAPSULOTOMY IN PSYCHIATRIC SURGERY

Björn A. Meyerson
Per Mindus

In 1947, Spiegel and Wycis first reported the application of stereotactic techniques to psychiatric surgery [29]. A few years later, such treatment was used systematically by Leksell [16] in Sweden and Talairach [31] in France. It was more than another decade before stereotactic technique was recognized widely as the preferred way to perform psychiatric surgery.

Modern psychiatric surgery employs stereotactic technique exclusively. It has been fostered mainly by British investigators such as Knight [10] who developed an operation called *subcaudate tractotomy*. The lesion target is the substantia innominata, located in the medial posterobasal part of the frontal lobes. Subsequently, this operation was redefined with inclusion of a new target region in the anterior cingulum. This combined approach has been called *limbic leucotomy*. In the mid-1970s, the practice of psychiatric surgery was particularly active in Great Britain with major contributions reported by Kelly [8, 9], a psychiatrist. Other pioneers in stereotactic psychiatric surgery include Craw and co-workers. (Bristol, Great Britain), Ballantine [1] (Boston, MA), and Sano (Tokyo); see [14] and [30] for additional information.

Many target regions have been used in stereotactic psychiatric surgery. The question of whether particular brain targets should relate to particular psychiatric symptoms or syndromes has been discussed extensively. We know that the same symptom may be influenced by lesions placed in multiple targets, which suggests a lack of specificity [9]. Although it is true that most targets encroach upon fiber tracts and relays that are all connected (as within the limbic system), it is still possible that some degree of target specificity does exist. For example, depressive symptoms respond best to intervention in the cingulum [1], whereas obsessive-compulsive and anxiety states respond better to capsulotomy or limbic leukotomy [2, 12].

The frontal lobes have remained a focus of interest in psychiatric surgery [15, 27]. Frequently, the frontal lobes or systems with close functional and anatomical connections to them are chosen as stereotactic target sites. Early investigations recognized that surgery confined to the mediobasal portion of the frontal lobe avoided a subsequent "frontal lobe syndrome." Fulton, whose classical studies on chimpanzees served as a model for the early development of psychiatric surgery, claimed that lesions involving the lateral convexity of the frontal lobes were likely to produce a state of apathy. Conversely, lesions produced in the posterior part of the orbital cortex could result in emotional and behavioral disinhibition.

The fiber connections of the frontal lobes are exceedingly complex and knowledge about their functional organization is still fragmentary. Nauta's pioneering research [24] described the intimate connections between the frontal lobes and limbic system; this work has been of paramount importance for understanding the morphological basis of the effects obtained by surgical lesions within these connections. The different target regions in the frontal lobe are not defined clearly, either in

L.D. Lunsford (ed.) *MODERN STEREOTACTIC NEUROSURGERY*. Copyright © 1988.
Martinus Nijhoff Publishing. Boston/Dordrecht/Lancaster. All rights reserved.

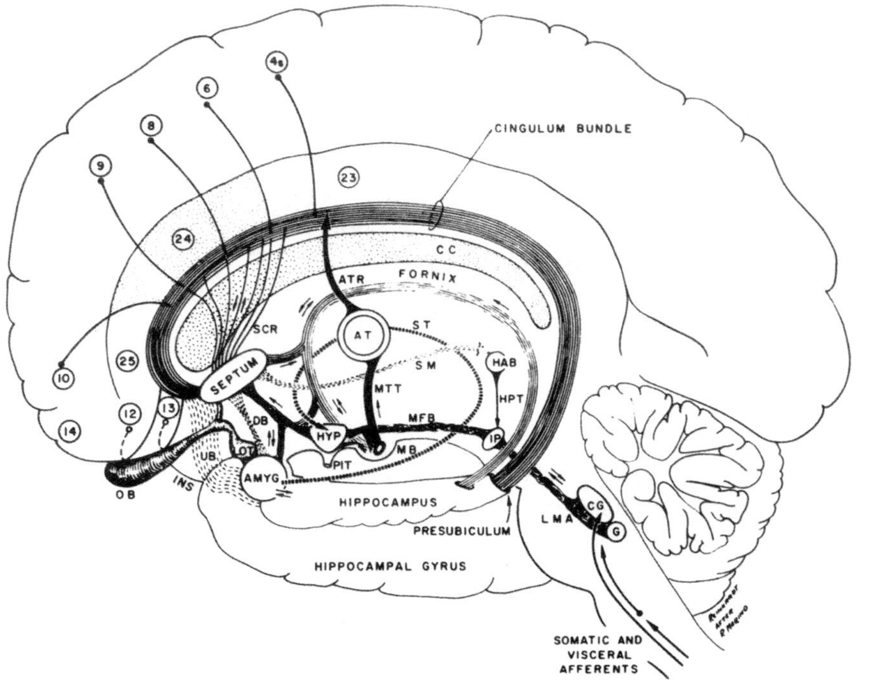

FIGURE 27–1. Organization of the limbic system: OB, olfactory bulb; LOT, lateral olfactory striae; INS, insula; UB, uncinate bundle; DB, diagonal band of Broca; AMYG, amydala; SCR, subcallosal radiations; HYP, hypothalamus; AT, anterior thalamus; MB, mammillary body; MTT, mammillothalamic tract (Vicq D'Azyr's tracts); ATR, anterior thalamic radiations; ST, stria terminalis; HAB, habenula; MFB, medial forebrain bundle; SM, stria medullaris; HPT, habenulointerpeduncular tract (fasciculus retroflexus of Meynert); IP, interpeduncular nucleus; LMA, limbic midbrain area of Nauta; G, nucleus of Gudden; CG, central gray; CCF, corpus callosum. (Reproduced with permission from Ballantine HT, Levy BS, Dagi TF, et al: Cingulotomy for psychiatric illness: Report of 13 years' experience. In Sweet WH, Obrador S, Martin-Rodriguez JG [eds]: *Neurosurgical Treatment in Psychiatry, Pain and Epilepsy*. Baltimore: University Park Press, 1977, pp 333–353.)

terms of stereotactic coordinates or as anatomical structures. Comparing the results obtained from intervention in each of these target regions is difficult. It is apparent that several of the target regions may overlap, and, consequently, the same fiber systems are likely to be partially involved by the various procedures. It is both plausible and important that frontal lobe projections to the limbic midbrain are located partly in the internal capsule. These projections interconnect the frontal lobes with the septo-hypothalamic-mesencephalic continuum (figure 27–1) as described by Nauta [23]. As a result of this organization, limbic functions can be modulated by inflow from the frontal lobes. (For an additional review, see [11].)

Even in the infancy of frontal lobe psychiatric surgery, postoperative effects were related to interruption of the frontothalamic fiber pathways. This knowledge led Talairach and colleagues [31] to make selective stereotactic lesions in the anterior limb of the internal capsule, an area that contains the frontothalamic fiber system. He reported that results were particularly favorable in patients with anxiety neuroses. The functional importance of the frontothalamic pathways was demonstrated indirectly by Meyer and Beck who performed autopsies on patients who had been subjected to different forms of lobotomy; they found that the best results occurred when the frontothalamic fibers were severed [18]. The report by Meyer and Beck was also the starting point for Leksell's innovations in psychiatric surgery. In 1952, Leksell used his recently developed stereotactic system to produce bilateral lesions in the frontothalamic fibers of the internal capsule. This operation later was referred to as *stereotactic bilateral anterior capsulotomy*. The first report on the long-term results of this new psychiatric surgical approach was published in 1961 by Herner [7]. In this study of 116 patients, Herner concluded that the best results were obtained in patients with anxiety and obsessive-compulsive states.

Indications

In the great majority of patients reported in the literature, the main indication for capsulotomy has been anxiety and obsessive-compulsive neuroses. In the *Diagnostic and Statistical Manual of Mental Disorders* (DSM III), these conditions are referred to as Phobic Disorders (300.20), Generalized Anxiety Disorders (300.20), or Obsessive-Compulsive Disorders (300.30). In relatively few patients, capsulotomy has been performed to alleviate symptoms of severe anxiety and obsessive-compulsive symptoms associated with chronic depression or schizophrenia (L. Laitinen, personal communication, 1984). These latter indications as yet are not established.

In addition to the diagnosis or the predominant symptom, several *inclusion criteria* must be considered before capsulotomy is performed:

1. The patient's condition must be classified as chronic, and surgery should be considered only when conventional psychiatric treatment modalities have proven ineffective.
2. The patient's illness should be severe and incapacitating.
3. The patient must be referred from a psychiatric clinic that also provides a post-operative rehabilitation program.
4. The patient should be evaluated by a psychiatrist who is knowledgeable about psychiatric surgery.
5. The patient's suitability for surgery should be decided jointly by the neurosurgeon and the psychiatrist.
6. The patient must agree to undergo surgery after having been informed fully about the likelihood of improvement and the risks or complications.

The following *exclusion criteria* should be noted:

1. The patient must not have an organic mental disorder, nor drug or alcohol abuse.
2. Patients should not have a personality disorder associated with dependency, passivity, or manipulative behavior.
3. Patients who are institutionalized against their will should not be considered for surgery.
4. Patients younger than age 20 in general should not be subjected to this operation. Although no absolute upper age limit exists, we believe that brain surgery is especially risky for patients older than age 70; capsulotomy should be considered only in exceptional cases.

Techniques

TARGET SITE

Anterior capsulotomy is designed to destroy the horizontally oriented fiber tracts that form the anterior portion of the internal capsule. The operation always is performed bilaterally. The location of the internal capsule in relation to the midline of the brain is variable [32] and partly related to the widths of the frontal horns. Axial computed tomography (CT) images demonstrate the capsule target at a level about 5 mm above the slice that corresponds to the foramen of Monro (figure 27–2). At this level, the frontal horns are relatively narrow. In the CT images that correspond to the most basal parts of the frontal horns, the internal capsule is less distinct, because capsular fibers are more dispersed. The target for anterior internal capsulotomy is in the anterior one-third of the capsule, 5 mm behind the anterior margins of the frontal horns of the ventricles; in this area, the fibers are funneled between the head of the caudate nucleus and the putamen [20]. In our experience, placement of the lesion in the anterior-posterior or longitudinal axis of the capsule does not influence the outcome of the operation. Care must be taken to ensure that the target is in the center of the low-

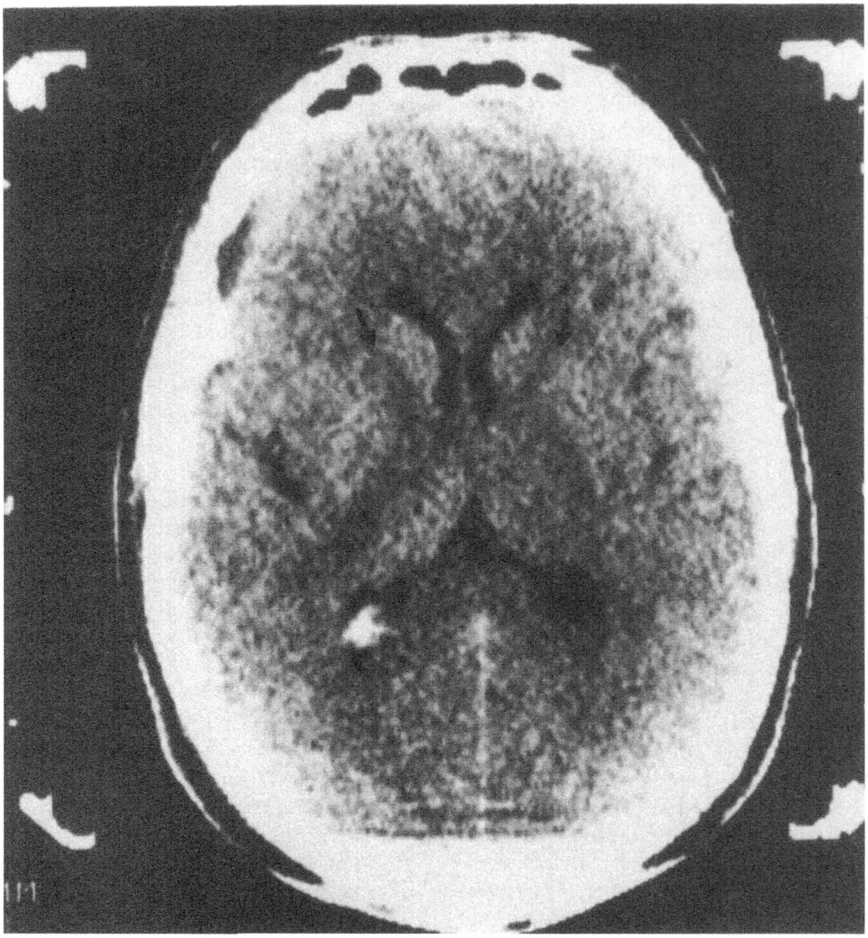

A

FIGURE 27–2. Axial CT image at the level of the foramen of Monro. Arrows indicate recommended target sites in the anterior limbs of the internal capsules (A). Corresponding section of a brain; target sites are marked by asterisks (B). (From Schaltenbrand G, Bailey P [eds]: *Introduction to Stereotaxis with an Atlas of the Human Brain*. New York: Grune and Stratton, 1959.)

attenuation zone on CT images, which corresponds to the capsular white matter (figure 27–3).

IMAGING

Before the era of modern imaging techniques, pneumoencephalography was used for target localization in stereotactic capsulotomy. Reference points were selected in the midline and the anterior extension of the intercommissural line. The target was located on the intercommissural line, approximately 13 mm anterior to the anterior commissure and 18–20 mm lateral to the midline. Because of the divergent course of the internal capsule in the horizontal plane, the lateral location of the target was critical. Meyerson and colleagues showed that dilation of the frontal horns during pneumoencephalography can cause considerable lateral dislocation of the capsule [20]. This unfortunate phenomenon, coupled with the inherent inaccuracies in localizing targets using remote reference points, made target determination difficult.

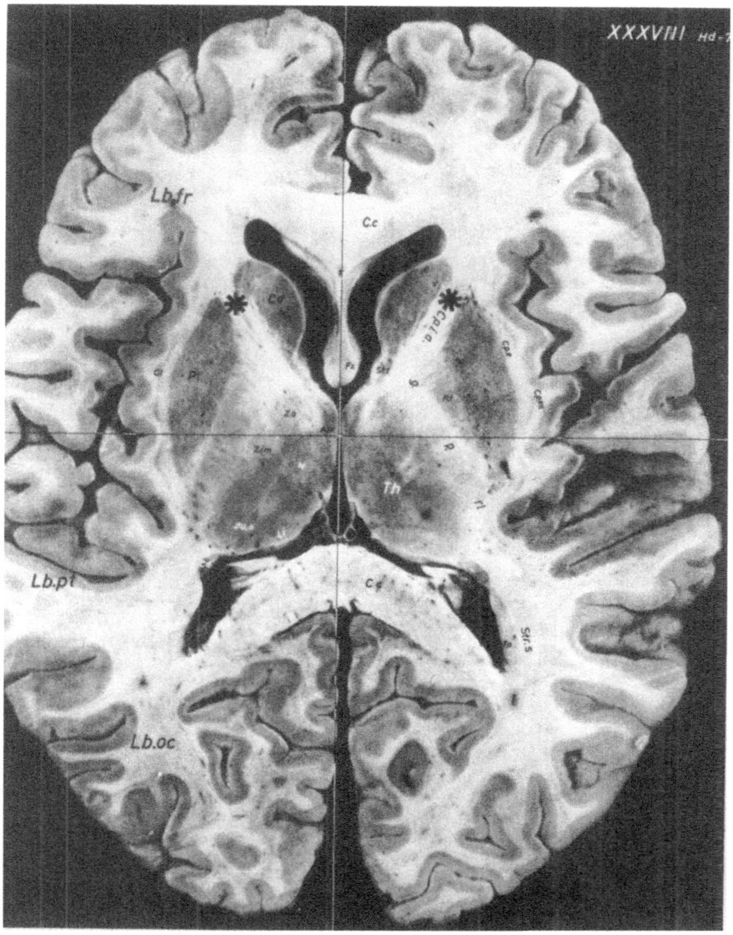

B

FIGURE 27–2. (cont.)

We believe that stereotactic CT localization should be used for this procedure, because CT allows direct visualization of the target area. Magnetic resonance imaging (MRI) can be used to directly visualize the target in the coronal plane and thus can be used to improve the precision of target localization.

ANESTHESIA

Local anesthesia is used whenever possible so that the neurosurgeon can observe the patient's neurological condition. Since patient cooperation is not required during the procedure, potent sedatives can be administered. We have observed that even patients who are incapacitated by anxiety (e.g., a tendency to have panic reactions) tolerate the strain of the procedure surprisingly well.

OPERATIVE TECHNIQUE

Bilateral burr holes are made slightly anterior to the coronal suture. With this approach, the trajectory of the lesion electrodes is perpendicular to the intercommissural plane. In both frontal reformatted CT images and in coronal MRI images, we confirmed that lower parts of the internal capsule are located closer to the midline than are upper parts. The electrode trajectory should be oriented 20° to the sagittal plane (figure 27–4). It is practical to position the electrode carrier so that the electrodes form an angle of about 20° and to mark the approximate location of the burr hole on the skin. Unless this precaution is taken, the burr hole will be placed too close to the midline.

To destroy the major part of the anterior internal capsule, the lesion must be 15–20 mm

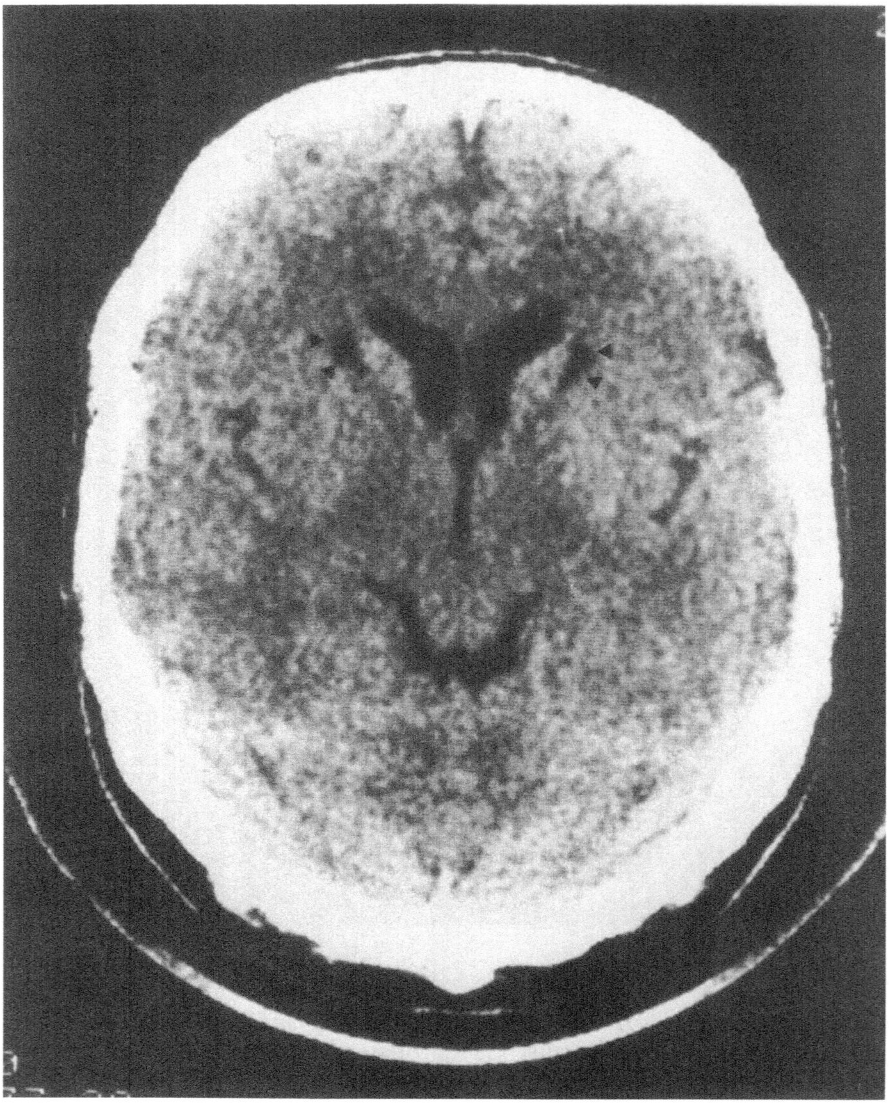

A

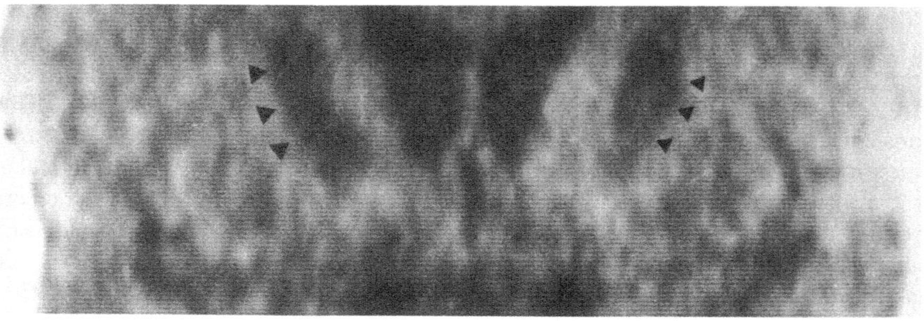

B

FIGURE 27–3. Axial (A) and coronal (B) reconstructed CT images showing the appearance of bilateral lesions (*arrows*) after capsulotomy.

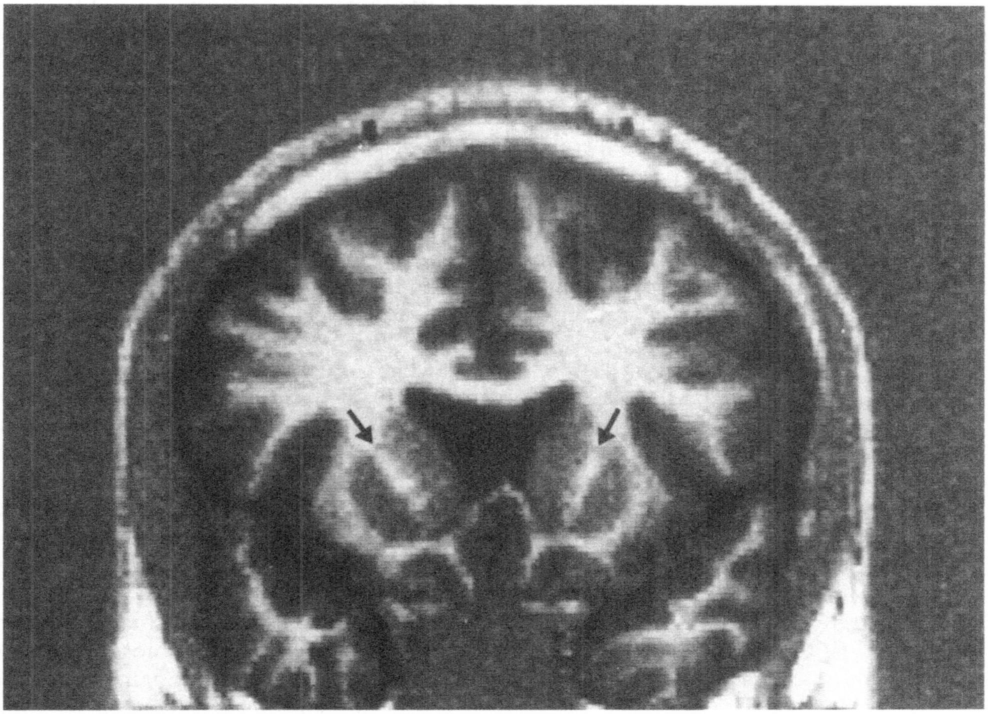

FIGURE 27–4. Appearance of the internal capsules (*arrows*) in a coronal magnetic resonance image.

high. We believe that the critical part of the target lies in the basal internal capsule [3, 19]. Lesion height possibly could be reduced to 10–12 mm if the center of the target was selected 5–7 mm below the standard CT section used for target localization. The change of target location in the superior-inferior internal capsule should be determined on the basis of coronal MRI visualization.

Whether the lesion is produced with monopolar or bipolar thermal radiofrequency electrodes does not seem critical. In the latter case, electrodes are spaced 3–6 mm apart and are oriented perpendicularly to the long axis of the capsule (figure 27–5). It is also possible to perform capsulotomy with stereotactic radiosurgery [16, 21, 26]. This method minimizes surgical complications but deprives the neurosurgeon of the opportunity to explore the target region electrophysiologically in order to elucidate the functional organization of the targeted pathways.

We do not perform electrical stimulation of the target region routinely because subjective responses to stimulation are only rarely produced [13]. Perhaps electrical impedance monitoring will help to verify correct placement of the electrode tip in the internal capsule white matter. To date, there has been no systematic study of the usefulness of impedance monitoring, but microelectrode recording has been used to identify the capsule [17].

Patients do not report subjective sensations during production of internal capsule lesions. Occasionally, some report feelings of release or relaxation immediately after the operation. While still in the operating room, approximately two-thirds of the patients develop confusion and disorientation with regard to time and space. Incoherent speech is also relatively common.

COMPLICATIONS

Capsulotomy is associated with few surgical complications. In our literature review, we encountered no reports of death in conjunction with this procedure. In our own series of 68 patients, two patients developed subcortical bleeding after insertion of the electrode; their symptoms were slight hemiparesis and somnolence. One patient had a hematoma in the target region and required temporary ventricular drainage. All three patients recovered completely without sequelae.

When psychiatric surgery was performed initially without stereotactic technique, epilepsy was a frequent late complication. After the introduction of stereotactic methods, postoperative epilepsy became exceedingly rare. In our series, only one of 68 patients subsequently developed epileptic symptoms that conceivably could be attributed to the operation.

ELECTROENCEPHALOGRAPHIC CHANGES

In a postoperative study performed on 35 capsulotomy patients, characteristic electroencephalographic (EEG) changes were demonstrated [4]. In the early postoperative period, bilaterally synchronous bursts of rhythmic slow waves dominated the frontal regions. Focal or epileptic abnormalities never were observed. At follow-up one to two years after the operation, the vast majority of the patients had the same EEG pattern they had preoperatively.

Early and Late Postoperative Course

After the operation, bed rest is imposed only during the first 24 hours. Because most patients are somewhat confused and disoriented during the first two to four postoperative days, they should be supervised. Urinary incontinence is relatively common. The state of confusion invariably disappears within a few days. Generally, medication with anxiolytics and similar drugs can be discontinued abruptly. Prophylactic anticonvulsant medication is not administered routinely.

During the second to fourth postoperative weeks, patients generally exhibit a marked decrease in initiative, and occupational therapy should be begun. Sometimes, this state of moderate lethargy lasts for a few months. Typically, the patient is reluctant to get up in the morning, lies passively in bed, takes excessive time to get things done, and misses appointments. In such cases, and active rehabilitation program is crucial. In our experience, most patients gain weight, generally less than 5 kg. Although some patients gain considerable weight postoperatively, such patients usually have had previous excessive weight problems. Patients and their families should be informed of this risk and encouraged to maintain their regular diet.

Results

To date, the results of anterior capsulotomy in approximately 300 patients has been reported by Herner [7], Burzaco [5], Bingley and co-workers [3], and others. The 1977 study by Bingley's group, working in Stockholm, has since been extended by a series of 30 consecutive patients treated between 1977 and 1985. Twenty-one additional patients underwent radiosurgical capsulotomy [21, 26]. Other studies on relatively small groups of patients have been published by Martinez and associates [17], Kullberg [12], Laitinen [13], and Fodstad and colleagues [6]. These different studies produced remarkably similar outcomes—about 70% of the patients benefiting from the operation.

Many reports on psychiatric surgery have been critized on methodological grounds, that is, retrospective study design, short duration of follow-up, and the use of subjective or unstandardized measures of outcome. Often, the physician in charge of both selection and treatment of the patients also performs the postoperative evaluation; the inherent bias problem is obvious. In recent years, important methodological advances in psychiatric research also have proven useful in psychiatric surgery. Internationally acknowledged diagnostic criteria and standardized symptom-rating procedures used prospectively by independent, trained observers may improve the reliability of outcome assessment considerably. It is particularly important that such methods be applied to the field of psychiatric surgery, as this type of treatment can easily evoke emotional reactions that bias the evaluation of outcome.

A recent prospective study illustrates the use of modern psychiatric research methods [22]. The study was performed on seven patients who had radiosurgical capsulotomies. The patients were examined before surgery and then both three and seven years after surgery. Psychiatric symptoms were rated by two psychiatrists who had not been responsible for selection or treatment of the patients. The Comprehensive Psychopathological Rating Scale (CPRS) was used. This scale has been shown to be highly sensitive to symptom changes induced

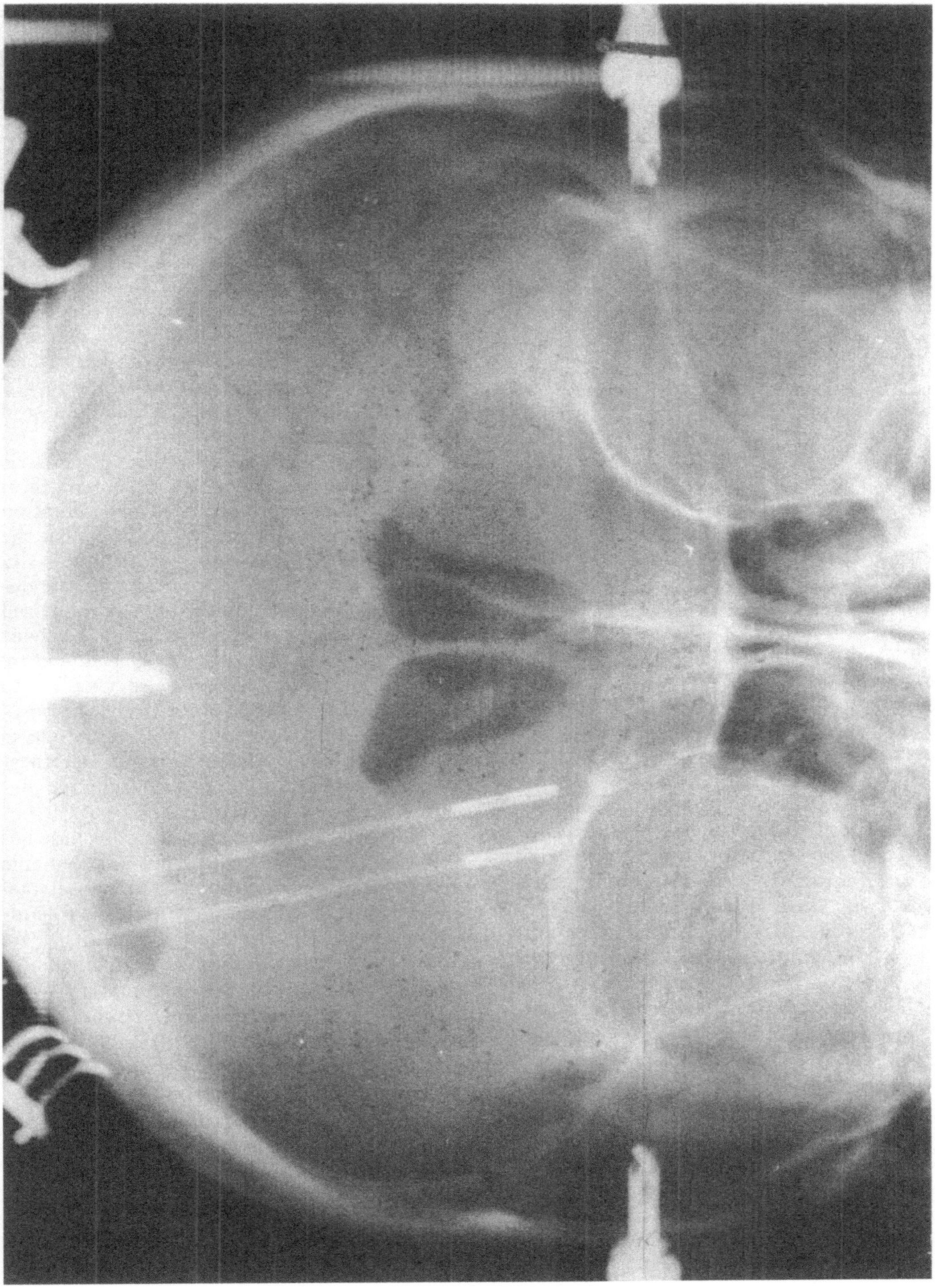

FIGURE 27–5. Intraoperative, stereotactic radiograph showing bipolar electrodes for lesion production in the internal capsule.

TABLE 27–1. Results of Anterior Internal Capsulotomy for Obsessive-Compulsive and Anxiety States[a]

Results	Series 1[b] (1970–1976)	Series 2[c] (1977–1985)
Symptom-free	19	14
Much improved	8	7
Slightly improved	11	2
Unchanged	0	7
Worse	0	0
Total patients	38	30

[a] Karolinska Hospital, Stockholm, Sweden.
[b] Duration of illness = 4–35 years, mean = 16 years, follow-up = 1½–5 years, mean = 3½ years.
[c] Duration of illness = 5–30 years, mean = 15 years, follow-up = 1–9 years, mean = 4 years.

by psychiatric treatment. Furthermore, it has high validity and both intra- and interrater reliability. The effect of the intervention on symptoms was studied by comparing pre- and postoperative CPRS scores. The interrater reliability was very high (product-moment correlation: 0.98). Symptom scores were reduced significantly. In addition to this symptom-oriented outcome measure, the patient's highest level of adaptive functioning was measured during the year before follow-up in three areas (social relations, occupational functioning, and use of leisure time), using the Axis V of the DSM III. The patients demonstrated great improvement in their level of adaptive functioning. Moreover, the evaluators jointly rated the patients on Pippard's five-graded rating scale [25], which is used widely in psychiatric surgery. This scale uses the following rating: (1) free from the symptoms that led to surgery; (2) much improved, with some symptoms remaining but considerably alleviated; (3) slight improvement, most symptoms remaining but somewhat reduced; (4) unchanged; (5) worse.

Data on the two consecutive series of patients treated in Stockholm are provided in table 27–1. Results in approximately 70% of the patients were judged successful, that is, the patients were free of symptoms or were much improved. This assessment of treatment outcome was based on regular postoperative examinations (generally once a year) by one or two psychiatrists. Reports were obtained from the referring psychiatrists who, as a rule, were responsible for postoperative rehabilitation. In most cases, the patient's relatives were interviewed, also. The patients were evaluated before and after the operation using several psychometric tests and personality inventories. No adverse effects on cognitive functions and no undesirable personality changes were detected postoperatively.

Examination of the results over time revealed no tendency toward relapse [19]. Recurrence of symptoms is most likely within the first postoperative year. Patients with such recurrence may benefit from a second operation. Burzaco reported that in 17 of 85 patients who underwent a second operation, half had long-term satisfactory results [5]. Patients with unsatisfactory results after surgery should undergo CT or MRI examinations to ensure that the lesion was not misplaced.

It should be emphasized that psychiatric surgery cannot achieve a favorable long-term outcome unless an intensive rehabilitation program is undertaken. It is our belief that the operation per se does not lead automatically to the elimination of symptoms. Despite decreased tension and anxiety, the patient still tends to maintain the maladaptive behavior pattern that was firmly established before surgery. The patient must be persuaded to accept exposure to situations that previously were likely to provoke fear. Without supportive and aggressive postoperative psychotherapy and behavioral training, maladaptive behavior patterns will persist.

Stereotactic anterior capsulotomy has become an established treatment for patients with chronic anxiety, phobias, and obsessive-compulsive states that are unresponsive to conventional management. The surgical risks are minimal and no undesirable permanent sequelae are likely to follow the operation. With the aid of CT or MRI, the target can be located with great precision. Despite the application of this technique only to those patients who have not responded to other conventional therapies and who have been ill for many years, the results of anterior internal capsulotomy are very favorable.

References

1. Ballantine HT, Levy BS, Dagi TF, et al: Cingulotomy for psychiatric illness: Report of 13 years' experience. In Sweet WH, Obrador S,

Martin-Rodriguez JG (eds): *Neurosurgical Treatment in Psychiatry, Pain and Epilepsy*. Baltimore: University Park Press, 1977, pp 333–353

2. Bartlett J, Bridges P, Kelly D: Contemporary indications for psychosurgery. *Br J Psychiatry* 138:507–511, 1981
3. Bingley T, Leksell L, Meyerson BA, et al: Long-term results of stereotactic anterior capsulotomy in chronic obsessive-compulsive neurosis. In Sweet WH, Obrador S, Martin-Rodriguez JG (eds): *Neurosurgical Treatment in Psychiatry, Pain and Epilepsy*. Baltimore: University Park Press, 1977, pp 287–299
4. Bingley T, Persson A: EEG studies on patients with chronic obsessive-compulsive neurosis before and after psychosurgery (stereotaxic bilateral anterior capsulotomy). *Electroencephalogr Clin Neurophysiol* 44:691–696, 1978
5. Burzaco J: Stereotactic surgery in the treatment of obsessive-compulsive neurosis. In Perris C, Struwe G, Jansson B (eds): *Biological Psychiatry 1981*. Proceedings of the Third World Congress on Biological Psychiatry. Amsterdam: Elsevier, 1981, pp 1103–1109
6. Fodstad H, Strandman E, Karlsson B, et al: Treatment of chronic compulsive states with stereotactic anterior capsulotomy or cingulotomy. *Acta Neurochir* (Wien) 62:1–23, 1982
7. Herner T: Treatment of mental disorders with frontal stereotaxis thermolesions. *Acta Psychiatr Neurol Scand* 36 [Suppl 158]:140, 1961
8. Kelly D: *Anxiety and Emotions: Physiological Basis and Treatment*. Springfield, IL: Thomas, 1980, p. 402
9. Kelly D: Psychosurgery in the 1970s. *Br J Hosp Med* 16:165–174, 1976
10. Knight G: Stereotactic tractotomy in the surgical treatment of mental illness. *J Neurol Neurosurg Psychiatry* 28:304–310, 1965
11. Kuhar MJ: Neuroanatomical substrates of anxiety: A brief survey. *Trends Neurosci* 9:307–311, 1986
12. Kullberg G: Differences in effect of capsulotomy and cingulotomy. In Sweet WH, Obrador S, Martin-Rodriquez JG (eds): *Neurosurgical Treatment in Psychiatry, Pain and Epilepsy*. Baltimore: University Park Press, 1977, pp 301–308
13. Laitinen L: Emotional responses to subcortical electrical stimulation in psychiatric patients. *Clin Neurol Neurosurg* 81–83:148–157, 1979
14. Laitinen L: Psychosurgery. In Kisker KP, et al (eds): *Psychiatrie der Genenwart*. Berlin, Heidelberg: Springer, 1980, pp 352–378
15. Le Beau J: *Psycho-Chirurgie et Fonctions Mentals*. Paris: Masson, 1954, p 429
16. Leksell L: *Stereotaxis and Radiosurgery*. Springfield, IL: Thomas, 1971, p 69
17. Martinez SN, Bertrand C, Molina-Negro P, et al: Alteration of pain perception by stereotactic lesions of fronto-thalamic pathways. *Confin Neurol* 37:113–118, 1975
18. Meyer A, Beck E: *Prefrontal Leucotomy and Related Operations*. Edingburgh, London: Oliver and Boyd, 1954, p 60
19. Meyerson BA: Stereotactic anterior capsulotomy in the treatment of obessive-compulsive neurosis. In Carrea R, (ed): *Neurological Surgery*. International Congress Series No 433. Amsterdam: Exerpta Medica, 1977, pp 307–312
20. Meyerson BA, Bergström M, Greitz T: Target localization in stereotactic capsulotomy with the aid of computed tomography. In Hitchcock ER, Ballantine HT, Meyerson BA (eds): *Modern Concepts in Psychiatric Surgery*. Amsterdam: Elsevier, 1979, pp 217–224
21. Mindus P, Bergström K, Levander S, et al: Clinical results and magnetic resonance findings in anxiety and obessive-compulsive disorders treated with psychosurgery: A prospective, multidisciplinary assessment. In Shagass C, et al (eds): *Biological Psychiatry*. Proceedings of the Fourth World Congress of Biological Psychiatry. New York: Elsevier, 1985, pp 1370–1372
22. Mindus P, Levander SE, Nyman H, et al: Long-term outcome of psychosurgical intervention in anxiety disorders—a prospective, multidisciplinary, independent evaluation. (Submitted to Acta Psychiatr Scand)
23. Nauta WJH: Connections of the frontal lobe with the limbic system. In Laitinen LV, Livingston KE (eds): *Surgical Approaches to Psychiatry*. Lencester, Eng: MTP Publications, 1973, pp 303–314
24. Nauta WJH: The problem of the frontal lobe: A reinterpretation. *J Psychiatr Res* 8:167–187, 1971
25. Pippard J: Rostral leucotomy: A report on 240 cases personally followed up after 1½ to 5 years. *Br J Psychiatry* 118:141–154, 1955
26. Rylander G: Stereotactic radiosurgery in anxiety and obsessive-compulsive states: Psychiatric aspects. In Hitchcock ER, Ballantine HT, Meyerson BA (eds): *Modern Concepts in Psychiatric Surgery*. Amsterdam: Elsevier, 1979, pp 235–272
27. Smith JS, Kiloh LG: The psychosurgical treatment of anxiety. In Burrows GP, Davies B (eds): *Handbook of Studies on Anxiety*. Amsterdam: Elsevier/North-Holland Biomedical Press, 1980, pp 377–398
28. Spiegel EA, Wycis HT: Physiological and psychological results of thalamotomy. *Proc R Soc Med* 42 [Suppl]: 84–93, 1949
29. Spiegel EA, Wycis HT, Marks M, et al: Stereotactic apparatus for operations on the human brain. *Science* 106:349–350, 1947

30. Sweet WH: Neurosurgical aspects of primary affective disorders. In Youmans JR (ed): *Neurological Surgery*, Vol 6. Philadelphia: Saunders, 1982, pp 3927–3946
31. Talairach J, Hecaen H, David M: Lobotomie préfrontale limitée par électrocoagulation des fibres thalamo-frontales à leur émergence du bras anterieur de la capsule interne. In IV Congress Neurologique International. Paris: Masson, 1949, p 141
32. Van Buren JM, Borke RC: *Variations and Connections of the Human Thalamus* (Vol 2). Berlin, New York: Springer, 1972, p 116

28. STEREOTACTIC CHEMICAL HYPOPHYSECTOMY

Allan B. Levin

The role of hypophysectomy in the treatment of cancer pain has been debated for several years. Although transcranial hypophysectomy for the treatment of malignant tumors was first described in 1952 [24, 29], it was originally conceived as a means of achieving objective regression of metastatic prostate and breast carcinoma. This procedure was a logical extension of the hormonal manipulation by gonadectomy and/or adrenalectomy pioneered by Charles Huggins [10]. It was soon found that hypophysectomy, like its antecedent operations, produced pain relief in cases of metastatic breast and prostate carcinoma more consistently than it caused objective tumor regression [26, 30]. With the advent of stereotactic and open transsphenoidal hypophysectomy, pituitary ablation could be accomplished with greater safety. Similarly, the introduction of chemical hypophysectomy by Moricca in 1963 [22] offered another nonoperative route for pituitary destruction. These types of surgery and their variations then became a practical option for providing pain relief, not only for patients who were too debilitated by advanced cancer to undergo craniotomy, but also for patients who were candidates for craniotomy.

Pain Relief Following Chemical Transsphenoidal Hypophysectomy

Chemical hypophysectomy has been used for pain relief in metastatic tumors of many types, including hormone-independent tumors [15, 17–19, 22]. In this technique, a hypophyseal lesion is produced by injecting alcohol into the sella turcica via a transsphenoidal route. The volume injected varies among surgical centers, ranging from 1–5 ml. Up to a point, the volume of injected alcohol must correlate with degree of hypophyseal damage. There is, however, inadequate endocrinological and anatomical (postmortem) data, correlated with pain relief, to serve as a guide in determining how much to inject. Surgeons who have used volumes of 1–2 ml [17–19, 22] have sometimes found it necessary to repeat alcohol injections because inadequate relief has been obtained at the first sitting.

Levin and Katz introduced the stereotactic approach to chemical hypophysectomy because of a desire to improve the technique of chemical hypophysectomy in two specific areas [14]. In surgical transsphenoidal hypophysectomies, the risk of cerebrospinal fluid (CSF) leaks without closing the floor of the sella turcica is relatively high. This is especially true in patients in whom a portion of the sella turcica may be filled with a cystic extension of the subarachnoid space or in patients in whom the diaphragma sellae is incompetent. By using a small-gauge needle to prevent large holes in the floor of the sella turcica, the chance of CSF leakage and subsequent infection are minimized.

Second, the stereotactic approach allows a large quantity of alcohol to be deposited with one needle insertion. It is anticipated that most of the alcohol remains in the pituitary gland and its extension. However, adequate pituitary destruction necessitates initially the instillation and adequate diffusion of the alcohol. Further destruction of pituitary tissue is accomplished by the compressive effects of fluid forced into a confined space. The stereotactic approach allows for the use of just one insertion of the needle and the more accurate depositing of this quantity of alcohol within the pituitary gland,

L.D. Lunsford (ed.) *MODERN STEREOTACTIC NEUROSURGERY*.

Martinus Nijhoff Publishing. Boston/Dordrecht/Lancaster.

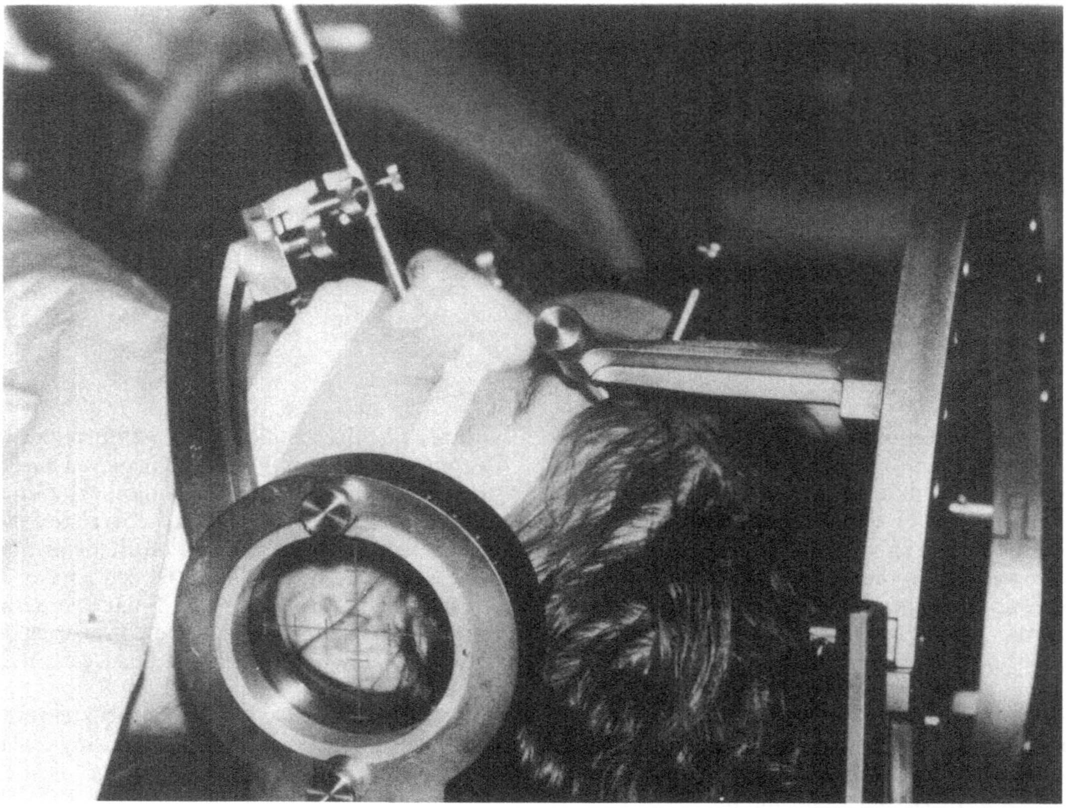

FIGURE 28–1. Patient in stereotactic head holder with needle guide in place.

thereby limiting the incidence of adverse side effects specifically related to the visual system. The injection dosage usually runs between 4 and 6 ml of alcohol injected in 2–3 aliquots as the needle is being withdrawn through the sella turcica. Postmortem studies have shown that this procedure accomplishes complete destruction of the pituitary gland.

Operative Technique

The actual operative procedure has not varied significantly from the initial descriptions [14, 15]. A light plane of general endotracheal anesthesia is established, and the patient is positioned in a Todd-Wells stereotactic head holder, utilizing a transverse quadrant assembly (figure 28–1). Under fluoroscopic lateral control and x-ray anterior-posterior control, the target is set for the posterior superior aspect of the sella turcica below the level of the posterior clinoid processes in the midline (figure 28–2). Either nostril can be used, and selection may be determined by deviated septum or size of the nasal turbinates. Four-percent cocaine is initially applied topically to produce vasoconstriction of the nasal mucosa. The nasal passage is then prepared with an organic iodine solution, and the needle guide is placed into the nostril. The needle guide is passed as far back as possible towards the superior aspect of the nasal passage. The angle of the transverse quadrant is adjusted so that the needle will have the greatest penetration through the pituitary gland on its way to the target. The mucosa at the tip of the guide is infiltrated with approximately 1 ml of 1% lidocaine with 1:100,000 epinephrine. Next, an 18-gauge, 6-inch spinal needle is passed through the floor of the sphenoid sinus, which is then thoroughly irrigated with a bacitracin solution (5,000 units/100 ml of saline). The 18-gauge needle is removed and a 6-inch,

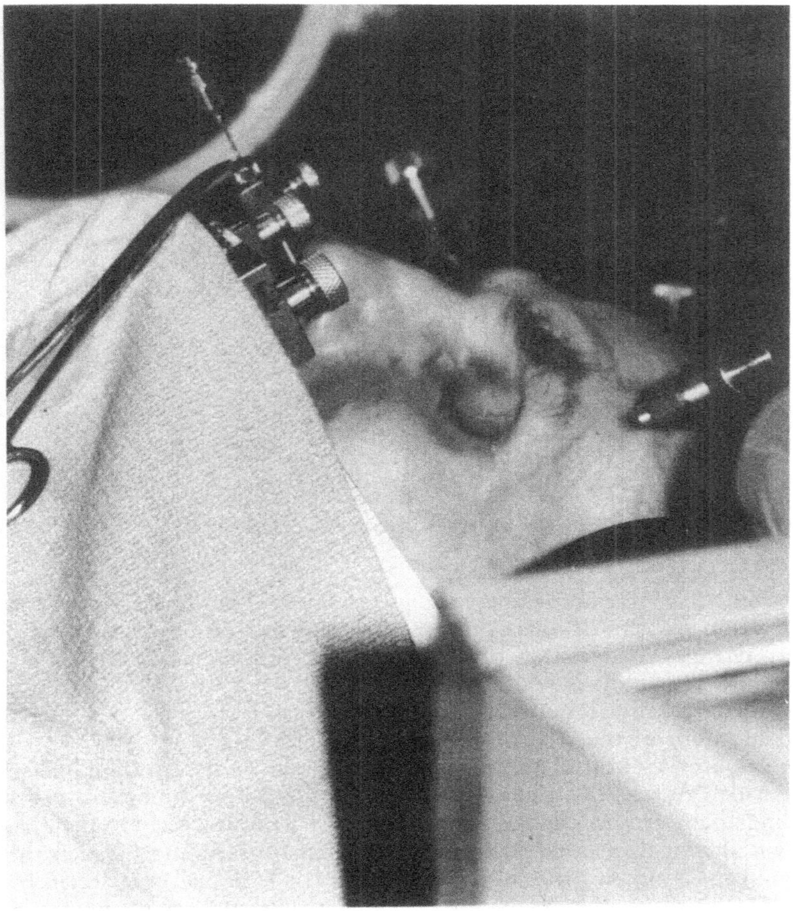

FIGURE 28-2. Twenty-gauge needle passed through needle guide into sella turcica.

20-gauge spinal needle is passed through the guide and gently inserted through the floor of the sella turcica. The anteroposterior (AP) x-rays and lateral fluoroscopy of the route of the 18-gauge needle should show that it has reached the floor of the sella turcica without any deviation from its path (figure 28-3). Likewise, upon entry of the 20-gauge spinal needle into the sella turcica, AP x-rays should confirm that the needle has not deviated from its path toward the midline target. Once this has been confirmed, further advancement of the needle under lateral fluoroscopy will verify its approach to the target. Once the needle has reached the target, confirmatory AP and lateral x-rays are made (see figure 28-2). Only in rare cases has it been difficult for the 18-gauge and 20-gauge needles to penetrate the appropriate bony pathway. In such cases, a small hole is drilled, using a Kirschner wire. The diameter of the Kirschner wire is just slightly larger than that of the spinal needle.

Once the position of the needle at the target is confirmed, the stylet is withdrawn, and up to 2 ml of absolute alcohol is deposited at the target. Injection under adequate fluoroscopic monitoring allows the surgeon to actually see the small air bubbles that have been entrapped within the needle entering the sella turcica. The pupils are checked after injection. Although it is believed that the alcohol stays within the sella turcica, rapid enlargement of the pituitary gland from the quantity of fluid injected can cause the pituitary to swell laterally and compress the nerves to the extraocular muscles lying within the cavernous sinus. Upward ex-

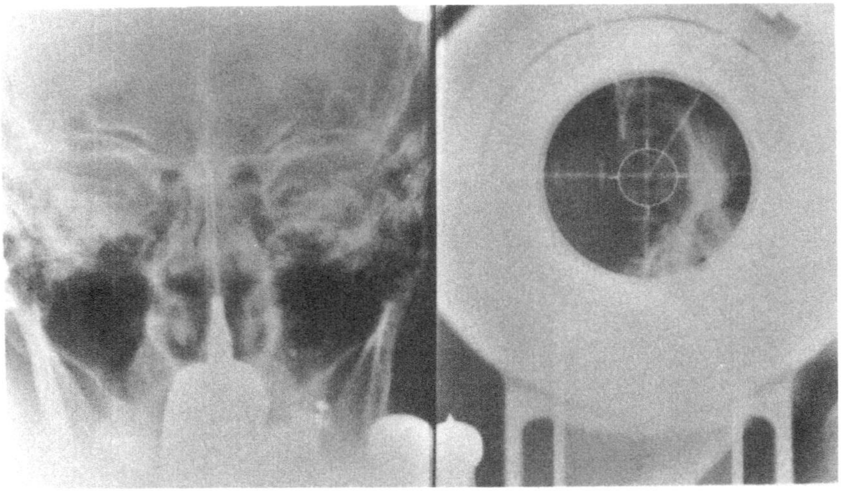

FIGURE 28–3. Left: Lateral view of needle at target. Right: Anterior-posterior view of needle at target.

tension of the swelling may also occur, thereby compressing the optic chiasm. If there have been no pupillary changes or deviation of the eyes from the midline, the needle is withdrawn to a point approximately halfway between the initial target and the floor of the sella turcica, and a second injection of 1–2 ml of the absolute alcohol is made. Again, the pupils are checked. Providing there are no changes, the needle is again withdrawn to a point halfway between the second injection and the floor of the sella turcica and a third injection of 1–2 ml of absolute alcohol is made. The needle is then withdrawn to just above the floor of the sella turcica, and approximately 1/2 ml of alpha-ethyl cyanoacrylate (slow polymerizing) is injected through the needle as it is withdrawn through the floor of the sella turcica. This allows for sealing of the single hole made in the floor of the sella turcica. At this point, the needle is withdrawn through the needle guide, and the needle guide is then withdrawn from the nostril. If there is any evidence of bleeding from the nasal passage, the nasal passage used for the needle guide is packed with petrolatum-impregnated gauze. If there is no significant bleeding, no nasal packing is used. The patient is awakened, extubated, and followed carefully over the next 24–48 hours for the onset of diabetes insipidus. Patients are routinely placed on hydrocortisone supplementation. Diabetes insipidus that cannot be controlled by oral intake is controlled with DDAVP (1-desamino-cysteine-8-D-arginine vasopressin). Thyroid supplementation is also started several days into the postoperative period.

Complications

We have had only one CSF leak in our series of 117 patients undergoing this procedure. In that patient, who was early in the series, the tumor had metastasized and invaded the floor of the sella. The CSF leak was sealed by an injection of alpha-ethyl cyanoacrylate into the sella turcica. Since then, with the routine use of alpha-ethyl cyanoacrylate, there have been no additional CSF leaks. Other complications have included six ocular nerve palsies, with four clearing completely. There were four patients with bilateral or unilateral temporal field loss, all of whom had associated ocular nerve palsies. One of these cleared completely, and two cleared partially. It is interesting to note that all but one of the complications occurred in the first 40 patients. Only one ocular nerve palsy has occurred since the first 40 patients, and there have been no procedure-related deaths in the entire series.

Results

By 1978, Miles and his colleagues had performed chemical hypophysectomy on 122 patients with all forms of cancer, 56% of which were cancer of either breast or prostate [19].

TABLE 28–1. Pain Relief Following Chemical Hypophysectomy in 110 Cancer Patients

Type of Cancer	No. of Patients	No. (%) of Patients with Good Results	No. (%) with Good Results Who Had Transient Exacerbation
Prostate	52	44 (85)	13 (30)
Breast	32	31 (97)	5 (16)
Lung, kidney, and other tumors	26	19 (73)	5 (26)
Total	110	94 (85)	23 (24)

Of the 122 patients, 42% obtained excellent pain relief, and an additional 33% (for a total of 75%) acquired sufficient relief to be able to discontinue narcotic analgesics. To achieve these results, 30% of patients required a second injection and 9% required a third injection. The mean duration of pain relief was between two and three months. Duration of pain relief did not correlate significantly with the type of cancer. The period of survival was not reported. Madrid had treated 329 patients with this technique by January 1978 [18]. Patients with metastatic breast and prostate carcinoma constituted 80% of his cases. Of the total number of patients, 67% had complete relief, and an additional 27% had partial relief. To realize these results, 25% of patients required a second injection, and 3% needed a third injection. No data were given correlating relief to tumor type, and no information was available on either duration of relief or postoperative survival. Moricca's rate of success appears to be good, but details correlating tumor type to pain relief, the role of multiple injections, and duration of relief are not available [22].

To date, we have performed stereotactic chemical hypophysectomy on 110 cancer patients. Breast and prostate cancer account for 76% of the cases; lung, kidney, and other tumors constitute the remainder. Preoperatively, all patients were unable to achieve acceptable pain control, despite large doses of parenteral narcotics. The results of chemical hypophysectomy are presented in table 28–1. Good results were obtained in 85% of cases. This category represents patients who reported either satisfactory pain control with no analgesics or the ability to achieve such control with nonnarcotic analgesics or codeine. Seven patients (four with prostatic and three with mixed) cancers transiently obtained good pain relief (lasting at least one month) but later required cordotomy (six patients) or reinjection of alcohol (one patient) to achieve longer-lasting pain relief. These seven patients are not included in the good result category. There were no significant differences ($p > 0.1$) in the response rates among the prostatic, breast, or mixed series. For most patients who could be followed carefully, duration of relief was limited not by recurrence of pain but by death due to underlying neoplastic disease. The mean postoperative survival was five months. The postoperative level of pain relief was not constant from day to day. Frequently, there were minor variations in the level of relief, necessitating nonnarcotic analgesics or codeine some days, whereas no drugs were required on other days. In 24% of the patients, there was occasional transient exacerbation of a more substantial nature, which would typically last one to five days before spontaneously remitting. In one-third of the patients involved, these exacerbations were multiple, occurring about once a month. The cause of the transient exacerbation is unknown, but it may be due to the development of new metastases or enlargement of already-present metastases.

In summary, chemical hypophysectomy has produced relief from pain caused by both hormone-dependent and hormone-independent tumors. The number of useful published studies is insufficient to permit rigid conclusions. Few reports have provided a definition of pain relief. Independent observers rarely have been used [17]. Although no systematic attempt has been made to provide detailed information on the type of pain that can be relieved by hypophysectomy, some investigators suspect that the pain most susceptible to relief is that from bone metastases [15]. In chemical hypophysectomy, the initial success rate appears slightly better than that reported following surgical hypophysectomy for breast and prostate cancer. However, the duration of both relief and survival seem to be shorter following chemical hypophysectomy. This may be explained by inadequate numbers of clinic reports. It may also be a reflection of far-advanced disease present at the time of neurosurgical referral.

Thalamic Pain

In 1977, the technique of stereotactic chemical hypophysectomy was extended to include pain considered to be of thalamic or central origin [16]. This technique was one of several alternatives for pain management offered to our patients with this pain syndrome. All seven patients had been evaluated previously at other medical centers where the diagnosis of thalamic pain syndrome had been made and where both conservative and surgical management had been ineffective. All post–chemical hypophysectomy patients have been followed either in our outpatient neurosurgical clinic or by correspondence. Six of the seven patients had good relief at first, and one patient initially had what he considered to be 50%–60% relief. Approximately six months after injection, one patient began to reexperience pain and was placed on tricyclic antidepressants and other medication without notable results. In considering a possible repeat hypophysectomy, pituitary function studies were performed that revealed that there had been no return of pituitary function. No further therapy was offered. The patient who obtained only partial relief continued to have intermittent exacerbations that became almost as severe as the initial pain approximately four months after injection. Approximately six months after injection, he developed hydrocephalus and was treated locally with an external ventriculostomy, which subsequently became infected, causing ventriculitis. He was treated and made an adequate recovery, again showing transient improvement followed by periodic exacerbation of his pain syndrome. His symptomatology was not entirely that of a thalamic pain syndrome because he also had signs of pontine involvement. The longest follow-ups have been approximately five years for two patients. Neither patient experienced recurrent symptoms.

The mechanism of relief in chemical hypophysectomy seems as mysterious as that following transsphenoidal hypophysectomy. Advocates of chemical hypophysectomy have proposed that the effect is due to concomitant hypothalamic injury and have suggested that this operation may be qualitatively different than transsphenoidal hypophysectomy [15, 19, 22].

Mechanism of Action: Pituitary

The mechanism by which pain is relieved in either chemical or surgical hypophysectomy is unknown. Unlike either cingulotomy or subcaudate frontal leucotomy, hypophysectomy does not produce relief primarily by allaying psychological suffering. Moreover, hypophysectomy does not alter normal sensitivity to pinprick, or the appreciation of pain due to acute injury [22, 31]. This argues against the theory that pain relief may be related to changes in peripheral pain receptor sensitivity [19]. The successful use of chemical hypophysectomy in patients with thalamic pain is additional evidence against such a theory.

Humoral or neural modulation of central pain-inhibiting neurons is a more plausible mechanism of action. According to this proposition, pain relief may result from excitation of central pain-suppressor mechanisms by means of either a humoral agent distributed by the CSF [19, 32] or by a direct neural stimulus. Hypophysectomy, it is reasoned, either eliminates a hormone responsible for pain augmentation produced by the pituitary or induces (possibly by elimination of feedback suppression) a neural or humoral response, originating from the hypothalamus, which is responsible for pain suppression.

It has long been recognized that oophorectomy [12], adrenalectomy, and orchiectomy yield prompt relief of pain usually within hours in some patients suffering from metastatic breast or prostate carcinoma. This relief begins long before objective remission; it may occur without objective remission, and relief seems to begin at about the same time as it does after hypophysectomy. These observations imply that there is a mechanism of pain relief common to all four operations that is also distinct from pain relief attendant on tumor regression. Such a mechanism might be a hypothalamic pain-suppressing response activated by the elimination of hormonal feedback.

The foregoing raises the possibility that pain

relief after hypophysectomy may be more directly the result of stimulation of hypothalamic function rather than the elimination of pituitary function. There is additional support for this view. Several lines of evidence cast doubt on the notion that pain relief from hypophysectomy is directly related to the expected fall in levels of *known* pituitary hormones: 1. Pain relief occurs in cases of malignancies not known to be hormone-dependent [15, 18] and in patients with breast and prostate carcinoma that is unresponsive to hormone manipulation [11]. 2. Although there exists some minimal level of hypophyseal damage sufficient to produce pain relief, beyond this point, pain relief does not appear to be correlated with the completeness of ablation of known pituitary endocrine function [15, 17, 19, 32, 34]. 3. Patients may derive relief despite failure to achieve an objective remission [5, 11]. 4. Pain relief may occur promptly following oophorectomy [12], orchiectomy, or adrenalectomy, which would then increase the level of the appropriate pituitary trophic hormones. 5. Pain relief occurs after stalk section [13], a procedure which normally elevates prolactin blood levels [33]. 6. Pain relief occurs with administration of L-dopa [20], a procedure that normally stimulates human growth hormone secretion [3].

Mechanism of Action: Hypothalamus

The belief that pain relief after hypophysectomy could be unrelated to the hypophysectomy led some investigators to look for concomitant damage in other neural structures. Lipton provided evidence that alcohol injected into the sella extends up the pituitary stalk into the hypothalamus and third ventricle, where damage has been found on postmortem examination [17]. Levin performed postmortem examinations in four cases of alcohol hypophysectomy for cancer pain [15]. These examinations revealed subependymal gliosis along the floor of the third ventricle, considerable cell loss in the supraoptic and paraventricular nuclei and damage to the median eminence. Our further investigation of pathways of alcohol in chemical hypophysectomy revealed that the alcohol enters not only the pituitary stalk and third ventricle, but that the alcohol refluxes under pressure into the portal hypophyseal vascular system. The importance of the posteromedial hypothalamus in pain control has been emphasized by the work of Sano [28] and Fairman [4]. These investigators demonstrated that lesions in the posterior inferior peri-third ventricular area produced good relief in more than 70% of patients whose pain was due to malignant tumor.

Despite the apparent success of posteromedial hypothalamic lesions in relieving the pain of malignancy, good pain relief has also been reported in 70%–90% of patients following open transsphenoidal microsurgical hypophysectomy for metastatic prostate and breast cancer [5, 11, 32], in which the likelihood of direct hypothalamic injury would be small. Daniel and Prichard examined the hypothalamus and pituitary stalk of 59 patients who had undergone one of three pituitary ablative procedures: transfrontal pituitary stalk section, transfrontal hypophysectomy, or transsphenoidal hypophysectomy [2]. They reported significant cell loss in both the supraoptic (SON) and paraventricular (PVN) nuclei due to retrograde degeneration. Other nuclei of the hypothalamus, however, did not show any obvious postoperative abnormalities. Regardless of which operative procedure was used, the only hypothalamic abnormalities observed lay anteriorly.

The relationship of anterior hypothalamic dysfunction to pain relief has not received extensive consideration in the literature. Our knowledge comes in part from studies examining the relationship between diabetes insipidus and pain relief, such as Lipton's series, which found no correlation [17]. As previously mentioned, we performed chemical hypophysectomy in seven patients with thalamic pain and six achieved good relief [16]. Our patients recovered from diabetes insipidus within a year (three patients recovered within six months), yet pain relief persisted. The failure of pain relief to correlate with this aspect of anterior hypothalamic dysfunction contradicts earlier speculation [15] of such correlation in a study of 29 patients with cancer pain. The life expectancy of the patient population in that earlier study apparently was too short to permit observations on pain relief that persisted after recovery from diabetes insipidus.

It would appear that overt hypothalamic damage, apart from retrograde cell loss in PVN and SON, may not be required to obtain prompt pain relief. Hypophysectomy, even when anatomically [23] and endocrinologically [13, 15, 17] incomplete, seems to be sufficient. Therefore, we must ask whether chemical hypophysectomy is a unique neuroablative technique or simply a variant of other forms of hypophysectomy, all of which act by a similar mechanism. The success of stereotactic chemical hypophysectomy on hormone-independent tumors may encourage the use of stereotactic thermal and cryohypophysectomy for tumors heretofore treated by open transsphenoidal hypophysectomy. The comparison of results could settle the question.

Mechanism of Action: Endogenous Opiate

Naloxone, a specific antagonist for morphine and its analogues, was administered in an attempt to restore pain in patients whose pain was relieved by hypophysectomy. The object was to determine whether hypophysectomy, like stimulation-induced analgesia [1, 8], produces pain relief by augmenting endogenous opiate release. Thus far, the evidence does not favor an opioid-mediated mechanism, but this evidence is preliminary. In studies by Levin, naloxone failed to reverse the pain relief achieved by chemical hypophysectomy in 29 patients with cancer and three with thalamic pain [15, 16]. In Miles's series of 12 patients who had undergone chemical hypophysectomy for cancer, eight failed to experience restoration of pain following administration of naloxone [19]. Misfeldt administered naloxone to a patient following transsphenoidal hypophysectomy for metastatic prostate and renal carcinoma [21]. Naloxone did not cause the pain to return. An extensive trial of naloxone testing after surgical hypophysectomy has not been published. In addition, there are several different classes of opiate receptors, each of which has varying affinity for naloxone [7], making naloxone studies difficult to interpret. Naloxone insensitivity could be a reflection of limited affinity rather than an argument for a nonopioid mechanism. Failure to demonstrate restoration of pain with naloxone may not rule out an opiate-mediated effect.

However, studies in humans and rats offer additional evidence that opioid mechanisms may not serve an important role in this form of pain inhibition. Miles assayed met-enkephalin and beta-endorphin in human lumbar CSF before, immediately after, and five hours after chemical hypophysectomy and failed to show elevation of either endogenous opiate [19]. Hypophysectomy in rats diminishes plasma levels of beta-endorphin [6, 9] and may either have no demonstrable effect on brain tissue beta-endorphin levels [9, 27] or may actually decrease the beta-endorphin content of mediobasal hypothalamus [34] and periventricular tissue [25].

Other Uses of Stereotactic Hypophysectomy Technique

The stereotactic technique utilized in stereotactic chemical hypophysectomy can also be used to approach lesions that might lie in the suprasellar area above the planum sphenoidale or just behind the dorsum sellae. These lesions usually represent cystic masses, either craniopharyngiomas or dermoids, which need intermittent evacuation. We have had the opportunity to treat four patients by such method. Three patients had recurrent cystic craniopharyngiomas, having previously undergone craniotomy for therapy. Drainage procedures preceded radiotherapy, and in one case, two subsequent drainage procedures occurred during the course of radiotherapy. One patient presented with a dermoid cyst that had been treated with a craniotomy (a transsphenoidal approach) and then x-ray therapy (figures 28–4 and 28–5). Despite the previous transsphenoidal surgery, no untoward problems or complications arose from the stereotactic procedures. In all cases, water-soluble contrast material was injected into the cyst at the time of needle insertion to outline the cyst and document its collapse.

Conclusion

The technique of stereotactic chemical hypophysectomy is accurate and technically simple. In the debilitated patient and in patients with conditions requiring ablation of the pituitary gland, this method of hypophysectomy should be considered. It should also be considered as a method of access to lesions in the suprasellar region.

References

1. Akil H, Richardson DE, Hughes J, et al: Enkephalin-like material elevated in ventricular cerebrospinal fluid of pain patients after analgesic focal stimulation. *Science* 201:463–465, 1978

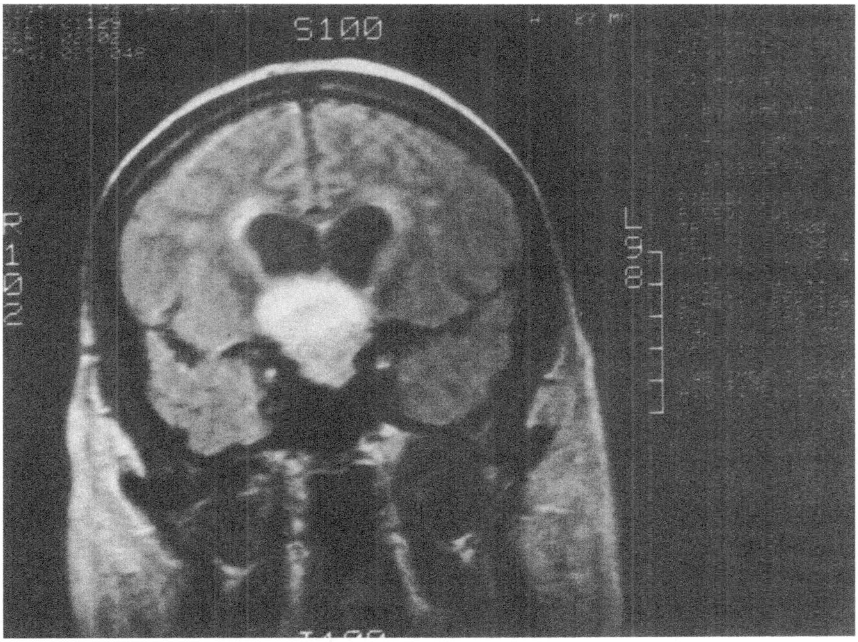

A

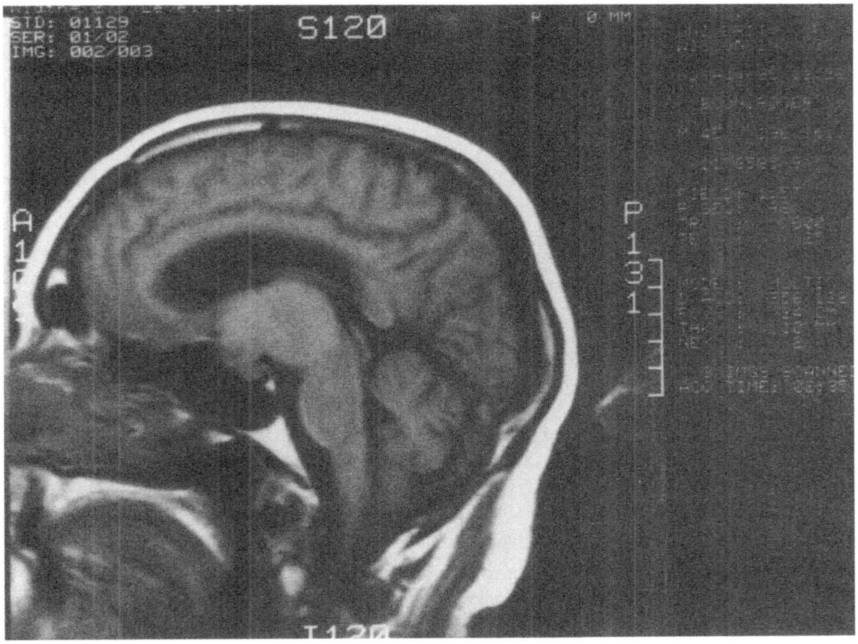

B

FIGURE 28–4. (A and B) Magnetic resonance imaging (MRI) of a suprasellar recurrent dermoid cyst.

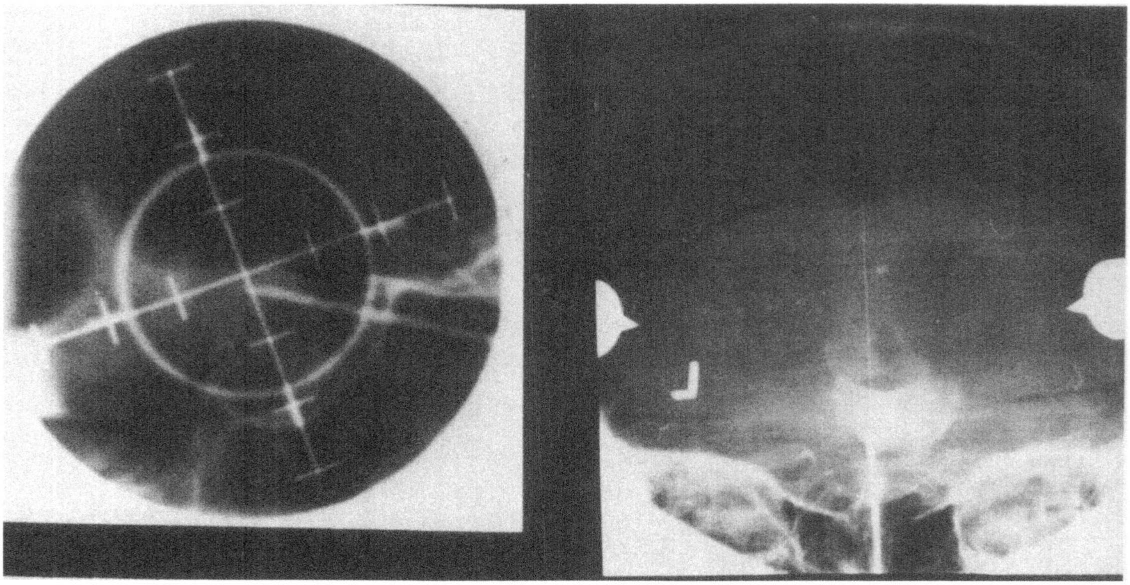

FIGURE 28–5. A: Lateral view of needle in a dermoid cyst (water-soluble contrast media outlining cyst). B: anterior-posterior view of needle in a dermoid cyst (water-soluble contrast media outlining cyst).

2. Daniel PM, Prichard MML: The human hypothalamus and pituitary stalk after hypophysectomy or pituitary stalk section. *Brain* 95: 813–824, 1972
3. Eddy RL, Gilliland PF, Ibana JD Jr, et al: Human growth hormone release: Comparison of provocative test procedures. *Am J Med* 56: 179–185, 1974
4. Fairman D: Hypothalamotomy as a new perspective for alleviation of intractable pain and regression of metastatic malignant tumors. In Fusek I and Kunc Z (eds): *Present Limits of Neurosurgery*. Prague: Avicenum, 1972, pp 525–528
5. Gros C, Frerbeau P, Privat JM, et al: Place of hypophysectomy in the neurosurgical treatment of pain. In Penzholz H, Brock M, Hamer J, Klinger M, Spoerri O (eds): *Advances in Neurosurgery*, Vol 3. Heidelberg: Springer-Verlag, 1975, pp 264–272
6. Guillemin R, Vargo T, Rossier J, et al: Beta-endorphin and adrenocorticotropin are secreted concomitantly by the pituitary gland. *Science* 197:1367–1369, 1977
7. Hill RG: The status of naloxone in the identification of pain control mechanisms operated by endogenous opioids. *Neuroscience Lett* 21: 217–222, 1981
8. Hosobuchi Y, Adams JE, Linchitz R: Pain relief by stimulation of the central gray matter in humans and its reversal by naloxone. *Science* 197:183–186, 1977
9. Houghten RA, Swann RW, Li CH: Beta-endorphin: Stability, clearance behavior, and entry into the central nervous system after intravenous injection of the tritiated peptide in rats and rabbits. *Proc Natl Acad Sci USA* 77:4588–4591, 1980
10. Huggins C: Endocrine induced regression of cancers: Nobel prize lecture 1966. *Cancer Res* 27:1925–1930, 1966
11. Kapur TR, Dalton GA: Transsphenoidal hypophysectomy for metastatic carcinoma of the breast. *Br J Surg* 56:332–337, 1969
12. Kennedy BJ: Hormonal therapy of mammary carcinoma. In Pack GT, Ariel I (eds): *Treatment of Cancer and Allied Disorders, Vol 4: The Breast, Chest, and Esophagus*. New York: Harper, 1960, pp 178–204
13. LaRossa JT, Strong MS, Melby JC: Endocrinologically incomplete transethmoidal, transsphenoidal hypophysectomy with relief of bone pain in breast cancer. *N Engl J Med* 298:1332–1335, 1978
14. Levin AB, Katz J: Treatment of diffuse cancer pain by instillation of alcohol into the sella turcica. *Anesthesiology* 46:115–121, 1977
15. Levin AB, Katz J, Benson RC, et al: Treatment of pain of diffuse metastatic cancer by stereotactic chemical hypophysectomy: Long term results and observations on mechanism of action. *Neurosurgery* 6:258–262, 1980
16. Levin AB, Ramirez LF, Katz J: The use of stereotaxic chemical hypophysectomy in the

treatment of thalamic pain syndrome. *J Neurosurg* 59:1002–1006, 1983

17. Lipton S, Miles J, Williams N, et al: Pituitary injection of a alcohol for widespread cancer pain. *Pain* 5:73–82, 1978
18. Madrid JL: Chemical hypophysectomy. In Bonica JJ, Ventafridda V (eds): *Advances in Pain Research and Therapy*, Vol 2. New York: Raven Press, 1979, pp 381–391
19. Miles J: Chemical hypophysectomy. In Bonica JJ, Ventafridda V (eds): *Advances in Pain Research and Therapy*, Vol 2. New York: Raven Press, 1979, pp 373–380
20. Minoto JP, Bronn DG, Kibbey WE: L-dopa effect in painful bony metastases. *N Engl J Med* 294:340, 1976 (Letter)
21. Misfeldt DS, Goldstein A: Hypophysectomy relieves pain not via endorphins. *N Engl J Med* 297:1236–1237, 1977
22. Moricca G: Neuroadenolysis for diffuse unbearable cancer pain. In Bonica JJ, Albe-Fessard D (eds): *Advances in Pain Research and Therapy*, Vol 1. New York: Raven Press, 1976 pp 863–866
23. Norrell H, Albes AM, Winternitz WW, et al: A clinicopathologic analysis of cryohypophysectomy in patients with advanced cancer. *Cancer* 25:1050–1060, 1970
24. Perrault M, Lebeau J, Klotz B, et al: L'hypophysectomie totale dan le traitment du cancer sein: Premier cas francais: avenir de la method. *Therapie* 7:290–300, 1952
25. Przewlocki R, Millan MJ, Gramsch CH, et al: The influence of selective adeno- and neurointermedio-hypophysectomy upon plasma and brain levels of beta-endorphin and the response to stress in rats. *Brain Res* 242:107–117, 1982
26. Ray BS, Pearson OH: Hypophysectomy in the treatment of disseminated breast cancer. *Surg Clin North Am* 42:419–433, 1962
27. Rossier J, Vargo TM, Minnick S, et al: Regional dissociation of beta-endorphin and enkephalin content in rat brain and pituitary. *Proc Natl Acad Sci USA* 74:5162–5165, 1977
28. Sano K: Intralaminar thalamotomy and posteromedial hypothalamotomy in the treatment of intractable pain. *Prog Neurolog Surg* 8:50–103, 1977
29. Scott WW: Endocrine management of disseminated prostate cancer, including bilateral adrenalectomy and hypophysectomy. *Trans Am Assoc Genito-Urinary Surgeons* 44:101–104, 1952
30. Scott WW, Schirmer HKA: Hypophysectomy for disseminated prostatic cancer. In *On Cancer and Hormones*. Chicago: University of Chicago Press, 1962, pp 175–204
31. Sweet WH: Central mechanisms of chronic pain. In Bonica JJ (ed): *Pain Research Publications*: New York: Raven Press, 1980, ARNMD 58, pp 287–303
32. Tindall GT, Payne NS, Nixon DW: Transsphenoidal hypophysectomy for disseminated carcinoma of the prostate gland. *J Neurosurg* 50:275–282, 1979
33. Turkington RW, Underwood LE, Van Wyk JJ: Elevated serum prolactin levels after pituitary stalk section in man. *N Engl J Med* 285:707–710, 1971
34. Vermes I, Mulder GH, Berkenbosch F, et al: Release of beta-lipotropin and beta-endorphin from rat hypothalami in vitro. *Brain Res* 211:248–254, 1981

29. POSTEROMEDIAL HYPOTHALAMOTOMY FOR BEHAVIORAL DISTURBANCES AND INTRACTABLE PAIN

Yoshiaki Mayanagi
Keiji Sano

The hypothalamus, a continuation of the central periaqueductal gray matter, comprises the center of the neuroendocrine system; it surrounds the third ventricle with groups of neurons anteriorly and central gray matter posteriorly. The periventricular fibers, the medial forebrain bundle, and the dorsal longitudinal fasciculus are important fiber tracts that pass through the region. Relevant to the third ventricle because of its location, the posterior hypothalamus lies between the midcommissural point and the posterior commissure, below the anterior commissure–posterior commissure (AC–PC) line and includes the area 5–6 mm from the midline.

Stereotactic surgery directed at this level of the brain's longitudinal axis was reported first by Spiegel and Wycis [35]. To treat psychosis, they made a small lesion in the lateral hypothalamus, which they usually combined with dorsomedial thalamotomy. In 1962, Sano originated a new stereotactic operation on the medial part of the posterior hypothalamus to ameliorate certain behavioral disturbances, particularly those characterized by aggression or violence; he named it *posteromedial hypothalamotomy* [26]. Sano examined the close relationship between such behavioral disturbances and hypersympathetic autonomic reactions and proceeded to make a small coagulation lesion in the most sympathetic area of the diencephalon. Sixty cases of the same condition underwent surgery between the first successful operation in 1962 and 1977 [12, 13, 24, 25, 27–31].

In 1971, Fairman reported the application of this technique for pain control [9]. He produced small circumscribed coagulation lesions in the paraventricular nucleus of the hypothalamus in 12 patients with intractable pain due to metastatic malignant tumors, expecting pain relief and reduction in tumor growth. The pain relief was dramatic in 10 patients; tumor growth was reduced in two; and appetite improved in six. No serious endocrine deficits occurred. In 1971, Yoshioka, Yoshimasu, and others in our group performed stereotactic posteromedial hypothalamotomy for relief of intractable pain in two patients with malignant tumors and obtained remarkable pain control [40]. Later, similar surgery was performed on 28 patients with pain of various causes. This procedure gradually evolved into stimulation-produced analgesia (SPA) in the same region [14, 15]. Along with these clinical studies, several basic experimental studies were conducted to clarify the central mechanism of pain relief obtained with this procedure. This chapter examines the significance of the posterior hypothalamus in the treatment of both behavioral disturbances and intractable pain, based on our experience with 100 cases over the past 20 years.

Posteromedial Hypothalamotomy

General endotracheal anesthesia was used in operations for behavioral disturbances and local anesthesia in procedures for intractable pain. Initially, Sano's stereotactic apparatus

L.D. Lunsford (ed.) *MODERN STEREOTACTIC NEUROSURGERY*.

was used; since 1975, we have used the Todd-Wells apparatus. A frontal burr hole was made, and a fine catheter was inserted into the anterior horn of the lateral ventricle, with the tip placed near the foramen of Monro. Ventriculography was performed with air or a small amount of a positive contrast agent. If the tip of the ventricular catheter entered the third ventricle easily, a small amount of cerebrospinal fluid (CSF) was taken for analysis. Using the AC and PC as a guide for measurement, we inserted a fine concentric bipolar electrode (1 mm in outer diameter with an interpolar distance of 0.5 mm) through a frontal burr hole into the target point in the posterior hypothalamus.

The target for behavioral disturbances was 2 mm below the midcommissural point and 2 mm lateral to the third ventricular wall; for intractable pain, various targets in the posterior hypothalamic area were selected. We monitored electroencephalograms (EEGs), electrocardiograms, electromyograms of the neck muscles, blood pressure, and respiration. Electrical stimulation was performed with parameters of 10–100 Hz and 10–20 V using square-wave pulses 1–2 msec wide.

Responses caused by high-frequency stimulation of the target point can be summarized as follows:

1. **Autonomic responses, mainly sympathetic:**
   Elevation of blood pressure
   Increase of pulse rate
   Respiratory suppression followed by hyperpnea or tachypnea
   Mydriasis
   Flushing of the face
2. **Somatomotor responses:**
   Rotatory movement (downward or inward) of the eye ball on the stimulated side
   Lateral flexion of the neck toward the stimulated side
3. **EEG responses:**
   Diffuse slow-wave burst of 2–3 Hz (with light general anesthesia)
   Diffuse desynchronized low-voltage fast waves (with local anesthesia)
4. **Endocrinological responses:**
   Elevated plasma levels of pituitary hormones, catecholamines, and nonesterified fatty acids (NEFAs)
   Elevation of CSF level of beta-endorphins

Figure 29–1 shows typical responses to high-frequency stimulation, registered by an EEG and a polygraph. The area in which definite sympathetic responses were obtained forms a small "ergotropic triangle" on the lateral plane of the posterior hypothalamus: the triangle is formed by lines connecting the midcommissural point, the PC, and the mammillary body (figure 29–2). In the frontal plane, this area is 2–5 mm lateral to the wall of the third ventricle.

Elevation of blood pressure was the most reliable response to confirm that the target point had been reached because it usually was elicited in the most narrow area of the posterior hypothalamus (as shown in figure 29–2). If the electrode tip was inserted more medially or laterally, the stimulation usually resulted in hypotension. These results suggested a three-layer organization of the posterior hypothalamus from medial to lateral: a medial parasympathetic area, a middle sympathetic area, and a second, lateral parasympathetic area [29]. When surgery was performed with the patient awake and locally anesthetized, blood pressure rarely decreased. Instead, elevated blood pressure was elicited by stimulating a wide area of the posterior hypothalamus. In the awake state, patients reported a very unpleasant sensation during stimulation. Although weak stimulation produced a warm sensation throughout the body, strong stimulation resulted in a feeling of fear or horror accompanied by dizziness and a sensation of spinning. In patients with cancer pain, weak stimulation was followed by pain relief. After confirming the proper placement of the electrode at the target point by radiological and stimulation studies, electrocoagulation was performed with either the same bipolar stimulating electrode or a newly inserted thermocontrol electrode (diameter of 2 mm, exposed tip of 2 mm). The lesion was performed using high-frequency current of 2–4 W for 30 seconds at 70°C. The coagulation lesion was 3–4 mm in diameter; this size was confirmed when autopsies were performed.

If necessary, surgery on the contralateral side was performed two to three weeks later by the same technique. Except for a temporary somnolent state, no neurological deficits developed postoperatively. Additional details of the operative procedure and the responses to stimulation are described elsewhere [29, 31].

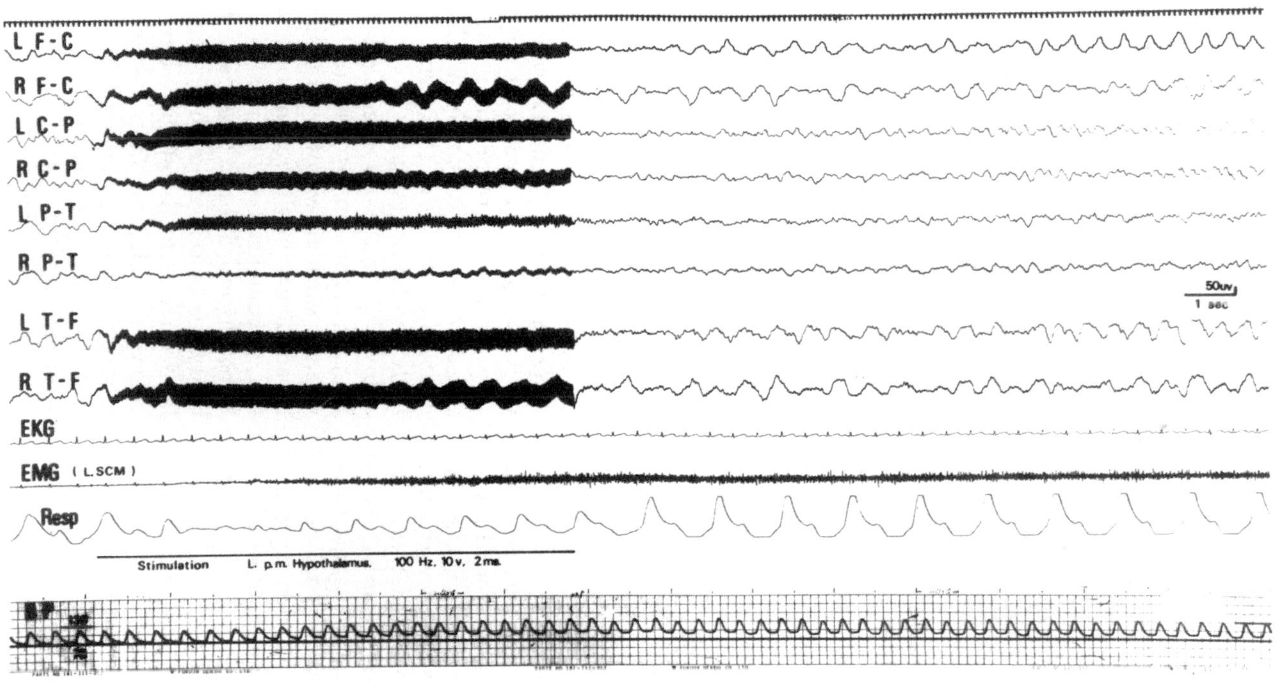

FIGURE 29–1. Electroencephalogram and polygraph recordings show responses caused by high-frequency stimulation in the left posterior hypothalamus of a patient who was given general anesthesia. F = frontal; C = central; P = parietal; T = temporal; L = left; R = right; EKG = electrocardiogram; EMG = electromyogram recorded from the left sternocleidomastoid muscle; Resp = respiration rhythm recorded on the chest; BP = blood pressure from the right radial artery.

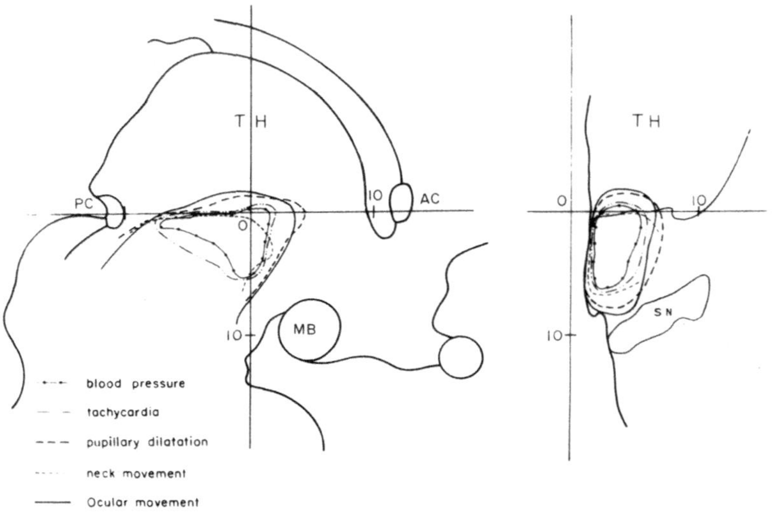

FIGURE 29–2. Summary of autonomic and somatomotor responses obtained by high frequency stimulation of the posterior hypothalamus. Blood pressure line indicates elevation of blood pressure upon stimulation, AC = anterior commissure; MB = mammillary body; O = midcommissural point; PC = posterior commissure; SN = substantia nigra; TH = thalamus (compare [29]).

Behavioral Disturbances

CLINICAL FEATURES

Sixty patients underwent surgery between 1962 and 1977. Prior to developing behavioral problems, most of the patients had experienced epileptic seizures, usually associated with some degree of mental retardation. These features indicated that the behavioral disturbances in these patients were the result of organic cerebral dysfunction. Pneumoencephalography often revealed diffuse ventricular enlargement, but porencephaly or focal abnormalities of the frontal lobes rarely were seen. The types of behavioral disturbances we treated can be classified into three categories: (1) aggressive behavior (usually against a particular member of the family or community, occasionally in the form of self-mutilation), (2) rage attacks (breaking objects, attacking any nearby person), (3) restless behavior (constant moving, running, jumping, leaping, or other hyperkinetic activity). Surgery was indicated only when the behavioral problem became so severe that isolating the patient was necessary to reduce the danger to other persons.

RESULTS

Of these 60 patients (44 males and 16 females), 29 (22 males and 7 females) were less than 15 years of age at the time of surgery. Two patients underwent reoperation, and one operative death occurred from hemorrhage. Follow-up studies in 1969, 1977, and 1985 yielded fairly consistent results.

By 1985, follow-up extended between 8 and 23 years. Thirteen patients (22%) had died: three of suicide; two of status epilepticus; two by accidental drowning; and one each of hepatitis, pneumonia, renal failure, lung cancer, and hematological disease. One patient died of an unknown cause. Although no deaths were related directly to the surgical intervention, we believe this high mortality rate is more likely related to the overall reduced life expectancy of these handicapped patients. The most recent assessment of the operation's effect upon behavioral disturbances and the current condition of 32 patients is summarized in table 29–1. Precise information on many aspects of their daily life was gathered from interviews with family members and health professionals who were involved in their care for a long time.

TABLE 29–1. Posterior Hypothalamotomy for Behavioral Disturbances: Patient Status at Follow-up

Effect on Behavioral Disturbances	Living With Family			Living in Centers for the Handicapped		Hospitalized at Psychiatric Institution	Total
	Part-time Job	Household Helping	Self-Care Only	Vocational Training	Unable to Work		
Excellent	3	8	1	4	0	0	16 (50%)
Good	2	4	0	1	1	2	10 (31%)
Fair	0	1	0	0	3	0	4 (13%)
Poor	0	0	1	0	0	1	2 (6%)
Total	5	13	2	5	4	3	
		20 (63%)		9 (28%)		3 (9%)	32 (100%)

Sixteen patients (50%) showed excellent results: in these patients, no violent or aggressive behavior occurred postoperatively, and the patients became cooperative enough to establish familial and social adaptation. Ten patients (31%) had good results; in these patients, no violent or aggressive behavior was noted, but the patients remained easily excited. In total, the results in 26 patients (81%) were considered to be satisfactory. In four other patients, fair results were obtained; these patients exhibited aggressive behavior occasionally. Two patients had poor results with no apparent clinical improvement.

The living condition of these patients varies, depending mainly upon both postoperative behavioral problems and the degree of preexistent mental retardation or epileptic seizures. Twenty patients (63%) live with their families. Five patients were especially gratifying, as they were able to be employed, even though their part-time jobs failed to generate enough income for them to live independently. Nine patients (28%) stay at centers for the physically handicapped; however, five work at the occupational training section in the centers. Three patients (9%) remain admitted to psychiatric institutions because of their poor social adaptation and severe mental retardation.

The results of this follow-up study are quite similar to the results of previous studies performed in 1969 and 1977. In 1977, 50% had excellent results and 34% had good results. The calming effects of the operation, once established, appear to be stable and consistent for as long as ten years. Long after surgery, special education and care are required to restore the familial and social adaptation of these patients. Other authors have reported on small series of patients treated in this way [4, 6, 23, 33, 34, 36]. The results are similar to our study, with satisfactory clinical improvement in more than 80% of the patients.

As a consequence of the operation, memory disturbances and decreased spontaneity were reported in a few patients. Intelligence quotient (IQ) scores usually improved postoperatively because the patients were able to concentrate better on the tasks. In some cases, the epileptic seizures were controlled more easily by anticonvulsants after the operation. We also noted a general tendency toward spontaneous remission of seizures, probably in line with the natural course of epilepsy.

ENDOCRINOLOGICAL RESULTS

Because the target for surgical intervention in this procedure is close to the neuroendocrinological center of the hypothalamic-pituitary system, we carefully studied the effects of various pituitary hormones on the plasma levels. Although stimulation of the posterior hypothalamus may cause a temporary elevation of pituitary hormone levels, especially prolactin and luteinizing hormone, no significant changes were noted postoperatively [12, 13]. Several patients developed relatively low levels of urine 11-hydroxy-corticosteroid (11-OHCS) and 17-ketosteroids (17-KS), but substitutional treatment was not required. Postoperative physical development curves could be made from the data of ten patients, all of whom had surgery

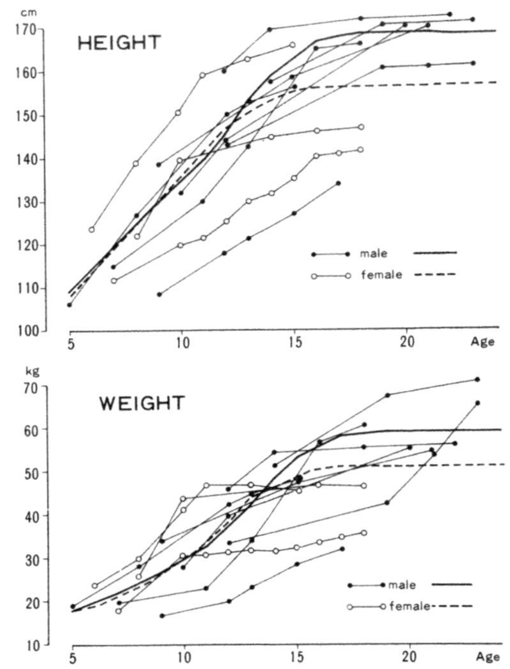

FIGURE 29–3. Physical development curves of pediatric patients after posteromedial hypothalamotomy. Each curve begins at the time of surgery. The solid and broken lines represent the standard Japanese development curve.

during childhood. Although a few patients tended to gain weight after the operation, no serious developmental problems were found (figure 29–3). The appearance of secondary sexual characteristics was normal. Menarche occurred between ages ten and 13 in female patients. In seven patients, follow-up dynamic stimulation tests of pituitary hormone release were performed to measure growth hormone, ACTH, luteinizing hormone, follicle-stimulating hormone, thyroid-stimulating hormone, and prolactin levels. The results were within the normal range, indicating that the hormonal regulatory system was not impaired even after bilateral posteromedial hypothalamotomies. The plasma level of NEFA in these patients was relatively high in comparison with the normal subjects. The stimulation of the posterior hypothalamus caused a temporary elevation of NEFA levels in the plasma. Postoperatively, the fasting level of NEFA returned to normal. These findings most likely are related to changes in sympathetic responses in these patients. The preoperative adrenaline test or Mecholyl test showed a state of sympathicotonia, which usually was normalized after the operation.

DISCUSSION

According to Hess, the diencephalon can be divided into two functional sectors, namely, the ergotropic sector and the trophotropic sector [10]. Connected to these two sectors are two functional circuits, ergotropic and trophotropic, which pass through the prosencephalon. Although these two circuits may take the same anatomical pathways in the central nervous system, particularly in the limbic system or neocortical system, they seem to separate in parts of the diencephalon and the brain stem. Based upon our hypothesis that behavioral disturbances result from imbalance between these two functional systems (i.e., exaggeration of the ergotropic system), surgical intervention was directed at the most sympathetic zone, located in the posterior hypothalamus. The various autonomic responses obtained by electrically stimulating different areas of the posterior hypothalamus suggested that separation of these two functional circuits is most apparent there. Ban studied the functional organization of the autonomic system in the diencephalon in rabbits; he proposed that the three-layer medial-to-lateral organization of the hypothalamus extends from the posterior to the anterior regions [5]. Ban described the dorsal longitudinal fasciculus as the structure most responsible for the sympathetic zone of the hypothalamus.

Tokizane and colleagues reported that the cat's hypothalamic region strongly activates the limbic system structures, that is, the archicortex is activated by the posterior hypothalamus, and the paleocortex by the anterior hypothalamus [38]. The posterior hypothalamus also exerts an influence on the neocortical system via the reticular formation. Consequently, posteromedial hypothalamotomy results in decreased activation of the posterior hypothalamus, the archicortex of the limbic system, and the neocortex. This profoundly influences emotional and behavioral mechanisms.

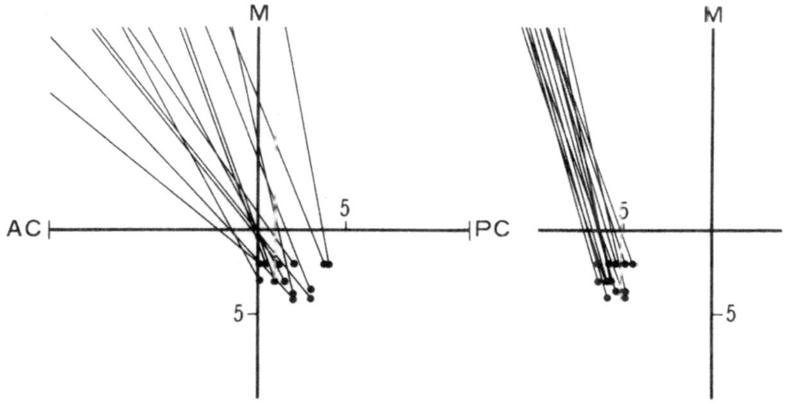

FIGURE 29–4. Lateral (*left*) and anteroposterior (*right*) view of electrode tracts and target points of 13 posteromedial hypothalamotomies for intractable pain (coagulation method). AC = anterior commissure; PC = posterior commissure; M = midcommissural point (*left*) and midline (*right*) (compare [13]).

TABLE 29–2. Results of Posteromedial Hypothalamotomy for Intractable Pain

	Total	Excellent	Good	Poor	Lost to Follow-up
Malignant pain[a]	18	11	5	0	2
Benign pain[b]	10	2	3	3	2

[a] Survival period: 1–12 months (average = 4 months).
[b] Follow-up period: 6 months to 6 years (average = 4 years, 2 months).

Intractable Pain

LESION TECHNIQUE

Posteromedial hypothalamotomy for pain control was performed first in 1971 and relied upon Fairman's initial experience [9]. Until 1977, 28 patients with pain of different origins underwent surgery by this technique. Satisfactory pain relief was obtained after a unilateral operation in 20 patients; in eight patients, surgery on the other side was required two or three weeks later. Figure 29–4 shows the trajectories for electrode insertion and corresponding target points in 13 operations. In the last 11 cases, the electrode was inserted at a larger angle from the AC–PC line in order to place the tip more posteriorly than in the earlier cases. This change was designed to avoid potential damage to the mammillothalamic fibers. Despite posterior shifting of the target point, the same pain control was achieved. Table 29–2 summarizes the results of posterior hypothalamic coagulation in patients with intractable pain. In 18 patients with cancer pain, surgery controlled pain during the comparatively short period of postoperative survival. Most of the patients were discharged so that they might spend the last several months of their lives at home. Some patients who survived for extensive periods after surgery had recurrent pain shortly before death. We treated ten other patients with "benign" pain including some with anesthesia dolorosa due to brachial plexus injuries, causalgia, postherpetic neuralgia, and thalamic pain. The pain relief in these ten cases was not as satisfactory as it was for cancer pain.

Immediate postoperative improvement frequently was limited; pain recurred in about half of the patients. Two patients, however, did have remarkable pain relief lasting several years after surgery.

STIMULATION TECHNIQUE

Prior to coagulation, patients often were aware of reduced spontaneous pain during trial stimulation designed to confirm the threshold for autonomic responses [14]. Subsequently, we studied the stimulation thresholds necessary to produce autonomic responses and to obtain pain relief (figure 29–5). This study indicated that less stimulation was required to reduce pain than to cause sympathetic responses. We were confronted with a paradoxical phenomenon: in the same posterior hypothalamic area, pain relief could be obtained by both stimulation and coagulation. Although the mechanism of this phenomenon remains unclear, our observations suggested that the clinical application of SPA in the posterior hypothalamic region would enable us to obtain pain relief without producing an electrocoagulation lesion. A commercially available deep-brain stimulation (DBS) apparatus (Medtronic, Inc., Minneapolis, MN) was utilized for the following cases.

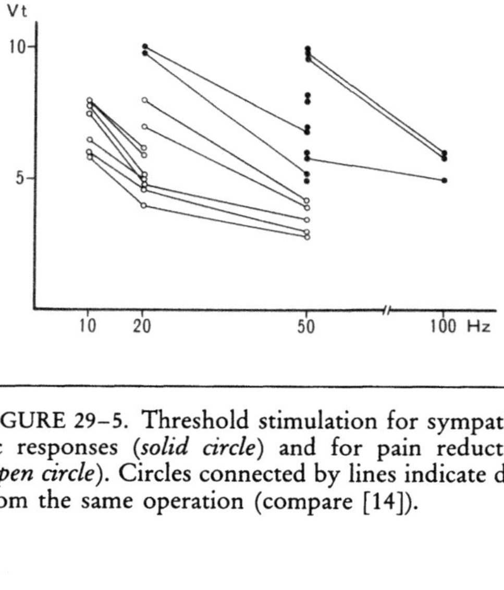

FIGURE 29–5. Threshold stimulation for sympathetic responses (*solid circle*) and for pain reduction (*open circle*). Circles connected by lines indicate data from the same operation (compare [14]).

Patients undergoing this surgical procedure were given local anesthesia. After obtaining satisfactory pain relief and sympathetic responses by electrostimulation with a concentric bipolar electrode, a four-pole platinum-wire electrode was implanted. Accurate placement of the wire-electrode tip was confirmed, the wire was fixed to the skull and the wound was sutured, leaving the end of the wires on the epicranium. Repetition of the test stimulation during the first postoperative week enabled us to select the most effective pair of electrodes. General anesthesia was given for the second operation, which allowed us to lead the wires under the skin to the right anterior chest region. The total system was internalized subcutaneously after the wires were connected to a receiving apparatus. To initiate stimulation, a coil from the external-stimulation apparatus was placed over the receiver to send signals from outside. Because analgesia produced by 10–60 minutes of stimulation usually lasted for several hours, intermittent stimulation several times a day provided satisfactory pain relief.

Posterior hypothalamic SPA was used for nine patients (Table 29–3). It was most effective in a 57-year-old woman who developed lumbosacral arachnoiditis after lumbar disc surgery. Hypothalamic SPA was performed to reduce pain that recurred two years after an open thoracic cordotomy. Effective control of severe left lower extremity pain was maintained during the next four years. Five patients had cancer pain; satisfactory pain relief was

TABLE 29–3. Results of Deep Brain Posterior Hypothalamic Stimulation for Chronic Pain[a]

Condition	Total Cases	Results		
		Excellent	Good	Poor
Malignant pain[b]	5	3	2	
Arachnoiditis[c]	1	1		
Myelopathy	1			1
Thalamic pain	2			2

[a] N = 9.
[b] Survival period, 3–7 months (average, 5 months).
[c] Four-year follow-up period.

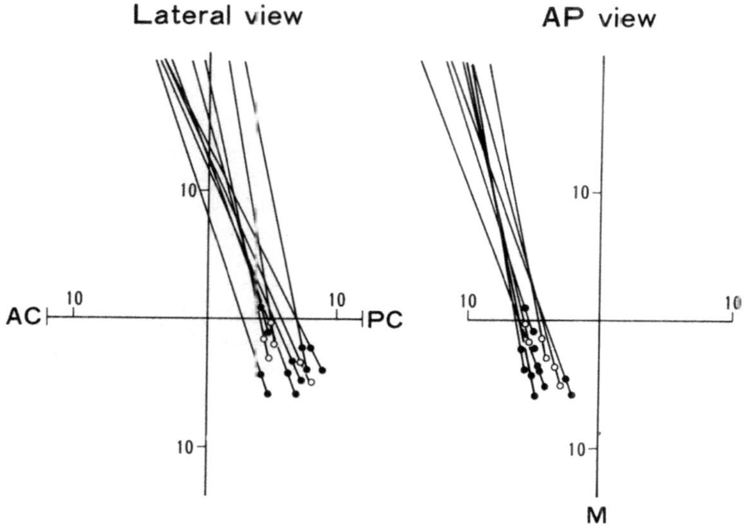

FIGURE 29–6. Tracts and placements of indwelling pair electrodes for intractable pain (stimulation method). Solid circles are effective cases; open circles, noneffective cases. AC = anterior commissure; M = midline; PC = posterior commissure.

obtained during the average five-month survival period. Both patients with thalamic pain failed to have pain relief; in fact, the pain was increased by electrical stimulation. In one case of spinal pain, relief was insufficient. Figure 29–6 shows the trajectories and positions of the bipolar stimulating electrodes. The final placement of the electrodes did not differ significantly between patients with effective and patients with ineffective relief. Based on these results, we concluded that the posterior hypothalamic stimulation is effective for pain originating from the peripheral nervous system, but it is not effective for pain resulting from destruction of the afferent nerve pathways (deafferentation pain).

BETA-ENDORPHIN MEASUREMENT

Pain research in the 1970s was enhanced by the discovery of endogenous brain opiates. Pain relief by acute or chronic electrical stimulation of the periaqueductal gray matter has been described [20, 21]. Various investigators reported that these opiate substances are released into the spinal or ventricular fluid during brain stimulation [2, 11]. We also studied the changes in the beta-endorphin level of the third ventricular fluid in patients undergoing hypothalamotomy [37]. In six patients, beta-endorphins in third ventricular fluid had risen from undetectable levels to 300–1,300 pg/ml; analgesic effects and increases in blood pressure were noted (figure 29–7). When gradual weak DBS was not associated with blood pressure increase, beta-endorphin elevation was found in only half of the trials. Further details of the study are described in a previous report.

Richardson described the successful reduction of pain after stimulation of the beta-endophin pathway in humans; this area includes the anterior hypothalamus, the arcuate area around the third ventricle, and the mesencephalic raphe nuclei [20]. He found the posterior hypothalamus to be the most favorable region to stimulate, producing few negative side effects such as autonomic responses. Our experience is quite similar to Richardson's. Further studies are required to clarify the relationship between analgesic effects and opiate substances such as beta-endorphins. In clinical studies, the concentration of these substances in CSF should be used as an indirect

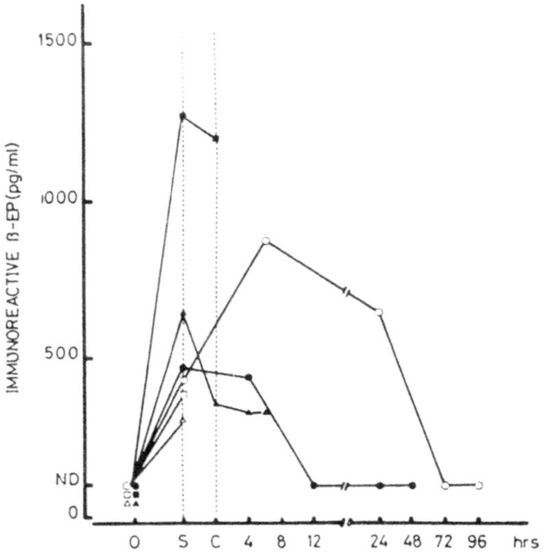

FIGURE 29–7. Effects of stimulation (S) and coagulation (C) in the posterior hypothalamus on immunoreactive beta-endorphin values in third ventricular fluid. ND = nondetectable level. (Compare [37].)

indicator; it still is not clear how accurately the movement of these substances in the brain tissue is reflected in the surrounding fluid.

In the posterior hypothalamic pain-control system, analgesia is the result of either electrical stimulation or coagulation lesion production. SPA has been found to be effective whether in the thalamus, mesencephalon, central gray matter, posterior hypothalamus, or internal capsule. All these structures are adjacent to the ascending pain pathway, which suggests that SPA may be dependent upon the negative feedback system inherent in the pain-transmitting system.

EXPERIMENTAL STUDIES

The posterior hypothalamus plays an important role in the pain-control mechanism of the central nervous system. Dafny reported that many neurons in the posterior hypothalamus of the cat respond to various modalities of sensory stimulation [8]. Currently, the spinothalamic tract and the spino-reticulo-thalamic pathway are recognized as the two major pain-transmitting systems; only the branches of these pathways are believed to reach to the posterior hypothalamus. Yamada and Otani proposed a third important ascending pain system [41]. This tract originates at different levels of the spinal cord, separates from the paleospinothalamic tract, and enters the central gray substance at the level of the hypoglossal nucleus, the nucleus coeruleus, the quadrigeminal plate and the nucleus of Darkshevitch. They named this system the spinoperiventricular fiber system or the spinohypothalamic fiber system, because the rostral end of this system reaches the periventricular gray substance of the posterior hypothalamus. If this spinohypothalamic fiber system proves to be an important pain-transmitting system, the posterior hypothalamus will be acknowledged as the most important segment of the ascending pain pathway.

Since Reynolds' report was published [19], experimental studies have described the analgesic system of the central gray matter. A descending inhibitory pain system has been defined, but the role of the posterior hypothalamus has been less well detailed [3, 16]. Carstens reported that medial hypothalamic stimulation inhibited posterior horn neuron responses to noxious skin heating in the cat [7]. Using this same experimental cat model, Watanabe and co-workers compared the effects of conditioned stimulation of the posterior hypothalamus and the periaqueductal gray matter (PAG) [39]. In 12 cats, 36 neurons of the posterior horn of the lumbar spinal cord were identified and found to respond to thermal and mechanical stimulation of the leg; 29 (80%) of these neurons were suppressed equally by conditioned stimulation of the posterior hypothalamus or the (PAG). The remaining neurons were affected more strongly by PAG stimulation than by posterior hypothalamic stimulation. Twenty-four neurons responded to tactile stimulation or joint movements; none of these neurons were inhibited by stimulation of either the PAG or the posterior hypothalamus. Thalamic stimulation did not produce inhibitory activity.

Recently, Satoh and his associates infused an analgesic drug (cyclazocine) into the dorsal hypothalamus in rats to study its descending inhibitory effect on the posterior spinal horn neurons [32]. The inhibitory effect was reversed by naloxone.

The medial forebrain bundle and the dorsal longitudinal fasciculus may be the main descending pain control pathways from the diencephalon to the mesencephalon and to the spinal cord; opiate-activated systems and monoamine-activated systems are interwined [1, 17, 18]. A direct downward pathway from the hypothalamus to the spinal cord has been confirmed also.

Summary

Our experience with approximately 100 stereotactic operations involving the posterior hypothalamus suggests that this small region has many complex and important functions, related to autonomic, emotional, and pain sensation. The development of stereotactic brain surgery enabled us to approach this deepest structure of the brain. Besides the clinical benefits in the fields of behavioral disturbances and intractable pain, posteromedial hypothalamotomy has given us the rare opportunity to understand many neuronal mechanisms involving this particular region. The distribution of sympathetic and parasympathetic zones in the human hypothalamus is now clearer. The close relationship between the emotional and autonomic functions has been demonstrated. Clinical observations during pain surgery helped to define the role of the posterior hypothalamus in both the pain-transmitting and the pain-controlling systems. Questions about the integration of many functional systems in the posterior hypothalamus are still unanswered. We plan further investigations into neuronal organization of the posterior hypothalamus and the role of various neurotransmitters in the hypothalamus.

References

1. Akil H, Liebeskind JC: Monoaminergic mechanisms of stimulation-produced analgesia. *Brain Res* 94:279–296, 1975
2. Akil H, Richardson DE, Hughes J, et al: Enkephalin-like material elevated in ventricular cerebrospinal fluid of pain patients after analgetic focal stimulation. *Science* 201:463–465, 1978
3. Balagura S, Raloh T: The analgesic effect of electrical stimulation of the diencephalon and mesencephalon. *Brain Res* 60:369–379, 1973
4. Balasubramaniam V, Kanaka TS: Amygdalotomy and hypothalamotomy—A comparative study. *Confin Neurol* 37:195–201, 1975
5. Ban T: The septo-preoptico-hypothalamic system and its autonomic function. In Tokizane T, Schade JP (eds): *Progressive Brain Research 21A*. Amsterdam: Elsevier, 1966, pp 1–43
6. Black P. Uematsu S, Walker AE: Stereotaxic hypothalamotomy for control of violent aggressive behavior. *Confin Neurol* 37:187–188, 1975
7. Carstens E: Inhibition of spinal horn neuronal responses to noxious skin heating by medial hypothalamic stimulation in the cat. *J Neurophysiol* 48:808–822, 1982
8. Dafny N, Bental E, Feldman S: Effect of sensory stimuli on single unit activity in the posterior hypothalamus. *Electroencephalogr Clin Neurophysiol* 19:256–263, 1965
9. Fairman D: Hypothalamotomy as a new perspective for alleviation of intractable pain and regression of metastatic malignant tumors. In Fusek I, Kunc Z (eds): *Present Limits of Neurosurgery*. Prague: Avicenum Czechoslovakian Medical Press, 1972, pp 525–528
10. Hess WR: *Das Zwischenhirn. Syndrome, Lokalisationen, Funktionen*. Basel: Schwabe, 1949
11. Hosobuchi Y, Rossier H, Bloom FE, et al: Stimulation of human periaqueductal gray for pain relief increases immunoreactive β-endorphin in ventricular fluid. *Science* 203:279–281, 1978
12. Mayanagi Y, Hori T, Sano K: The posteromedial hypothalamus and pain-behavior, with special reference to endocrinclogical findings. *Appl Neurophysiol* 41:223–231, 1978
13. Mayanagi Y, Sano K: Long-term follow-up results of the posteromedial hypothalamotomy. In Hitchcock ER, Ballantine HT Jr, Meyerson BA (eds): *Modern Concepts in Psychiatric Surgery*. Amsterdam: Elsevier–North Holland Biomedical Press, 1979, pp 197–204
14. Mayanagi Y, Sano K, Suzuki I, et al: Stimulation and coagulation of the posteromedial hypothalamus for intractable pain, with reference to beta-endorphins. *Appl Neurophysiol* 45:136–142, 1982
15. Mayanagi Y, Teramoto A, Hanamura T, et al: A study on stimulation producing analgesia in the hypothalamus and thalamus. In Tsubokawa T (ed): *Brain Stimulation and Neural Plasticity*. Tokyo: Neuron Press, 1985, pp 97–100
16. Mayer DJ, Liebeskind JC: Pain reduction by focal electrical stimulation of the brain: An anatomical and behavioral analysis. *Brain Res* 68:73–93, 1974
17. Oliveras JL, Guibaud G, Besson JM: A map of serotoninergic structures involved in stimulation producing analgesia in unrestrained freely moving cats. *Brain Res* 164:317–322, 1979
18. Oliveras JL, Hosobuchi Y, Guibaud G, et al: Analgesic electrical stimulation of the feline nucleus rephe magnus: Development of tolerance and its reversal by 5-HTP. *Brain Res* 146:404–409, 1978
19. Reynolds DV: Surgery in the rat during electri-

cal analgesia induced by focal brain stimulation. *Science* 164:444–445, 1969
20. Richardson DE: Analgesia produced by stimulation of various sites in the human beta-endorphin system. *Appl Neurophysiol* 45:116–122, 1982
21. Richardson DE, Akil H: Pain reduction by electrical brain stimulation in man. Part 1. Acute administration in periaqueductal and periventricular sites. *J Neurosurg* 47:178–183, 1977
22. Richardson DE, Akil H: Pain reduction by electrical brain stimulation in man. Part 2. Chronic self-administration in the periventricular gray matter. *J Neurosurg* 47:184–194, 1977
23. Rubio E, Arjona V, Rodriguez-Burgos F: Stereotactic cryohypothalamotomy in agressive behavior. In Sweet WH, et al (eds): *Neurosurgical Treatment in Psychiatry, Pain and Epilepsy*. Baltimore: University Park Press, 1977, pp 439–444
24. Sano K: Aggressiveness. In Schaltenbrand G, Walker AE (eds): *Stereotaxy of the Human Brain*. New York: Thieme-Stratton, 1982, pp 617–621
25. Sano K: Posterior hypothalamic lesions in the treatment of violent behavior. In Fields WS, Sweet WH (eds): *Neural Bases of Violence and Aggression*. St. Louis: WH Green, 1975, pp 401–420
26. Sano K: Sedative neurosurgery with special reference to posteromedial hypothalamotomy. *Neurol Med Chir* (Tokyo) 4:112–142, 1962
27. Sano K: Sedative stereoencephalotomy: fornicotomy, upper mesencephalic reticulotomy and postero-medial hypothalamotomy. In Tokizane T, Schade JP (eds): *Progressive Brain Research 21B*. Amsterdam: Elsevier, 1966, pp 350–372
28. Sano K: Surgery of the hypothalamus—in commemoration of Otfrid Foerster. In Sano K, Ishii S (eds): *Recent Progress in Neurological Surgery*. Amsterdam: Excerpta Medica, 1974, pp 210–218
29. Sano K, Mayanagi Y, Sekino H, et al: Results of stimulation and destruction of the posterior hypothalamus in man. *J Neurosurg* 33:689–707, 1970
30. Sano K, Sekino H, Hashimoto T, et al: Posteromedial hypothalamotomy in the treatment of intractable pain. *Confin Neurol* 37:285–290, 1975
31. Sano K, Sekino H, Mayanagi Y: Results of stimulation and destruction of the posterior hypothalamus in cases with violent, aggressive or restless behavior. In Hitchcock E, et al (eds): *Psychosurgery*. Springfield, IL: Thomas, 1972, pp 57–75
32. Satoh M, Kawajiri S, Takagi H: Activation of dorsal hypothalamus-spinal dorsal horn descending inhibitory system by cyclazocine, an analgesic drug. In Fields HL, et al (eds): *Advances in Pain Research and Therapy*, Vol 9. New York: Raven Press, 1985, pp 487–492
33. Schvarcz JR: Results of stimulation and destruction of the posterior hypothalamus: A long-term evaluation. In Sweet WH, et al (eds): *Neurosurgical Treatment in Psychiatry, Pain and Epilepsy*. Baltimore: University Park Press, 1977, pp 429–438
34. Schvarcz JR, Driollet R, Rios E, et al: Stereotactic hypothalamotomy for behavior disorders. *J Neurol Neurosurg Psychiatry* 35:356–359, 1972
35. Spiegel EA, Wycis HT, Freed H, et al: Thalamotomy and hypothalamotomy for treatment of psychoses: Psychiatric treatment. *Res Publ Assoc Res Nerv Ment Dis* 31: 379–391, 1953
36. Sranja M, Nadvornik P: Surgical complication of posterior hypothalamotomy. *Confin Neurol* 37:193–194, 1975
37. Tari A, Miyachi Y, Tanaka K, et al: Elevated immunoreactive β-endorphin level in ventricular fluid after analgesic electrical stimulation of posteromedial hypothalamus. *Endocrinol Jpn* 30:747–752, 1983
38. Tokizane T, Kawamura H, Imamura G: Hypothalamic activation upon electrical activities of paleo- and archicortex. *Neurol Med Chir* (Tokyo) 2:63–76, 1960
39. Watanabe E, Mayanagi Y, Sano K: Influence of periaqueductal gray matter and posterior hypothalamic area on neuronal activity of the spinal dorsal horn. *Brain Nerve* (Jpn) 33:1031–1036, 1981
40. Yoshioka M, Yoshimasu N, Yamada R, et al: Stereotactic posteromedial hypothalamotomy for relief of intractable pain. *Neurol Med Chir* (Tokyo) 12:372–373, 1972
41. Yamada J, Otani K: The spinoperventricular fiber system in the rabbit, rat and cat. *Exp Neurol* 61:395–406, 1978

30. TRANSPLANTATION TO THE BRAIN

Erik-Olof Backlund

This chapter is a brief presentation of the encounter between a fast-growing research field, transplantation to the mammalian central nervous system (CNS), and stereotactic brain surgery. The author deliberately has confined this discussion to recent efforts designed to develop a new type of surgical therapy for patients with Parkinson's disease.

It is generally agreed that parkinsonian patients with tremor as the predominant symptom are those most suitable for stereotactic thalamotomy. When rigidity or hypokinesia dominate the clinical picture, thalamotomy is less rewarding and thus less commonly indicated. To date, patients in these latter categories have relied on medication only. In recent years, L-dopa and dopamine agonists have become the preferred medications. However, results from a wide range of animal experimentation now have opened new perspectives.

For many years, rats with 6-hydroxydopamine (6-OHDA)–induced selective nigrostriatal degeneration have been used as a model for experimental studies of movement disorders [24]. The pathological motor behavior of such animals is stereotyped, can be measured quantitatively [25], and shows typical changes after pharmacological provocation. Interestingly, transplantation of monoamine-producing grafts to the striatum of these animals counteracts their pathological movement patterns [19]. This animal model has been explored extensively, and various types of grafted tissue have been studied, including homologous fetal substantia nigra, autologous adrenal medulla, and, recently, suspensions of heterologous fetal substantia nigra cells, derived from aborted human fetuses.

Despite these experiments, the mechanisms behind the observed effects on the motor system remain obscure. It is clear that such grafts do not influence the neuronal interplay in the recipient area by developing authentic neuronal connections or by synapse formation. Histochemical preparations show a wide halo of catecholamines around the transplanted tissue and this halo greatly exceeds the size of the graft, itself. This "internalized" monoamine supply seems to be sufficiently great to explain some of the rewarding effects observed.

The spectacular discovery of the specific noxious effect of (N-methyl–4-phenyl–1,2,3,6-tetrahydropyridine) MPTP upon the nigrostriatal system in humans and other primates [10] led to experiments in monkeys similar to those described with rats. After the administration of MPTP, monkeys exhibited symptoms typical of parkinsonism [4]. These animals were "cured" after substantia nigra tissue from fetuses of the same species was transplanted to the striatum of the recipient [21].

Rationale for Clinical Trials

Prior to primate experiments, Olson, in 1970, showed that adrenal medullary chromaffin cells in rodents were transformed into neuron-like cells after transplantation to brain tissue [16]; subsequently, Olson described a tendency of such cells to innervate the recipient area [18]. Moreover, the pathological motor behavior of animals with 6-OHDA–induced lesions was counteracted by the transplantation of either catecholamine-producing neural tissue or cells from the adrenal medulla [17, 23]. Even adult (nonfetal) tissue could be used for successful grafting [16]. These findings stimulated our ultimate initiation of a clinical project. For a neurosurgeon familiar with thalamotomy as

L.D. Lunsford (ed.) *MODERN STEREOTACTIC NEUROSURGERY*.

a tremor-alleviating operation, it was logical to consider these results when designing a stereotactic operation for patients with rigidity and hypokinesia. In 1979, the author initiated and originally reported the first clinical study of transplantation to the brain based on these principles [2]. We chose to use the patient's own catecholamine-producing tissue (adrenal medulla or sympathetic ganglion). After unilateral transplantation of autologous adrenal medulla to the caudate nucleus, in two initial cases, subtle but short-lasting improvement was shown, providing an impetus for continuation of the project [3].

Because it is beyond the scope of this chapter to discuss extensively the theoretical grounds of brain transplantation, the reader is referred to excellent reviews in the rapidly growing literature [6, 14, 20]. This chapter is intended to provide technical aspects of the surgical procedure.

Target Selection

In the animals with 6-OHDA–induced lesions, the transplanted cells were introduced most often into the central area of striatum. In rodents, this nuclear complex is dominated by the head of the caudate nucleus. Thus, this structure also was chosen arbitrarily as the target site for the first human operations. Subsequent postmortem studies of brains from other Parkinson's disease patients indicate that the putamen is more depleted of dopamine than is the caudate nucleus [15]. Further, when positron emission tomography studies were performed with dopamine-receptor ligands in normal patients, the putamen was found to have the highest density of dopamine receptors (as compared with the rest of the striatum); the opposite seems to be the rule in parkinsonian patients [5].

Systemically administered L-dopa probably reaches all regions of the CNS. In normal patients, it is likely that areas rich in dopaminergic terminals, such as the putamen, synthesize dopamine from L-dopa given orally. Thus, we reasoned that the putamen would be a more suitable recipient region for dopamine-producing grafts than the caudate nucleus.

We used the van Buren and Borke stereotactic atlas [26] to select target coordinates. The caudate target was 10 mm from the midline, 10 mm anterior to the anterior commissure, and 10 mm above the horizontal intercommissural plane. Two targets were chosen for putaminal implantation: one located 20 mm from the midline, 5 mm anterior to the anterior commissure and 5 mm above the intercommissural plane; the other in the same horizontal plane but at the level of the anterior commissure (in the anteroposterior direction) and 25 mm from the midline.

Graft Preparation

Because cells of the human adrenal medulla are very difficult to dissociate, we prepared grafts that were composed of a number of 1-mm medullary fragments and that were carefully dissected from the adrenal cortex. Under normal conditions, the adrenal cortex stimulates monoamine synthesis in the medulla to produce adrenaline. In contrast, in cortex-free medullary fragments, adrenaline production is inhibited in favor of a greater production of noradrenaline and possibly dopamine. A specially designed cannula was developed to introduce the graft fragments into the brain. The cannula tip accommodates a 2 × 15-mm steel spiral, used to hold the graft (figure 30–1). Although we use this spiral additionally as a radiographic marker, a transplant also can be introduced easily without this holder/marker.

Operative Procedure

The operation begins at the computed tomography (CT) laboratory with the application of the stereotactic frame under local anesthesia. CT stereotactic localization [11] is performed with the thin-slice technique and reformatted imaging [8] and the anterior and posterior commissures are identified. The anterior limb of the internal capsule, usually quite distinct on CT images, serves as a further reference structure for the identification of striatal anatomy (figure 30–2). After the coordinates are calculated, general anesthesia is induced and (part of) one of the patient's adrenal glands is removed. The graft, prepared as previously described, then is introduced into the predetermined target(s) in the brain via a burr hole placed in the bregma region.

Future Aspects

Experience from the first clinical trials has provided guidelines for further improvements in

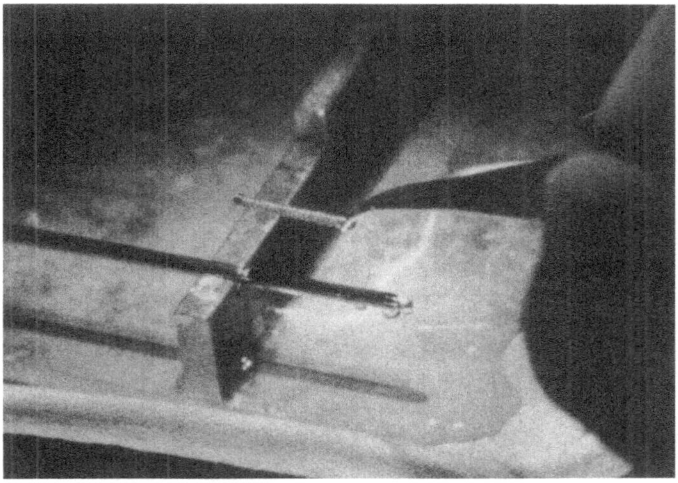

FIGURE 30–1. The small steel spiral holders harboring the adrenal medullary tissue fragments is placed in the transplantation cannula. The whole preparation procedure is performed under completely sterile conditions, under an operation microscope; the suprarenal gland specimens are irrigated/cooled continuously with Ringer's solution mixed with serum from the patient.

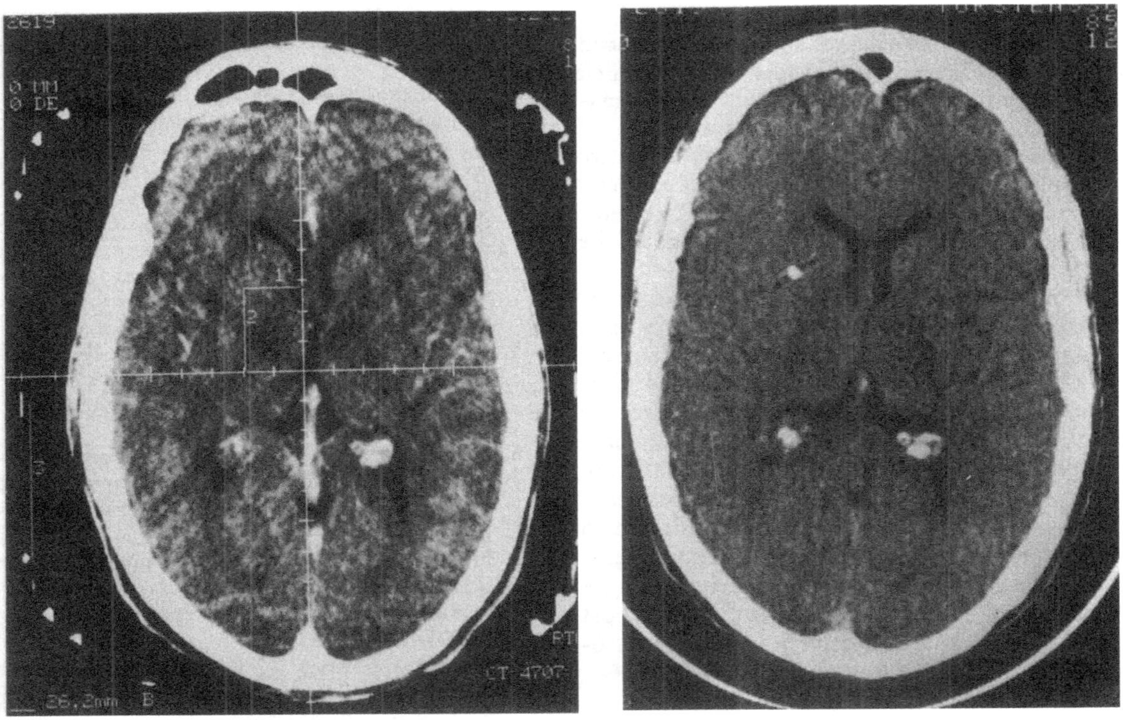

A B

FIGURE 30–2. Coordinates for a target in the putamen are determined by stereotactic CT (Leksell technique). The origin of the scanner's grid and the center of the stereotactic frame coincide, making the measurements very simple (A). Causing small artifacts on the image, the spiral marker is seen in the predetermined position on a postoperative CT image (B).

the operative technique. It is possible to monitor the local neurohumoral effects of the graft in the recipient area. This can be done using a microdialysis probe [28], as elegantly demonstrated in recent animal experiments [27]. In our initial patients who had transplantations, the rewarding effects were fairly short-lived, perhaps related to limited survival of the transplanted cells or to glial scar formation. Recent experimental evidence suggests that nerve growth factor or gangliosides should be administered after transplantation [1, 23]. Such factors could be delivered either by a microdialysis probe or by an implanted pump for long-term therapy [7].

Stereotactic technique allows the neurosurgeon the option of performing the entire transplantation procedure under local anesthesia if the adrenalectomy technique is redesigned, or if other graft sources are used. If one s willing to sacrifice the elegance of the autologous donor approach, well-defined catecholamine-producing cell lines would be potential sources [9]. The brain is considered an immunologically "privileged site," with reduced host-graft reactions; it remains to be clarified whether immunosuppression will be mandatory if nonautologous transplants are used. If the patient were awake during the entire transplantation procedure, sophisticated perioperative electrophysiological and biochemical exploration of the target region could be performed.

Monoamine-producing brain tissue (substantia nigra) from aborted human fetuses is a tempting alternative source of transplantable tissue. However, the serious ethical implications must be analyzed thoroughly before this method is chosen [12, 13]. Nonetheless, some hospitals already have obtained approval from their ethics committees. An unbiased decision in this crucial question is especially difficult to make; intriguing ongoing animal experiments have revealed that human fetal neuroblasts have remarkable vitality and plasticity in the host (rat) brain and effectively counteract 6-OHDA–induced motor dysfunction [22].

Conclusion

When the first transplantation to a patient's brain was performed, an essentially new therapeutic modality was founded. In addition to Parkinson's disease, other classic problems in the clinical neurosciences are now subjects for concentrated research related to transplantation to the CNS: spinal cord injury, Alzheimer's disease, and Huntington's chorea, among others. Joint efforts by basic neurobiologists and modern neurosurgeons doubtlessly will open new therapeutic prospects during the ensuing years.

References

1. Agnati LF, Fuxe K, Calza L, et al: Gangliosides increase the survival of lesioned nigral dopamine neurons and favour the recovery of dopaminergic synaptic functions in striatum of rats by collateral sprouting. *Acta Physiol Scand* 119:347–363, 1983
2. Backlund EO, Granberg PO, Hamberger B, et al: Transplantation of adrenal medullary tissue to striatum in parkinsonism: First clinical trials. *J Neurosurg* 62:169–173, 1985
3. Backlund EO, Olson L, Seiger Å, et al: Towards a transplantation therapy in Parkinson's disease: a progress report from continuing clinical experiments. In Azimita EC, Björklund A (eds): Cell and tissue transplantation into the adult brain. *Ann NY Acad Sci*, Vol 495, 1987, pp 658–673.
4. Burns RS, Chieuh CC, Markey SP, et al: A primate model of parkinsonism: Selective destruction of dopaminergic neurons in the pars compacta of the substantia nigra by N-methyl-4-phenyl-1,2,3,6-tetrahydropyridine. *Proc Natl Acad Sci USA* 80:4546–4550, 1983
5. Garnett ES, Nahmias C, Firnau G, et al: Central dopaminergic pathways in hemiparkinsonism examined by positron emission tomography. *Can J Neurol Sci* 11:174–179, 1984
6. Gash DM, Collier TJ, Sladek JR: Neural transplantation: A review of recent developments and potential applications to the aged brain. *Neurobiol Aging* 6:131–150, 1985
7. Harbaugh RE, Coombs DW, Saunders RL, et al: Implanted continuous epidural morphine infusion system: Preliminary report. *J Neurosurg* 56:803–806, 1982
8. Hardy TL, Koch J, Lassiter A: Computer graphics with computerized tomography for functional neurosurgery. *Appl Neurophysiol* 46:217–226, 1983
9. Hefti F, Hartikka J, Schlumpf M: Implantation of PC12 cells into the corpus striatum of rats with lesions of the dopaminergic nigrostriatal neurons. *Brain Res* 348:283–288, 1985

10. Langston JW, Ballard P, Tetrud JW, et al: Chronic parkinsonism in humans due to a product of meperidine-analog synthesis. *Science* 219:979–980, 1983
11. Leksell L, Jernberg B: Stereotaxis and tomography: A technical note. *Acta Neurochir* (Wien) 52:1–7, 1980
12. Murphy PJ: Moral perspectives in the use of embryonic cell transplantation for correction of nervous system disorders. *Appl Neurophysiol* 47:65–68, 1984
13. Neville RC: Ethics in medical donations. *Appl Neurophysiol* 47:73–76, 1984
14. Nottebohm F (ed): *Hope for a New Neurology*. New York: New York Academy of Science, 1985
15. Nyberg P, Nordberg A, Wester P, et al: Dopaminergic deficiency is more pronounced in putamen than in nucleus caudatus in Parkinson's disease. *Neurochem Pathol* 1:193–1202, 1983
16. Olson L: Fluorescence histochemical evidence for axonal growth and secretion from transplanted adrenal medullary tissue. *Histochemie* 22:1–7, 1970
17. Olson L, Backlund EO, Sedvall G, et al: Intrastriatal chromaffin grafts in experimental and clinical parkinsonism: First impressions. In Usdin E, Carlson A, Dahlstrom A, et al (eds): Catecholamines. Part B: Neuropharmacology and central nervous system—theoretical aspects. *Neurology and Neurobiology*, Vol 8B. New York: Alan R Liss, 1984, pp 195–201
18. Olson L, Seiger Å, Freedman R, et al: Chromaffin cells can innervate brain tissue: Evidence from intraocular double grafts. *Exp Neurol* 70:414–426, 1980
19. Perlow MJ, Freed WJ, Hoffer BJ, et al: Brain grafts reduce motor abnormalities produced by destruction of nigro-striatal dopamine system. *Science* 204:643–647, 1979
20. Sladek JR, Gash DM (eds): *Neural Transplants: Development and Function*. New York, London: Plenum Press, 1984
21. Sladek JR, Collier TJ, Haber SN, et al.: Reversal of parkinsonism by fetal nerve cell transplants in primate brain. In Azimita EC, Björklund A (eds): Cell and tissue transplantation into the adult brain. *Ann NY Acad Sci*, Vol 495, 1987, pp 641–657
22. Strömberg, I, Bygdeman M, Goldstein M, et al: Human fetal substantia nigra grafted to the dopamine-denervated striatum of immunosuppressed rats: Evidence for functional reinnervation. *Neurosci Lett*, (In press)
23. Stromberg I, Herrera-Marschitz M, Ungerstedt U, et al: Chronic implants of chromaffin tissue into the dopamine-denervated striatum: Effects of NGF on survival, fiber growth and rotational behaviour. *Exp Brain Res* 60:335–349, 1985
24. Ungerstedt U: 6-Hydroxydopamine-induced degeneration of the nigro-striatal dopamine pathway: The turning syndrome. *Pharmacol Ther* 2:37–40, 1976
25. Ungerstedt U, Arbuthnott G: Quantitative recording of rotational behaviour in rats after 6-hydroxydopamine lesions of the nigro-striatal dopamine system. *Brain Res* 24:485–493, 1970
26. Van Buren, Borke RC: *Variations and Connections of the Human Thalamus*, Vol 2: *Variations of the Human Diencephalon*. New York: Springer, 1972
27. Zetterström T, Brundin P, Gage FH, et al: In vivo measurement of spontaneous release and metabolism of dopamine from intrastriatal nigral grafts using intracerebral dialysis. *Brain Res* 362:344–349, 1986
28. Zetterström T, Sharp T, Marsden CA, et al: In vivo measurement of dopamine and its metabolites by intracerebral dialysis: Changes after D-amphetamine. *J Neurochem* 41:1769–1773, 1983

31. DEEP BRAIN STIMULATION FOR CHRONIC PAIN: LONG-TERM RESULTS AND COMPLICATIONS

Robert M. Levy
Sharon Lamb
John E. Adams

Electrical stimulation of brain structures in an attempt to produce analgesia in humans was first reported by Heath in 1954 [6] and by Pool and co-workers in 1956 [15]. Acute thalamic stimulation was reported to suppress the aversive properties of pain in patients with facial postherpetic neuralgia [26] and in patients with anesthesia dolorosa [9]. Based upon the hypothesis that chronic stimulation of denervated thalamic neurons would suppress deafferentation pain, further clinical trials of deep brain stimulation (DBS) for pain relief were undertaken. Hosobuchi, Adams, and co-workers [9] in the United States and Mazars and colleagues [12] in Europe published the first reports on the relief of deafferentation pain with chronic electrical stimulation of sensory thalamic nuclei. The technique of DBS for chronic pain was expanded after the observation that central gray matter stimulation in animals initiated the release of endogenous opioid peptides and resulted in analgesia [2, 13, 17]. Soon thereafter, Hosobuchi and associates and Richardson and Akil [19, 20] reported that chronic pain in humans was believed by long-term electrical stimulation of the periaqueductal gray matter.

Since these initial reports, several groups have confirmed the observation that electrical stimulation of sensory thalamic nuclei or endorphin-containing areas such as the periaqueductal gray matter (PAG) or periventricular gray matter (PVG) can relieve chronic pain. Only recently, however, has the efficacy of DBS for specific pain states or its long-term effectiveness been reported [3, 7, 12, 14, 16, 18, 19, 23–25, 27]. At the University of California, San Francisco, between 1972 and 1984, approximately 300 patients underwent placement of deep-brain–stimulating electrodes in an attempt to relieve chronic pain. We report here the initial and long-term results and complications of 304 operations performed on 141 of these patients, all of whom were operated on by Dr. Adams. This study represents both the largest reported series of such patients and the longest duration of follow-up.

Dr. Levy is supported in part by a research fellowship from the Research Foundation of the American Association of Neurological Surgeons.

Theoretical and Technical Concerns

On the basis of its character and response to pharmacological intervention, chronic pain can be categorized as either deafferentation or nociceptive in nature. Nociceptive pain arises from the interaction of painful stimulation with peripheral nociceptors, which then activates an intact central nociceptive system. Nociceptive pain is often described as sharp or aching in character. Common nociceptive states seen by the neurosurgeon are chronic low back pain, including some cases of the postsurgical "failed low back syndrome," and pain caused by the invasion of cancer. Nociceptive pain is often responsive to opiate analgesics.

Deafferentation pain, on the other hand, is

L.D. Lunsford (ed.) *MODERN STEREOTACTIC NEUROSURGERY*.

defined as pain that follows damage to the nervous system. The resultant degeneration of nerve cells and fibers presumably leads to loss of input to central pain pathways. Through a mechanism that is not well understood, this deafferentation can result in profound pain. The site of injury can occur at virtually any level of the peripheral or central nervous system. Causes include damage to peripheral nerves, resulting in painful peripheral neuropathies; damage to the spinal cord, causing paraplegic pain; and damage to the brain in cerebrovascular accidents, which can then produce a "thalamic pain syndrome." Deafferentation pain is often described as burning or aching in character; clinical signs of deafferentation pain include allodynia, hyperpathia, and hyperalgesia. These pain states are typically unresponsive to opiates and to pharmacological therapy, although some success has been had with tricyclic antidepressants.

Based on the concept that there are distinct mechanisms responsible for deafferentation and nociceptive pain, two separate areas of the brain have been used as sites for electrical brain stimulation. Stimulation of sensory thalamic nuclei has been used most often in treating deafferentation pain states because of the previously described effects of acute sensory thalamic stimulation on facial postherpetic neuralgia pain [26] and anesthesia dolorosa [1, 9]. As there is a clear representation of the body within the nucleus ventralis posterolateralis (VPL) and of the face within the nucleus ventralis posteromedialis (VPM), stimulation is administered within that area that represents the part of the body where the pain is felt. Appropriate electrode placement is confirmed by test stimulation in the operating room.

Although the mechanism of sensory thalamic stimulation–induced pain suppression is not fully clear, it appears that this stimulation is inhibitory and prevents the pathological spread of painful stimuli. Gerhart and co-workers [5] demonstrated that the inhibitory effect of thalamic stimulation upon lamina-I neurons was eliminated by bilateral lesions of the dorsolateral funiculi and the ventral part of the ipsilateral lateral funiculus. They concluded that thalamic stimulation may exert its analgesic effect either via a thalamocortical-corticofugal pathway or by antidromic stimulation of spinothalamic tract neurons. We believe that when sensory thalamic stimulation suppresses deafferentation pain, it may do so by activation of this nonopioid descending inhibitory system.

At about the time of the empirical observation that deafferentation pain was relieved by sensory thalamic stimulation, animal studies were performed that revealed that electrical stimulation of the mesencephalic central gray matter in rats could produce acute analgesia [13, 17]. Soon thereafter came the discovery of endogenous opioid peptides [10] and the observation that naloxone, a specific opiate antagonist, could at least partially block analgesia induced by PVG stimulation [2]. It was postulated that electrical stimulation of the PVG resulted in activation of an endogenous opioid system, which produced analgesia. Although it has since been attempted for all chronic pain states, stimulation of the PVG or the adjacent PAG would theoretically be most effective in those pain states that are responsive to exogenous opiates. Thus, for nociceptive pain states, stimulation of brain regions that contain and release endorphins is preferred.

As might be expected with any chronic pain problem, the clinical picture is seldom as clear as its theoretical construct. Thus, many patients present with pain syndromes that appear to possess features of both deafferentation and nociceptive pain. Attempts are then made to implant electrodes into both the PVG/PAG and sensory thalamic systems. Although in the past, chronic stimulation was limited to a single electrode, the advent of multichannel systems has made it possible to simultaneously provide activation of both systems.

Despite the described indications for the differential stimulation of sensory thalamic or PAG/PVG sites for deafferentation or nociceptive pain, respectively, we did not always adhere to these indications in this study. During the early years of the study, several other stimulation sites were tested; most commonly tested was the internal capsule when thalamic stimulation produced no acute response. These sites were ultimately abandoned due to the greater efficacy of sensory thalamic or PAG/PVG stimulation. For a short time after the discovery of the analgesic potential of PAG/PVG stimulation, PAG/PVG sites were stimulated for all pain syndromes. Again, PAG/PVG stimulation for deafferentation pain was later abandoned as it became clear that sensory thalamic stimulation was more effective.

TABLE 31–1. Preoperative Status of Patients with Deafferentation Pain States

Diagnosis	No. of Patients (N = 84)	Mean Age (years)	Mean Pain Duration (months)	Mean Prior Operations
Thalamic pain	25	54.4	39.8	0
Peripheral neuropathy	16	47.9	71.1	3.9
Anesthesia dolorosa	12	52.3	102.9	2.8
Paraplegia pain	11	50.1	95.9	2.3
Postcordotomy dysesthesia	5	55.8	100.6	0.4
Phantom limb pain	5	58.6	142.6	2.2
Thoracic neuralgia	4	50.3	49.8	2.5
Miscellaneous	6	48.2	87.7	2.8

TABLE 31–2. Preoperative Status of Patients with Nociceptive Pain States

Diagnosis	No. of Patients (N = 57)	Mean Age (years)	Mean Pain Duration (months)	Mean Prior Operations
Cancer pain	6	41.0	35.5	0.8
Low back and skeletal pain	51	50.9	153.6	4.4

Materials and Methods

PATIENT CHARACTERISTICS AND SELECTION

From 1972 until 1984, 141 patients with chronic pain underwent implantation of DBS electrodes. A total of 304 surgical procedures were performed on these patients. All patients had severe, chronic intractable pain, and all other available medical and surgical therapies had failed them. The patients had experienced their pain for an average of 65 months prior to DBS.

Eighty-four patients suffered from deafferentation pain syndromes. These included thalamic pain (25 patients), painful peripheral neuropathies (16), facial anesthesia dolorosa (12), paraplegic pain (11), postcordotomy dysesthesia (5), phantom limb pain (5), and thoracic neuralgias (4). Peripheral neuropathies were secondary to prior operation (6 patients), ischemia (3), trauma (3), degenerative neurological illness (2), and diabetes (1). Table 31–1 summarizes the preoperative status of these chronic pain patients by their specific diagnosis. The mean age of these patients was 52 years. The incidence by sex was roughly equal, although some pain states clearly were associated with a sexual predominance. Nine of 12 patients with facial anesthesia dolorosa, for example, were female, whereas all five of the patients with phantom limb pain were male. The interval between the onset of pain and the first DBS trial ranged from 40 months for those patients with thalamic pain syndrome (reflecting the fact that there is no other effective treatment for this difficult pain syndrome) to 143 months for the patients with phantom limb pain. A similar variation in the number of prior pain-directed surgical procedures was noted: no patient with thalamic pain had had prior surgery, but patients with peripheral neuropathies had undergone an average of 3.9 prior pain-directed procedures.

Fifty-seven patients underwent DBS for nociceptive pain states; their preoperative status is detailed in Table 31–2. Most of these patients (51) were treated for chronic low back and skeletal pain, including patients with the failed low back syndrome. Six patients were treated for pain secondary to invasive cancers.

The mean age of those with low back and skeletal pain was 51 years; the patients with pain from invasive cancer were, on the whole, much younger (mean 41 years). The duration of pain prior to DBS reflected the chronicity of the primary disease; cancer pain patients had suffered their pain for a mean of 36 months prior to surgery, whereas those with low back pain had had their pain for a mean of 154 months. Although prior surgical approach had been attempted on only one cancer patient, those with low back pain, in addition to exhausting medical therapies, had undergone an average of 4.4 prior surgical procedures directed at their pain. These procedures included repeat laminectomy, fusion, and scar resection as well as attempts at spinal dorsal column stimulation.

Screening tests were not consistent over the 12-year span. Many patients underwent both morphine intravenous infusions and provocative naloxone testing. This latter test has been well-described elsewhere [4, 8]. The results were not used to determine whether or not the procedure should be attempted, but rather they were used in combination with the patient's clinical presentation to delineate the appropriate target for stimulation. Those who responded well to low doses of morphine and had reversal of pain relief with naloxone were felt to be candidates for PVG/PAG stimulation. Patients whose pain was unresponsive to morphine and whose clinical syndrome was compatible with deafferentation pain underwent sensory thalamic stimulation.

Although formal neuropsychiatric evaluation was performed in selected patients, it was not used routinely. Patients with gross psychiatric illness or with intellectual handicaps that would prevent them from being able to comply with testing or self-stimulation procedures were excluded. Patients with more subtle psychiatric problems, including reactive depression, anxiety, and somatization, were not necessarily excluded from surgery; there is some evidence to suggest that these disorders do not negatively effect surgical outcome [22].

SURGICAL PROCEDURE

Local anesthesia was administered to patients undergoing electrode implantation. After application of the Leksell stereotactic frame, one or more parasagittal frontal burr holes were placed. A ventricular cannula was advanced into the lateral ventricle, and contrast/air ventriculography was performed.

The target coordinates were then calculated using coordinates from the Schaltenbrand and Bailey human stereotactic atlas [21]. For facial deafferentation pain, electrodes were directed at the VPM, with initial coordinates 8 mm posterior to, 8 mm lateral to, and 1–3 mm above the midpoint of the anterior commissure-posterior commissure (AC-PC) line. For extremity deafferentation pain, VPL electrodes were initially placed 9 mm posterior to, 10–12 mm lateral to and 2–5 mm above the mid-AC-PC line. A 1-mm diameter monopolar electrode was first used to stimulate the target point. The electrode position was adjusted until paresthesias were obtained within the region of pain. The temporary electrode was then removed and a four-pole platinum electrode introduced at these final coordinates. Test stimulation was then repeated to confirm electrode placement.

For PVG/PAG stimulation, four-pole platinum electrodes were implanted directly, with the most distal pole 1 mm caudal to and 1 mm below the posterior commissure and 2–3 mm lateral to the lateral wall of the third ventricle. Proper electrode location was indicated when stimulation with 5–6 mA produced a sensation of bodily warmth, oscillopsia, loss of upward gaze, or pain relief. Bilateral PAG/PVG electrodes were placed in several patients; both sensory thalamic and PVG/PAG electrodes were placed in the patients with mixed nociceptive/deafferentation pain. For testing, electrode leads were externalized through a separate stab wound.

All possible bipolar combinations of the four poles of the electrode were surveyed in the immediate postoperative period. Over the following several days, we performed stimulation trials of the most promising electrode pairs, varying the length, pulse interval, frequency, and intensity of stimulation. Stimulation of PAG/PVG was at a low frequency (10 Hz ± 5 Hz), whereas the frequency of sensory thalamic stimulation varied (20–100 Hz). The voltage threshold for PAG/PVG stimulation was usually 1–5 V; a higher threshold (3–8 V) was noted for VPM/VPL stimulation. Both standard continuous and ramped voltage stimulation were tested. Patients rated their pain on a subjective scale (0–10) before, during, and after stimulation. At the end of this trial period, ranging from one to several days, the elec-

TABLE 31–3. Initial and Long-Term Results of Deep Brain Stimulation for Deafferentation Pain States

Diagnosis	No. of Patients	No. of Patients with Initial Success (%)	No. of Patients with Long-Term Success (%)
Thalamic pain	25	14 (56)	6 (24)
Peripheral neuropathy	16	11 (69)	8 (50)
Anesthesia dolorosa	12	8 (67)	2 (17)
Paraplegia pain	11	4 (36)	0
Postcordotomy dysesthesia	5	3 (60)	2 (40)
Phantom limb pain	5	4 (80)	1 (20)
Thoracic neuralgia	4	3 (75)	1 (25)
Miscellaneous	6	4 (67)	4 (67)
Total	84	51 (61%)	24 (29%)

trodes were either removed, cut of at the scalp, or the most effective combination was internalized. Internalization was accomplished by attaching the electrode to a receiver implanted subcutaneously in the chest wall in the region of the pectoral muscles. The patients could then initiate their own stimulation using an inductive transmitter with an antenna overlying the subcutaneous receiver.

FOLLOW-UP AND DATA EVALUATION

Initial follow-up was performed by the primary surgeon within six weeks of operation. At this time, "initial success" was established if the patients were using their stimulators at regular intervals and reported that they were obtaining pain relief. Although the use of such an operational definition is not very restrictive, it may help to eliminate inaccuracies such as those introduced by surgeon's bias and patient's dishonesty with respect to their intake of analgesic medications. Thus, initial failure was designated as occurring in all patients who either did not have a response sufficient to warrant internalization of the electrode or did not report regular use and pain relief at their first follow-up.

Although most patients returned for medical follow-up with the primary surgeon, for the purposes of this study, the last follow-up, upon which our results are based, was obtained by a clinician (a neurosurgeon or neurosurgical nurse specialist) other than the operating surgeon. A 10-page questionnaire was completed either by consultation with the patient or, (rarely) if the patient was unavailable, from the patient's medical record. In all possible cases, direct or telephone contact was made for follow-up; if no such contact was made, the patient was grouped as "lost to follow-up." Follow-up ranged from two years to 14 years (mean 6.8 years). Long-term success was operationally defined as continued regular use of the stimulator with reported pain relief from stimulation.

Initial and Long-Term Results

The results of DBS for patients with deafferentation pain syndromes are detailed in Table 31–3.

THALAMIC PAIN SYNDROME

Patients with thalamic pain syndrome (25) usually underwent placement of sensory thalamic electrodes. Of the 14 implanted VPL electrodes, nine (64%) produced sufficient analgesia to be internalized. Of the 11 VPL electrodes that produced appropriate paresthesias in the operating room, nine (82%) were implanted. Internal capsule electrodes were implanted in six patients; two of these produced appropriate paresthesias, and one of these was internalized. Three patients had PAG/PVG electrodes implanted; although two of the three produced intraoperative oscillopsia with high-voltage stimulation, none produced sufficient analgesia to warrant internalization. The overall initial success rate was 56%. Six patients (24%) have continued to obtain pain relief on long-term follow-up.

In four patients, we were unable to induce paresthesias in the area of pain. This failure may have resulted from the degeneration of thalamic target cells secondary to the central nervous system lesion that itself was responsible for the patient's pain.

PERIPHERAL NEUROPATHY

Eight patients (of 16) with painful peripheral neuropathies underwent placement of sensory thalamic electrodes; six electrodes (75%) were internalized. Thirteen PAG/PVG electrodes were implanted, most in patients with postoperative sciatic neuropathies combined with low back pain; five patients (39%) underwent internalization of their electrodes. The overall initial success rate was 69%; at follow-up, eight patients (50%) had persistent pain relief with stimulation.

ANESTHESIA DOLOROSA

Of 12 patients with anesthesia dolorosa, nine patients underwent placement of sensory thalamic electrodes. Seven electrodes produced intraoperative paresthesias in the area of pain; six of these were internalized. Seven PAG/PVG electrodes were implanted, but only two (29%) were internalized. As in some patients with thalamic pain syndrome, three of these patients were thought to have loss of target cells as both a cause of their pain and an explanation for the inability to induce paresthesias. Although the initial success rate was high (67%), only two patients continued to use their stimulators at follow-up (18%).

PARAPLEGIA PAIN

Fourteen electrodes were implanted in 11 patients with pain secondary to spinal cord injury; these included seven sensory thalamic and seven PAG/PVG electrodes. Two each of these electrodes were internalized (36%). No patients obtained persistent pain relief with DBS.

POSTCORDOTOMY DYSESTHESIAS

Six sensory thalamic and two PAG/PVG electrodes were implanted in these five patients. Two VPL electrodes and one PAG/PVG electrode were internalized; three patients (60%) had overall initial success. One patient had spontaneous pain resolution that was not thought to be related to the DBS, and two patients continue to obtain pain relief with self-stimulation.

PHANTOM LIMB PAIN

Five sensory thalamic and two PAG/PVG electrodes were implanted in the five patients with phantom limb pain. Four of the thalamic electrodes were internalized; none of the PAG/PVG electrodes afforded pain relief. Despite the initially high success rate (80%), only one patient (20%) has had persistent pain relief with chronic stimulation.

THORACIC NEURALGIAS

All of these patients (four) underwent placement of PAG/PVG electrodes only; three (75%) obtained initial pain relief. Follow-up examination found one patient continuing to use self-stimulation for pain relief.

MISCELLANEOUS DEAFFERENTATION PAIN SYNDROMES

Various other pain syndromes treated with DBS included two cases of atypical facial pain and one case each of postherpetic neuralgia, brachial plexus avulsion, deafferentation perineal pain, and extremity pain secondary to Friedreich's ataxia. Three sensory thalamic electrodes were implanted; one evoked paresthesias in the area of pain and was internalized. Four PAG/PVG electrodes were implanted, and three subsequently were internalized. All patients in whom electrodes were internalized (67%) have had persistent pain relief and continue to use stimulation.

Nociceptive Pain States

The initial and long-term success rates for patients with nociceptive pain states are listed in Table 31–4.

CANCER PAIN

In six patients with pain secondary to the invasion of cancer, three sensory thalamic electrodes and five PAG/PVG electrodes were implanted. One VPL electrode and two PAG/PVG electrodes were internalized (initial success rate = 50%). Two patients continued to have profound pain relief until their deaths.

LOW BACK AND SKELETAL PAIN

Forty-seven PAG/PVG electrodes were implanted in 51 patients; 28 of these provided sufficient pain relief and were internalized. One of six sensory thalamic electrodes also was internalized. The overall initial success rate was 57%. Within a mean follow-up period of 6.8 years, 32% of all patients maintained self-stimulation and obtained relief from their chronic pain.

TABLE 31–4. Initial and Long-Term Results of Deep Brain Stimulation for Nociceptive Pain States

Diagnosis	No. of Patients	Patients with Initial Success (%)	Patients with Long-Term Success (%)
Cancer pain	6	3 (50)	2 (33)
Low back and skeletal pain	51	29 (57)	16 (31)
Total	57	32 (56)	18 (32)

TABLE 31–5. Major Complications of Deep Brain Stimulation for Chronic Pain in 141 Patients

Complication	No. of Occurrences	Frequency (%)
Infection	17	12.1
Erosion of hardware	10	7.1
Foreign body reaction	7	5.0
Intracranial hemorrhage	5	3.5
Intracerebral	3[a]	
Epidural	1	
Periventricular	1	
Psychosis	3	2.1

[a] 1 death.

Complications of Therapy

The major complications of DBS for chronic pain in this series of 141 patients are listed in Table 31–5.

INTRACRANIAL HEMORRHAGE

The most significant complication was intracranial hemorrhage, which occurred in five patients (3.5%). Although this complication is common to all stereotactic surgery, two intracerebral hematomas produced upon the removal of electrodes were unique to stimulation procedures. There were three cases of intracerebral hemorrhage and one case each of epidural and periventricular hematomas; one patient died, two were left with a significant neurological deficit, and two had complete resolution of their deficits.

INFECTION

As with the implantation of any foreign body, the occurrence of infection is a major concern with DBS. A total of 23 infections occurred in 17 patients (12.1%). Almost exclusively, the site of infection was a skin wound, including 17 scalp wounds through which the electrode was implanted, three chest wall wounds through which the receiver was inserted, and one neck wound through which the wire connecting the electrode to the receiver was passed. Two cases of stitch abscess were also noted. In contrast to these 23 local infections, only one case of meningitis occurred (0.7%).

TABLE 31–6. Infectious Complications of Deep Brain Stimulation for Chronic Pain: Causative Organisms in 20 Cultured Infections

Staphylococcus epidermidis	9
Staphylococcus aureus	6
Propionibacterium acnes	2
Enterobacter cloacae	1
Group B streptococci	1
Micrococcus species	1

There was a fairly even division between infections occurring soon after electrode implantation (less than 30 days after, 12 cases) and those occurring late (more than 30 days, 10 cases). No correlation between the time of externalization of the electrode for testing and the time of infection was detected.

The causative organisms of these infections, listed in table 31–6, were as expected given the sites of infection. Of the 20 cultured infections, 15 were caused by staphylococcal species (nine *Staphylococcus epidermidis* and six *Staphylococcus aureus*). Two infections were caused by

Propionibacterium acnes and one infection each was caused by group B streptococci, *Micrococcus*, and *Enterobacter cloacae*.

Several modes of therapy were undertaken to cure these infections. Because several patients had excellent pain relief, we made several attempts to cure infection without electrode removal. The use of antibiotics alone failed in all but one case, that being a minor wound infection with *Staphylococcus epidermidis*. Antibiotics combined with local debridement successfully treated the two stitch abscesses but failed all six times that they were used for more serious infections. Use of antibiotics combined with the total removal of hardware was successful in all 11 cases. We cured eight infections by combining parenteral antibiotics with the removal of a unilateral electrode, leaving in place other electrodes and hardware. Thus, removal of all hardware is not necessary, and functioning electrodes not near the site of infection can be spared.

EROSION

With bulky hardware implanted underneath a scalp already thinned by previous surgery, the risk of skin breakdown becomes significant. Erosion of the scalp without infection occurred in 10 patients (7.1%) over the 14 years of study. Five patients had nonfunctioning DBS systems removed, and in five patients, successful reimplantation of the hardware and reclosure of the wound was accomplished without antibiotic therapy and without further complication.

FOREIGN BODY REACTIONS

Five patients (3.5%) experienced a total of seven episodes of foreign body reaction stimulated by the presence of their hardware. This reaction was characterized by local pain, inflammation, and erythema, with occasional systemic generalization of an immunological reaction. Marked eosinophilia was noted in peripheral blood smears. One patient spontaneously resolved these symptoms, and four required the complete removal of their DBS systems.

MECHANICAL COMPLICATIONS

Although mechanical problems were once a major cause of failure of neurostimulation procedures, technical innovations over the 14 years of this study have significantly decreased their incidence. Migration of the electrode, resulting in failure of stimulation to provide pain relief, occurred 20 times in 14 patients (9.9%). After the original electrodes were redesigned, this complication essentially was eliminated. Current leakage into soft tissues, usually resulting from fractures in electrical insulation, occurred 14 times in 12 patients (8.5%). There were six additional cases of hardware failure (4.3%), which were corrected by replacement of specific components.

PSYCHIATRIC ILLNESS

Three patients (2.1%) had psychotic reactions after DBS implantation. Prolonged psychiatric hospitalization was required for two patients; unreported polypharmacy abuse both prior to and during hospitalization was implicated in both cases. One patient had no such history, but the postsurgical psychotic symptoms nonetheless occurred.

MINOR COMPLICATIONS AND SIDE EFFECTS OF THERAPY

Minor complications were defined as results that either were undetected by the patient or were considered insignificant; also included were those complications that resolved by the time of discharge from the hospital. Side effects were considered to be results that were unpleasant for the patient but were expected and time-limited phenomena related to the surgery.

Headaches were the most common of these problems, occurring in 72 patients (51.5%). In most cases, headaches resulted directly from the cranial surgery and resolved by the time of discharge. Eight patients, however, had persistent headaches requiring further analgesic therapy for varying periods.

Side effects of air/contrast ventriculography and PAG/PVG stimulation were also frequent. These included diplopia (14.2%), nausea (10.6%), vertical gaze palsies (9.9%), blurred vision (9.2%), horizontal nystagmus (4.3%), and persistent oscillopsia (3.5%). With refinement of stimulation parameters, these symptoms almost invariably resolved completely by the time of discharge.

The complications of therapy are listed in table 31–7. Those occurring more than 5% of the time included temporary and completely resolving hemiparesis or monoparesis (8.5%), confusion (7.8%), lethargy (6.4%), dysphagia (5.7%), and local pain with stimulation (5.0%).

TABLE 31–7. Complications of Deep Brain Stimulation for Chronic Pain: Minor or Resolved at Discharge

Complication	No. of Patients	Frequency (%)
Hemiparesis or monoparesis	12	8.5
Confusion	11	7.8
Lethargy	9	6.4
Dysphasia	8	5.7
Persistent headache	8	5.7
Local pain	7	5.0
Seizures	6	4.3
Urinary incontinence	5	3.5
Cranial nerve palsies	5	3.5
Ptosis	4	2.8
Urinary retention	4	2.8
Bronchospasm	2	1.4
Hypesthesia (facial or hemi-body)	2	1.4
Hallucinations	2	1.4
Photophobia	2	1.4
Memory loss	2	1.4
Hypotension	2	1.4
Facial pain	2	1.4
Hypertension	1	0.7
Shortness of breath	1	0.7
Dysphoria	1	0.7
Thrombophlebitis	1	0.7
Stimulation-induced sleep	1	0.7

A particularly peculiar complication occurred in one patient: upon the initiation of stimulation, the patient immediately fell asleep. Thus, despite excellent pain relief, the system was unusable for this patient.

Discussion and Conclusions

The relief of chronic pain and the treatment of the patient with chronic intractable pain are major challenges. The neurosurgeon is often consulted after nonsurgical therapies (pharmacotherapy, psychiatric intervention, physical therapy, transcutaneous nerve stimulation, acupuncture, and biofeedback) have been exhausted. When conventional surgical approaches to pain have been rejected or have failed, patients have been referred for consideration of DBS in a last-ditch attempt to control their chronic pain. This selection process results in a group of the most difficult pain patients, those in whom the success rate of many prior therapies has been zero. It is in light of this patient population that the efficacy of DBS for chronic pain must be assessed.

The overall initial success rate, that is, the number of patients who had sufficient relief to warrant electrode internalization and who obtained good pain relief at their first outpatient examination, was approximately 59%. After an average of 6.8 years, 31% of all patients in whom electrodes were implanted were still using their stimulators regularly for pain relief. This figure represents a long-term success rate of nearly 52% of those patients in whom electrodes were internalized.

Some types of pain appear to be more responsive to this mode of treatment than others. Peripheral neuropathies, including painful postoperative sciatic neuropathy and diabetic and ischemic neuropathies, are quite responsive, with initial and long-term success rates of 69% and 50%, respectively. Other syndromes, such as anesthesia dolorosa or pain arising from spinal cord injury and paraplegia, are very unresponsive to DBS, and have long-term success rates of only 18% and 0%, respectively. Patients with other types of pain have intermediate response rates as detailed in tables 31–3 and 31–4. Based on these findings, we now only rarely consider DBS for some of these pain problems, most notably paraplegia pain and facial anesthesia dolorosa.

The advent of other neurosurgical techniques for the treatment of chronic pain has also limited our application of this technique. For example, the installation of epidural or intrathecal opiates for the treatment of pain from cancer invasion has been so successful that we no longer consider DBS for these patients.

The overall incidence of serious complications in our series, including infections, intracranial hemorrhage, and unexplained psychosis, was 16.3%. Serious infections were treated effectively with the removal of the infected electrode. In those patients with multiple electrodes, the noninfected electrodes could be maintained. Erosion of the hardware without accompanying infection was easily treated by wound revision only. The potential for infection increases during the period in which wires are externalized for electrode testing. New multichannel transmitter systems are capable of transcutaneous multipolar stimulation surveys and thus allow for internalization of the entire DBS system in one procedure, which should decrease the incidence of this complication.

Intracranial bleeding was seen in five patients; two patients recovered without sequelae, two were significantly debilitated, and one died. Two of these hemorrhages occurred after removal of the electrodes. Because of this, the intracranial portion of the electrodes was not removed in later patients unless absolutely necessary.

The persistent postimplantation headaches that occurred appeared to have a strong vascular component; they were predominantly unilateral and throbbing in nature and were not correlated with the presence or absence of stimulation. Interestingly, many of these patients responded to the intravenous infusion of dihydroergotamine, an ergot derivative used for the treatment of acute migraine headaches. These patients have been maintained on antimigraine medications, which has provided good relief of their headache pain.

Several investigators have reported the results of their long-term experience using DBS for chronic intractable pain [3, 12, 14, 16, 18, 19, 23, 25–7]. Comparison of these data is difficult because the definition of success or failure is not consistent and because cases are not always clearly reported with respect to specific pain syndromes and stimulation sites. Tables 31–8 and 31–9 summarize the long-term results of DBS for deafferentation and nociceptive pain states, respectively; the data have been normalized for purposes of comparison. Successful cases were those in which pain relief was reported to be good or excellent or greater than 50% of the baseline pain rating. If these were not specifically reported, the authors' own criteria of success or failure were employed.

Eleven studies reported on 628 patients who underwent implantation of deep-brain electrodes for deafferentation pain states. There was no consistent use of sensory thalamic or PVG electrodes for deafferentation pain states; three studies used exclusively VPL electrodes, and two used exclusively PAG/PVG electrodes. The remaining six studies used combinations of the two stimulation sites. The range of follow-up time was reported in nine studies and the mean follow-up time in five. The shortest follow-up period was one month and the longest was 168 months; mean follow-up times ranged from 10–80 months. Initial success rates, reported in seven of these studies, ranged from 29% to 82%. The overall long-term success rate was 47% (296/628).

Table 31–9 summarizes the results of DBS reported for 337 patients with nociceptive pain. PAG/PVG electrodes were used exclusively in three of nine studies; both VPL and PAG/PVG electrodes were used in five. Mazars and co-workers [12] reported their experience with only sensory thalamic stimulation for nociceptive pain in 22 patients; no patients obtained satisfactory pain relief. Initial success rates, available for five of the remaining studies, ranged from 40% to 98%. The overall long-term success rate was 60% (201/337).

The results of the authors' study suggest a somewhat lower efficacy of DBS for chronic pain, with long-term success rates of 30% for deafferentation pain and 32% for nociceptive pain states. In patients for whom electrodes were initially successful, long-term success rates were 49% (deafferentation pain) and 57% (nociceptive pain). The reason for the discrepancy between this report and others is un-

TABLE 31–8. Results of Deep Brain Stimulation for Deafferentation Pain

Author	Year	No. of Patients	Initial Success (%)	Long-Term Success (%)	Follow-up Mean (range) in months	Electrodes
Adams	1986	84	56 (67)	25 (30)	80 (14–168)	VPL/IC/PVG
Hosobuchi	1986	76	52 (68)	44 (58)	(14–168)	VPL/PVG
Siegfried	1985	96	67 (70)	49 (51)	(9–56)	VPL
Young	1985	17	14 (82)	10 (59)	20 (2–60)	VPL/PVG
Plotkin	1982	18		10 (56)	(6–42)	VPL/PVG
Dieckmann	1982	41	31 (76)	9 (22)	(6–54)	VPL/PVG
Turnbull	1980	18	14 (78)	13 (72)	10 (1–47)	VPL
Ray	1980	9		7 (78)	14 (1–33)	PVG
Mazars	1979	99		83 (84)		VPL
Meyerson*	1979	160	47 (29)	42 (26)		VPL/IC/PVG
Richardson	1977	10		4 (40)	18 (1–46)	PVG
Total		628		296 (47%)		

* International Cooperative Study includes 56 patients operated upon by Hosobuchi or Adams; compare [24].
VPL = sensory thalamic electrodes; PVG = periaqueductal or periventricular gray electrodes; IC = internal capsule electrodes.

TABLE 31–9. Results of Deep Brain Stimulation for Nociceptive Pain

Author	Year	No. of Patients	Initial Success (%)	Long-Term Success (%)	Follow-up Mean (range) in months	Placement of Electrodes
Adams	1986	57	32 (56)	22 (32)	80 (24–168)	PVG/VPL
Hosobuchi	1986	65	64 (98)	50 (77)	(24–168)	PVG/VPL
Young	1985	31	29 (94)	25 (81)	20 (2–60)	PVG/VPL
Plotkin	1982	42		34 (81)	(6–42)	PVG
Dieckmann	1982	5	2 (40)	1 (20)	(6–54)	PVG/VPL
Ray	1980	19		14 (74)	14	PVG
Meyerson[a]	1979	76	50 (66)	41 (54)		PVG/VPL
Mazars	1977	22				VPL
Richardson	1977	20		14 (70)	18 (1–46)	PVG
Total		337		201 (60%)		

[a] International Cooperative Study includes 56 patients operated upon by Hosobuchi or Adams; compare [24].
VPL = sensory thalamic electrodes; PVG = periaqueductal or periventricular gray electrodes.

clear. However, our study differs from some others in that our patients were followed by someone other than the primary operating surgeon, and follow-up lasted considerably longer. We believe that our study provides a more objective evaluation of surgical response and a longer period of follow-up; these features explain why our success rate of this procedure is somewhat lower. In addition, during the evolution of our study, very broad patient selection criteria were employed. As there appear to be several categories of patients who do not respond well, including those with some specific pain states, those with psychiatric problems, and those involved in litigation, more careful screening of patients may lead to greater long-term success rates.

Analysis of our study reveals several important predictors of success with this procedure. Therapy for all patients with thalamic pain syndrome, for example, produced a long-term success rate of 24% (6/25). In patients with thalamic pain syndrome in whom the sensory thalamus was stimulated, the success rate was 42.8% (6/14). If consideration is limited to patients in whom intraoperative sensory thalamic stimulation produced paresthesias within the area of pain, the long-term success rate further increases to 54.5% (6/11). This last figure may more accurately reflect the current potential of DBS for the treatment of chronic deafferentation pain.

Based on our experience, there are several factors that might lead to even better surgical results in the future. These include proper patient selection criteria, careful selection of stimulation targets based on the nature of the pain syndrome, and accurate electrode placement using the results of intraoperative stimulation as a guide. There may be a role for magnetic resonance imaging coupled with stereotactic procedures; not only would this provide greater anatomical detail than other stereotactic techniques, but the possible side effects of air/contrast ventriculography might be avoided.

Also of possible importance to the future use of DBS for chronic pain are advances in the use of intraoperative electrophysiological techniques. Somatosensory evoked potentials can be used to more accurately position subcortical electrodes in those thalamic subnuclei subserving specific body regions. This technique may be particularly valuable in anxious or poorly compliant patients as well as those with prior infarction in whom the isolation of specific target cells is difficult.

Several technical advances may also further decrease surgical morbidity. Improvement in electrode design has already led to a significant decrease in the number of electrode migrations necessitating reoperation. The advent of multichannel stimulation systems has made possible the immediate internalization and in situ testing of deep-brain-stimulating electrodes, thus minimizing the risk of infection. Smaller and lighter hardware may prevent irritation, minimize foreign body reactions, and make the systems more comfortable for patients. Improved design of hardware connectors and insulation materials may also lessen the possibility of hardware failure and current leakage.

In light of our results, we believe that DBS should be considered in those patients with chronic severe pain who have failed to achieve pain relief with other modes of therapy. Our success rate has improved considerably over the past few years; from this experience we believe that careful patient selection and operation by neurosurgeons experienced with this technique are two critical variables for the successful application of this procedure to pain patients. We continue to believe that there are patients in whom DBS can have a significant impact on chronic pain problems.

References

1. Adams JE, Hosobuchi Y, Fields HL: Stimulation of internal capsule for relief of chronic pain. *J Neurosurg* 41:740–744, 1974
2. Akil H, Mayer DJ, Liebeskind JC: Antagonism of stimulation-produced analgesia by naloxone, a narcotic antagonist. *Science* 191:961–962, 1976
3. Dieckmann G, Witzmann A: Initial and long-term results of deep brain stimulation for chronic intractable pain. *Appl Neurophysiol* 45:617–172, 1982
4. Dionne RA, Muller GP, Young RF, et al: Contrast medium causes the apparent increase in beta-endorphin levels in human cerebrospinal fluid following brain stimulation. *Pain* 20:313–321, 1984
5. Gerhart KD, Yezierski RP, Fang ZR, et al: Inhibition of primate spinothalamic tract neurons by stimulation in ventral posterior lateral (VPL) thalamic nucleus: Possible mechanisms. *J Neurophysiol* 48:496–422, 1983
6. Heath RG: *Studies in Schizophrenia.* Cambridge, MA: Harvard University Press, 1954
7. Hosobuchi Y: Subcortical electrical stimulation for control of intractable pain in humans. *J Neurosurg* 64:543–553, 1986
8. Hosobuchi Y, Adams JE, Linchinz R: Pain relief by electrical stimulation of the central gray matter in humans and its reversal by naloxone. *Science* 197:183–186, 1977
9. Hosobuchi Y, Adams JE, Rutkin B: Chronic thalamic stimulation for the control of facial anaesthesia dolorosa. *Arch Neurol* 29:158–161, 1973
10. Hughes J: Isolation of an endogenous compound from the brain with pharmacological properties similar to morphine. *Brain* 88:295–308, 1975
11. Mayer DJ, Wolfle TL, Akil H, et al: Analgesia from electrical stimulation of the brain stem of the rat. *Science* 174:1351–1354, 1971
12. Mazars GJ, Merienne L, Cioloca C: Comparative study of electrical stimulation of posterior thalamic nuclei, periaqueductal gray and other midline mesencephalic structures in man. In Bonica JJ (ed): *Advances in Pain Research and*

Therapy, Vol 3. New York: Raven Press, 1979, pp 541–546
13. Mazars GJ, Merienne L, Cioloca C: Stimulations thalamiques intermittentes antalgiques: Note preliminaire. *Rev Neurol* (Paris) 128:273–279, 1973
14. Plotkin R: Results in 60 cases of deep brain stimulation for chronic intractable pain. *Appl Neurophysiol* 45:173–178, 1982
15. Pool JL, Clark WK, Hudson P, et al: *Hypothalamic-Hypophysial Interrelationships.* Springfield, IL: Thomas, 1956
16. Ray CD, Burton CV: Deep brain stimulation for severe, chronic pain. *Acta Neurochir [Suppl]* (Wien) 30:289–293, 1980
17. Reynolds DV: Surgery on the rat during electrical analgesia induced by focal brain stimulation. *Science* 164:444–445, 1969
18. Richardson DE: Long-term follow-up of deep brain stimulation for relief of chronic pain in the human. In Brock M (ed): *Modern Neurosurgery.* Berlin: Springer-Verlag, 1982, pp 449–453
19. Richardson DE, Akil H: Long term results of periventricular gray self-stimulation. *Neurosurgery* 1:199–202, 1977
20. Richardson DE, Akil H: Pain reduction by electrical brain stimulation in man. Part I. Acute administration of periaqueductal and periventricular sites. Part II. Chronic self-administration in the periventricular gray matter. *J Neurosurg* 47:178–194, 1977
21. Schaltenbrand G, Bailey P: *Introduction to Stereotaxis with an Atlas of the Human Brain,* Vol 2. New York: Grune & Stratton, 1959, plates 38–47
22. Shulman R, Turnbull IM, Diewold P: Psychiatric aspects of thalamic stimulation for neuropathic pain. *Pain* 13:127–135, 1982
23. Siegfried J: Long-term results of intermittent stimulation of the sensory thalamic nuclei in 67 cases of deafferentation pain. In Lazorthes Y, Upton ARM (eds): *Neurostimulation: An Overview.* Mt Kisko, NY: Futura Publishing, 1985, pp 129–143
24. Sweet WH: Intracerebral electrical stimulation for the relief of chronic pain. In Youmans JR (ed): *Neurological Surgery,* Vol 6 (2nd ed). Philadelphia: Saunders, 1982, pp 3739–3748
25. Turnbull IM, Shulman R, Woodhurst W: Thalamic stimulation for neuropathic pain. *J Neurosurg* 52:486–493, 1980
26. White JC, Sweet WH: *Pain and the Neurosurgeon: A 40-Year Experience.* Springfield IL: Thomas, 1969
27. Young RF, Kroening R, Fulton W, et al: Electrical stimulation of the brain in treatment of chronic pain. *J Neurosurg* 62:389–396, 1985

32. DEEP BRAIN STIMULATION FOR THE TREATMENT OF MOTOR DISORDERS

Jean Siegfried
G. L. Rea

Since the 1950s, electrical stimulation of deep brain structures has been used to localize the thalamic nuclei during stereotactic surgery for extrapyramidal movement disorders [19]. More recent evidence suggests that chronic deep brain stimulation effectively relieves the symptoms of some motor disorders. However, because this use of deep brain stimulation is currently a surgical procedure with an unknown mechanism of action and no clear clinical guidelines, its use should be examined rigorously [20]. This chapter reviews the literature regarding deep brain stimulation for movement disorders, presents the experience of the University of Zurich with thalamic stimulation, and examines the theories regarding the mode of action of this procedure. Its use and indications also are reexamined.

Literature Review

Hassler and colleagues (1960) reported the effects of stimulating various deep-brain structures during stereotactic surgery [12]. They found that stimulating the basal parts of the ventral lateral nucleus (VL) of the thalamus caused some increase in tremor amplitudes followed by a pause. This increase in amplitude depended upon the phase of the tremor when the stimulation occurred. Even when not present, tremor may be evoked by a stimulus rate of 4–8 impulses per second. Stimulating the medial part of the oral ventral nucleus during cases of torsion dystonia frequently leads to slow torsion movements of the head, shoulder, and arm. Stimulation of the pallidum with higher frequencies primarily reduces the intensity of tremor and may even lead to complete arrest of tremor and to synergy of flexion. In patients with athetosis and torsion dystonia, stimulation with low frequencies (4–8 per sec) during spontaneously occurring abnormal movements elicits the typical hyperkinetic pattern in the contralateral extremities. Higher stimulus frequencies and strengths can augment or suppress an existing spontaneous hyperkinesia.

The first modern study of chronic therapeutic deep brain stimulation in human movement disorders appeared in several articles by Bechtereva and colleagues between 1972 and 1975 [2–4]. They reported that chronic stimulation had favorable effects in patients who had tremor associated with Parkinson's disease, Wilson's disease, and dystonia musculorum deformans. Unfortunately, information regarding the number of patients, the techniques for electrode placement, and the proposed target was not divulged.

Mundinger was the first to describe in detail beneficial effects on abnormal motor behavior when chronic stimulation was performed in specified deep areas, such as the thalamus, pulvinar, and dentate nucleus [15]. In a 1982 review of patients with dystonia, spasticity, and spasmodic torticollis, Mundinger emphasized the importance of stimulation-induced paresthesias overlying the affected area and of a programmed pattern of stimulation to select the optimal parameters for each patient [16]. He found that seven of eight cases improved; improvement was greater in patients with hemispasticity and infantile cerebral paresis and less in patients with torsion dystonias.

L.D. Lunsford (ed.) *MODERN STEREOTACTIC NEUROSURGERY*. Copyright © 1988.

Brice and McLellan initially treated three female patients with multiple sclerosis; all had severe intention tremor when the subthalamic area was stimulated (20 mm behind the anterior commissure, 6–8 mm below the intercommissural plane, and 10 mm from the midline) [5]. Good results were obtained in two patients with the use of stimulation parameters of 75–100 Hz, square wave pulses of 0.5–1 mA and 200–400 m sec duration. In an attempt to decrease the total time of stimulation, the transmitter was controlled by a switching device triggered by electromyography (EMG) signals in the deltoid muscle of the appropriate arm. Although these investigators postulated some initial "thalamotomy effect" on the abnormal movements (resulting from the trauma of electrode placement), the long-term improvement in two patients was ascribed to stimulation.

The sensory thalamic ventral posterolateral nucleus (VPL) was stimulated by Mazars and associates to alleviate deafferentation pain; they found that stimulation also controlled associated abnormal movements [14]. They stressed the significance of stimulation-induced paresthesias affecting the involved portion of the body. Both pain and abnormal movements ceased after one to three minutes of stimulation but returned 6–28 hours later. Mazars and co-workers also attempted stimulation in patients with Parkinson's disease, congenital choreoathetosis, Wilson's disease, and action tremor, but without success. These authors concluded that for stimulation to be successful, the dyskinesias had to be associated with sensory deafferentation and that stimulation acted as a substitute for sensory information delivered to VPL.

Cooper has reported the largest series of patients with involuntary movement disorders treated by deep stimulation [6, 7]. In a group of 49 patients with movement disorders of various types and causes, he stimulated the posterior thalamus, internal capsule, and zona incerta; 27 were improved. This method appeared to be most effective in patients with spasticity secondary to cerebral palsy. Thalamic somatosensory responses were recorded to aid in electrode placement and to obtain optimal stimulation parameters.

The thalamic area surrounding the ventral intermedial nucleus (V.i.m.), the centromedian nucleus (CM), and the parafascicular nucleus (PF) was stimulated in nine patients by Andy [1]. The motor problems in these patients consisted of congenital, traumatic, or parkinsonian tremor; torticollis; and facial spasm. He reported the results in six patients as good to excellent and in three patients (with parkinsonian tremor) as fair to good.

This review of the literature indicates that thalamic and subthalamic stimulation can favorably affect patients with various disorders of motor control. However, the areas stimulated, the types of motor disorders treated, and the results in each type of disorder all have varied. These factors, plus the lack of a solid physiological explanation for the reported efficacy, made us quite reluctant to use this technique, even though it has been used for pain control at the University of Zurich since 1977. Despite these misgivings, observations of patient responses to stimulation during stereotactic procedures convinced us that the primary sensory nucleus of the thalamus plays an important role in motor behavior [21].

Patient Population

Four patients had thalamic pain syndrome and associated severe dyskinetic movements, and two patients had deafferentation pain with associated severe spasticity after traumatic paraplegia. All six underwent surgery primarily for treatment of deafferentation pain. The four patients with thalamic pain following cerebral infarction had unilateral electrodes placed in the VPL nucleus of the thalamus (3 mm anterior to the posterior commissure, 1–2 mm below the intercommissural line, and 13 mm from the midline). Bilateral electrodes were placed 3 mm more laterally in the paraplegic patients. We used an electrode of a flexible monopolar design (Avery) with a central rigid stylet. Its helical shape provides high resistance to fatigue fracture and allows it to "move" with the brain. It is fixed in place by a specially designed titanium screw that also provides a watertight seal of the burr hole [18]. For each patient, the electrode was connected to a percutaneous extension. When pain was controlled sufficiently, a programmable totally implanted system (ITREL®-Medtronic) was placed subcutaneously in the upper thorax region.

Results

In all four patients with thalamic pain syndrome, stimulation with impulses of 1–2 mA, 200 m sec, and 33 Hz yielded satisfactory areas of paresthesia and almost instantly suppressed involuntary movements. Suppression of the dyskinesias was complete, but they reappeared after one to two minutes when the stimulation was stopped. The implants then were programmed to stimulate for one of every two minutes. With this technique, complete relief of involuntary movements has lasted for one to two years of follow-up.

In the patients who had pain following paraplegia, the results were similar. There was virtually immediate control of pain and clonus with bilateral stimulation. After stimulation was discontinued, the clonus reappeared within two to three minutes. These bilateral systems also were programmed for one minute of stimulation every two minutes. Relief has endured for these patients.

Discussion

Although both the literature and our experience indicate that deep brain stimulation can alleviate some motor symptoms, the mechanism of its action remains unknown. Two broad theories exist: that stimulation inhibits sensory activity, or that stimulation supplies or augments sensory activity. Although these theories admittedly ignore some of the complexities involved, they do provide a simple beginning upon which to base further information.

Cooper (1982) [6] and Andy (1983) [1] ascribed the beneficial effects of thalamic stimulation to a functional ablation of the discharging systems. Cooper supported this argument with early experimental work and theorized that motor symptoms may be the result of an inhibitory-facilitory imbalance. He stated that lesions or stimulation in the posterior VL suppress a posterior VL sensory funnel and lessen the imbalance.

Mazars [14], Cooper [8], and the present authors favor the theory that stimulation supplies decreased or no "sensory input" to the thalamus. The thalamus in turn relays input to the motor cortex; alternatively, stimulation input may pass directly to the motor cortex. The importance of the VL and especially VPL input to the motor cortex is indicated by the fact that 70% of all thalamocortical connections are from the VPL, and 95% are from oral and caudal parts of the VL and the oral part of the VPL [17]. The physiological importance of the thalamus as a receiver of information from the basal ganglia and a projector of revised information onto the motor and premotor cortex has been emphasized by others [9–11, 13]. This physiologically demonstrated capability of thalamic output to modify motor behavior has two well-known clinical correlates in patients with movement disorders: the inability of athetotic patients to control their movements without the help of sensory input and the "geste antagoniste" phenomenon, which occurs when a patient is able to modify torticollis by lightly placing an index finger on the chin.

Although recent physiological data and clinical corelations are intriguing, no solid rationale for thalamic stimulation in movement disorders has been developed to date. Thus, surgeons must be quite cautious in proposing such procedures and must review carefully the available literature to assess which patients might benefit and what methods and sites of stimulation should be used.

The most uniformly successful results are in patients who suffer sensory loss and deafferentation pain in addition to abnormal motor behavior. Those patients without sensory loss have shown a more varied response. It also appears that tremor, spasticity, and dystonic movements tend to respond somewhat more consistently than other abnormal movements. One should also be wary of using the procedure in patients with diseases such as multiple sclerosis, which can fluctuate, making evaluation virtually impossible. The ideal patient would have a sensory and motor abnormality due to a fixed deficit and would be clinically disturbed by tremor and/or spasticity. Regardless of whether a patient fits this description, the specific symptom altered (tremor, spasticity, dystonia, total function) and the extent of the effect must be examined closely.

According to available anatomical physiological, and most consistent clinical data, the site of stimulation is the primary sensory nucleus, VPL. Tasker has indicated that V.i.m. might also have some stimulation efficacy [22]. It is essential to elicit paresthesias that include the site of motor disability. Failure to achieve appropriate paresthesias may reflect an unavoidable failure in technique rather than a failure in the general concept of deep brain stimulation.

Conclusion

Although deep brain stimulation has been proven efficacious in both our small group of patients and in limited other clinical reports, many questions remain. In this chapter, we have tried to address these questions, but at this time, we remain very cautious in our evaluation. Although we do not doubt the potential efficacy of thalamic stimulation for motor disorders, we are concerned that the safety and ease of the procedure coupled with the lack of alternative treatments could lead to its use in patients with little hope for improvement, and thus it could lose its credibility as a treatment in appropriate patients.

References

1. Andy OJ: Thalamic stimulation for control of movement disorders. *Appl Neurophysiol* 46: 107–111, 1983
2. Bechtereva NP, Bondartchuk AN, Smirnov VM, et al: Method of electrostimulation of the deep brain structures in treatment of some chronic diseases. *Confin Neurol* 37:136–140, 1975
3. Bechtereva NP, Bondartchek AN, Smirnov VM, et al: Therapeutic electrostimulation of the deep brain structures. *Vopr Neurokhir* 1:7–12, 1972
4. Bechtereva NP, Kombarova DK, Smirnov VM, et al: Using the brain's latent abilities for therapy: chronic intracerebral electrical stimulation. In Sweet WH, Obrador S, Martin-Rodriquez JG (eds): *Neurosurgical Treatment in Psychiatry, Pain and Epilepsy*. Baltimore, London, Tokyo: University Park Press, 1975, pp 581–613
5. Brice J, McLellan L: Supression of intention tremor by contingent deep brain stimulation. *Lancet* 1:1221–1222, 1980
6. Cooper IS: A general theory of caution and reversibility of involuntary movement disorders. *Appl Neurophysiol* 45:317–323, 1982
7. Cooper IS, Upton ARM, Amin I: Chronic cerebellar stimulation and deep brain stimulation in involuntary movement disorders. *Appl Neurophysiol* 45:209–217, 1981
8. Cooper IS, Upton ARM, Amin I: Reversibility of chronic neuralgic deficits: Some effects of electrical stimulation of the thalamus and internal capsule in man. *Appl Neurophysiol* 43:244–258, 1980
9. Delong MR, Georgopoulos A: Motor functions of the basal ganglia. In Brookhard JM, et al (eds): *The Nervous System*. Bethesda, MD: American Physiological Society, 1979, pp 1017–1061
10. Delong MR, Georgopoulos AP, Crutcher MD, et al: Functional organization of the basal ganglia: Contributions of single cell recording stuides. In *Functions of the Basal Ganglia*, Ciba Foundation Symposium 107. London: Pitman, 1984, pp 103–107
11. Evarts EV, Wise SP: Basal ganglia outputs and motor control. In *Functions of the Basal Ganglia*, Ciba Foundation Symposium 107. London: Pitman, 1984, pp 83–102
12. Hassler R, Riechert T, Mundinger F, et al: Physiological observations in stereotaxic operations in extrapyramidal motor disturbances. *Brain* 83:339–350, 1960
13. Kitai ST: Electrophysiology of the corpus striatum and brain stem integrating system. In Brookhart JM, et al (eds): *The Nervous System*. Bethesda, MD: American Physiology Society, 1979, pp 997–1013
14. Mazars G, Merienne L, Cioloca G: Control of dyskinesia due to sensory deafferentation by means of thalamic stimulation. *Acta Neurochir [Suppl]* (Wien) 30:239–243, 1980
15. Mundinger F: Neue stereotaktisch-funktionelle Behandlungsmethode des Torticollis spasmodicus mit Hirnstimulatoren. *Med Klinik* 72:1982–1986, 1977
16. Mundinger F, Neumuller H: Programmed stimulation for control of chronic pain and motor lisease. *Appl Neurophysiol* 45:102–111, 1982
17. Porter R: Basal ganglia links for movement, mood and memory (General Discussion I). In *Functions of the Basal Ganglia*, Ciba Foundation Symposium 107. London: Pitman, 1984, pp 103–107
18. Siegfried J, Comte R, Meier RR: Intracerebral electrode implantation system. *J Neurosurg* 59:356–359, 1983
19. Siegfried J, Hood T: Brain stimulation procedures in dystonic, hypertonic, dyskinetic and hyperkinetic conditions. In Eccles JC, Dimitrijevic M (eds): *Recent Advances in Restorative Neurology*. New York, Basel: Karger, 1985, pp 79–90
20. Siegfried J, Lazorthes Y, Sedan R: Indications and ethical considerations of deep brain stimulation. *Acta Neurochir [Suppl]* (Wien) 30:266–274, 1980
21. Siegfried J, Pamir MC: Electrical stimulation in humans of the sensory thalamic nuclei and effects on dyskinesias and spasticity. In Strupler A, Weindl A (eds): Berlin: Springer, 1985, in press
22. Tasker RR, Organ LW, Hawrylyshyn P: Investigation of the surgical target for alleviation of involuntary movement disorders. *Appl Neurophysiol* 45:261–274, 1982

33. EPILEPSY: DEEP BRAIN ELECTRODES

David W. Roberts

Electroencephalographic recording from subcortical structures has been performed since the 1930s. Because it is useful in a variety of laboratory and clinical settings, this technique is valued in the investigation of the epileptic patient.

In the evaluation of seizure disorders, scalp electroencephalography has an established diagnostic role; this role has been extended to defining potentially resectable pathology in the surgical candidate. There are obvious limitations to scalp recording, however. Among these are the attenuation of the signal by bone and scalp, the presence of artifacts, and the inability to record adequately the electrical activity of certain important regions. Recording from electrodes placed directly into the brain significantly reduces these difficulties, providing greater sensitivity in the region of interest. Such recording also has limitations and disadvantages, the most obvious of which are the greater difficulty of electrode placement and the increased risks imposed on the patient. Only through a full appreciation of these strengths and weaknesses can depth recording be most judiciously and optimally employed.

Historical Background

Within a few years of Hans Berger's 1929 report of electroencephalogram (EEG) usage [7], the laboratory technique of recording from subcortical structures was widely practiced [8, 22, 33, 46, 50]. Foerster's cerebellar electrocorticographic investigations [21] also were performed at this time, but it was not until the late 1940s that repeated investigations with depth electrodes were carried out in the clinical setting [10, 25, 42, 50, 52].

Early studies of seizure disorders involved acute exploration of the basal ganglia or thalamus and were oriented more toward general neurophysiological inquiry than surgical planning [33]. The subsequent refinement of chronic depth recording paralleled progress in the clinical neurosurgical fields of psychosurgery and epilepsy surgery. In seeking to understand the electrical phenomena associated with psychopathological states, several researchers established a method for more routine use of the modality [9, 15, 16, 26, 27, 33, 41, 51]. With the rapidly expanding interest in cortical resection and temporal lobectomy for intractable epilepsy, that method found a more secure application and was advanced by a number of investigators [3, 7, 12, 15, 16, 28].

The logical integration of this technique with stereotaxy addressed the requirement for precision in electrode placement and reached elegant execution in the stereoelectroencephalographic investigations of Talairach and Bancaud [4, 47, 48]. Depth recording is evolving in step with stereotactic surgery, particularly with the incorporation of multiple-imaging modalities and computer capabilities, as illustrated by the work of Olivier [35].

Indications

Given both the individualized nature of each seizure disorder and the number of independent epilepsy centers, it is not surprising that no current consensus exists for specific indications for depth electrode investigation. Several general principles are widely acknowledged however. Foremost among these is that the technique should be reserved for patients who are being seriously considered for operative intervention. Associated risks are not warranted in others. Surgical candidacy, of course, implies medical intractability, acceptable anesthetic and surgical risk, and potential benefit from surgi-

L.D. Lunsford (ed.) *MODERN STEREOTACTIC NEUROSURGERY*.

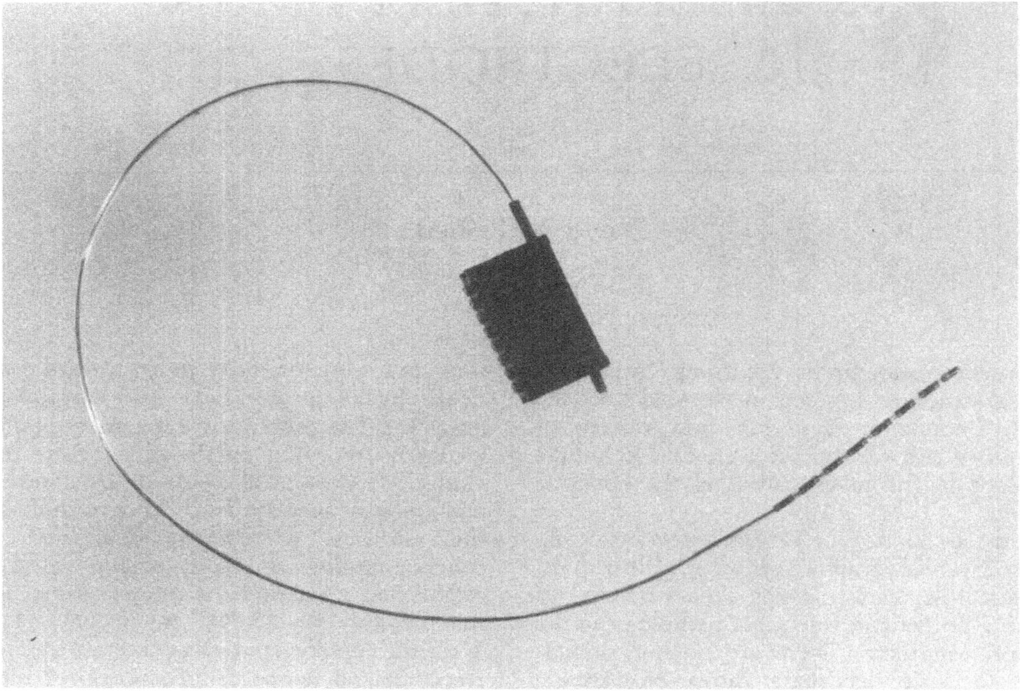

FIGURE 33–1. Eight-contact depth electrode (manufactured by the PMT Corporation, Hopkins, MN); 2-mm contacts are separated by 3-mm intervals; the outer diameter is 1 mm.

cal treatment. By determining the type, site, or extent of surgical treatment, depth electrode study should be used to aid either patient selection or operative planning. The strongest rationale for using a supplemental invasive procedure such as depth recording to identify and localize the epileptogenic focus exists when noninvasive studies provide insufficient or inconsistent information. Examples include clinical situations in which (1) scalp (and sphenoidal or nasopharyngeal) EEG fails to demonstrate either ictal or interictal epileptiform activity, and other evidence strongly implicates a seizure disorder; (2) scalp and basal EEGs demonstrate bilateral epileptiform activity; (3) scalp and basal EEGs demonstrate both temporal and frontal epileptiform activity; (4) scalp and basal EEG information conflicts with knowledge derived from clinical seizure manifestations, neurological examination, psychometric testing, or studies other than EEG; and (5) interictal and ictal EEG data are inconsistent. (DW King, American Epilepsy Society Annual Course, New York, NY, December 1, 1985.)

The confidence in and reliance upon information obtained without depth recording varies considerably among epilepsy centers. Although some reports support frequent use of invasive recordings [14, 44, 45], others contend that it is possible to extract more information than conventionally believed from noninvasive studies [34]. Specific indications remain the judgment of the individual epilepsy team.

Materials and Methods

ELECTRODES

Early investigators employed reusable, rigid, multicontact probes, but concern about transmissible disease prompted the adoption of tresses consisting of thin wire strands [33]. The majority of investigators currently use flexible, multicontact electrodes [17] and restrict them to a single use. A number of electrodes are available commercially (figures 33–1, 33–2), although many institutions prefer to make their own. Typical electrodes have 4 to 18 contact points, 2–10 mm apart.

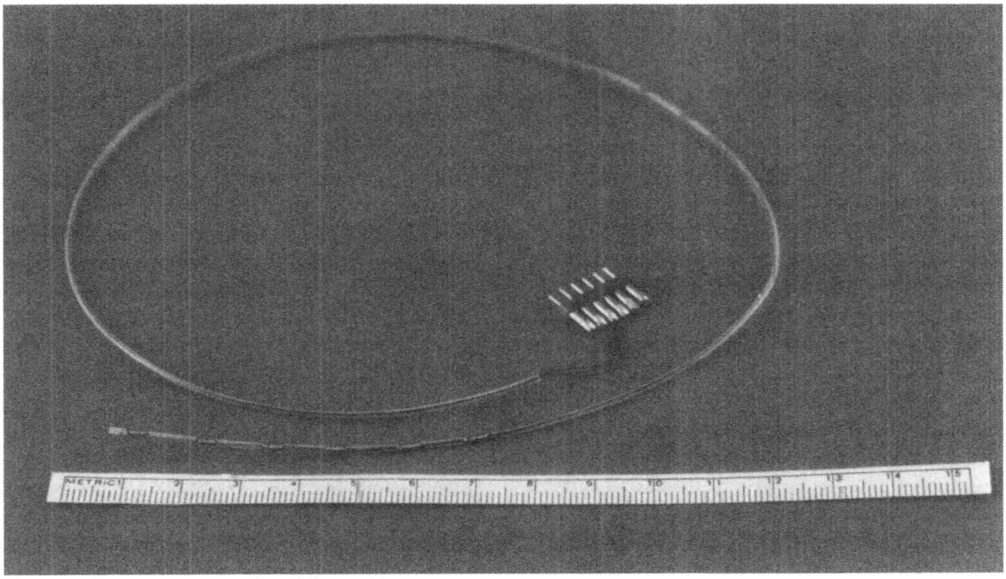

FIGURE 33–2. Six-contact depth electrode (manufactured by Rochester Electro-Medical, Minneapolis, MN); 3-mm contacts are separated by 9-mm intervals; the outer diameter is 1 mm.

INSERTION TECHNIQUE

A recent survey by Engel indicated that 91% of centers using depth electrodes placed them stereotactically, and 31% used computed tomography (CT) guidance [17]. Probe delivery is dictated largely by probe design. The most common techniques are insertion and withdrawal of a central stylet; use of an insertion instrument, the tip of which attaches to a small loop at the end of the electrode (leaving it behind as it is withdrawn); and use of a double cannula through which the electrode can be positioned before the outer cannula is withdrawn.

ARRAY

The type of electrode array must be suited to the goal of the depth electrode study. An array used to identify laterality in a patient with bilateral anterior temporal lobe activity on a scalp EEG may well differ from one used to tailor the extent of hippocampal or temporal lobe resection in a patient with already-established laterality. Engel found that 83% of centers implanted symmetrical arrays and approximately equal numbers used radial and orthogonal approaches [17].

One standard approach for temporal lobe investigation was described by Flanigin [20] and Joseph Smith (personal communication, February 24, 1986). Electrodes are inserted through parasagittal frontal burr holes and placed bilaterally into the amygdala and hippocampus; mesial frontal lobe placement is used when necessary. A modified Todd-Wells frame is used, and coordinates (standard X and Y) are generated from conventional film, the bottom of the sella turcica serving as a reference landmark. The lateral (standard Z) coordinate is generated from a CT scan (usually 20 mm from the midline for the amygdala and 25 mm from the midline for the hippocampal target, which is 20 mm posterior to the amygdala).

An alternative approach to the temporal lobe was reported by Dennis Spencer (meeting of the American Association of Neurological Surgeons [AANS], Boston, MA, 1981). Exploration along the longitudinal axis of the temporal lobe is provided by an additional electrode placed from an occipital entry site. In this manner, recording along the major length of the hippocampus allows detection of the posterior hippocampus focus. The typical array for this technique consists of three electrodes per hemisphere, each directed towards the same reference landmark, 20–25 mm lateral to the tip of the posterior clinoid process (approximating the junction of the amygdala and the hippocampus). The frontal electrodes are inserted 1 cm from the midline and pass anterior to the cingulate and through the subcallosal gyri. The middle temporal electrodes enter 25 mm from the midline and 10 mm anterior to the coronal suture. The posterior electrodes described previously enter within 1 cm of the lambdoid suture, 20–25 mm from the midline, and are angled 3° medially (Dennis Spencer, personal communication, February 23, 1986).

The most extensive explorations thus far are those of the Talairach stereoelectroencephalography school [4, 11, 32, 40, 47, 48]. Incorporating multiple neuroradiological studies (including pneumoencephalography and angiography) into a common stereotactic system, these investigators perform highly individualized explorations to delimit the epileptogenic and related areas as thoroughly as possible. Although not restricted to orthogonal approaches, the Talairach stereotactic frame facilitates the insertion of multiple electrodes, which most often are inserted laterally.

A similar approach, updated to incorporate CT, magnetic resonance imaging (MRI), and digital subtraction angiography, was developed by Olivier and colleagues [35–37]. Their localization process has moved away from CT-generated coordinates to a technique in which angiographic localization of the medial temporal lobe structures (primarily the anterior choroidal artery) determines a plane of interest; a corresponding MRI plane is then obtained. Laterally inserted electrodes record from the amygdala, 22–24 mm from the midline; from the anterior hippocampus, 12 mm posterior to the amygdala electrode and 24–25 mm from the midline; and from the hippocampus, 24 mm posterior to the amygdala electrode and 25–26 mm from the midline. Additional electrodes are placed in an array designed for the individual patient's requirements.

OPERATIVE PROCEDURE

The surgical technique of electrode placement varies as much as the arrays employed. For illustrative purposes, the procedure used at Dartmouth-Hitchcock Medical Center will be described. We have used symmetrical arrays similar to those of Flanigan [20] and Dennis Spencer (personal communication, February 23, 1986; data presented at AANS meeting, Boston, MA, 1981). These arrays were modified for a special group of patients to allow recording from medial callosal radiations [38] (figure 33–3). The CT-adapted Leksell stereotactic system (AB Elekta Instrument, Stockholm, Sweden) has been used for all patients. Semiflexible four- and six-contact single-use electrodes (figure 33–2) have proven reliable.

The stereotactic frame is affixed to the head, and coordinates for electrode placement are generated on a GE 8800 CT scanner (General Electric Medical Systems, Milwaukee, WI). Unenhanced fine scans through the temporal and inferior frontal lobes are sufficient to target the amygdala and fronto-orbital cortex. Anteroposterior and lateral coordinates in the plane of the CT image are well-defined; the lateral coordinate for the amygdala electrode generally lies 20–24 mm from the midline. We have generated that coordinate from CT information, acknowledging that the resolution in the axis of the images is not perfect (and that Olivier has achieved better accuracy [35, 36]).

From the CT suite, the patient is brought to the operating room and placed in either a supine position for frontal and lateral trajectories or a sitting position for occipital approaches. Following repreparation of the scalp and frame, the scalp is infiltrated with 1% lidocaine, and the stereotactic arc and probe guide are positioned for the first electrode. Frontal and anterior temporal electrodes usually are placed through separate entry sites, approximately 2.5 cm from the midline and anterior to the coronal suture. The occipital entry sites approximate those used by Spencer. Through a 3-mm incision, a small craniotomy is made with an air-powered drill and a 3/16-inch Steinmann pin through the bushing guides of the stereotactic frame. The dura is coagulated and perforated with the central stylet of a Backlund biopsy needle (AB Elekta Instrument, Stockholm, Sweden). A cut-off, 14-gauge intravenous catheter (Becton, Dickinson & Co., Rutherford, NJ) is placed over the stylet for insulation of all but the tip.

A modified outer cannula of a Backlund biopsy needle is inserted with the original central stylet to the target coordinates. The cannula is cut away on one side, allowing insertion of electrodes already soldered to connectors. The stylet then is withdrawn, and the electrode is advanced the length of the needle. The connector end of the electrode is brought through the

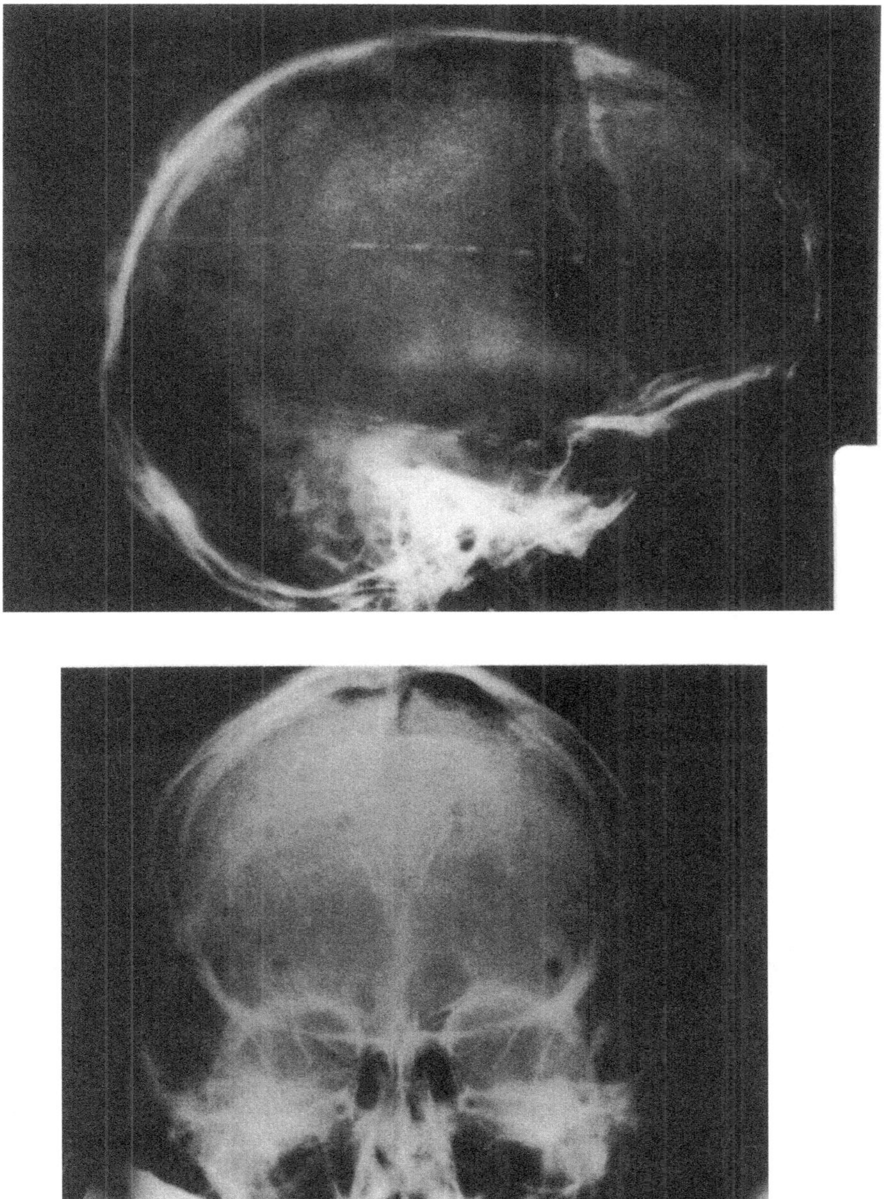

FIGURE 33-3. Symmetrical array of temporal and frontal electrodes. Additional electrodes in the callosal radiations were placed in this patient who was being considered for a corpus callosum section.

side cut, and then the outer cannula is withdrawn, leaving the electrode properly positioned. A single suture closes the incision and secures the electrode. This sequence is repeated for each electrode.

Recording and evaluation of electrode placement take place the same day; actual depth recording usually is begun the following day. We leave electrodes in place from several days to a week and a half and often continue depth recording throughout subsequent seizure surgery and the initial postoperative period

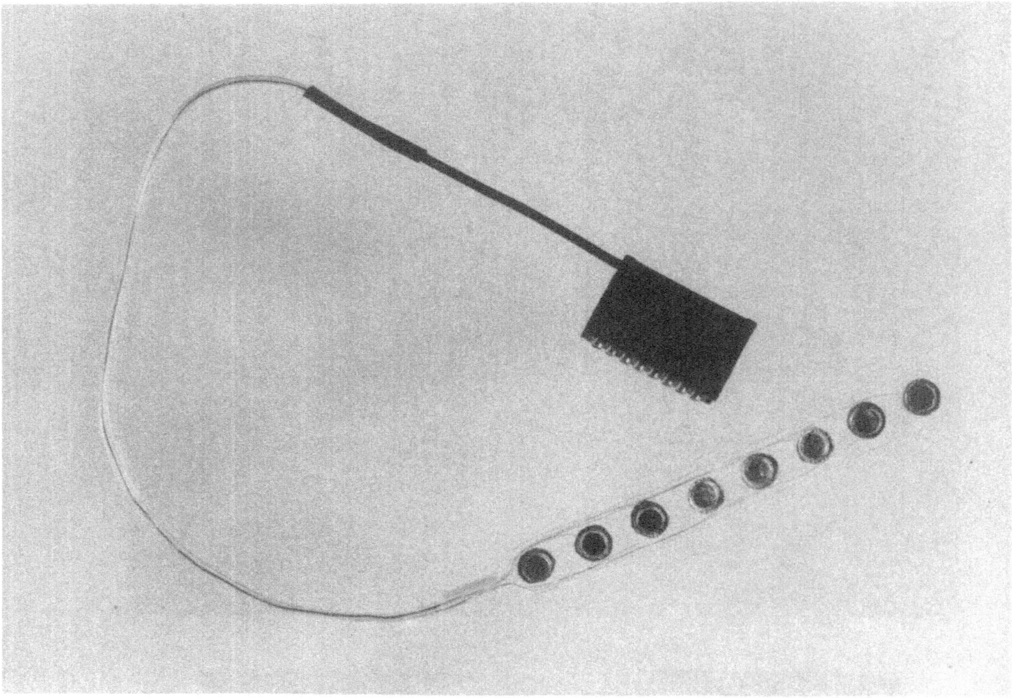

FIGURE 33–4. Eight-contact strip electrode (manufactured by PMT Corporation, Hoskins, MN). The exposed contact surface is 4 mm in diameter; contact centers are 10 mm apart.

without experiencing difficulty. Others have reported recording for as long as six weeks [20]. Electrodes are removed on the neurosurgical ward.

SUBDURAL AND EPIDURAL RECORDING

Subdural placement of multicontact probes has been advocated by Lueders [30, 31], Lesser [29], Rosenbaum [39], and Wyler [53]; epidural placement has been reported by Goldring [23, 24]. Although distinct from depth electrodes placed intraparenchymally, electrode strips and grids warrant mention by virtue of their degree of invasiveness and their similar purpose.

Large grid arrays, which require formal craniotomy for placement, provide broad sampling over considerable cortical surfaces, particularly over the convexities and along the base. Although less satisfactory than depth electrodes in recording subcortical activity, they are superior in recording from the cortical territory they overlie. In addition, physiological mapping through evoked responses or stimulation can be obtained as an aid in the planning of resective surgery, and can at least partially replace mapping and electrocorticography at the time of resection.

Multicontact electrode strips (figure 33–4) can be placed through either burr holes [39, 53] or a larger craniotomy and do not require stereotactic technique. Their advantage over depth electrodes lies in their preservation of parenchymal integrity and their ability to monitor a region of the convexity or basal cortex. They achieve the latter less well than grids, but they suffice when lateralization rather than precise localization is the goal, and their insertion is easier.

Results

Given the intuitively apparent advantages of depth recording, a number of centers advocated the practice early on. Initial comparisons with noninvasive electroencephalography supported the superiority of depth studies, citing both its ability to detect activity absent on the scalp (or additional foci) and its greater precision in lateralizing abnormal activity projected bilaterally on noninvasive recording [1, 2, 6,

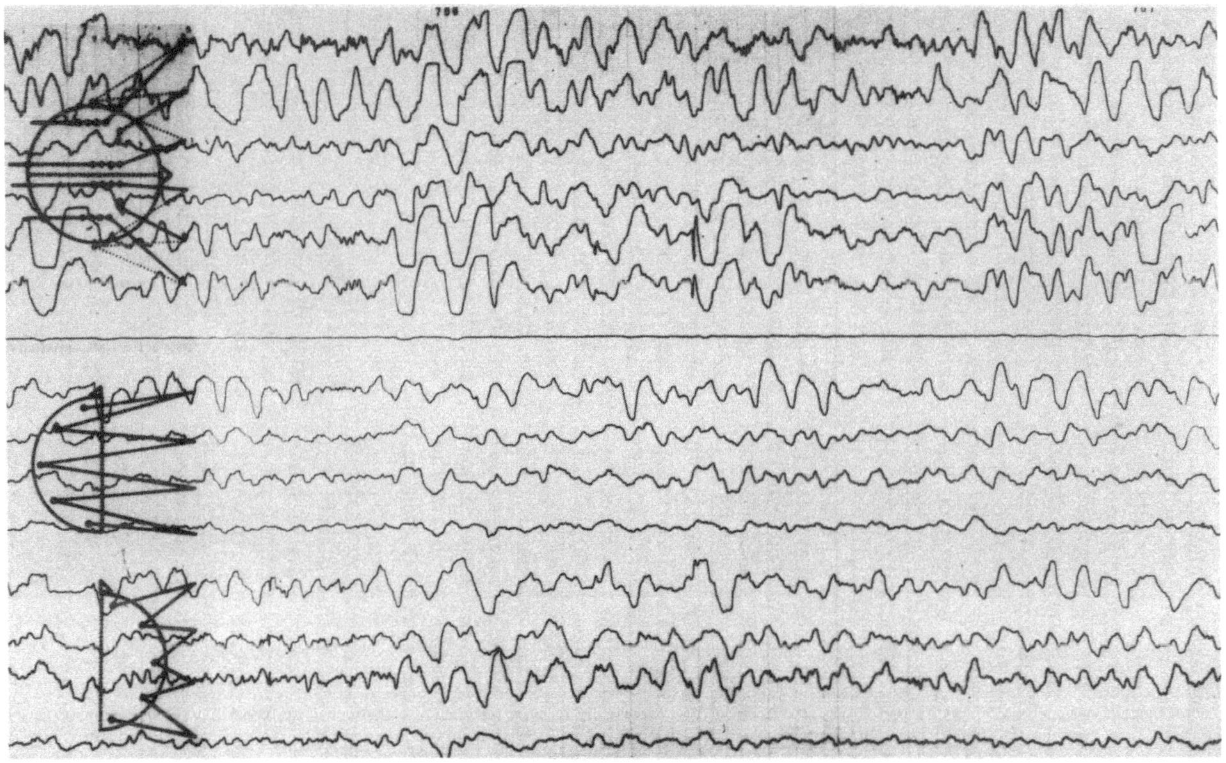

FIGURE 33–5. Scalp and depth (temporal, frontal, callosal) EEGs. At top, the greater sensitivity of the depth recording is evident.

13, 14, 44]. Figure 33–5, a recording of concurrent scalp and depth recording, illustrates this heightened sensitivity.

A review of surgical series at centers using depth recording and those using only noninvasive studies reveals a comparable range of success in seizure improvement for both groups. Although this might appear to contradict the popular opinion that results can be improved when such additional EEG information is available, a review of such series by Susan Spencer suggests that the two groups see different patient populations [44]. Based on data extracted from those reports, she calculates that depth electrode investigation could have enabled an additional 36% of patients to benefit from seizure surgery (by identifying a resectable epileptogenic focus not detected by scalp EEG). Depth electrode studies also could have demonstrated a different or additional focus in an additional 18% of patients and thus spared them an unsuccessful operation. A subsequent report from Yale University confirmed the value of depth recording. Depth studies of 16 patients with nonlocalizing scalp EEGs found three to have a definable focus; depth studies of 15 patients with abnormalities localized by scalp EEG found three to have multiple foci; in four other patients, a different localization was demonstrated by that technique [45]. Spencer's earlier finding of poorer surgical results in patients whose posterior hippocampal focus was not resected remains significant and provocative (data presented at AANS meeting, Boston, MA, 1981).

Engel and colleagues correlated the results of 14 preoperative studies that included scalp and depth EEGs as well as various tests of functional deficits [19]. They found that the most reliable criterion for localization of epileptic foci was depth recording at the site of ictal onset. Interestingly, tests of focal functional deficits, such as thiopental-induced fast activity, intracarotid amobarbital testing, and positron emission tomography (PET) scanning, frequently provided confirmatory evidence of the seizure focus.

The goal of collecting sufficient data from noninvasive testing to avoid depth implantation remains attractive. Engel points out that patients whose scalp recording and other noninvasive tests are consistent in localization may not require depth studies [19]. Although ictal EEG information may fail to localize or may be misleading because of rapid propagation properties, functional tests, when results are abnormal, may be more reliable. This fundamental observation has stimulted enthusiasm for metabolic studies by PET [17–19]. The varying enthusiasm for depth recording corresponds to the degree of confidence in extracting reliable information from noninvasive studies. Ojemann contended that sufficient data usually are present without depth recording [34].

In addition to the benefits derived from depth recording, it is critical to consider the associated complications. Van Buren recently collected such information from 13 centers with a combined experience of 2,674 implantations. These centers reported no mortality, 10 infections, five hemorrhages with permanent deficits, five hemorrhages without permanent deficits, and two cases of Jakob-Creutzfeldt transmission [49]. Another eight centers with 245 implantations of subdural or epidural strips had one infection and one contusion without deficits; nine centers reported 288 implantations of subdural or epidural grids with three infections, one hemorrhage without deficits, one aseptic necrosis of the bone falp, four instances of increased intracranial pressure, and one case of hemiparesis [49]. Individual centers report complications ranging from 1%–8%, with the most frequent and serious morbidity related to hemorrhage and infection [20, 32, 40].

Conclusions

Since the earliest reports of depth electrode recording, the frequent ability of the technique to provide valuable localizing information has been demonstrated repeatedly. At the same time, the technology for depth implantation, recording, and analysis has improved significantly in terms of both accuracy and safety. As an increasing number of neurosurgical departments acquire stereotactic capability, the ability to surgically implant depth electrodes is becoming widespread. The associated electroencephalographic and epilepsy resources, an essential part of the exercise, are almost certainly less prevalent. The technological advances that have facilitated depth recording have also improved or developed complementary studies, and the increasing ease of using implanted electrodes has been balanced by the growing contributions of the noninvasive studies. PET [17–19] magnetoencephalography [5], and newer mathematical methods of scalp EEG analysis that may reliably localize deep abnormalities [43] continue to evolve and potentially decrease dependence on depth EEG.

Whether and how to use depth electrodes remain a decision of the individual epilepsy team. Despite their variation in protocols, most centers would agree that at least some epileptic patients benefit from the investigation. The details of how the technique is used must depend on each center's resources, experience, and judgment.

References

1. Adams JE, Rutkin BB: Diagnostic telemetry from depth electrodes in epilepsy. *Confin Neurol* 34:363–367, 1972
2. Ajmone Marsan C, Abraham K: Considerations on the use of chronically implanted electrodes in seizure disorders. *Confin Neurol* 27:95–110, 1960
3. Angeleri F, Ferro-Milone F, Parigi S: Electrical activity and reactivity of the rhinencephalic, pararhinencephalic and thalamic structures: prolonged implantation of electrodes in man. *Electroencephalogr Clin Neurophysiol* 16:100–129, 1964
4. Bancaud J, Albe-Fessard D, Rayport M, et al: Stereoelectroencephalography. *Handbook Electroencephalogr Clin Neurophysiol* 10B:1–65, 1975
5. Barth DS, Sutherling W, Engel J Jr, et al: Neuromagnetic localization of epileptiform spike activity in the human brain. *Science* 218:891–894, 1982
6. Bates JAV: Special investigation techniques—Indwelling electrodes and electroencephalography. In Hill D, Parr G (eds): *Electroencephalography*. New York: Macmillan, 1963, pp 429–479
7. Berger H: Ueber das Elektrenkephalogram des Menschen. *Arch Psychiatr* 87:527–570, 1929
8. Bickford RG: The application of depth electrography in some varieties of epilepsy. *Electroencephalogr Clin Neurophysiol* 8:526–527, 1956
9. Bickford RG, Uihlein A, Petersen MC: Electrical rhythms recorded from the depth of the frontal lobes during operations on psychotic patients. *Proc Staff Meet Mayo Clin* 28:135–143, 1953
10. Bishop GH, Clare MH: Responses of the cortex to direct electrical stimuli applied at different depths. *J Neurophysiol* 16:1–19, 1953
11. Bouvier G, Mercier C, St. Hilaire JM, et al: Anterior callosotomy and chronic depth electrode recording in the surgical management of some intractable seizures *Appl Neurophysiol* 46:52–56, 1983
12. Brazier MAB: Depth recordings from the amygdaloid region in patients with temporal lobe epilepsy. *Electroencephalogr Clin Neurophysiol* 8:532–533, 1956
13. Crandall PH: Developments in direct recordings from epileptogenic regions in the surgical treatment of partial epilepsies. In Brazier MAB (ed): *Epilepsy, Its Phenomena In Man*, Vol 17. New York: Academic Press, 1973, pp 287–310
14. Crandall PH, Walter RD, Rank RW: Clinical applications of studies on stereotactically implanted electrodes in temporal-lobe epilepsy. *J Neurosurg* 20:827–840, 1963
15. Delgado J: Use of intracerebral electrodes in human patients. *Electroencephalogr Clin Neurophysiol* 8:528–530, 1956
16. Dodge HW, Bailey AA, Bickford RG, et al: Neurosurgical and neurologic application of depth electrography. *Proc Staff Meet Mayo Clin* 28:188–191, 1953
17. Engel J Jr: Approaches to lateralization. In *Proceedings of the International Conference on the Surgical Treatment of Epilepsy* (Palm Desert, CA, February 20–24, 1986). New York: Raven Press (In press)
18. Engel J Jr, Kuhl DE, Phelps ME, et al: Comparative localization of epileptic foci in partial epilepsy by PCT and EEG. *Ann Neurol* 12:529–537, 1982
19. Engel J Jr, Rausch R, Kuhl DE, et al: Correlation of criteria used for localizing epileptic foci in patients considered for surgical therapy of epilepsy. *Ann Neurol* 9:215–224, 1981
20. Flanigan H: Depth electrode implantation. In *Proceedings of the International Conference on the Surgical Treatment of Epilepsy* (Palm Desert, CA, February 20–24, 1986). New York: Raven Press (In press)
21. Foerster O, Altenburger H: Elektrobiologische Vorgange an der menschlichen Hirnrinde. *Deutsche Ztschr f Nervenk* 135:277–288, 1935
22. Gerard RW, Marshall WH, Saul LJ: Electrical activity of the cat's brain. *Arch Neurol Psychiatr* 36:675–738, 1936
23. Goldring S: Epilepsy surgery. *Clin Neurosurg* 31:369–388, 1983
24. Goldring S: Extradural grids. In *Proceedings of the International Conference on the Surgical Treatment of Epilepsy* (Palm Desert, CA,

February 20–24, 1986). New York: Raven Press (In Press)

25. Hayne RA, Belison L, Gibbs FA: Electrical activity of subcortical areas in epilepsy. *Electroencephalogr Clin Neurophysiol* 1:437–445, 1949
26. Heath RG: Correlation of electrical recordings from cortical and subcortical regions of the brain with abnormal behavior in human subjects. *Confin Neurol* 18:305–315, 1958
27. Heath RG, Peacock SM, Miller W: Induced paroxysmal electrical activity in man recorded simultaneously through subcortical and scalp electrodes. *Trans Am Neurol Assoc* 78:247, 1953
28. Kellaway P: Depth recording in focal epilepsy. *Electroencephalogr Clin Neurophysiol* 8:527–528, 1956
29. Lesser R, Dinner B, Lueders H, et al: Differential diagnosis and treatment of intractable seizures. *Cleve Clin Q* 51:227–240, 1984
30. Lueders H: Invasive EEG recording: Discussion. In *Proceedings of the International Conference on the Surgical Treatment of Epilepsy* (Palm Desert, CA February 20–24, 1986). New York: Raven Press (In press)
31. Lueders H. Hahn J, Lesser RP, et al: Localization of epileptogenic spike foci: Comparative study of closely spaced scalp electrodes, nasopharyngeal, sphenoidal, subdural, and depth electrodes. In Akimoto H, Kazamatsuri H, Seino M, et al (eds): *Advances in Epileptology:* XIIIth Epilepsy International Symposium. New York: Raven Press, 1982, pp 185–189
32. Munari C: Depth electrode implantation. In *Proceedings of the International Conference on Surgical Treatment of Epilepsy* (Palm Desert, CA, February 20–24, 1986). New York: Raven Press (In press)
33. Niedermeyer E: Depth electroencephalography. In Niedermeyer E, da Silva FL: *Electroencephalography: Basic Principles, Clinical Applications, and Related Fields.* Baltimore: Urban and Schwartzenberg, 1981, pp 519–536
34. Ojemann G: Invasive EEG recording. In *Proceedings of the International Conference on the Surgical Treatment of Epilepsy* (Palm Desert, CA, February 20–24, 1986). New York: Raven Press (In press)
35. Olivier A: Depth electrode implantation. In *Proceedings of the International Conference on the Surgical Treatment of Epilepsy* (Palm Desert, CA, February 20–24, 1986). New York: Raven Press (In press)
36. Olivier A, Gloor P, Quesney LF, et al: The indications for and the role of depth electrode recording in epilepsy. *Appl Neurophysiol* 46:33–36, 1983
37. Peters TM, Olivier A, Bertrand G: The role of computed tomographic and digital radiographic techniques in stereotactic procedures for electrode implantation and mapping and lesion localization. *Appl Neurophysiol* 46:200–205, 1983
38. Roberts DW, Allen CD, Allen AH, et al: Depth electrode recording in patients undergoing corpus callosotomy for intractable epilepsy. *Appl Neurophysiol* 46:26–32, 1983
39. Rosenbaum T: Strip electrodes. In *Proceedings of the International Conference on the Surgical Treatment of Epilepsy* (Palm Desert, CA, February 20–24, 1986). New York: Raven Press (In press)
40. St. Hilaire JM: Depth electrode implantation. In *Proceedings of the International Conference on the Surgical Treatment of Epilepsy* (Palm Desert, CA, February 20–24, 1986). New York: Raven Press (In press)
41. Sem-Jacobson CW: *Depth Electrographic Stimulation of the Human Brain and Behavior.* Springfield, IL: Thomas, 1968
42. Shinners BM, Hamby WB, Krauss R: The electrical activity of the thalamus and cortical remnants in a case of schizencephaly. *Electroencephalogr Clin Neurophysiol* 1:522, 1949
43. Smith DB, Sidman RD, Flanigan H, et al: A reliable method for localizing deep intracranial sources of the EEG. *Neurology* 35:1702–1707, 1985
44. Spencer SS: Depth electroencephalography in selection of refractory epilepsy for surgery. *Ann Neurol* 9:207–214, 1981
45. Spencer SS, Spencer DD, Williamson PD, et al: The localizing value of depth electroencephalography in 32 patients with refractory epilepsy. *Ann Neurol* 12:248–253, 1982
46. Spiegel EA: Comparative study of the thalamic cerebral and cerebellar potentials. *Am J Physiol* 118:569–579, 1937
47. Talairach J, Bancaud J: Stereotaxic approach to epilepsy: Methodology of anatomo-functional stereotaxic investigations. In Krayenbuhl H, Maspes PE, Sweet WH (eds): *Progress in Neurological Surgery*, Vol 5, New York: S Karger, 1973, pp 297–354
48. Talairach J, Bancaud J: Stereotaxic exploration and therapy in epilepsy. In Vinken PJ, Bruyn CW (eds): *Handbook of Clinical Neurology*, Vol 15, *The Epilepsies.* Amsterdam: North Holland, 1974, pp 758–782
49. Van Buren J: Complications. In *Proceedings of the ____ International Conference on the Surgical Treatment of Epilepsy* (Palm Desert, CA, February 20–24, 1986). New York: Raven Press (In press)
50. Walker AE, Uematsu S, Niedermeyer E, et al: Depth recording. In Schaltenbrand G, Walker AE (eds): *Stereotaxy of the Human Brain: Ana-*

tomical, Physiological and Clinical Applications. New York: Thieme-Stratton, 1982, pp 661–668
51. Walter WG, Crow HJ: Depth recording from the human brain. *Electroencephalogr Clin Neurophysiol* 16:68–72, 1964
52. Williams D, Parsons-Smith G: The spontaneous electrical activity of the human thalamus. *Brain* 72:450–482, 1949
53. Wyler AR, Ojemann GA, Lettich E, et al: Subdural strip electrodes for localizing epileptogenic foci. *J Neurosurg* 60:1195–1200, 1984

34. STEREOTACTIC CT ATLASES

Tyrone L. Hardy

Computed tomography (CT) is well established as a valuable diagnostic and investigative imaging device and has revolutionized the evaluation and treatment of neurological conditions. The increasing applications and use of CT technology with stereotactic and functional neurosurgery are readily evidenced by the many articles dealing with this subject in published proceedings of stereotactic and functional neurosurgical societies [3, 17]. Advancing computer technology has been the basis upon which CT scanning technology has developed; this same technology is supporting the development of the newer digital angiographic and nuclear magnetic resonance (NMR) imaging systems.

The increased resolution afforded by CT and NMR scanning systems allows direct identification of brain structures that could only be inferred from conventional roentgenological techniques. Stereotactic surgery, being primarily a procedure performed without the aid of direct visualization, is dependent on sophisticated imaging techniques for its accurate execution. Therefore, it necessarily follows that as computer and imaging technology improve, so do the possibilities of stereotactic surgery. This chapter is primarily concerned with the use of computer-graphics techniques and CT scanning for generating composite CT brain-scan/atlas-map images to better aid the stereotactic neurosurgeon in localizing subcortical structures.

Historical Background

In the early 1970s, we developed a computer system that could display digitized diencephalic brain maps to the neurosurgeon during stereotactic thalamotomy for dyskinesias [4, 20, 21]. The software program for the system operated in a computer with a graphics display terminal that could be taken to the operating suite for interactive use by the neurosurgeon. The system had several important features:

1. It could display scaled digitized diencephalic maps (figures 34–1, 34–2), which could be adjusted to the size of the patient's diencephalon as determined from measurements (e.g., intercommissural distance, thalamic height, and third-ventricular width) taken from a stereotactic contrast encephalogram (figures 34–3, 34–4). Because the target position for diencephalic subnuclear structures generally is determined by proportional extrapolation from standardized atlas maps [18, 19], this particular feature allowed the atlas maps to be expanded or contracted to more closely fit a given patient's diencephalic measurements, thus increasing the accuracy of target size determination. The problems resulting from diencephalic anatomical differences were thereby considerably diminished.

2. The system corrected the complex three-dimensional geometric problems inherent in a precise stereotactic technique and presented an on-line graphic display of the position of stereotactic probes and electrodes superimposed on cross-sections of the human thalamus. This particular feature is important because the stereotactic technique is principally a blind surgical procedure reliant upon a coordinate system for anatomical localization of subcortical structures. Therefore, it is difficult for stereotactic surgeons to conceptualize the location of surgical probes inserted into deep brain structures; they must imagine the location of the probe while taking into account its forward and lateral angles, its distance from the

The author wishes to thank our project engineer and director, John McGuffin, and our engineers and systems programmers, Karl Kortkamp, Clark Tampsett, Mike Collier, and Kevin Stroup, for their tireless efforts in the development of this system.

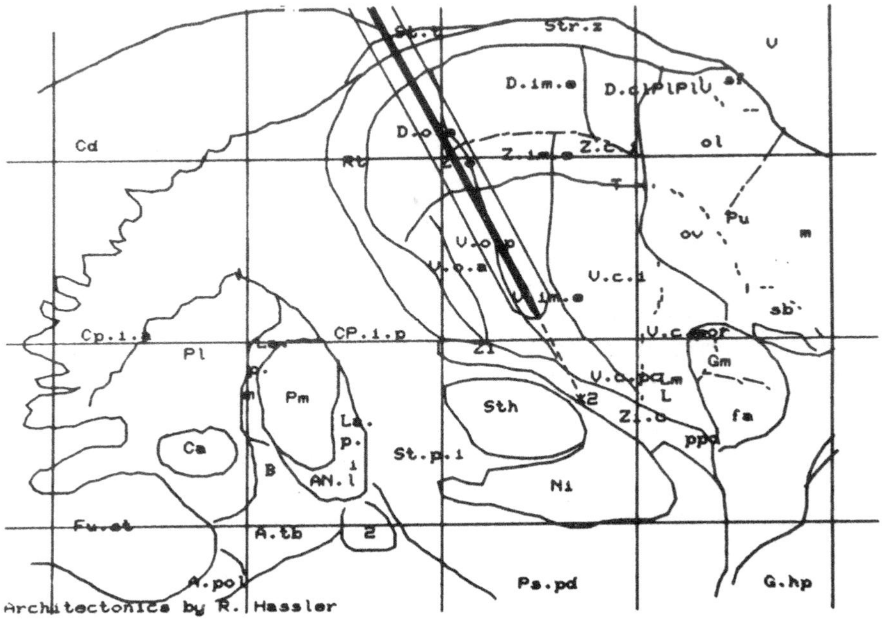

A

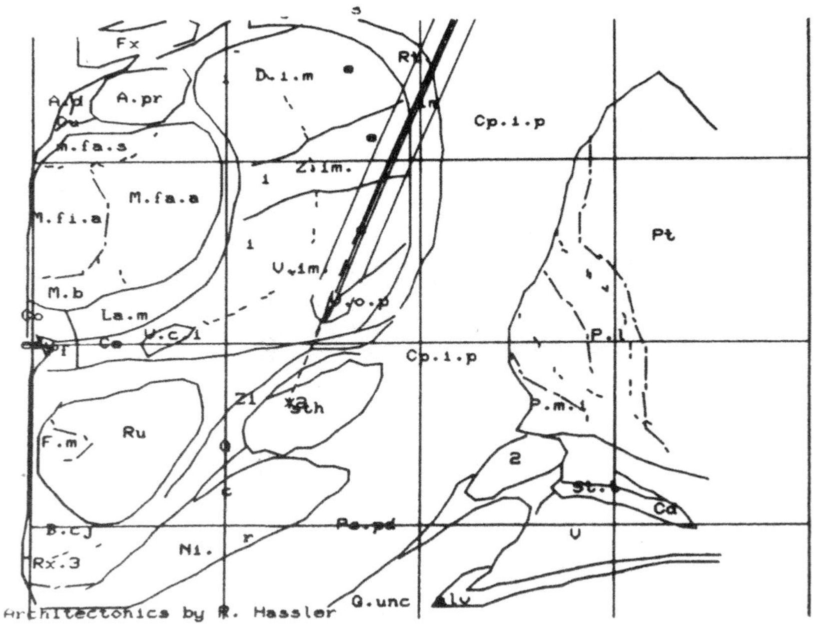

B

FIGURE 34–1. Sagittal (A), frontal (B), and horizontal (C) maps of the diencephalon (digitized from the Schaltenbrand and Bailey *Atlas* [18]). The probe is directed at a target structure and has its electrode (tip indicated by asterisk) projecting from its end. The dashed lines indicate the portion of the probe and/or electrode extending beyond the plane of the displayed map.

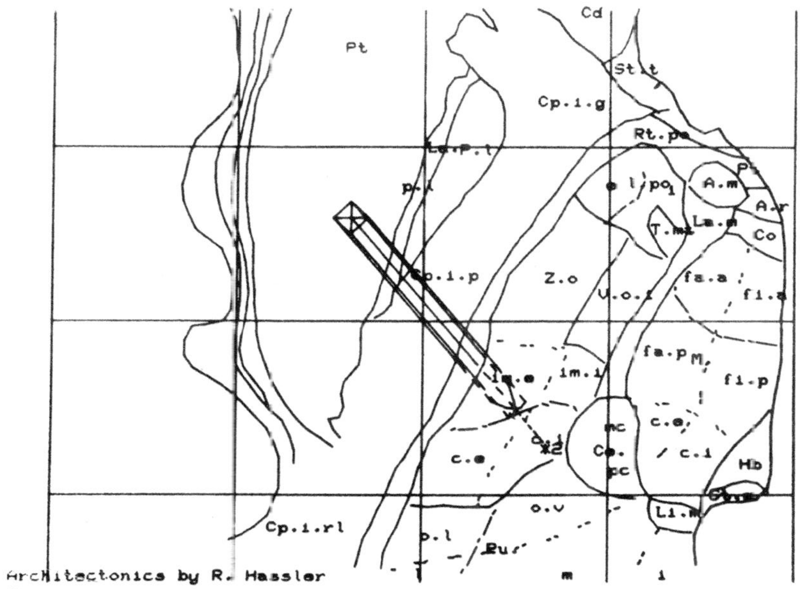

C

FIGURE 34–1. (cont.)

target, and the direction of any electrode extending from the probe (in cases in which curved exploratory electrodes are used). Misalignment of the stereotactic frame on the patient's head (i.e., collateral displacement and tilt, rotational and skew angulation) compound the potential for error in correctly placing the surgical probe [4, 5, 8, 21]. The software functions of the computer system corrected for these many variables and, by graphic simulation, helped the surgeon accurately envision the position of a probe or an electrode with respect to various subdivisions of the thalamus.

3. The system was able to store and selectively display the position of various coded electrophysiological responses found during exploratory diencephalic stimulation and recording (figures 34–5, 34–6). This capability was important because data gathered from various electrophysiological methods (e.g., exploratory stimulation and recording about the intended target site) could be stored in a disc-based file that could display selected response points from a large group of patients on a digitized map background. Data displayed in this manner aided in the more precise determination of nuclear zones and in the electrophysiological mapping of the diencephalon [4, 6, 7].

Computer-Assisted Stereotactic Surgery (CASS) System Development and Modifications

With the capabilities just described, we found the computer to be a useful adjunct to our stereotactic operative technique, as have other authors with similar techniques [1, 2]. Consequently, since its development, there have been numerous modifications of the original system [8–11]. These modifications have been concerned mainly with increasing the system's portability, improving its graphics capability, and adapting the system for use with the newer imaging technologies of CT and NMR scans.

The original system was designed to run on a Digital Equipment Corporation (Albuquerque, NM) PDP-12 computer with software written in assembly-level language. This system was very large and could not be taken into the operating room. The graphics display terminal, which could be taken separately into the operating room, had to be interfaced with the computer by long coaxial linkages. This method

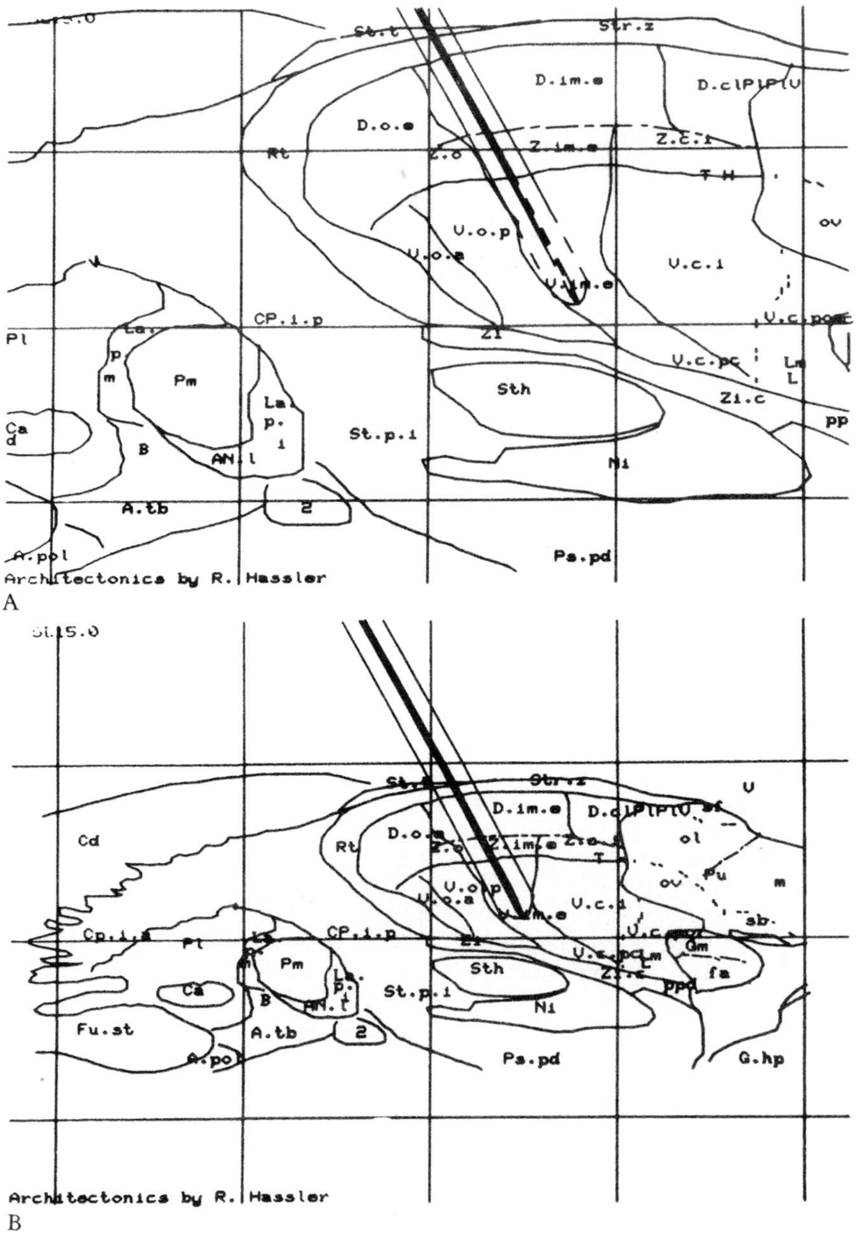

FIGURE 34–2. Example of two sagittal diencephalic maps demonstrating the computer's ability to change the size of the maps displayed. Map A has an "exaggerated" intercommissural distance (ICD) of 40 mm and a "normal" thalamic height of 19 mm. Map B has an "exaggerated" ICD of 40 mm and an unusually small thalamic height of 10 mm (maps from Schaltenbrand and Bailey Atlas [18]). By comparison, the sagittal map in figure 34–3 has an ICD of 23 mm and a thalamic height of 19 mm.

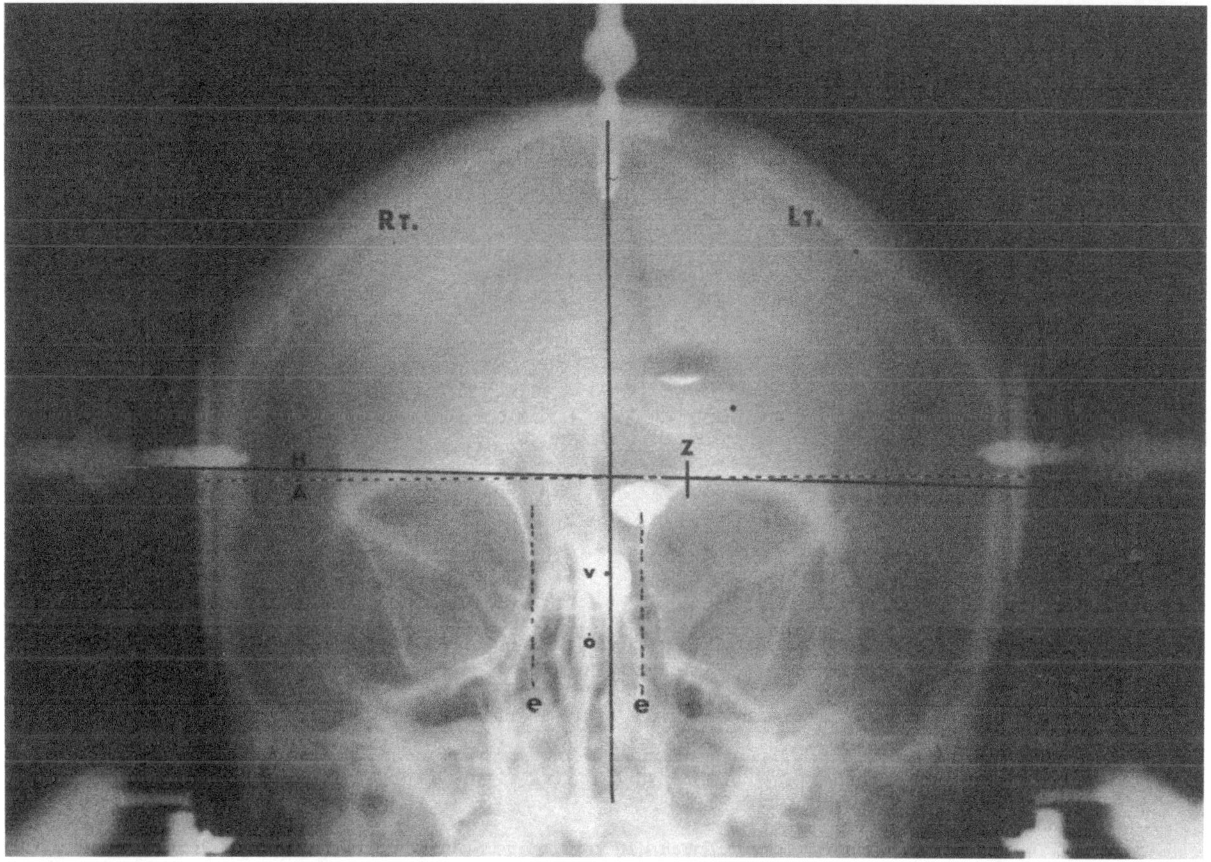

FIGURE 34–3. Anterior-posterior roentgenogram with central roentgen ray beam aligned in mid-vertical plane of frame. Z is in the target position for a left thalamotomy. The line H is the horizontal plane of the brain drawn parallel to the orbital roofs. Line A is the horizontal plane of the stereotactic frame intersecting H at the mid-vertical plane. The angle formed by the intersection of lines A and H is the *tilt* angle. V represents the center of the third ventricle. Dotted parallel lines (e) are tangent to the medial orbital walls. Point O is equidistant between lines e. The horizontal distance between O and V represents the displacement due to *rotational* angulation. There is no collateral (mediolateral) misalignment, because point V coincides with the mid-ventricular plane of the Leksell stereotactic frame.

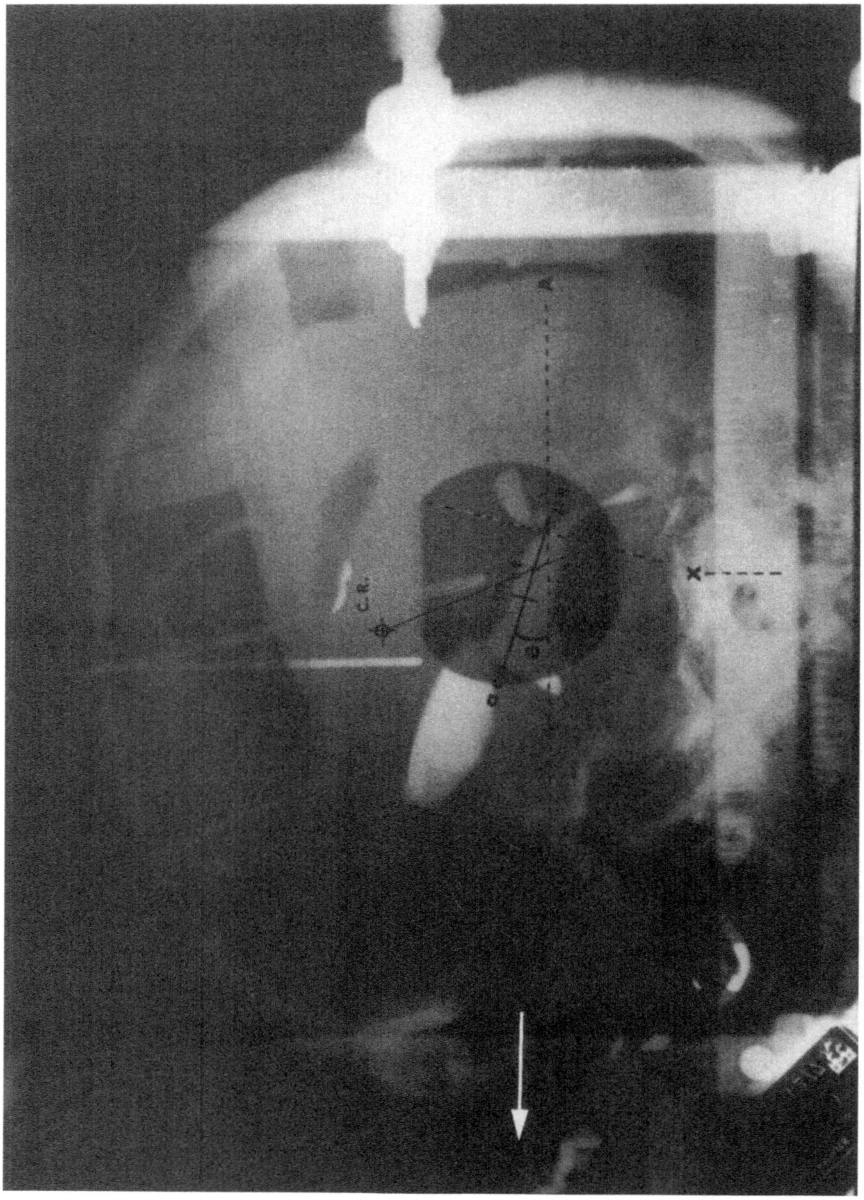

FIGURE 34–4. A lateral contrast encephalogram with a stylet in the frontal horn of the lateral ventricle. C.R. is the incidence point of the central roentgen ray beam on the roentgenogram. The radian from C.R. (*arrow*) is constructed to the target (T) on the anterior commissure-posterior commissure line (Leksell method [13]). The point along this radian above T is the corrected target position for magnification and distortion. X and Y (*white arrow*) are coordinates for this corrected target. Line A is the horizontal plane of the frame. Angle *e* represents the *skew* angle (Leksell stereotactic frame [4, 14]).

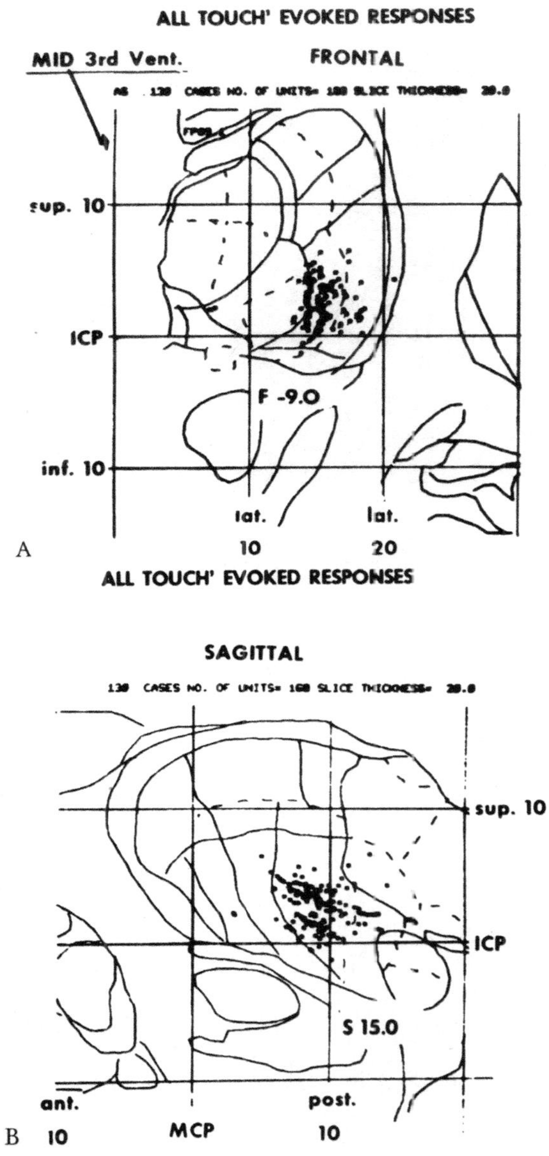

FIGURE 34–5. Computer maps on frontal (A) and sagittal (B) diencephalic map sections show the position of coded responses to light touch-evoked unit cellular responses found during microelectrode exploratory recordings. Map sections are from the Schaltenbrand and Bailey *Atlas* [18]). There are a total of 168 units obtained from 130 patients. Responses are plotted according to their true spatial coordinates with respect to a common midcommissural point (MCP) (see [7]). F − 9.0 = 9 mm posterior to MCP. S − 15.0 = 15 mm lateral to mid–third ventricle.

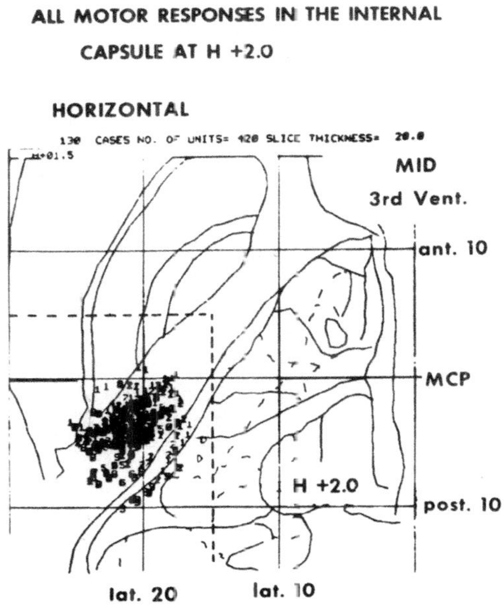

FIGURE 34–6. Horizontal diencephalic map from the Schaltenbrand and Bailey *Atlas* [18] at H + 2.0 (2 mm above the intercommissural plane) showing the position in 130 stereotactic procedures of 420 motor responses to exploratory stimulation in the posterior limb of the internal capsule. MCP is midcommissural plane (Reprinted with permission from *Applied Neurophysiol* 42:160–170, 1979.)

of operation was cumbersome but necessary, given the hardware constraints inherent in the computer design. When the considerably smaller and portable newer type of PDP-11 MINC computer was developed by Digital Equipment Corporation, we undertook the very extensive project of converting the software programs for the original system to run in Fortran on this smaller computer system, which we called CASS (computer-assisted stereotactic surgery). Some additional enhancements to the original computer software also were developed [8, 9]. As computer design has advanced we have integrated increasingly smaller and more sophisticated computer hardware systems for our use [10, 11].

The stereotactic brain maps of the diencephalon, with architectonics by R. Hassler [12], were digitized for use with the original system from the earlier Schaltenbrand and Bailey stereotaxic atlas [18]. Software routines

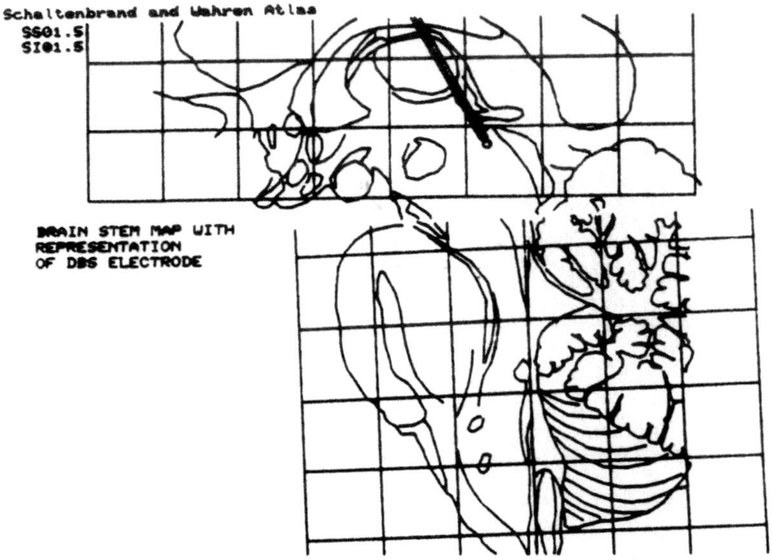

FIGURE 34–7. Sagittal diencephalic and brain-stem map. The tip of a stimulating electrode lies at the periaqueductal area (digitized from the Schaltenbrand and Wahren *Atlas* [19]) (see figure 34–14B). DBS = deep brain stimulation, simulation of a product from Medtronic, Inc. (Minneapolis, MN).

for modifying the computer displays of the brain maps were necessary to correct for deficiencies in anatomical sectioning (the horizontal sections vary 8° from the intercommissural plane) and for variations in the sizes of the atlas maps (the frontal maps were considerably smaller than the horizontal maps). The coordinate system for the digitized atlas map sections were based, as those of the anatomical atlas maps, on a brain coordinate system constructed about the third ventricular core; that is, an intercommissural line bisected by a midcommissural line and a horizontal line representing the basal plane of the brain.

The brain stem and cerebellar maps of the newer Schaltenbrand and Wahren atlas [19] afforded an opportunity to expand our computer mapping capabilities to include these rhombencephalic structures (figure 34–7) [9]. Incorporating these maps into our computer system required the development of a coordinate system that would allow the simultaneous display of diencephalic architectonics and the remaining brain stem and cerebellum (figure 34–8). Allowance was also required for variations in the angle of the junction of the diencephalon with the lower brain stem. For example, the angle of intersection will be closer to 90° in a patient with a brachycephalic brain in which brain-stem angulation is perpendicularly oriented. Both coordinate systems can be moved independently of each other; the size of the brain maps, including the brain-stem length, can be readily varied to match the patient's anatomical dimensions as determined from contrast ventriculograms, CT, or NMR scans. As noted in figure 34–8, this was accomplished by developing a method of intersecting an upper (diencephalic) coordinate system constructed about the third ventricular core, with a lower coordinate system constructed about the fourth ventricle. Adjustments for differences in brain-stem sizes were achieved by a software subroutine that could be prompted to expand or contract the digitized maps.

In recent years, advancing computer technology has resulted in the development of high-resolution, color-graphics raster display monitors that can interface with small computer systems. With improvements in this technology, it became possible to modify our comput-

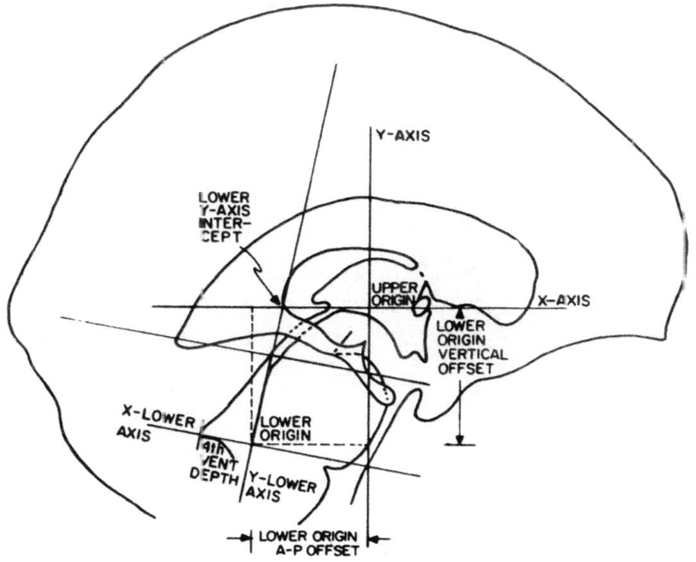

FIGURE 34–8. Upper and lower coordinate systems, modified from Schaltenbrand and Wahren [19] for use in the computer program. The upper origin is the midintercommissural point; the lower origin is the intersection of a perpendicular line from the apex of the fourth ventricle on a line tangent to the floor of the aqueduct and fourth ventricle. The upper and lower coordinate systems intersect along the X axis, which is an extension of the intercommissural line (lower Y-axis intercept). The angle formed by this intersection varies according to a patient's brain-stem angulation.

er system so that it could use such a monitor to display CT images and benefit from the addition of color graphics. The result was our first portable CT-CASS system [10, 11], which could store, manipulate, and selectively display CT images in the operating room independent of the CT scanner. Our previously digitized atlas maps also could be superimposed on CT sections of the diencephalon. This method of graphic operative simulation could serve as a valuable guide for using CT data in performing functional neurosurgery. The advantage of the CT-CASS system is that it avoids the extreme expense of a CT-dedicated stereotactic system or the cumbersome and cost-inefficient use of a nondedicated CT scanner for performing stereotactic surgery. As opposed to these CT-controlled stereotactic techniques, most stereotactic surgeons are inclined by circumstance to use a CT-guided method in which preoperative CT data is taken to the operating room for use during surgery. Our efforts, therefore, have been focused on improving this CT-CASS system, which is an enhanced CT-guided technique.

Hardware

The present hardware system (Medical Instrumentation and Diagnostics Corporation, MITDO, Albuquerque, NM) is based on the Motorola (Phoenix, AZ) 68000 Microprocessor (figure 34–9) and functions on a VME BUS at a clock rate of approximately 12.5 MHz. The system has a hard-disc drive sufficient in storage size to hold 20 CT (or NMR) images. A specially interfaced imaging board in the computer allows CT (or NMR) images to be directly loaded into the computer's memory for subsequent hard-disc storage. Digital image processing of up to 12 "bit planes" of graphics overlay is possible. A 19-inch color video monitor is used for image display and graphics. The monitor has a touch screen for ease of cursor functions and software menu manipulation. The system also has a 5¼-inch floppy-disc drive and a hard-copy unit. This hardware system is small, portable, and has sufficient memory and speed to efficiently execute software commands. CT or NMR images from any scanner can be captured by the system. This

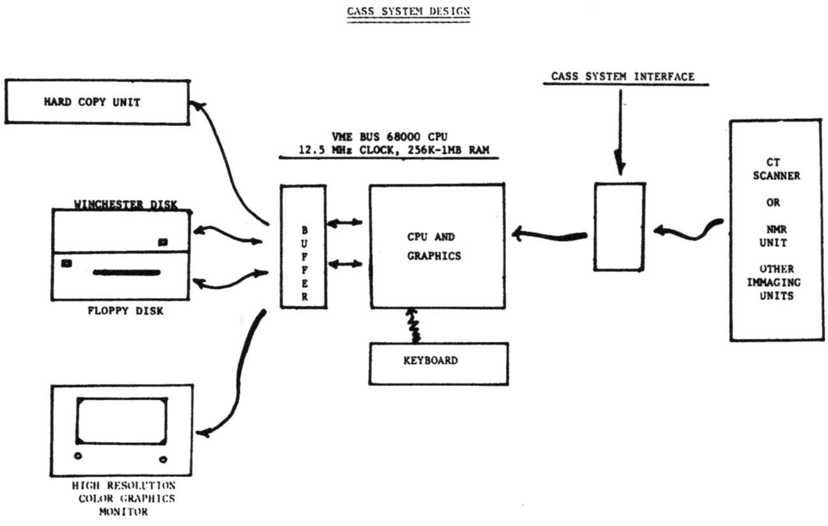

FIGURE 34–9. CASS system design.

particular feature is a considerable improvement over our previous system, which had to be programmed separately for each type of scanner [10].

Software Environment

CT (NMR)-CASS is written in Fortran under the Unix System V operating system (Bell Laboratories, Blue Bell, PA). The software environment is structured on a multiple modular bi-divisional foundation, which consists of a division for CT/NMR-image enhancement and manipulation and a division for graphics and user-specific functions. Each division can be entered via the main menu. Specific menus for divisional subroutines then can be selected for desired functions. The division for CT/NMR-image enhancement and manipulation includes modular software subroutines for (1) image capture, storage, and archiving; (2) pixel analysis for an entire image or user-defined areas of interest; (3) zoom and pan functions; (4) contrasting and filtering images with functions for smoothing, sharpening, Laplacian, and pseudocoloring; and (5) image editing.

The division for graphics and user-specific functions contains software modular subroutines that control (1) the manipulation and swapping of 110 diencephalic and brain-stem atlas maps in frontal, sagittal, and horizontal sections; (2) the manipulation of various probes and electrodes; (3) alphanumeric functions for demographic data and for coding, storing, and selectively displaying the position of various electrophysiological response points; and (4) measurement functions for determining stereotactic coordinates and other user-specific calculations.

The software routines are organized on a 12-bit plane (2^{12}) hardware overlay format (figure 34–10) for graphic simulation and composite image display. Each bit plane has been assigned specific software functions. CT/NMR images, for example, require eight bit planes (2^8) to display the standard 256 × 256 grayscale matrix of the average scanner. This particular feature is analogous to stacked transparent cellophane planes upon which different data or images can be written. The information on these planes is overlaid and, therefore, viewed as a composite picture on the video monitor. Software routines allow data on each plane to be manipulated separately. Thus, this particular hardware-software format allows the independent manipulation of CT/NMR images, brain maps, probes, electrodes, coordinate and map measurements, and coded physiological data points to produce various composite images for operative simulation during surgery.

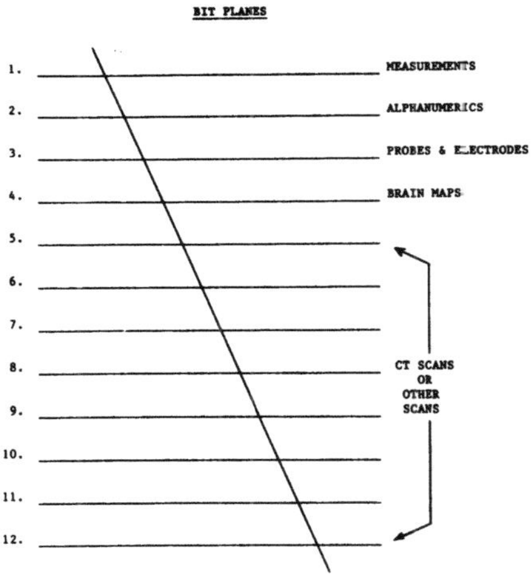

FIGURE 34–10. Computer graphics "bit-plane" format for composite image formation. Each horizontal line represents a "bit-plane." There are a total of 12 planes overlaid upon each other, each with a designated function.

Operation of CT-CASS

Most stereotactic surgeons regard the nucleus ventralis intermedius (V.i.m.) of the thalamus as the anatomical target site of choice for lesion production to treat dyskinesias. Others prefer to extend the lesion slightly into the dorsal subthalamic H-fields of Forel. The total target is small, approximately 6 × 4 × 4 mm. It is bounded by areas with important anatomical functions, e.g., motor fibers in the internal capsule laterally, the sensory nucleus posteriorly, the mammillothalamic bundle medially, and the subthalamic nucleus inferiorly. Therefore, lesion localization must be accurate; lesions should not extend into these surrounding areas. CT-scanning localization allows direct imaging of this target area, which could only be inferred from contrast encephalographic techniques. Although current CT-scanning technology cannot discern specific thalamic nuclei, it can demonstrate the thalamocapsular border that is the lateral limit of a thalamic lesion in V.i.m.

In our CT-guided technique, the base frame of the Leksell stereotactic instrument [13, 14] is attached to the patient's head, and then contiguous, small-increment CT images are taken in the region of the thalamus. For adequate reformatting purposes, CT images taken in 1.5-mm increments, approximately in the area 20–30 mm above the posterior clinoid process, generally will include both anterior and posterior commissures. Once images through the commissures are obtained, the thickness of the images can be increased. This will reduce scanning time and decrease the radiation dose to the patient. The area of smaller contiguous cuts then can be bracketed (above and below) by 4–5 mm slices. These scans then are used to obtain a reformatted midsagittal CT scan (figure 34–11).

The anterior and posterior commissures are identified on the midsagittal image, from which a reformatted horizontal CT image (figure 34–12) next is obtained. Latchaw and co-workers described a somewhat similar technique [15]. An image at this level is along the intercommissural plane and represents the maximal depth along the Z ordinate. (A probe placed much below this level could damage the subthalamic nucleus.) This and any other image parallel to the intercommissural plane can be stored in the CT-CASS computer. The patient and the computer then can be transported to the operating room for surgery, leaving the CT scanner for its regular use.

In the operating room, the computer system's software division for image enhancement and manipulation can be used to identify and further clarify the thalamocapsular border, which is the lateral boundary of the intended target area of V.i.m. for dyskinesia. In this regard, the computer's software routines for pixel analysis can sharpen the CT image, and, if desired, white matter and gray matter can be color-coded separately for even greater contrast (see figure 34–14A). The software routines for diencephalic map manipulation can be used next to create composite CT scan/map overlay images (figure 34–13) that will show the relative position of thalamic nuclear divisions. Measurement subroutines allow tentative determination of the target coordinates.

The mediolateral X ordinate and the anterior-posterior Y ordinate of the chosen target site can be determined very accurately by CT measurements. Z-ordinate determinations are not so accurate because they are dependent on scan-slice thickness. To avoid damage to the subthalamic nucleus, care must be taken to ensure that the depth of a stereotactic probe tip does not extend along the Z ordinate more than 1 mm below the intercommissural plane.

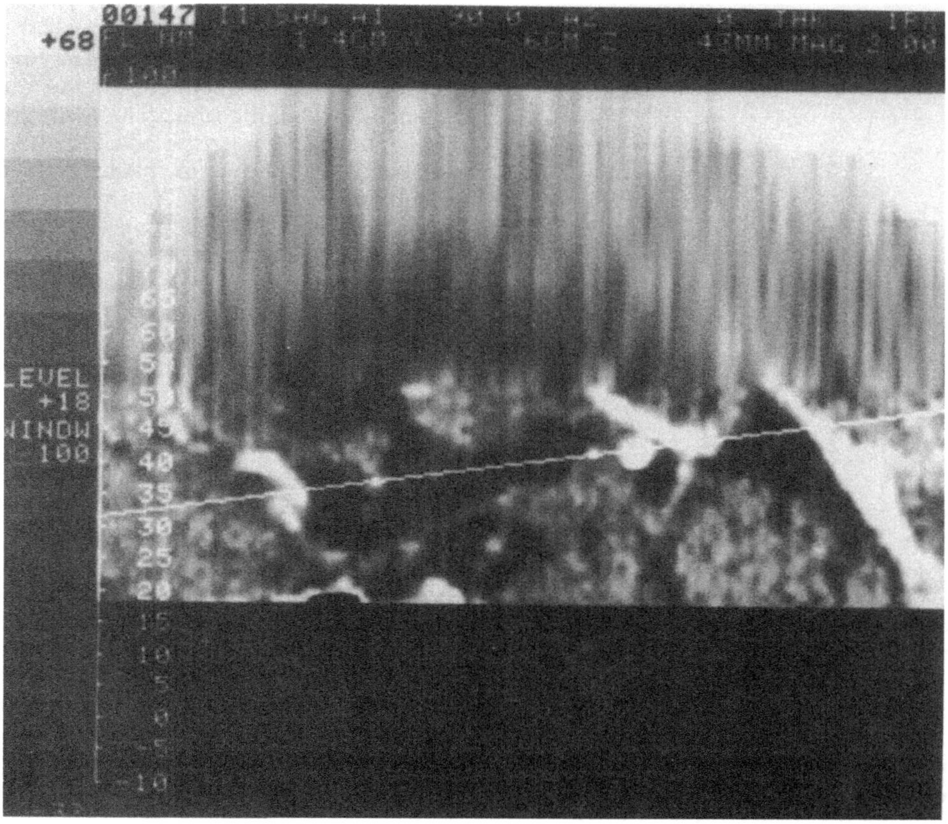

FIGURE 34–11. Reformatted sagittal CT image. A line runs through the anterior and posterior commissures.

After the coordinate measurements for the intended target site are determined, a trajectory for the stereotactic probe can be simulated for evaluation and manipulation prior to actual placement in the target area. The position of the probe that was determined by CT measurements can be confirmed in the operating suite by use of standard anterior-posterior and lateral roentgenograms; its position should correspond to the same frame coordinates. If desired, the position of the anterior and posterior commissures can be constructed on the lateral roentgenogram. This is also a way to verify the probe's position (Z ordinate) in relation to the intercommissural plane.

Although the use of coordinate measurements derived by CT-CASS to localize a particular target structure greatly aids in increasing the accuracy of the CT stereotactic technique for functional neurosurgery, it is important to remember that it does not completely eliminate error. The position of the diencephalic structure in any particular diseased brain cannot be exactly predicted by the surgeon [16]. The need for a neurophysiological test to confirm that a probe or an electrode is positioned in the proposed theraeutic target site long has been recognized as a necessary step in stereotactic surgery for dyskinesias. We use an exploratory stimulation and recording technique to confirm the limits of the target area before placing a therapeutic lesion [4, 6, 7].

The Future

The primary emphasis of our research and development has been directed towards producing a small, compact, and portable operating-room computer system that the stereotactic surgeon can use for both functional and morphological procedures. As currently designed, the system also can be used for tumor biopsies

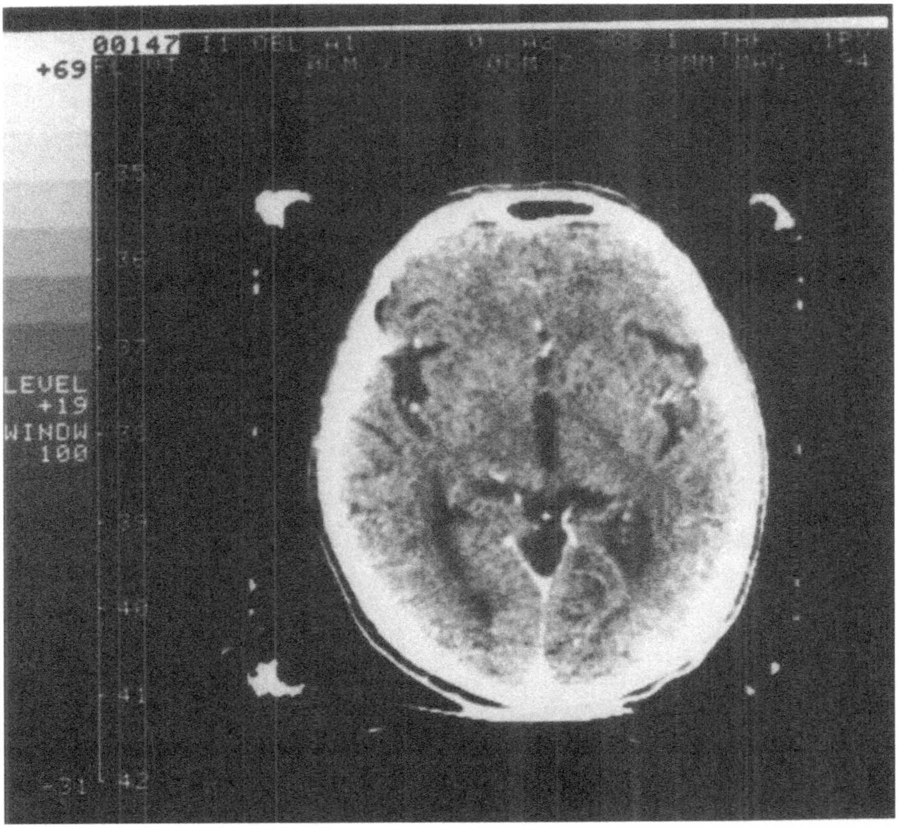

FIGURE 34–12. Reformatted horizontal CT image through the anterior and posterior commissures.

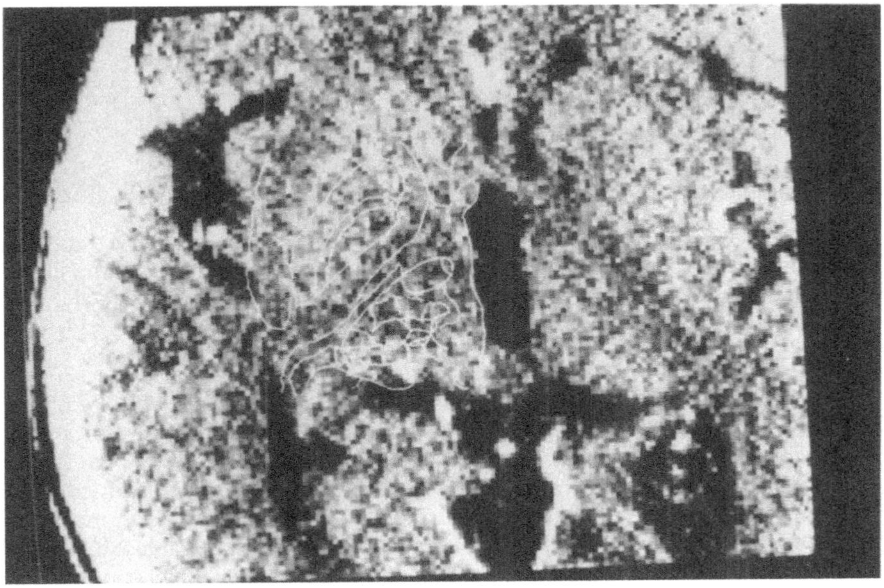

FIGURE 34–13. Magnified view of thalamic region (figure 34–12) with computer-graphic overlay of brain map.

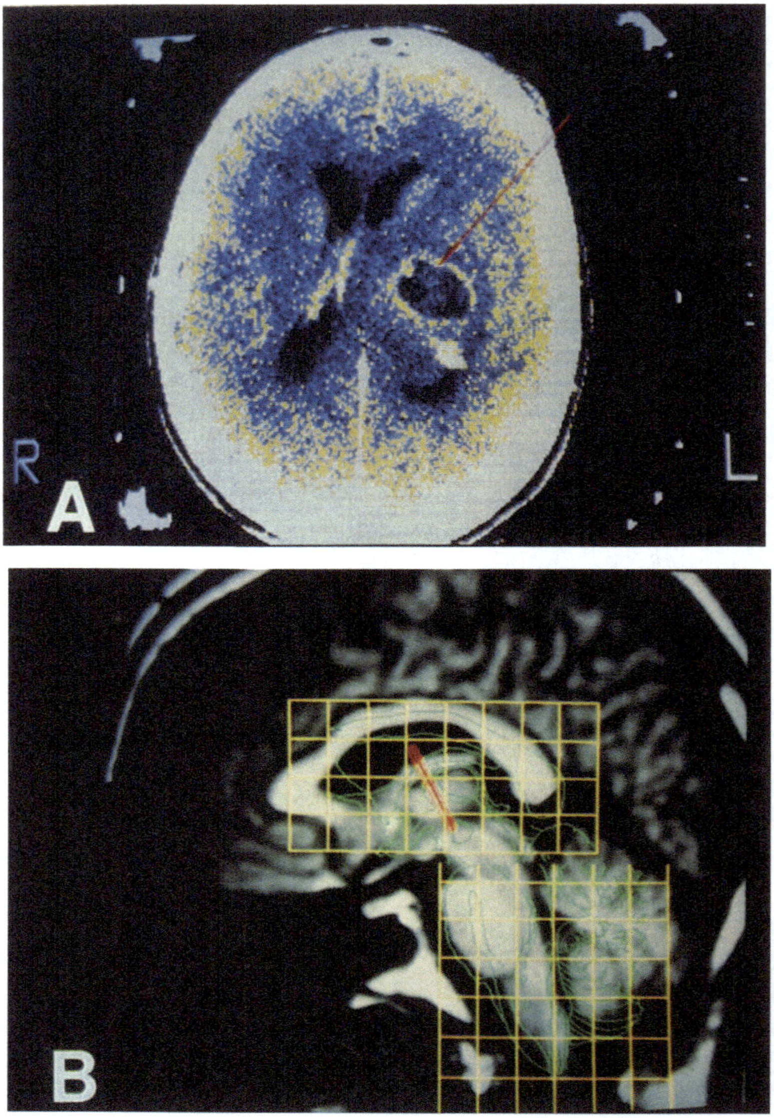

FIGURE 34–14. (A) Patient with cystic tumor in left deep central region. Biopsy probe's trajectory is simulated in red. Computer can be set to pseudocolor white matter in blue and gray matter in yellow. (Patient of Dr. L. Dade Lunsford, University of Pittsburgh School of Medicine.) (B) Midsagittal NMR image with digitized diencephalic and brain-stem maps (green) and graticules (yellow) superimposed on scan section. For demonstration purposes, probe (red) is directed toward the red nucleus.

[11] (figure 34–14A) and, with appropriate user-specific software routines, could be used to guide and simulate radioisotope implantations. With improvements in NMR-compatible stereotactic instruments, we plan to develop the system further to make use of this imaging technology. We now are able to superimpose diencephalic and brain stem maps on NMR sections (figure 34–14B). In the future, with increasing NMR resolution and contrast, the superimposition of these maps may not be necessary. The pixel-analysis capability of this computer system allows for an increase in contrast by either pseudocoloring and/or decreas-

ing or increasing the apparent density of certain pixels. With increased NMR contrast this feature may enable discernment of major thalamic subdivisions. Similar techniques can be applied now to CT images for increased contrasting.

Efficient, high-speed, vector-processor hardware that can handle very large data bases has been developed for small computer systems. With this technology, we are in the process of developing a hardware-software adjunct to our computer system that will permit three-dimensional, real-time image processing. This feature would bring an additional perspective to stereotactic imaging.

Given the system's capabilities of storing images displayed on any cathode-ray-tube screen, there are plans to develop software routines that will permit the superimposition of images from various sources (e.g., isotope brain scanning, CT scanning, NMR, digital angiography, stereotactic atlases, and ventriculography); this should result in more complete imaging information. Thus, data from many sources can be compared or combined to plan or execute a stereotactic operative procedure.

References

1. Birg W, Mundinger F: Computer programmes for stereotaxic neurosurgery. *Confin Neurol* 36:326–333, 1974
2. Birg W, Mundinger F, Klar M: A computer programme system for stereotaxic neurosurgery. *Acta Neurochir [Suppl]* (Wien) 24:99–108, 1977
3. Gybels J, Gildenberg PL and Siegfried J (eds): Technical advances: Part III of the Proceedings of the 8th Meeting of the World Society and the 5th Meeting of the European Society for Stereotactic and Functional Neurosurgery, Zurich, July 9–11, 1981. *Appl Neurophysiol* 45: 341–548, 1982
4. Hardy TL: Computer display of the electrophysiological topography of the human diencephalon during stereotaxic surgery. Master's Thesis, McGill University, Montreal, Canada, 1975
5. Hardy TL: A method for calculation of rotational angulation in stereotactic surgery. *Surg Neurol* 13:437–439, 1980
6. Hardy TL, Bertrand G, Thompson CJ: The position and organization of motor fibers in the internal capsule. *Appl Neurophysiol* 42:160–170, 1979
7. Hardy TL, Bertrand G, Thompson CJ: Touch-evoked thalamic cellular activity: The variable position of the anterior border of somesthetic SI thalamus and somatotopography. *Appl Neurophysiol* 44:302–313, 1981
8. Hardy TL, Koch J: CASS: A program for computer assisted stereotaxic surgery. In *Proceedings of the 5th Annual Symposium on Computer Application in Medical Care*. Washington, DC: 1981, pp 1116–1126
9. Hardy TL, Koch J: Computer-assisted stereotaxic surgery. *Appl Neurophysiol* 45:396–398, 1982
10. Hardy TL, Koch J, Lassiter A: Computer graphics with computerized tomography for functional neurosurgery. *Appl Neurophysiol* 46:217–226, 1983
11. Hardy TL, Lassiter A, Koch J: A portable computerized tomographic method for tumor biopsy. *Acta Neurochir* [Suppl] (Wien), pp 444, 1983
12. Hassler R: Anatomy of the thalamus. In Schaltenbrand G, Bailey P (eds): *Introduction to Stereotaxy with an Atlas of the Human Brain*, Vol 1. Stuttgart: Thieme, 1959, pp 230–290
13. Leksell L: *Stereotaxis and Radiosurgery: An Operative System*. Springfield, IL: Thomas, 1971, p 69
14. Leksell L, Jernberg B: Stereotaxis and tomography: A technical note with 6 figures. *Acta Neurochir* (Wien) 52:1–7, 1980
15. Latchaw RE, Lunsford LD, Kennedy WH: Reformatted imaging to define the intercommissural line for CT-guided stereotaxic functional neurosurgery. *AJNR* 6:429–433, 1985
16. Lichtenstein B: Abnormal topographical relations of the brain resulting from disease. In Schaltenbrand G, Bailey P (eds): *Introduction to Stereotaxis with an Atlas of the Human Brain*, Vol 1. Stuttgart: Thieme, 1959, pp 65–69
17. Nashold BS Jr, Gildenberg PL, Franklin PO (eds): Proceedings of the Meeting of the American Society for Stereotactic and Functional Neurosurgery, Durham, NC, April 29–May 1, 1983. *Appl Neurophysiol* 46:1–4, 1983
18. Schaltenbrand G, Bailey P: *Introduction to Stereotaxis with an Atlas of the Human Brain*. New York, Stuttgart: Thieme, 1959
19. Schaltenbrand G, Wahren W: *Atlas for Stereotaxy of the Human Brain* (2nd ed) Stuttgart: Thieme, 1977
20. Thompson CJ, Bertrand G: A computer program to aid the neurosurgeon to locate probes used during stereotaxic surgery on deep cerebral structures. *Comput Programs Biomed* 2:265–276, 1972
21. Thompson CJ, Hardy TL, Bertrand G: A system for anatomical and functional mapping of the human thalamus. *Comput Biomed Res* 19:9–24, 1977

35. COMPUTERIZED THREE-DIMENSIONAL STEREOTACTIC ATLASES

John K. Vries
Sean McLinden
Gordon Banks
Richard E. Latchaw

The goal of functional stereotactic surgery is to stimulate or ablate selected targets in the brain. The usual targets are subcortical nuclei and white matter tracts. To accomplish this goal, the three-dimensional coordinates of the target sites must be precisely determined. The traditional tool for this purpose has been the stereotactic atlas.

The application of computed tomography (CT) has led to a resurgence of interest in stereotactic surgery, creating a need for stereotactic atlases that take advantage of modern computer and neuro-imaging technology. This chapter reviews efforts to create computerized neuroanatomic databases and presents an experimental system for generating three-dimensional stereotactic atlases.

Conventional Stereotactic Atlases

In experimental animals such as the rhesus monkey and the cat, it is possible to determine the coordinates of neuroanatomical targets by reference to bony landmarks [22]. Stereotactic atlases for these animals have used a rectangular coordinate system based on a horizontal plane passing through the external auditory meatus and the inferior margins of the orbits, a vertical plane passing through the auditory meatus, and a midsagittal plane passing through the sagittal suture [8]. These standards cannot be applied to humans, however, because there is more variety among human brains than there is among the brains of laboratory animals. Spiegel and Wycis found a range of 16 mm in the distance between the pineal gland and the vertical interaural plane in humans [33]. Studies by Schaltenbrand and Wahren showed a 15-mm range for the distance from the midcommissural point to the vertical interaural plane [32]. This variety led to a search for stereotactic reference points based on intracranial structures.

In 1955, Talairach proposed that a line drawn from the anterior commissure to the posterior commissure (AC–PC line) might serve this purpose [35]. The AC–PC line is readily determined from ventriculograms, and its length shows minimal variation. The anterior commissure is also intimately related to stereotactic targets such as the putamen, the globus pallidus, the amygdala, and the anterior temporal lobe. In a study of 26 human brains, Talairach found the AC–PC line to average 25.5 mm in length, with a range of 23–28.5 mm. These figures were confirmed by Schaltenbrand and Wahren in a study of 31 human brains [32]. A variety of atlases for human stereotaxis constructed over the past three decades have used the AC–PC line as a reference. These include the atlases of Talairach, Van Buren and Maccubin, Andrew and Watkins,

This work is supported by the National Library of Medicine grant Neuro-Imaging Expert System SRC 1 RO 1 LM04431–01.

L.D. Lunsford (ed.) *MODERN STEREOTACTIC NEUROSURGERY*.

and Schaltenbrand and Bailey [2, 31, 36, 41]. One of the most popular recent atlases is that of Schaltenbrand and Wahren, which has a coordinate system based on three orthogonal planes that pass through the midpoint (midcommissural point) of the AC–PC line [32].

Atlases based on the AC–PC line have been effective for determining the coordinates of targets in the thalamus and basal ganglia that are in close proximity to the midline and the anterior or posterior commissures. Unfortunately, accuracy diminishes as a function of distance from the line. This effect is significant enough that the AC–PC line cannot be used to locate targets in the hypothalamus or the posterior fossa; other intracranial references, such as the outline of the anterior third ventricle or the position of the floor of the fourth ventricle, must be employed [1, 32].

The most significant deficiency in current stereotactic atlases is that the coordinates for neuroanatomical structures are based on a small number of specimens. The extensive variation of the thalamus and basal ganglia has been shown by numerous investigators [7, 25, 41]. Attempts to compensate or correct for these differences have had limited success because of the complex, nonlinear nature of the variation. It is also known that aging and ventricular size can markedly affect coordinate location.

Computerized Neuroanatomic Databases

With the advent of CT scans came the capacity to directly visualize pathological lesions and locate them in three-dimensional space. Moreover, many normal intracranial landmaks could be seen, such as the third ventricle and the internal capsule. These new capabilities spurred intense efforts to adapt stereotaxis to CT scanning. Older stereotactic frames (Leksell, Todd-Wells, Riechert-Mundinger) were modified for use in the CT scanner. New frames (e.g., Brown-Roberts-Wells) were designed specifically for CT use [6, 10, 16, 26]. The possibility of applying the principles of magnetic resonance imaging (MRI) to stereotaxis has also been explored. In theory, many subcortical nuclei of interest to the functional stereotactic surgeon can be seen on MRI scans. Major problems related to image distortion and accuracy remain, however.

Despite the advances in neuro-imaging, nuclei important for functional stereotactic surgery, such as the nucleus ventralis lateralis of the thalamus, cannot be visualized directly. Such regions can be differentiated from surrounding structures only by detailed microscopic studies of their architectonics. Their locations can be determined only by reference to stereotactic atlases or by direct neurophysiological recordings with microelectrodes [12, 13, 25, 37]. These problems have led to an interest in developing computer-resident atlases for functional CT stereotaxis. There also has been an interest in developing methods to compensate for anatomical variation, based on the identification of landmarks with fixed relationships to functional targets.

Lunsford and colleagues developed a method for reformatting CT images to define the AC-PC line so that the Leksell stereotactic frame coordinates could be related to Schaltenbrand and Wahren's atlas [27]. Olivier and Bertrand reported the use of a digitized Schaltenbrand atlas that could be scaled according to the length of the AC-PC line [5]. Hardy applied rectangular normalizing transformations to digitized structures from stereotaxic atlases and superimposed them on CT images [15]. Using a digitized atlas, Giorgi developed a three-dimensional display system that was capable of showing arbitrary views of subcortical nuclei and proposed probe tracts [11]. Kall and coworkers also devised a means for reformatting CT images in the axial plane of the Schaltenbrand and Wahren stereotactic atlas [24]. Their interactive user package allows the surgeon to outline structures of interest, such as the thalamus, in these reformatted images. Nuclear subgroups inside these structures are scaled in proportion to the relationship between their CT outlines and their outlines in the stereotactic atlas. This is accomplished with a system of polar coordinates originating at the center of gravity of the respective outlines. Utilities also are provided to label parent structures and subregions. The target coordinates determined by this system agree closely with targets calculated on the basis of ventriculography and microelectrode recordings.

Advances in Computer Graphics

Revolutionary advances have been made in computer graphics over the last few years.

VLSI technology has made high-resolution image processing computationally and economically feasible. Hardware advances have been paralleled by software advances. Efficient algorithms have been developed for most common graphics operations. These include procedures for translating, scaling, and rotating objects in two- and three-dimensional space; procedures for hidden surface elimination and shading; and user-friendly interactive systems based on window packages [9, 14, 23, 29, 39]. Industry-wide graphics standards such as the ACM SIGGRAPH Core Standard have also emerged.

Increasingly powerful computers have prompted numerous investigators to apply these techniques to the digital data from CT and MRI scans. Sungroff and Greenberg developed an interactive system that uses splines to generate three-dimensional images from CT scans [34]. Vries developed a similar system to display three-dimensional images of neuroanatomical structures from stereotactic atlases [42]. Herman and his co-workers have created extensive three-dimensional imaging packages based on boundary detection principles for use with commercial CT and MRI scanners [3, 4, 17–21, 38]. Meagher has developed a three-dimensional image-processing system based on hierarchical representation of images; this system is much faster than conventional techniques in performing graphical operations on CT data [28]. The principle of hierarchical representation has been combined with parallel processing in the Phoenix system to produce a CT graphics system that can rapidly manipulate solid three-dimensional objects.

Radiologic Automated Diagnosis (RAD)

For the past several years, the authors of this chapter have been involved in an effort to produce a system for the automated diagnosis of CT scans (RAD). Our approach involves comparing normalized three-dimensional neuroanatomic models with objects of interest that have been automatically extracted from CT images. As part of this effort, a series of programs has been developed for manipulating and displaying three-dimensional images. From these programs, an experimental image-processing system has been assembled that generates three-dimensional images from CT scans and stereotactic atlases. The RAD graphics system combines hierarchical data-representation techniques with homogeneous coordinate transformations. The system can normalize atlas components to individual CT scans, and it can correct for CT-scan obliquity. Three-dimensional atlas components can be stretched interactively in the X, Y, and Z axes. The user can construct three-dimensional images of arbitrarily combined atlas and CT components. These composite images can be rotated, scaled, and translated in three dimensions under user control. Three-dimensional representation of subcortical structures can also be mapped onto arbitrary two-dimensional CT projections in the axial, coronal, or sagittal planes. The system can be used to display targets and trajectories in stereotactic surgery. It can also be used for modeling neurosurgical procedures; for teaching neuroanatomy; and as a component in automated systems for classifying, diagnosing, and archiving neuro-images.

The Rad Graphics System

The representation of material objects in a manner that allows display and interpretation by computers requires substantial storage and processing resources. To reduce these requirements, RAD uses a data-representation technique known as "octree encoding." A CT image in the form of a threedimensional array of Hounsfield numbers is converted into a binary image by thresholding. A large parent cube serves as the bounding volume for this image. The image is then divided recursively into octants, forming a tree of order eight (octree). The process terminates when the "leaves" of the tree are either completely full or completely empty (figure 35–1).

The computational advantages of octrees for image representation are significant. Translation, scaling, and hidden surface elimination can be performed without the need for multiplication or division. Rotation in 90° increments can be accomplished by merely traversing the octree in a different order. Parallel traversal of two objects in octree format produces the logical AND or the logical OR of the objects in three-dimensional space. Individual octants also can be processed independently in parallel, providing the potential for real-time image manipulation.

Image files, generated from a General Elec-

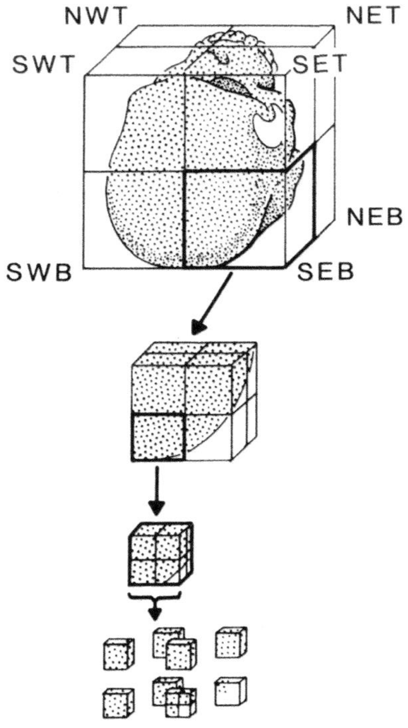

FIGURE 35–1. Diagram of octree encoding process.

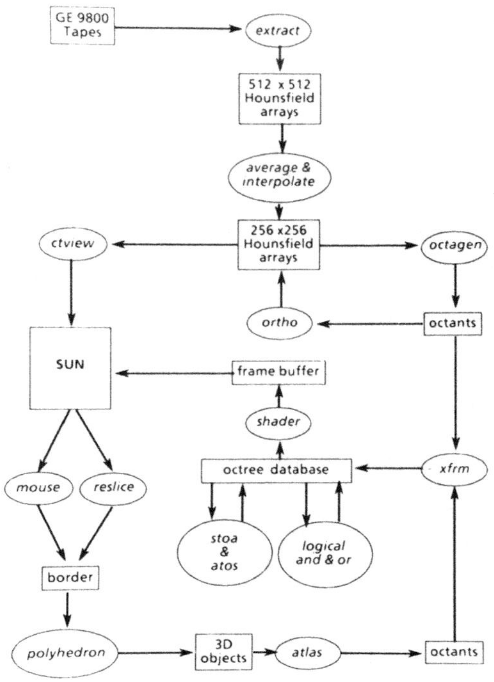

FIGURE 35–2. Organization of the RAD system using GE 9800 CT scanner (General Electric, Medical Systems, Milwaukee, WI).

tric 9800 CT scanner, are extracted from tape and converted into 512 × 512 arrays of Hounsfield numbers (figure 35–2). These arrays are averaged and interpolated to produce a 256 × 256 × 256 cube of 16-bit numbers. Arbitrary two-dimensional images in the axial, coronal, or sagittal planes can be obtained from this data structure with the ORTHO and CTVIEW routines. Octree data structures are generated from this cube with the recursive routines in OCTAGEN. Recursion stops when a "daughter" octant is entirely full or entirely empty. If this has not occurred by the time the octree is eight levels deep, the pixels are forced to be full or empty.

Octrees are created for each appropriate threshold range (bone, cerebrospinal fluid, white matter, etc.). Although average values for these ranges are known, individualized ranges can be obtained prior to octree generation by manually thresholding with CTVIEW.

The octree data structures are the basis for the remaining operations. The XFRM routine is used to translate, scale, and rotate the octree objects and to perform hidden surface elimination. The output of this routine is a 256 × 256 array of 16-bit numbers that represent the distance from the surface of the view plane to the object at each point (z-buffer). The SHADER routine uses this z-buffer data to generate pseudo three-dimensional shading. The z-buffer is interpreted as a contour map, and imaginary light vectors are bounced off its surface. The intensity of reflected light is calculated by the laws of geometrical optics. The distance information is contained in the low-order byte of the 16-bit numbers in the z-buffer. The upper byte is used to index into alternate color maps to permit multicolor pseudo three-dimensional shading. Color map indexing is controlled by the STOA and ATOS routines. Three-dimensional frontal, lateral, and cutaway axial views of the skull can be generated by RAD from a routine diagnostic CT scan (figure 35–3).

Composite images are generated with the

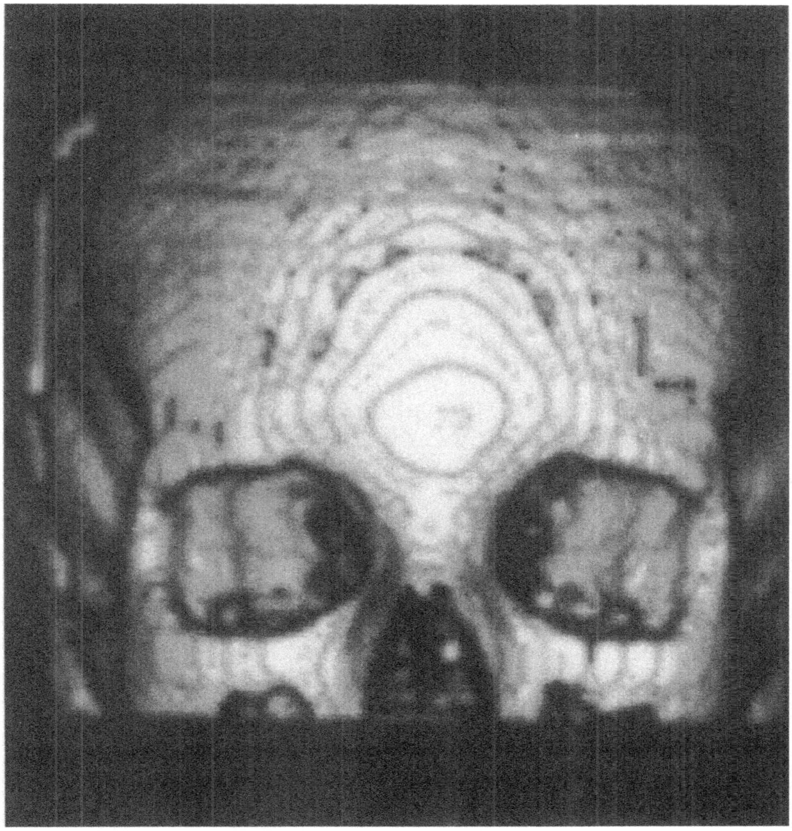

A

FIGURE 35–3. Three dimensional frontal (A), lateral (B), and axial (C) views of the skull. The lower images were obtained at 3-mm intervals, the upper images at 10-mm intervals. The ring artifact seen in the lateral view was produced by the coarseness of 10-mm images. The cutaway axial view reveals the detail that is possible with 3-mm images. Finer CT scanning would further improve the resolution.

LOGICAL_OR and LOGICAL_AND routines. These programs perform a parallel traversal of two objects in octree format to produce a third octree object that is the logical OR or logical AND of the original two objects.

Currently, the RAD system is written in the C programming language, and has the capacity to interface with artificial intelligence (AI) modules in Common Lisp language. The octree generation routines currently run on both a VA 11/780 computer and a Sun Microsystems Workstation*, the output device is the Sun, which is also the input device for the generation of atlas figures. The windows environment, which is the control mechanism for the RAD modules, is implemented in C via calls to the SunView windows system [40]. This system is patterned after the Xerox Cedar window environment, which was the model for the familiar MacIntosh computer windows.

* Sun Microsystems Inc., Mountain View, CA

Three-Dimensional Neuroanatomic Databases

The ability to manipulate and display three-dimensional brain models requires a computer-resident neuroanatomic database. The RAD system can be used to generate such databases from three different sources: conventional stereotactic atlases, CT scans displayed on video monitors, or interactive editorial operations on existing three-dimensional structures.

Digitized outlines of structures from stereotactic atlases are obtained by placing atlas

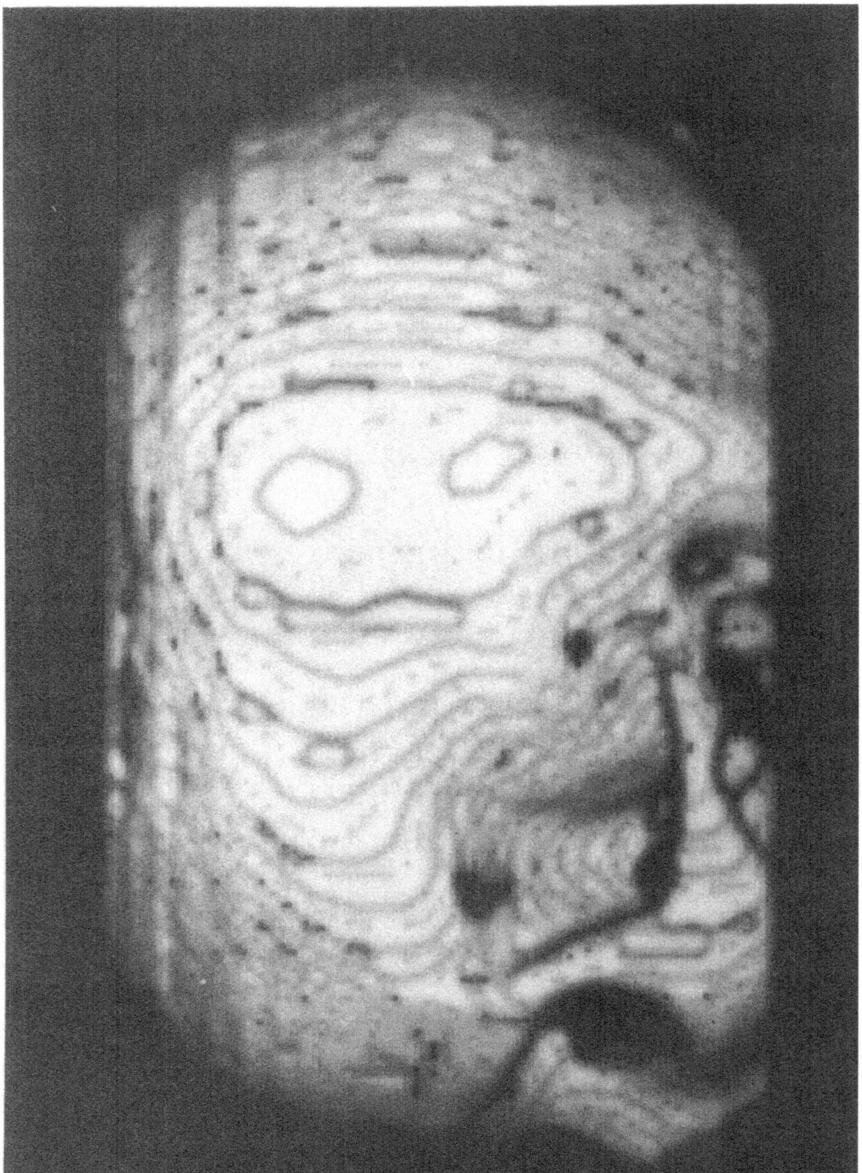

B
FIGURE 35–3. (cont.)

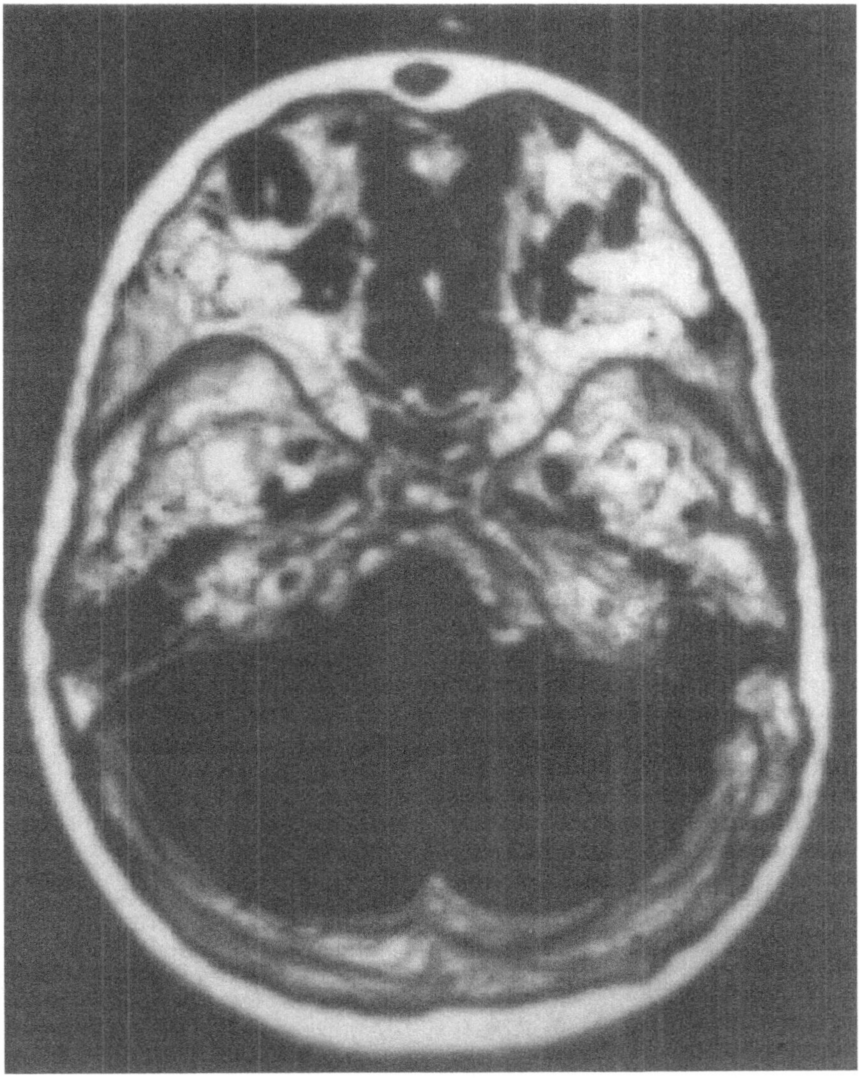

C
FIGURE 35-3. (cont.)

plates on a tablet known as a bitpad (HIPAD). The borders of the objects of interest are traced with a special input device. The position of the device on the surface of the plate is sensed by a grid of wire embedded in the bitpad. Figure 35-4 shows a flow chart of the program elements used to create three-dimensional outlines from these tracings.

Digitized outlines of objects in CT scans are obtained from appropriate CT images displayed on a video monitor. CT images in the axial, coronal, or sagittal planes are obtained by applying the ORTHO program to the interpolated three-dimensional CT cube. The borders of these objects are interactively traced with a mouse.

The method for performing interactive editorial operations on three-dimensional objects is the same as for tracing operations on CT scans. The only difference is that the images on the video monitor are two-dimensional back projections of three-dimensional objects. The method used to generate these back projections is described in the next section.

A database management program known as FM facilitates interactive database operations

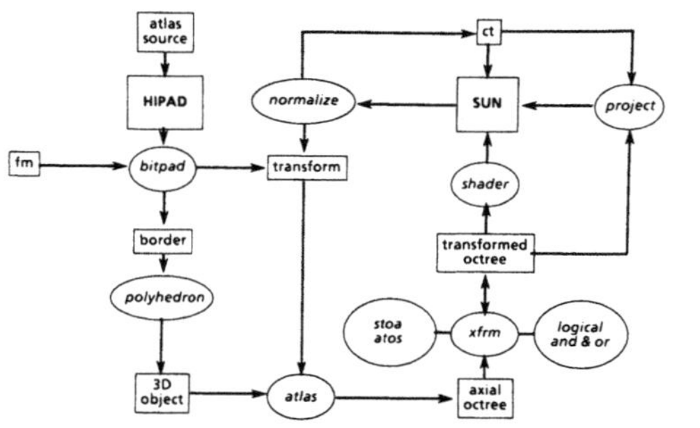

FIGURE 35–4. Flow chart of the program elements used to create three-dimensional outlines.

by performing a series of bookkeeping operations. This program keeps track of the atlas or CT projections used for tracing objects as well as the image numbers. It permits the interactive user to generate outlines in arbitrary order for any object at any time. It also provides a means for editing, replacing, or expanding existing sets of outlines.

Three-dimensional images are generated from two-dimensional outlines with the program called POLYHEDRON. A stack of two-dimensional outlines derived from an object are sorted by depth into ascending order. A process of linear interpolation is invoked to create a uniform series of outlines at 1-mm intervals from the bottom of the object to the top. The application of area scan conversion to the members of this stack generates a list of the X, Y, and Z coordinates for all the points inside the object [9, 29].

The list of three-dimensional X, Y, and Z coordinates thus generated is converted to octree format by the program called ATLAS. This program contains a function that takes the X, Y, and Z coordinate values for an arbitrary point in three-dimensional space and returns the octree representation for that point at 1-mm resolution. The resulting octree is then compacted by condensing terminal nodes that have components of equal value. The final result is an octree representation of the object that is identical in form to the octree representation used for the CT scan. All of the octree transformation operations used on CT scans can be used on these objects including scaling, translation, and rotation, as well as the logical OR and logical AND operations. The result of these operations on a database of thalamic outlines obtained from the Schaltenbrand and Wahren *Atlas* is shown in figure 35–5.

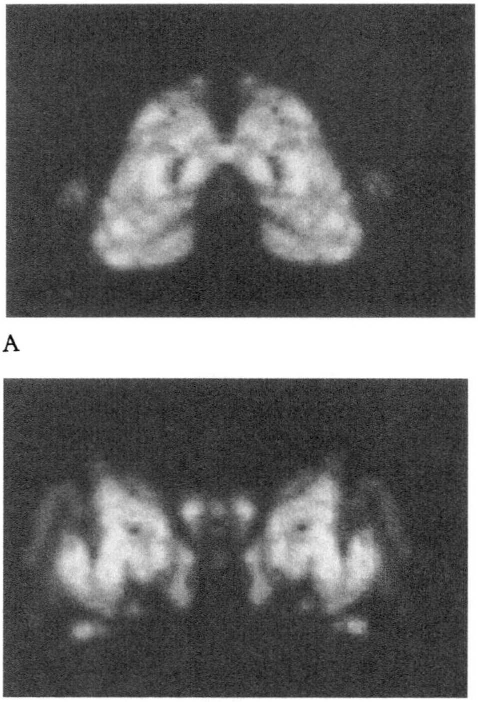

FIGURE 35–5. Thalamic outlines traced from axial plates using the bitpad. The mirror image of the thalamus was obtained by reflecting the thalamic database about the Y axis. The final image was created by generating right and left three-dimensional thalamic images in octree format and then logically "ORing" the result (A). A similar process has applied to axial, coronal, and sagittal plates of the caudate nucleus, thalamus, globus pallidus, and putamen to obtain the composite ganglionic mass (B).

Normalization of Atlas and CT components

In the RAD system, the three-dimensional representations of atlas and CT components are identical; therefore atlas and CT components could be combined, given a suitable method for normalization. This has been accomplished in RAD by combining octree encoding with homogenous coordinate transformation and a reference system based on the AC–PC line [9, 29, 30, 35].

The problem of normalization can be broken down into three parts. The first involves transforming the original interactively derived outlines into a standard projection. An outline of a structure such as the thalamus can be derived from a variety of projections, including sagittal, axial, and coronal views. The outline can also be taken from atlas plates or CT scans at different levels of magnification. In the database, however, the three-dimensional representation of the thalamus should be the same, regardless of origin. The second part involves relating components in a neuroanatomic database to structures in patient CT scans. This requires the establishment of stable reference points that are invariant from patient to patient and that can be related to the database. The third part involves correction in three dimensions for the obliquity of CT scans, which results from imperfect alignment at the time of scanning.

Mathematically, normalization involves the application of a sequence of translations, scaling, and rotations to a set of three-dimensional coordinates. Although these operations could be performed in octree format, they are awkward to program. This is particularly true for rotations at angles that are not multiples of 90°.

In computer graphics, the most widely used method for three-dimensional manipulation is homogeneous coordinate transformation [9, 29, 30]. Basically, this involves mapping the coordinates into the next (higher) dimension. Complex sequences of translations, scalings, and rotations can then be carried out as matrix multiplications. A single transform matrix representing a transform sequence of arbitrary length and complexity is obtained. The application of such a transform to the coordinates of a structure results in a transformed set of points that is easily mapped back to the original dimension.

Homogeneous coordinate transformations have excellent qualities for programming normalization sequences, but they are considerably slower than octree transforms. The data sets of three-dimensional objects in neuroanatomic databases, however, are much smaller than the data sets of three-dimensional CT scans. If structures from the neuroanatomic database were normalized with respect to CT scans, rather than the CT scans being normalized with respect to neuroanatomy, the loss of speed associated with homogeneous coordinate operations would be minimized.

The ideal time to use homogeneous coordinate transformations is in the ATLAS program, just before the use of the function that converts the X, Y, and Z coordinates of points to octree format. The octree data structure then reflects the entire sequence of normalization operations, which permits stereotactic atlas components to be combined in three dimensions with CT scans.

To normalize for the various orientations of the stereotactic atlas plates or CT scan projections that are used to generate the neuroanatomic database, the axial view as seen from the top was defined as the standard view. Defining the orientation of the atlas plates for the ATLAS program (i.e., axial, coronal, sagittal) automatically generates the transform matrix for conversion to the standard view.

The normalization of structures from the neuroanatomic database to CT scans is based on the AC–PC line. The general principles involved are presented in the introduction to this chapter. To determine the AC–PC line, the midline sagittal CT image is obtained from the interpolated three-dimensional CT scan with the ORTHO program. This view is displayed on the video monitor and a mouse is used to mark the position of the anterior and posterior commissures. The midpoint of the AC–PC line determines the origin of the X and Y coordinates. The Z coordinate is determined by the image selected to represent the midline in the sagittal plane. Figure 35–6 shows the AC–PC line ascertained in this fashion from a CT scan. The transform matrix necessary to normalize the neuroanatomic database with respect to the origin of the X, Y, and Z coordinate system in the CT scan is automatically created when the AC–PC line is marked.

Correction for obliquity involves the determination of an orientation vector in the sagittal, coronal, and axial planes. In the case of the sagittal view, the orientation of the AC–PC line is used. When the Schaltenbrand and Wahren atlas is used, an additional correction of 7° is made to compensate for the inclination of the axial plates in that atlas. The orientation vector for the coronal plane is determined by using the ORTHO program to obtain a coronal view showing the third ventricle. With the mouse, the bottom and the top of the ventricle are marked. The line connecting these two

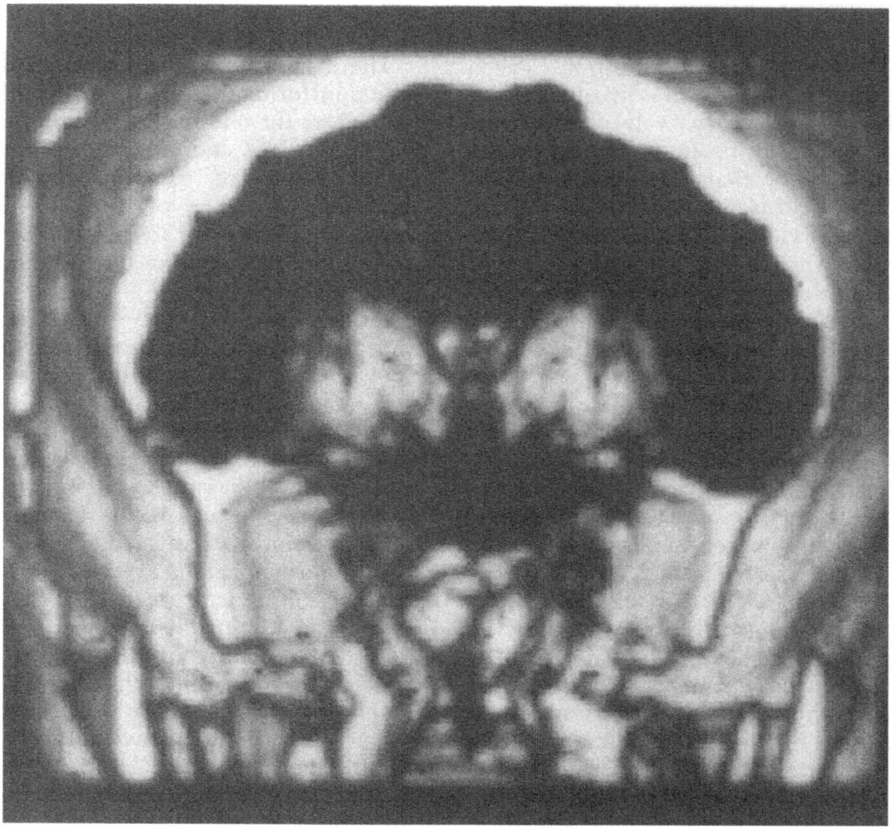

FIGURE 35-6. Three-dimensional image of the normalized basal ganglia projected onto a cutaway frontal view of the skull.

points is the coronal orientation vector. The axial orientation vector is obtained in a similar fashion by selection of an axial view that contains the third ventricle and the aqueduct of Sylvius. A point connecting the anterior third ventricle to the aqueduct constitutes the orientation vector. Information from these three is sufficient to calculate the obliquity correction matrix.

It is also possible to interactively manipulate the transform matrices. The X, Y, and Z axes can be scaled independently to expand or contract a three-dimensional object. The scaling parameters in the transform matrices also can be given negative values, which creates a mirror image of an object about the axis in question. When all orientation, normalization, correction, and interactive parameters have been selected, a final transform matrix is calculated by matrix multiplication.

Applications to CT Stereotaxis

The graphics capabilities of RAD can be applied to CT stereotaxis in several different ways. Using the logical OR and normalization routines, three-dimensional images of target structures such as the thalamus can be viewed relative to their external landmarks (see figure 35-6).

One of the most important features of the RAD system is its ability to use back projection to superimpose outlines of three-dimensional objects into the sagittal, coronal, or axial planes of arbitrary CT images. This permits direct comparison of the normalized

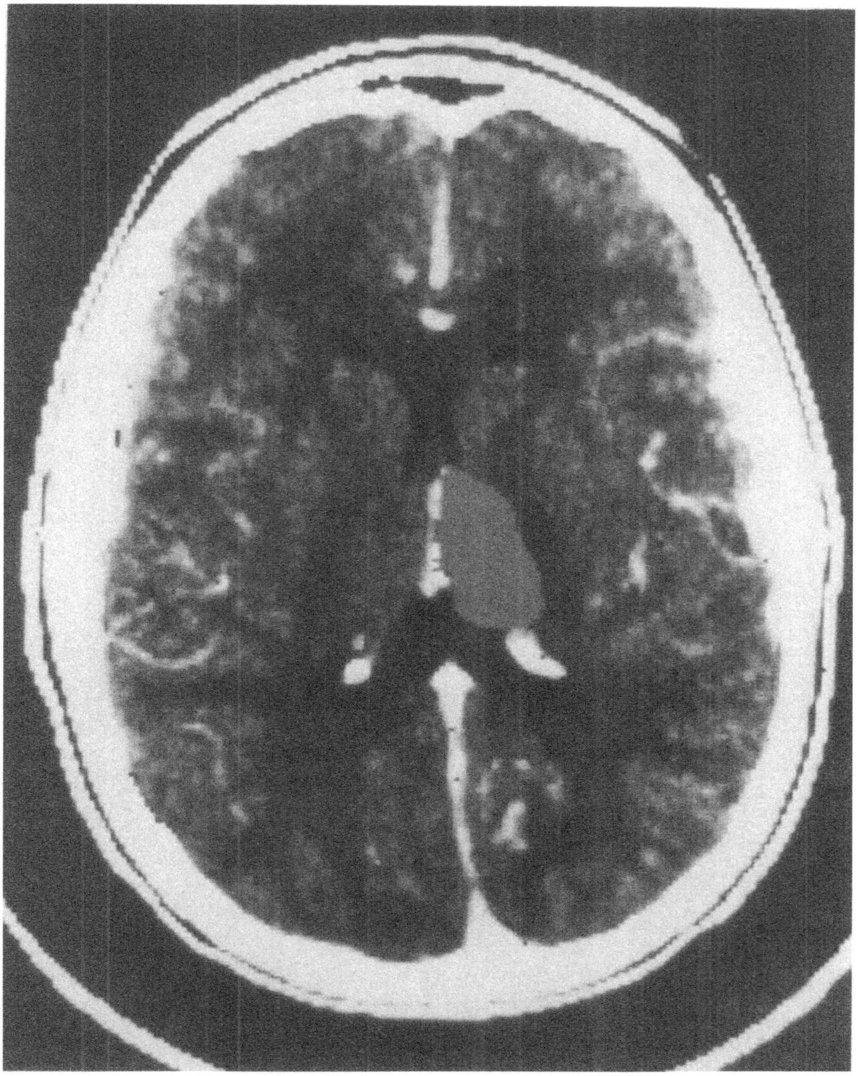

FIGURE 35–7. Back projection outline of a thalamus from the Schaltenbrand and Wahren *Atlas* in an axial CT scan. The outline compares favorably with the real thalamus on the opposite side.

models of brain structures in the neuroanatomic database and their real counterparts as seen on CT scans (figure 35–7). Figure 35–8 further illustrates back projections of ganglionic structures. The nuclear subgroups of neuroanatomical structures such as the thalamus also are contained in the database; therefore, it is possible to display targets for functional stereotactic surgery that are not directly visible in CT images (figure 35–9).

Because direct comparisons of structures visible by CT and their models in the neuroanatomic database are possible, scaling factors for the X, Y, and Z axes can be derived also. These scaling factors can be used to generate corrected three-dimensional models. If the same correction parameters are employed throughout the neuroanatomic database, all structures and their subnuclei are proportionately transformed.

Because the normalized coordinates of any structure in the database are known, the system can directly provide the target coordinates for any type of stereotactic frame. The user need

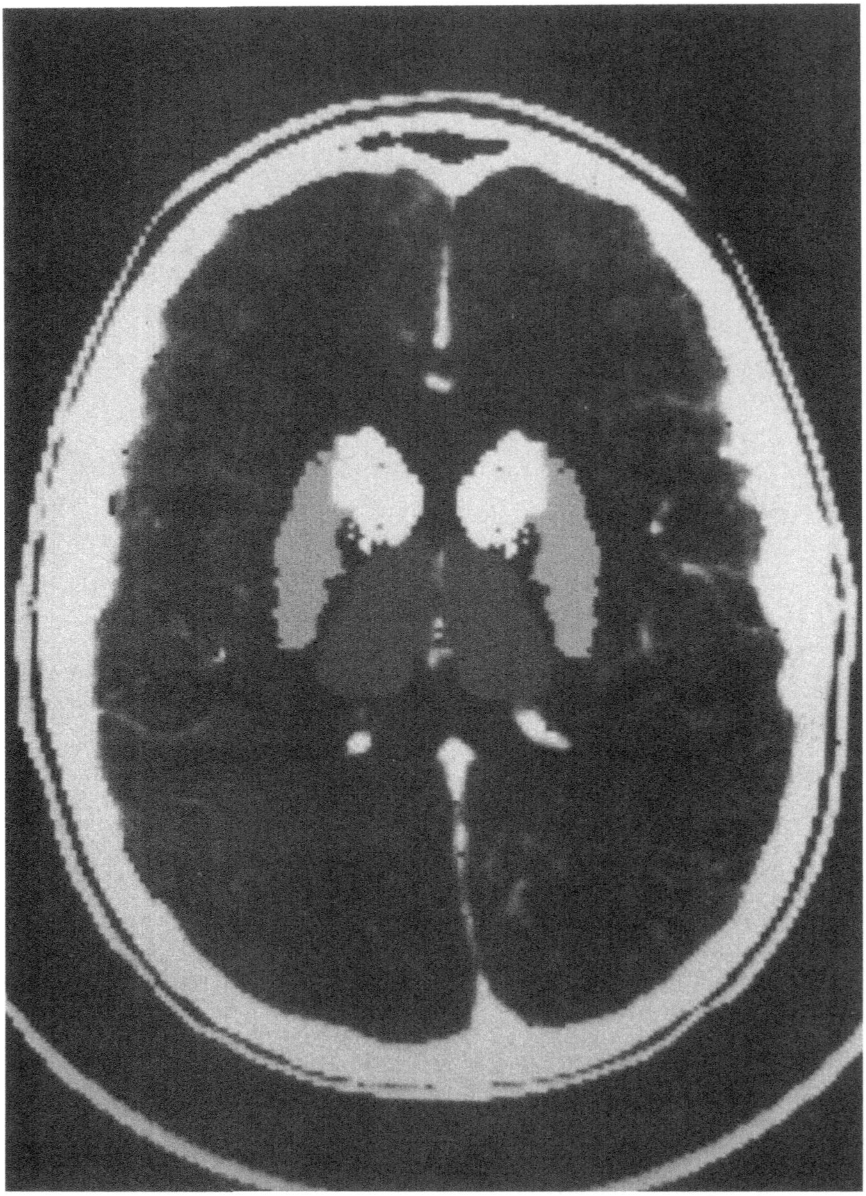

A

FIGURE 35–8. Back projections of ganglionic structures in axial (A), coronal (B), and parasagittal (C) planes.

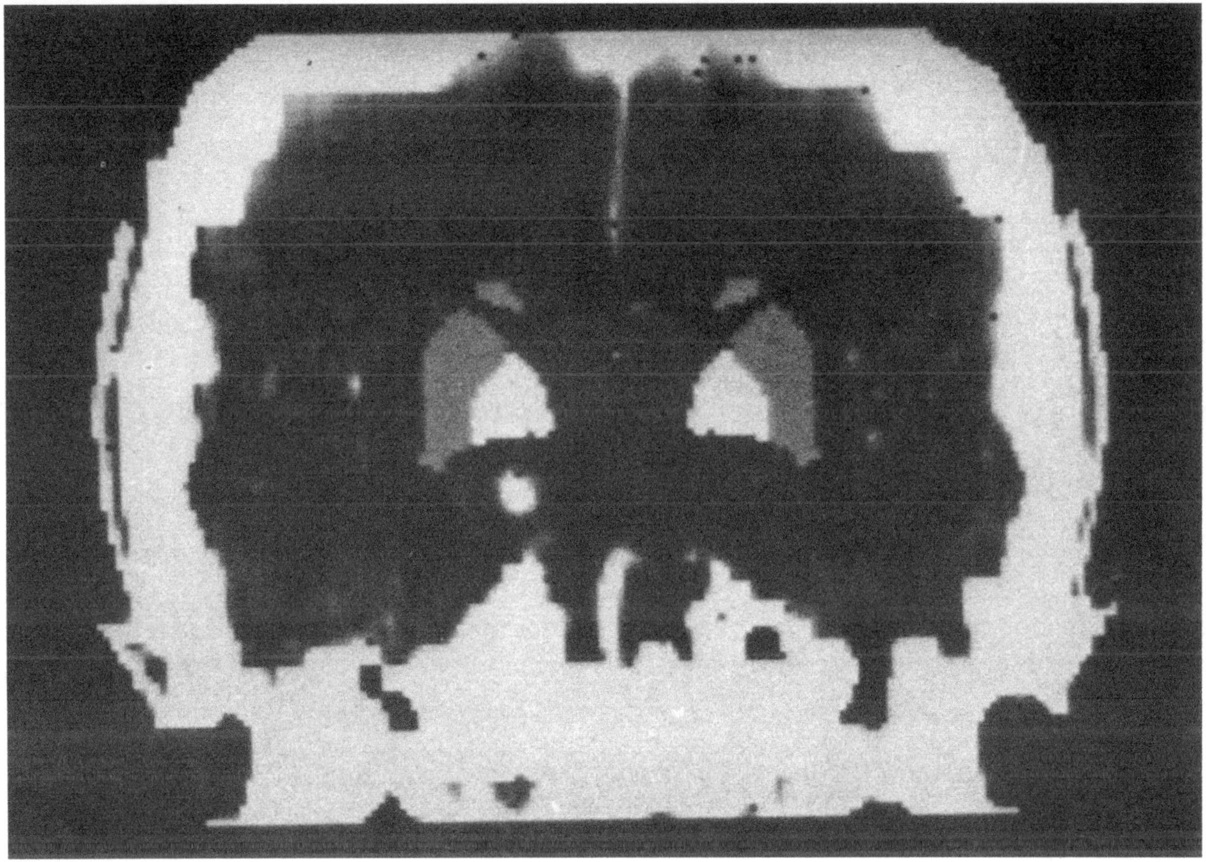

B
FIGURE 35–8. (cont.)

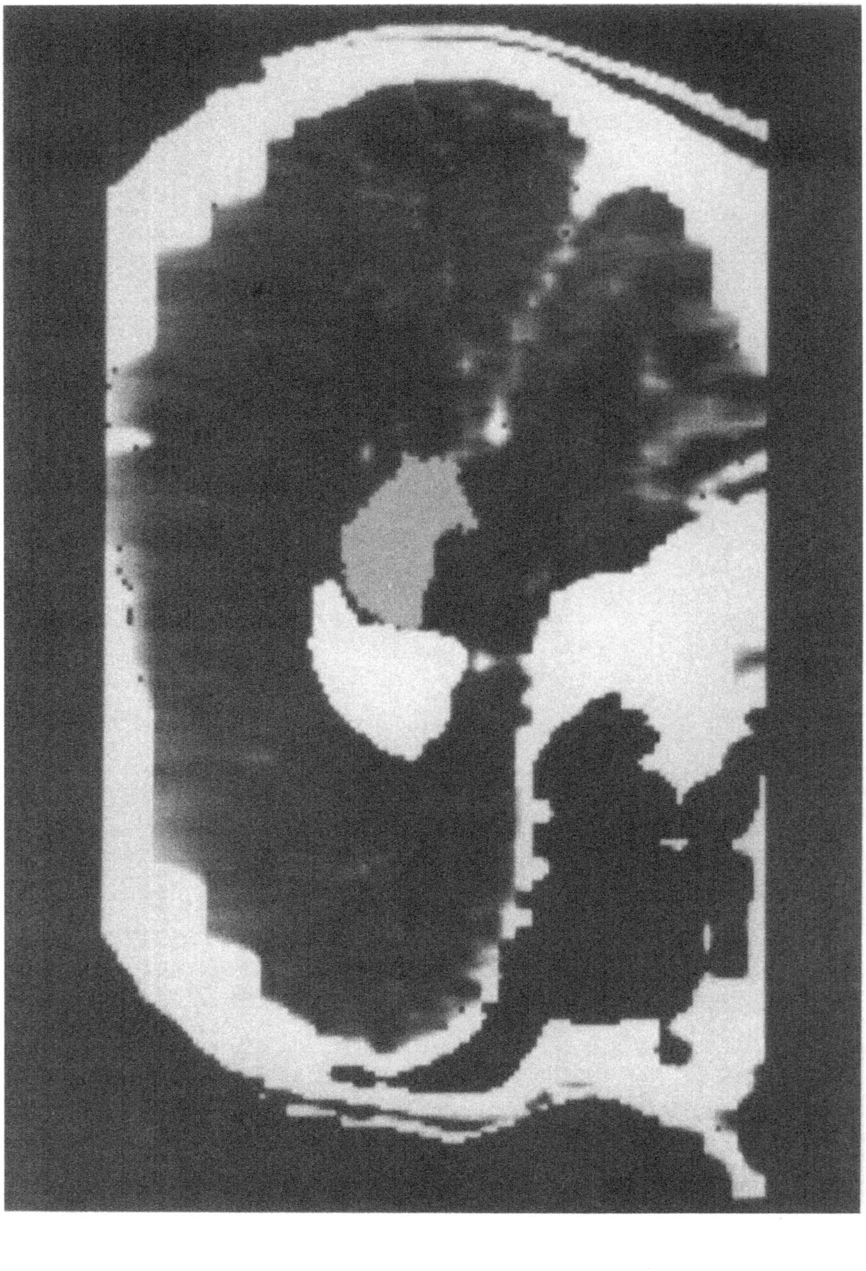

C
FIGURE 35–8. (cont.)

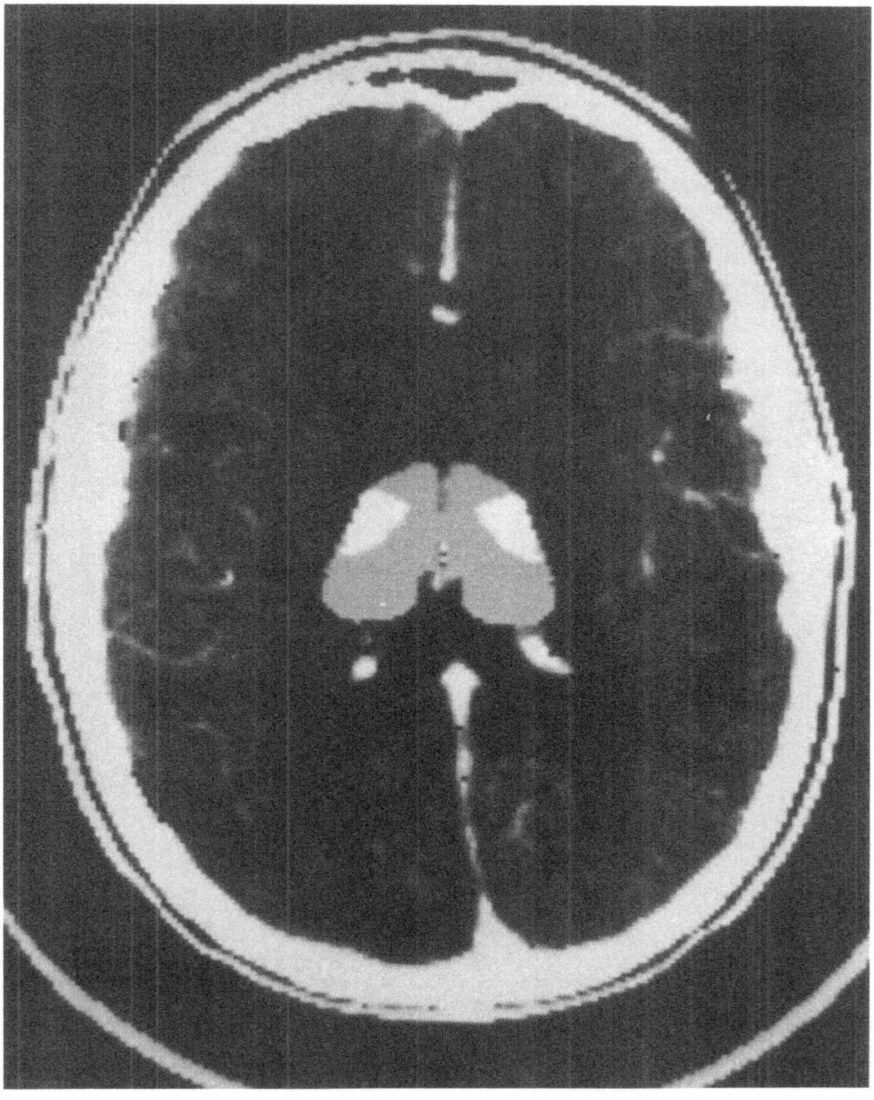

A

FIGURE 35–9. Back-projected nucleus ventralis lateralis in axial (A), coronal (B), and parasagittal (C) planes.

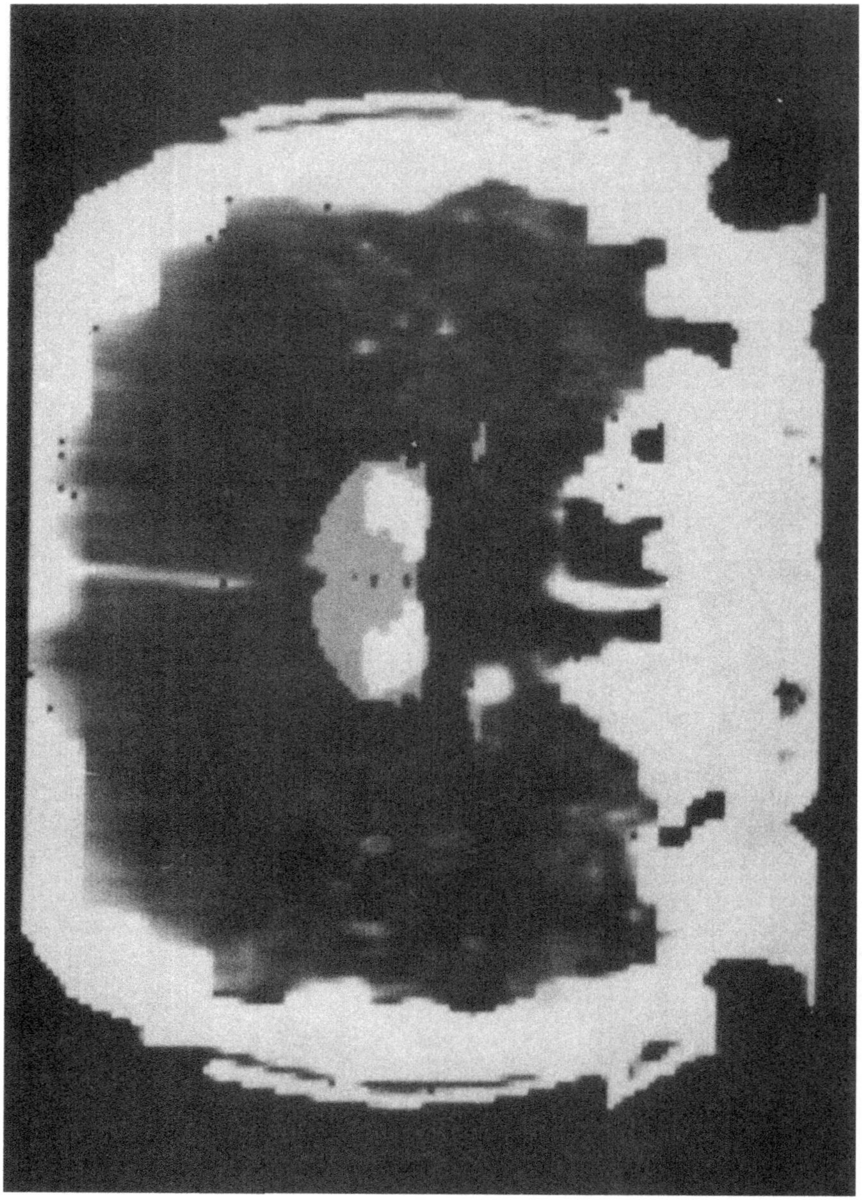

B
FIGURE 35–9. (cont.)

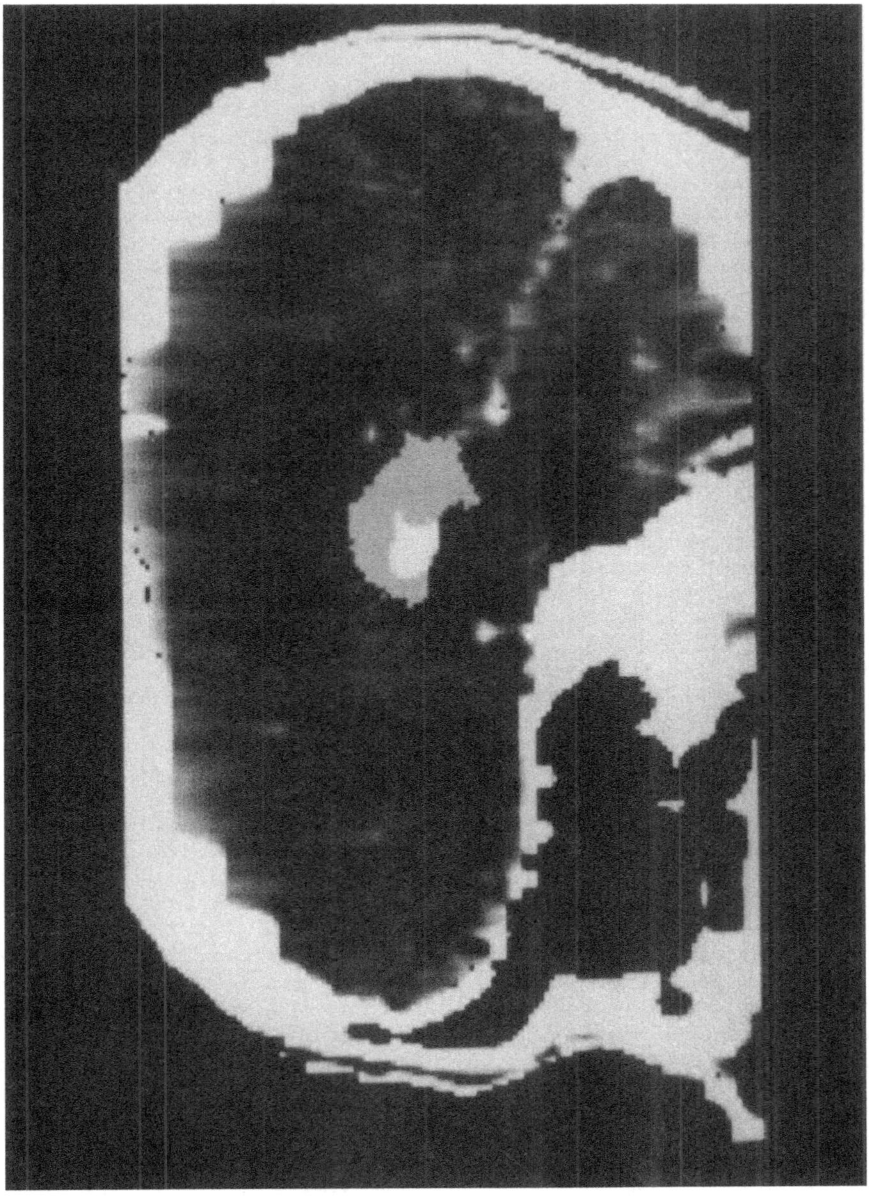

C
FIGURE 35–9. (cont.)

only interactively supply the translation and rotation parameters for the transform matrix necessary to convert the target coordinates into frame coordinates.

References

1. Afshar F, Watkins ES, Yap JC: *Stereotaxic Atlas of the Human Brainstem and Cerebellar Nuclei.* New York: Raven Press, 1978
2. Andrew J, Watkins ES: *A Stereotaxic Atlas of the Human Thalamus and Adjacent Structures.* Baltimore: Williams & Wilkins, 1969
3. Artzy E, Frieder G, Herman GT: The theory, design, implementation and evaluation of a three-dimensional surface detection algorithm. *Comput Graphics Image Proc* 15:1–24, 1981
4. Artzy E, Herman GT: Boundary detection in three dimensions with a medical application. *Comput Graphics* 15:92–123, 1981
5. Bertrand G, Olivier A: Computer display of stereotaxic brain maps and probe tracts. *Acta Neurochir* (Wien) 21:235–243, 1974
6. Boethius J, Bergstrom M, Greitz J: Stereotaxic computerized tomography with a GE 8800 scanner. *J Neurosurg* 52:794–800, 1980
7. Brierley J, Beck E: The significance in human stereotactic brain surgery of individual variation in the diencephalon and globus pallidus. *J Neurol Neurosurg Psychiatry* 22:286–298, 1959
8. Clarke RH, Henderson EE: Atlas of photographs of the frontal sections of the cranium and brain of the rhesus monkey. In *Investigation of the Central Nervous System.* Baltimore: Johns Hopkins Hospital, 1920
9. Foley JK, Van Dam A: *Fundamentals of Interactive Computer Graphics.* New York: McGraw-Hill, 1979
10. Gildenberg PL: Stereotactic neurosurgery and computerized tomographic scanning. *Appl Neurophysiol* 46:170–179, 1983
11. Giorgi C, Gartibotto G, Garozzo S, et al: Three-dimensional processing of a stereotactic brain atlas. *Appl Neurophysiol* 45:419–425, 1982
12. Guiot GA: Procedes de controle neurophysiologique pour la thalamotomie stereotaxique. *Neurochirurgie* 15:557–586, 1968
13. Guiot G, Hardy J, Albe-Fessard D: Delimitation precise des structures sous-corticales et identification de noyaux thalamiques chex l'homme par l'electrophysiologie stereotaxique. *Neurochirurgie* (Stuttg) 5:1–18, 1962
14. Hall EL: *Computer Image Processing and Recognition.* New York: Academic Press, 1979
15. Hardy T, Koch J: Computer-assisted stereotactic surgery. *Appl Neurophysiol* 45:396–398, 1982
16. Heilbrun MP, Roberts TS, Apuzzo ML, et al: Preliminary experience with Brown-Roberts-Wells (BRW). *J Neurosurg* 59:217–222, 1983
17. Herman GT: *Image Reconstruction from Projections: The Fundamentals of Computerized Tomography.* New York: Academic Press, 1980
18. Herman GT: Three-dimensional imaging from tomograms. In Hohne KH (ed): *Digital Image Processing in Medicine.* Berlin: Springer, 1981, pp 93–118
19. Herman GT, Liu HK: Display of three-dimensional information in computed tomography. *J Comput Assist Tomogr* 1:155–160, 1977
20. Herman GT, Liu HK: Three-dimensional display of human organs from computed tomograms. *Comput Graphics Image Proc* 9:1–21, 1979
21. Herman GT, Udupa JK, Kramer DM, et al: Three-dimensional display of nuclear magnetic resonance images. *Optical Eng* 21:923–926, 1982
22. Horsley VA, Clarke RH: The structure and function of the cerebellum examined by a new method. *Brain* 31:45–124, 1908
23. Kak A, Rosenfeld A: *Digital Picture Processing* (2nd ed). New York: Academic Press, 1982
24. Kall BA, Kelly PJ, Goerss S, et al: Methodology and clinical experience with computed tomography and a computer-resident stereotactic atlas. *Neurosurgery* 17:375–379, 1985
25. Kelly PJ, Derome P, Guiot G: Thalamic spatial variability and the surgical results of lesions placed with neurophysiologic control. *Surg Neurol* 9:307–315, 1978
26. Leksell L, Jernberg B: Stereotaxis and tomography: A technical note. *Acta Neurochir* (Wien) 52:1–7, 1980
27. Lunsford LD, Latchaw RE, Vries, JK: Stereotactic implantation of deep brain electrodes using computed tomography. *Neurosurgery* 13:280–286, 1983
28. Meagher D: Geometric modelling using octree encoding. *Comput Graphics Image Proc* 19: 129–147, 1982
29. Newman RF, Sproull WM: *Principles of Interactive Computer Graphics* (2nd ed). New York: McGraw-Hill, 1979
30. Roberts LG: Homogeneous matrix representation and manipulation of N-dimensional constructs. Ms no 1405. Cambridge, MA: MIT Lincoln Laboratory, 1982
31. Schaltenbrand G, Bailey P: *Introduction to Stereotaxis with an Atlas of the Human Brain.* New York: Grune and Stratton, 1959
32. Schaltenbrand G, Wahren W: *Atlas for Stereotaxy of the Human Brain.* Stuttgart: Thieme, 1977
33. Spiegel EA, Wycis HT: *Stereoencephalotomy.* New York: Grune and Stratton, 1952, p 176
34. Sungroff A, Greenberg D: Computer generated

images for medical applications. *Comput Graphics* 12:196–202, 1978
35. Talairach J: In VI Congreso Latin-Americano de Neurocirugia. Montevideo, 1955, pp 865–925
36. Talairach J, David M, Tournoux R: In *Atlas d'Anatomie Stereotaxique*. Paris: Masson, 1957
37. Tasker RR, Organ CW, Hawrylyshyn PA: In *The Thalamus and Midbrain of Man. A Physiologic Atlas Using Electrical Stimulation*. Springfield, IL: Thomas, 1982
38. Udupa JK: Display of 3D information in discrete 3D scenes produced by computerized tomography. *Proc IEEE* 71:420–431, 1983
39. Udupa J, Srihari SN, Herman GT: Boundary detection in multidimensions. IEEE Trans Pattern Anal Mach Itell Pami 4:41–50, 1982
40. SunView Programmer's Guide, Revision A: Sun Microsystems, Inc., Mountain View, CA, February 17, 1986
41. Van Buren J, Maccubbin D: An outline atlas of human basal ganglia and estimation of anatomic variants. *J Neurosurg* 19:811–839, 1962
42. Vries JK, Sclabassi RJ: An image processing system for use in neurosurgery. *Clin Neurosurg* 31:75–89, 1983

IV. STEREOTACTIC RADIOSURGERY

36. STEREOTACTIC BRAGG PEAK PROTON BEAM THERAPY

Raymond N. Kjellberg
Masamitsu Abe

Stereotactic Bragg peak proton beam therapy has been performed in more than 2,000 procedures during the past 25 years at the Harvard Cyclotron Unit. This technique was developed as particle beam surgery, in which the terminal energy peak of protons (Bragg peak) is directed to an intracranial target by the stereotactic method. Proton beams are not electromagnetic radiation but share with it the ability to induce ionization in biologic systems. There is no exit dose of radiation beyond the target. The dose (rad) of a single beam is two to four times greater than the path dose at the Bragg peak [6]. The Bragg peak of the proton beam is biologically more effective than are the plateau portion of the proton beam, cobalt-60 rays, or roentgen rays at the same physical dose [7, 13]. If a number of such beams are converged upon a brain target, the dose within the target may be many times greater than the dose along any path. For example, if 12 proton beams from different directions are focused upon a pituitary tumor, the dose within the tumor is more than 25 times as great as any path dose.

Preparatory Radiographic Studies

Marker films: Anteroposterior (AP), lateral, and base-view roentgenograms are taken orthogonally to correct for the magnification of the films and to measure the thickness of bone and soft tissue for angiograms and other conventional radiograms. Plastic strips (metric scales) with lead spots at 10-mm intervals are used as markers. These are placed parallel to Reid's base line, coronally vertical to Reid's plane, and parasagittally parallel to the midplane, so that the plane of each marker passes through the therapeutic target. The thickness of bone and the amount of soft tissue (brain and skin) between the surface and the target center can be measured along the course of proton beam paths.

The path length through soft tissue is 4% shorter than through a water phantom. Passing through bone, the penetration is shortened according to the equation arrived at by experimentally determined figures [9]. The values for soft-tissue and bone shortening of the beam path are recorded on a worksheet. These values are critical to the placement of the Bragg peak at the intended site. For arteriovenous malformations (AVM) of the brain, three-vessel angiography is performed in the position just described for marker films.

Computed tomography (CT) scans: Reconstructed CT scans are used primarily to detect tumors and some vascular abnormalities that angiograms fail to locate. Thin images of the sellar region are necessary for reconstruction of pituitary adenomas. Thin slices around the lesion and all slices from the first cervical vertebra to the top of the head are required for fine para-axial sagittal reconstruction of other tumors. The site of the lesion in the para-axial sagittal image is transposed to the midline sagittal image so that a lesion can be located in the lateral view.

Magnetic resonance imaging: MRI currently is used for vascular abnormalities that cannot be located with angiography. Lateral parasagittal images are used in the same way as reconstructed CT scans.

Polytomographic cisternography (with metrizamide) and CT scans are performed for pituitary adenomas to establish the position of the diaphragma sellae, the optic nerves, and the optic chiasm.

Digital subtraction angiography of the caver-

L.D. Lunsford (ed.) *MODERN STEREOTACTIC NEUROSURGERY*.

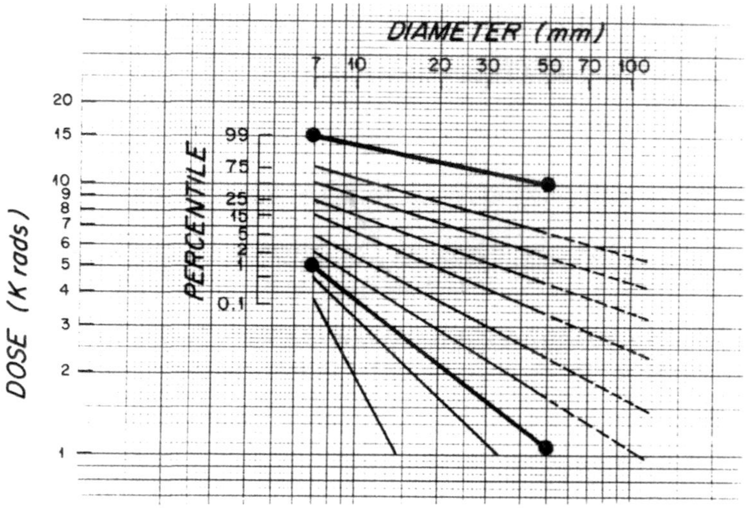

FIGURE 36–1. The dose (Krad) plotted against proton beam diameter can be used to determine the relative risk of brain necrosis. The safe dose for normal brain is below the first percentile.

nous portion of the internal carotid artery is performed for pituitary adenomas to determine the width of the contents of the sella turcica.

Isoeffective Dose Parameters

The biological effect of a single session of proton beam therapy cannot be evaluated by the dose parameters ordinarily employed in conventional fractionated roentgen-ray therapy. We have used the following parameters when planning the dose delivery [1].

SINGLE VERSUS FRACTIONATED RADIATION

Radiation delivered in a short interval requires a significantly lower dose to produce the effect achieved by radiation administered over a long period. Strandqvist proposed this principle in relation to radiation of skin tumors with roentgen rays [12], and Lindgren later applied it to brain necrosis [10]. According to Lindgren's curve, radiation delivered over 30 days should be kept below 4,500 rad to avoid brain necrosis; but if delivered in a single session, it must be kept below 1,200 rad. This effect is also important in determining the dose for a patient who has had previous radiation therapy.

THE RADIUS OF VOLUME IRRADIATED

Small volumes require proportionately larger radiation doses than large volumes. Data from several sources support this principle. The term *isoeffective dose* is used to recognize this difference from the physical dose as measured in rads. When plotted as log radius versus log dose, doses that cause brain necrosis over a range (from about 0.02–80-mm radii) approximate straight lines (figure 36–1). We use the segment between beams 7 mm in diameter and beams 100 mm in diameter as a guide to treatment. The data points in this figure were established from our measurements in experimental animals and in humans [1, 7, 11]. For example, 7-mm beams produce necrosis over a range of 5,000–15,000 rad. Fifty-millimeter beams produce necrosis over a range of 1,050–10,000 rad. A one percentile line is established between 5,000 rad for a 7-mm beam to 1,050 rad for 50-mm beam. A 99 percentile line is established between 15,000 rad for a 7-mm beam and 10,000 rad for a 50-mm beam. Other percentile lines between these two extremes also have been determined. As individual patients vary substantially in their sensitivity to necrosis, safe practices require the radiation dose to normal brain to be sufficiently below the one percentile isoeffective dose line. A dose high

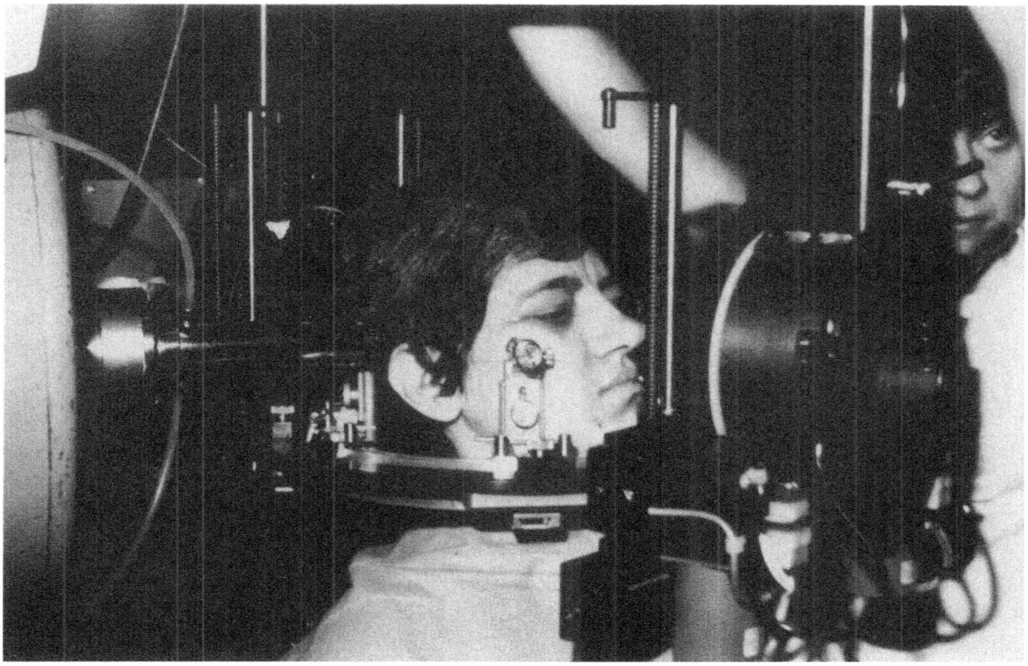

FIGURE 36-2. Stereotactic instrument developed for use with the Harvard 160-MeV proton beam unit.

enough to produce central necrosis should be administered to pituitary tumors and certain other benign tumors.

RELATIVE BIOLOGICAL EFFECTIVENESS
The relative biological effectiveness (RBE) of Bragg peak has not been clearly determined. Although in practice, we have considered the RBE to be 1.0, a recent experimental study reported proton beam RBE values to be 1.09–1.32, compared with cobalt-60 rays [13].

Stereotactic Instrument

The stereotactic device currently used is of the senior author's design, based on some features of the Leksell device. It has a vertical axis of rotation and a right angle intersecting the horizontal axis of rotation. The patient's head is held firmly in the stereotactic instrument by skeletal fixation (figure 36-2). The head can be moved vertically, horizontally, and laterally to superimpose the therapeutic target center exactly on the intersection of the vertical and horizontal axes of rotation.

In the calibration of the stereotactic instrument with respect to the Bragg peak of the proton beam, the Bragg peak is superimposed on the intersection of the axes. The radiography apparatus is aligned via superimposed cross hairs and proton beam spot to ensure precise orthogonal films in the AP and lateral views.

Cyclotron Proton Beam

The proton beam is generated at the 160-MeV Harvard cyclotron. The beam is extracted, focused, directed, and then absorbed to leave a 12-cm working range. Three brass collimators make the rays of the beam nearly parallel (figure 36-3). The beam passes through a variable water absorber that, when applied to the side of the head, automatically compensates for individual portal paths.

Stereotactic Procedure

Local anesthesia is used except in young children. It is infiltrated into the skin of the external auditory canals and into the sites of the drill-rod skeletal fixation.

On the circular head frame, ear bars and four drills are mounted (figure 36-4). Ear bars are introduced into the external auditory canals for stabilization. Drill-rod mounts are aligned to the maxillary eminences and occipital cranium.

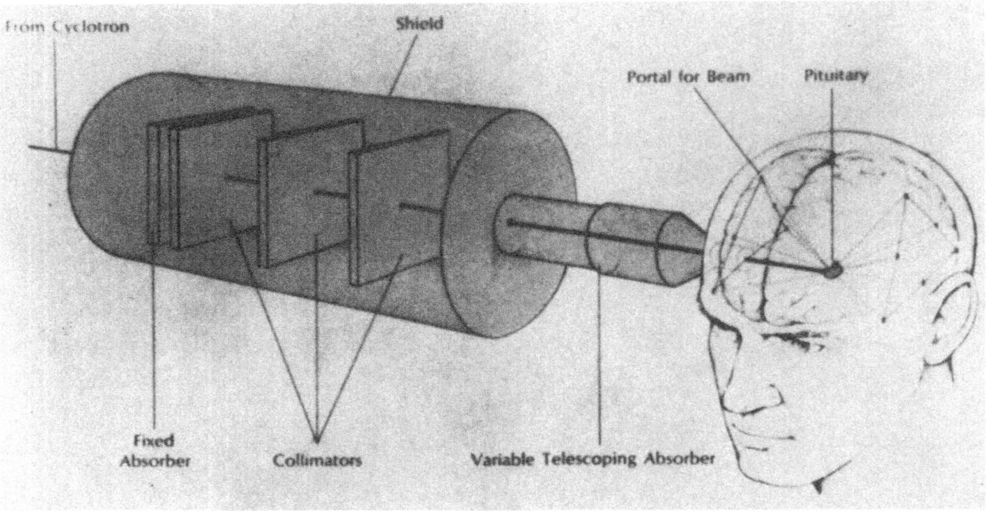

FIGURE 36–3. The proton beam generated by the cyclotron is focused, directed, and absorbed to leave a 12-cm working range.

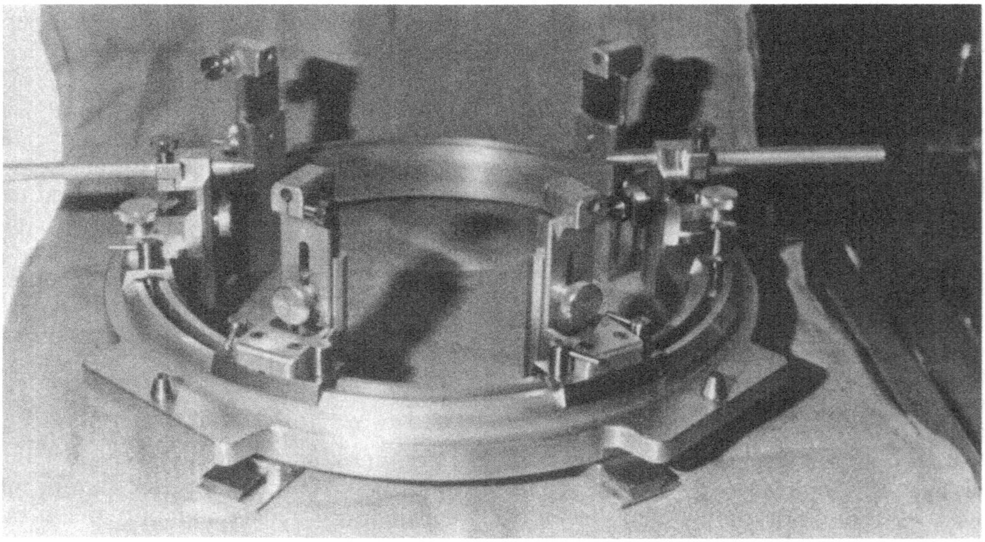

FIGURE 36–4. The stereotactic instrument is attached to the head by steel pins.

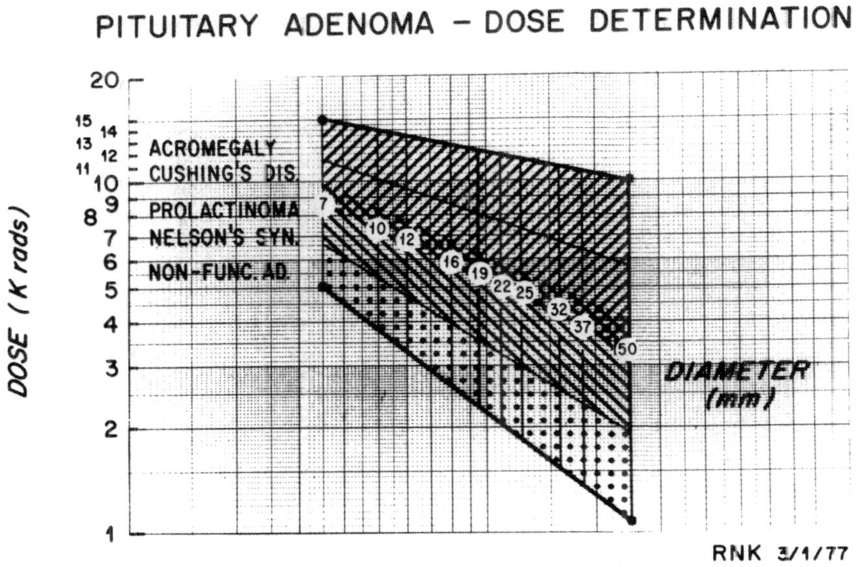

FIGURE 36–5. Dose determination used for secretory and nonsecretory pituitary tumors depending upon beam size selected.

The skin is punctured, and the drill rods passed 2–3 mm into the bone. The ear bars then are removed, and the head frame is attached to the overhead-mounted stereotactic instrument.

TARGET DETERMINATION

With the patient positioned in the stereotactic instrument, an initial pair of AP and lateral roentgenograms are taken. The patient's head is moved vertically, horizontally, and laterally to bring the intracranial target in correct relation to the proton beam spot and the cross hairs of the horizontal axis of rotation. A second pair of roentgenograms is obtained to confirm target alignment accuracy.

Proton Therapy

Beam diameters from 7–50 mm are selected and modified to conform to the size and shape of the target volume. Isoeffective doses used for various beam diameters are shown in figure 36–1. The one-percentile level for ionization injury to normal brain varies from 5,000 rad for 7-mm beams to 1,050 rad for 50-mm beams; we depend on the linear relationship between the logarithm of the beam diameter and the logarithm of the dose. The beam size, central dose, target-edge dose, and dose distribution are determined with the aid of the chart in figure 36–1.

The entire proton beam procedure is conducted in a single session lasting normally about 90 minutes. Patients are discharged the day after treatment with instructions for lifetime follow-up.

Arrangement of Proton Beam and Practical Indications

PITUITARY ADENOMAS

Figure 36–5 shows the usual dose ranges for various diagnostic categories of pituitary adenomas and the corresponding beam diameters used [4]. Acromegaly and Cushing's disease require the largest isoeffective dose. To some extent, the degree of hyperfunction influences dosage: higher doses are chosen for greater hormonal hyperfunction. Central doses are often selected to produce ablative effects of radionecrosis. However, lower doses may be used to arrest tumor growth. The dose that will be delivered to the edge of the target or to nearby structures is calculable.

When 12 beams (portals) are used on both

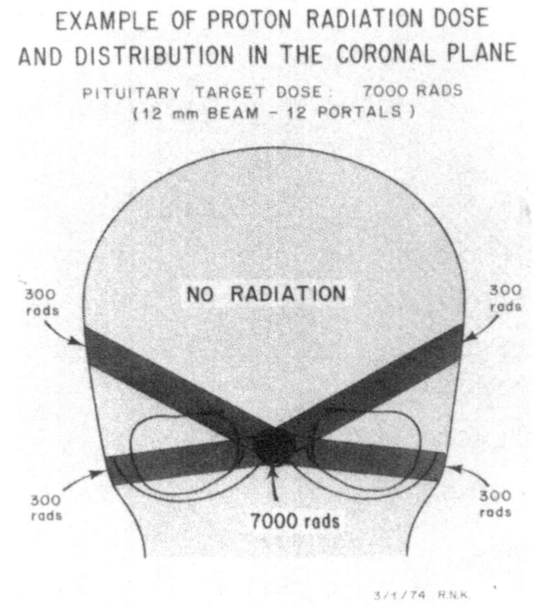

FIGURE 36–6. Example of proton (Bragg peak) radiation dose and distribution in the coronal plane of a patient receiving 7,000 rad to the pituitary fossa.

sides of the head, the target dose can be 20 to 25 times greater than a path dose (figure 36–6). Figure 36–7 shows an isodose curve for a pituitary target. The beam spot is situated to keep the optic nerve dose below 600 rad.

An intrasellar adenoma is the best candidate for stereotactic Bragg peak radiotherapy because a radiation dose sufficient to destroy the lesion can be used without risk of radiation damage of the optic nerves. Adenomas with suprasellar or lateral extensions cannot be given enough radiation to be ablated because of the high risk of optic-nerve damage or oculomotor disturbance. The treatment usually recommended for these lesions is a debulking procedure (surgical resection) followed by proton therapy or conventional radiation therapy. In selected patients, relatively low-dose proton therapy can suppress tumor growth without inducing tumor necrosis.

ARTERIOVENOUS MALFORMATIONS AND VASCULAR ABNORMALITIES

Vascular abnormalities we have treated include venous angiomas, cavernous angiomas, and angiographically occult vascular malformations [2, 3]. The AVM volume to be irradiated is established from angiograms. We seek to iden-

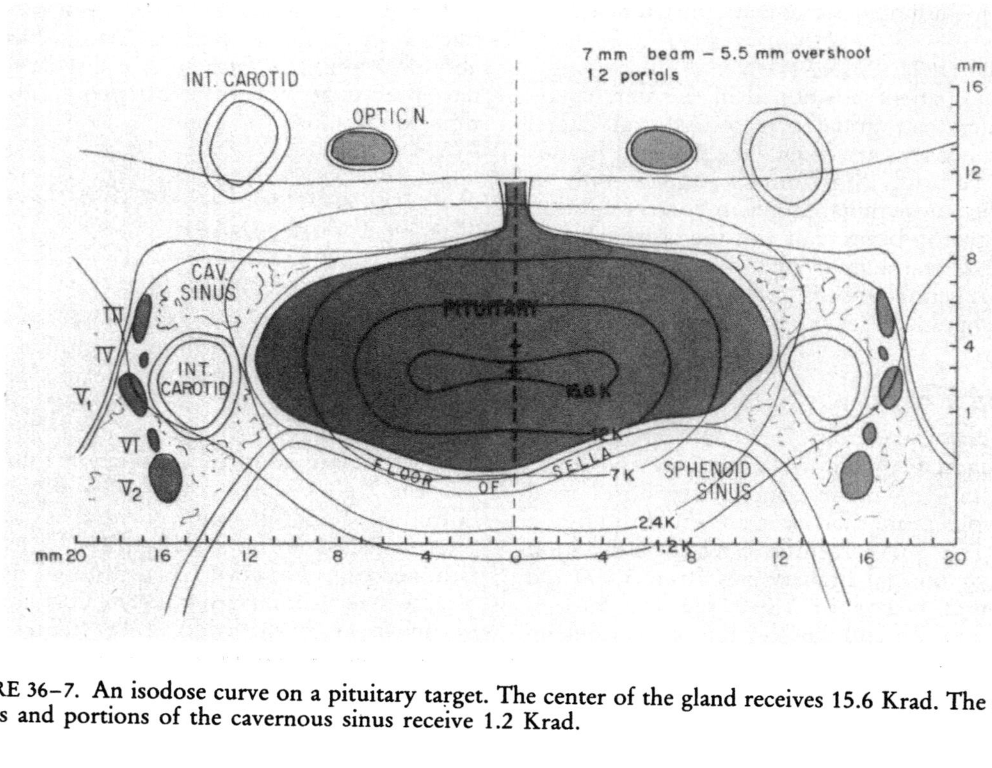

FIGURE 36–7. An isodose curve on a pituitary target. The center of the gland receives 15.6 Krad. The carotid arteries and portions of the cavernous sinus receive 1.2 Krad.

tify the "small vessel" component of the AVM as the target volume. CT scans and MRI also are used to locate vascular abnormalities.

Necrosis of the brain must be avoided in neurologically active regions. The radiation dose should be high enough to be effective on abnormal blood vessels but also low enough to spare brain that may surround the AVM. The isoeffective dose diagram shown in figure 36–1 helps in predetermining the radiation dose to an AVM. We currently choose a dose just below the 0.7 percentile isoeffective dose line, which means that the risk of radiation necrosis can be expected to be below 0.7%.

The Bragg peak is about 10 mm wide. Laminated beams are delivered to a lesion wider than 10 mm in the AP view to achieve homogeneous dose distribution. For large AVMs, a beam profile up to 105 mm is tailored and milled to the shape of the lesion.

Most of the patients selected for this therapy are considered unsuitable for open microsurgical excision or embolization. Physicians and patients may elect the comparatively low-risk alternative of proton therapy.

SELECTED BENIGN TUMORS

Proton beam treatment may be performed on meningiomas, acoustic neuromas, craniopharyngiomas, hemangioblastomas, or chordomas when attempts at open excision have failed or when initial open excision is considered unsuitable. Comparatively low doses of radiation can induce growth arrest and in some instances tumor regression. Higher doses delivered to the center of the tumor will induce radionecrosis in the central core of the tumor, but this inert radionecrotic mass may swell and require excision by craniotomy.

Results

Our experience with stereotactic Bragg peak proton beam therapy includes more than 2,000 produres in the categories shown in table 36–1. Most have been performed for pituitary adenomas and AVM of the brain.

PITUITARY ADENOMAS

Most patients with acromegaly begin to exhibit reversal of clinical features and reduction of growth hormone three to six months after therapy [8]. Clinical change and decrease in growth hormone are progressive thereafter. Cure (human growth hormone 5 ng/ml) occurred in 28% of our patients after two years, in 75% after 5 years, and in 93% after 20 years.

TABLE 36–1. Lesions Treated by Stereotactic Bragg Peak Proton Beam Therapy at the Harvard Cyclotron Unit*

Lesion	No. of Cases
Pituitary adenomas (N = 1,025)	
Acromegaly	551
Cushing's disease	163
Nelson's disease	33
Prolactinoma	123
Thyrotropin = secreting adenoma	1
Nonfunctioning adenoma	154
Vascular disease (N = 777)	
Arteriovenous malformation	749
Vascular abnormality	28
Other benign tumors (N = 59)	
Meningiomas	20
Acoustic neuromas	17
Craniopharyngiomas	5
Hemangioblastomas	4
Chordomas	3
Miscellaneous sellar tumors	10
Malignant Tumors	33
Normal pituitary suppression	219
Others	5
Total	2,118

*Through 1/1/86.

Patients with Cushing's disease respond similarly to patients with acromegaly [5]. Cure occurred in 55% of our patients after two years, in 80% after 5 years, and in 90% by 20 years.

No patient died as a result of therapy. Visual field disturbance occurred in 1.57% of patients with acromegaly and in one patient with Cushing's disease. Transient diplopia developed in a small number of treated patients. Hypopituitarism resulted from proton therapy in about 10% of patients with pituitary tumors. One acromegalic patient developed a brain sarcoma years after proton therapy. Recurrence of hyperfunction was nearly never seen and the therapy to date appears to be lifetime effective.

ARTERIOVENOUS MALFORMATIONS

No results occur immediately after treatment; effects require up to two years to develop [2]. In 841 patients studied by life-table analysis, the 20-year survival rate was 95%; most deaths from hemorrhage occurred within 2 years after therapy ("incubation interval"). Nonlethal hemorrhages after treatment rarely caused neurological deficits (1%). The complication rate fell to 0.5% in the last 800 patients we treated. Seizures, progressive neurological deficits, or headaches may or may not be improved. However, patients with these initial symptoms appear to be well protected from subsequent lethal hemorrhage after the two-year incubation period. Angiography showed reduction of AVM ranging from total obliteration (20%) to no obliteration (13%). In 56% of the remaining patients studied, the malformations were reduced by 50% or more. We believe that the prevention of lethal hemorrhage results from thickening of the abnormal vessel wall and subsequent narrowing or occlusion of vessel lumina by subintimal proliferation of collagen and hyalin.

Hospital stays varied from three to seven days for work-up and treatment. Patients were seen by staff the day after treatment and were free to return to work and other activities immediately thereafter. Patients were directed to contact their regular doctors for an annual follow-up for the rest of their lives.

Proton therapy is relatively safe; it appears to yield lifelong effective outcomes and is cost-effective. Short durations of hospitalization and treatment, absence of convalescent periods, and low complication rates contribute to the low costs associated with stereotactic Bragg peak proton beam therapy.

Patients from 50 countries have undergone proton beam therapy. Members of the medical and nuclear science communities are engaged in developing state-of-the-art accelerators to make this service more widely available.

References

1. Kjellberg RN: Isoeffective dose parameters for brain necrosis in relation to proton radiosurgical dosimetry. In Szikla G (ed): *Stereotactic Cerebral Irradiations.* Amsterdam: Elsevier, 1979, pp 157–166
2. Kjellberg RN, Davis KR, Lyons S, et al: Bragg peak proton beam therapy for arteriovenous malformation of the brain. In *Clin Neurosurg* 31: 248–290, 1983
3. Kjellberg RN, Hanamura T, Davis KR, et al: Bragg peak proton beam therapy for arteriovenous malformation of the brain. *N Engl J Med* 309:269–274, 1983
4. Kjellberg RN, Kliman B: Proton therapy for functioning pituitary adenoma. In Tinsdall GT, Collins WF (eds): *Clinical Management of Pituitary Disorders.* New York: Raven Press, 1979, pp 315–334
5. Kjellberg RN, Kliman B, Swisher B, et al: Proton beam therapy of Cushing's disease and Nelson's syndrome. In Black PM, et al (eds): *Secretory Tumors of the Pituitary Gland.* New York: Raven Press, 1984, pp 295–307
6. Kjellberg RN, Koehler AM, Preston WM, et al: Stereotactic instrument for use with the Bragg peak of a proton beam. In First International Symposium on Stereoencephalotomy. *Confin Neurol* 22:183–189, 1962
7. Kjellberg RN, Koehler AM, Preston WM, et al: Intracranial lesions made by a proton beam. In Haley TJ, Snider RS (eds): *Responses of the Nervous System to Ionizing Radiation.* Boston: Little Brown and Co., 1964, pp 36–53
8. Kliman B, Kjellberg RN, Swisher B, et al: Proton beam therapy of acromegaly: a 20 years experience. In Black PM, et al (eds): *Secretory Tumors of the Pituitary Gland.* New York: Raven Press, 1984, pp 191–211
9. Koehler AM, Dickinson JG, Preston WM: The range of protons in human skullbone. *Radiat Res* 26:334–342, 1965
10. Lindgren M: On tolerance of brain tissue and sensitivity of brain tumors to irradiation. *Acta Radiol [Suppl]* (Stockh) 170:1–73, 1958
11. Nielsen SL, Kjellberg RN, Asbury AK, et al: Neuropathologic effects of proton beam irradiation: intracranial neoplasm. *Acta Neuropathol* (Berl) 20:348–356, 1972
12. Standqvist M: Studien Uer die Kumulative Wirkung der Rontgenstrahlen bei franktionierung. *Acta Radiol [Suppl]* (Stockh) 55:1–300, 1944
13. Urano M, Verhey LJ, Goitein M, et al: Relative biological effectiveness of modulated proton beams in various murine tissues. *Int J Radiat Oncol Biol Phys* 10:509–514, 1984

37. ADAPTATION OF LINEAR ACCELERATORS TO STEREOTACTIC SYSTEMS

Arun-Angelo Patil

The "gamma knife" technique of radiosurgery has been used extensively in Sweden since its initial development by Leksell and co-workers [5, 7, 9, 14]. In this technique, which essentially is the stereotactic direction of external-beam radiation therapy, the target is placed at the center of a system toward which multiple radiation sources are directed. This results in a cumulative radiation dose at the focal point with only minimal radiation at the periphery. Such focused radiation permits delivery of very high doses of radiation at the target without undesirable effects on the surrounding tissue. Because the focal destruction of the target is similar to a surgical lesion, this technique has been called a "radiation knife." It has been used clinically for the treatment of malignant and benign tumors, including acoustic neuromas and pituitary tumors; for functional neurosurgery; and in the treatment of vascular lesions, including arteriovenous malformations (AVM). The results have been very encouraging in terms of the safety of the procedure and the control of the primary disease.

Linear accelerators have the unique capability of rotating along an arc and delivering radiation to the center of the arc, also known as the isocenter (figure 37–1). It is possible to vary the radiation dose from 0.5 to 5 rad per degree of rotation [2]. The table can be rotated around an axis which passes through this isocenter. Thus, multiple arcs of radiation can be directed toward the isocenter by rotating the table around this axis. If the target is placed precisely and firmly at the isocenter, an effect similar to gamma knife technique can be produced. Such precise placement of the target requires the use of a stereotactic system. With the introduction of computed tomography (CT) stereotaxis, this procedure has been simplified further, although few reports on this technique have been presented or published [1, 2, 11–14].

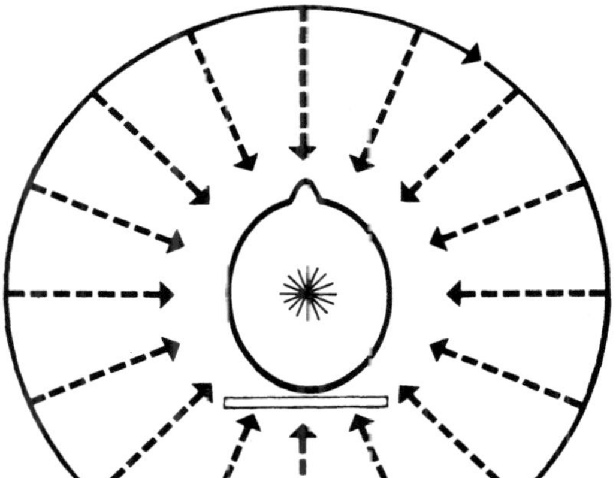

FIGURE 37–1. The concept of arc radiation at the isocenter.

Heifetz and colleagues conducted a study to determine whether it was possible to utilize conventional radiation therapy equipment to achieve the same results as the gamma knife [2]. Beams of 1 × 1 cm and 0.5 × 0.5 cm were used. Film density was measured using Kodak XV-A film in a phantom. The film was exposed in the phantom at a source-to-surface distance of 100 cm perpendicular to the radiation beam. Relative machine output and iso-

L.D. Lunsford (ed.) *MODERN STEREOTACTIC NEUROSURGERY*.

dose contours were determined from these film densitometer readings and from an Uptronix p 1000 rotating-drum film scanner. The isodose lines indicated that the dose was well restricted to a narrow field of 6.5 mm at the central area, using a beam of 1 × 1 cm. Field overlap can occur near the focus but can be greatly reduced when a beam 5 mm in diameter is used. In this chapter, various adaptations of linear accelerators are described along with a detailed description of such an adaptation to the Patil stereotactic system [10–12]. Clinical experience with this technique is presented.

The System

The Patil stereotactic system (Terhorst Technologies, Inc., 615 Burdick Expressway, Minot, ND 58701) is described in detail in chapter 8. Except for the base platform, the head holder, and one of the vertical bars carrying the circular attachments, the components of the system are removed for linear accelerator adaptation (figure 37–2, A). The movable vertical bar is mounted on the side of the base platform and can slide along its length. The movable circular attachment is mounted on the vertical bar and can be adjusted vertically (figure 37–2, B). The vertical movement of the circular attachment is calibrated in millimeters, with the zero starting point at the top of the base platform. A millimeter scale is fitted from side to side on the top surface of the base platform. The center marker (one edge of the groove in the middle of the base platform) serves as the zero starting point (figure 37–2, C). The base platform carries a head holder with four chromium-plated brass head pins and has easily detachable screws to secure it to the top surface of both the CT table attachment and the linear accelerator table.

TECHNIQUE

The system is affixed to the top of the CT table, perfectly parallel to its length, by means of the table attachment. The patient's head is held in the head holder with the head pins. With the CT gantry vertical, scans are obtained in the area of interest. On the CT picture containing the image of the target, the cursor is used to measure the X coordinate (the distance between the target and the center marker on the base platform (figure 37–3, A) and the Y coordinate (the distance between the target and the top surface of the base platform, figure 37–3, B). The vertical bar is moved along the length of the base platform to align the vertical cross marker on the circular attachment with the laser positioning light of the scanner; this indicates the CT plane of the target (see figure 37–2, A). This also brings the middle of the circular attachment into the CT plane of the target and adjusts the Z coordinate (the distance between the target and the base image). The circular attachment is then moved to a height equal to the Y coordinate distance.

With the patient's head in the head holder, the system is lifted from the table attachment of the CT table and moved to the linear accelerator room. There, the system and the patient are placed on the linear accelerator table. The base platform is attached to the table, perfectly parallel to its length, with screws that pass from the base platform to the accelerator table. The lateral laser cross-marker of the accelerator is aligned with the cross-marker of the circular attachment on the stereotactic system (see figure 37–2, B) by moving the table in the appropriate direction. This aligns the Z and Y coordinates of the isocenter of the accelerator with those of the target. The X coordinate is aligned next by moving the table from side to side in order to align the vertical marker of the accelerator with the point on the scale of the base platform indicating the X coordinate (see figure 37–2C). The target is now at the isocenter.

Next, the table is rotated 90°, and arc radiation is delivered. The table is rotated in 18° increments around an axis that passes through the isocenter. At each position, additional radiation is administered from the arc. There are 11 possible table positions, the final position being 270° (figure 37–4, A). At 180° ± 20°, the arc can be completely rotated (see figure 37–1). However, at 90° and at 270°, only half arcs are possible (figure 37–4, B and C). Arcs are designed to permit certain areas of the brain to be excluded from the radiation beam. For example, in the case of a third ventricular tumor, we have used an initial arc position just above the orbit to avoid irradiating the lens and the optic nerve.

The sizes of the photon radiation beams should be equal to the average diameter of the tumor, which is determined using CT images. The selected target is at the center of the tumor. Among all the axial images on which the target is visible, the middle image is chosen. An

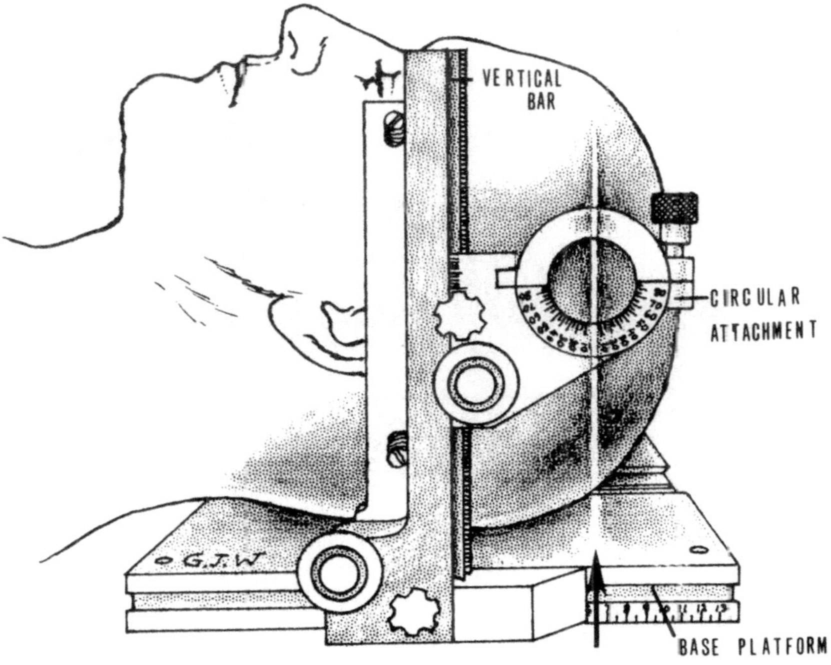

A

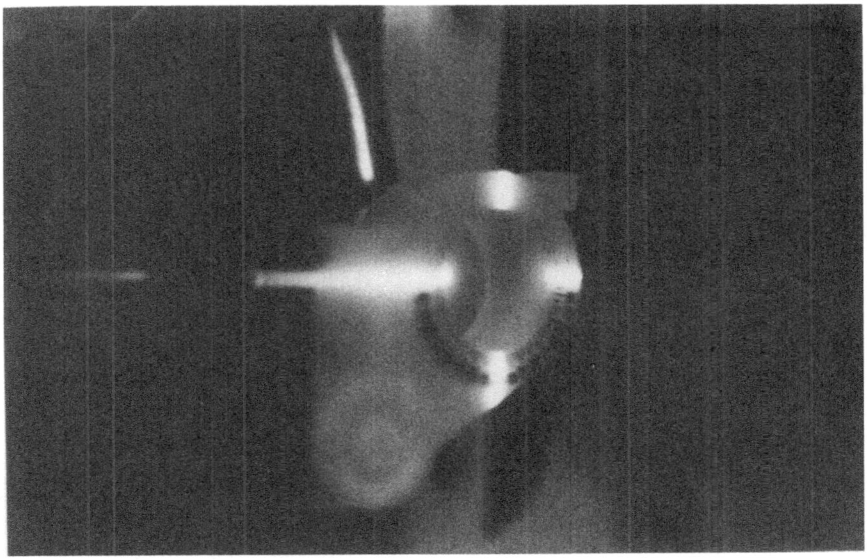

B

FIGURE 37–2. The Z coordinate is adjusted by aligning the laser positioning light of the scanner with the vertical mark on the circular attachment (*arrow*) (A). The laser positioning light of the linear accelerator is aligned with that of the cross mark on the circular attachment, (B). The vertical marker of the accelerator is aligned with the point on the scale on the top of the base platform marking the X coordinate (*large arrow*) (C).

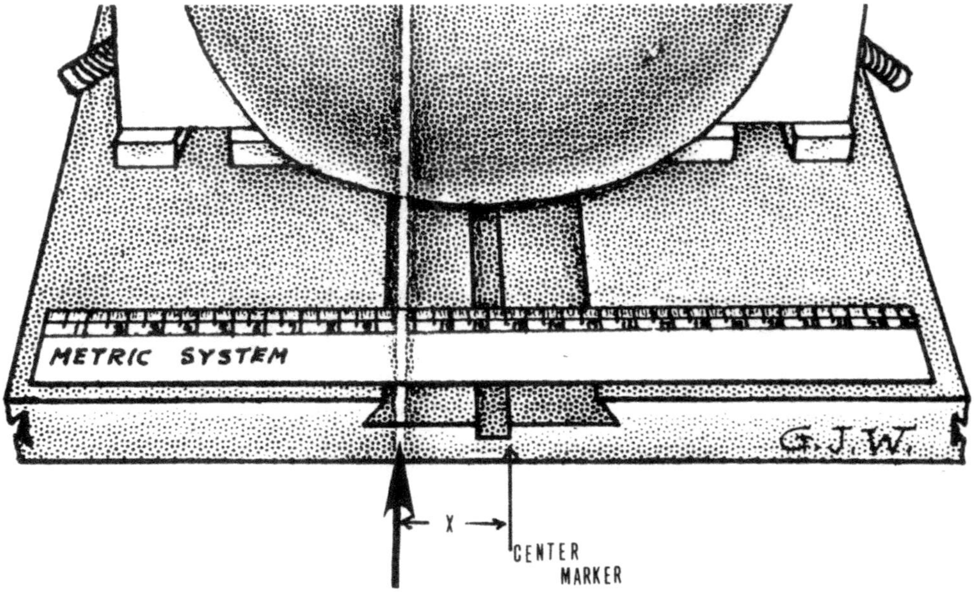

C

FIGURE 37–2. (cont.)

optimal rotational arc dose rate is computed for each patient depending on the geometry of the tumor. In cases of an oblong-shaped tumor, two targets can be planned in order to cover the entire lesion. The depth of tissue for each arc of radiation that must be passed is measured directly on the CT console by using the cursor.

Accuracy Testing

Before clinical trials were performed, the device was tested for accuracy. A thermolucent dosimeter (TLD) was placed at the center of a plastic block and was used as a target. Several TLD chips were placed around the target at various distances. Using the previously described technique (600 rad were delivered with a 1-cm photon beam through a Mevatron 74 (Siemen's Aktiengesellschaft, Medical Engineering Group, Erlangen, Federal Republic of Germany) at an energy level of 10 MeV. As Table 37–1 demonstrates, the radiation was concentrated mainly within the 1-cm target zone and the surrounding area received only a fraction of the amount delivered to the target.

Patients

Our initial experience consisted of seven patients with deeply seated malignant intracranial tumors (four metastatic, three primary) and one patient with a thalamic AVM. An average dose of 5,500 rad was delivered at one sitting. The patients with malignant tumors also were treated with fractionated conventional external-beam radiation to an additional dose of 3,000 rad over a period of three to three and one-half weeks.

Results

Within 24 hours, a definite reduction in tumor contrast enhancement was seen by CT scanning, followed by progressive decrease in the size of all but one tumor over the next four to five weeks (figures 37–5, 37–6). None of the patients developed any immediate side effects from this single-sitting large dose of radiation. Notably, in the postradiation CT scan, no evidence of significant swelling of the surrounding brain structure was detected. After a one-year follow-up of cases with malignant tumors, one

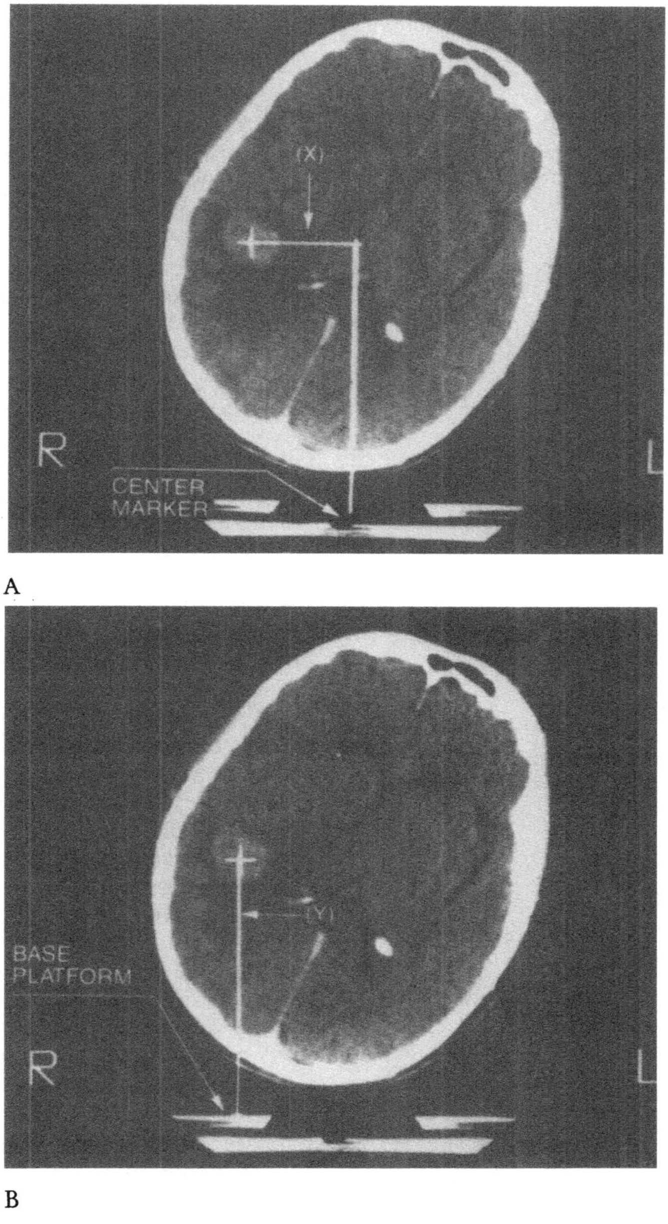

FIGURE 37–3. X coordinate (perpendicular distance of target from the midline center marker) (A). Y coordinate (perpendicular distance of the target from the top surface of the base platform) (B).

patient needed surgery because of continued tumor growth. In another case, after significant initial shrinkage, regrowth of the tumor occurred approximately eight months after radiation treatment. In the rest of the cases, there was no increased growth of the tumors before the patients died from their primary lesions outside the nervous system. In one case of primary brain tumor, the patient died from lung cancer. Our one patient with a thalamic AVM showed a slight decrease in size of the AVM six months after receiving radiation.

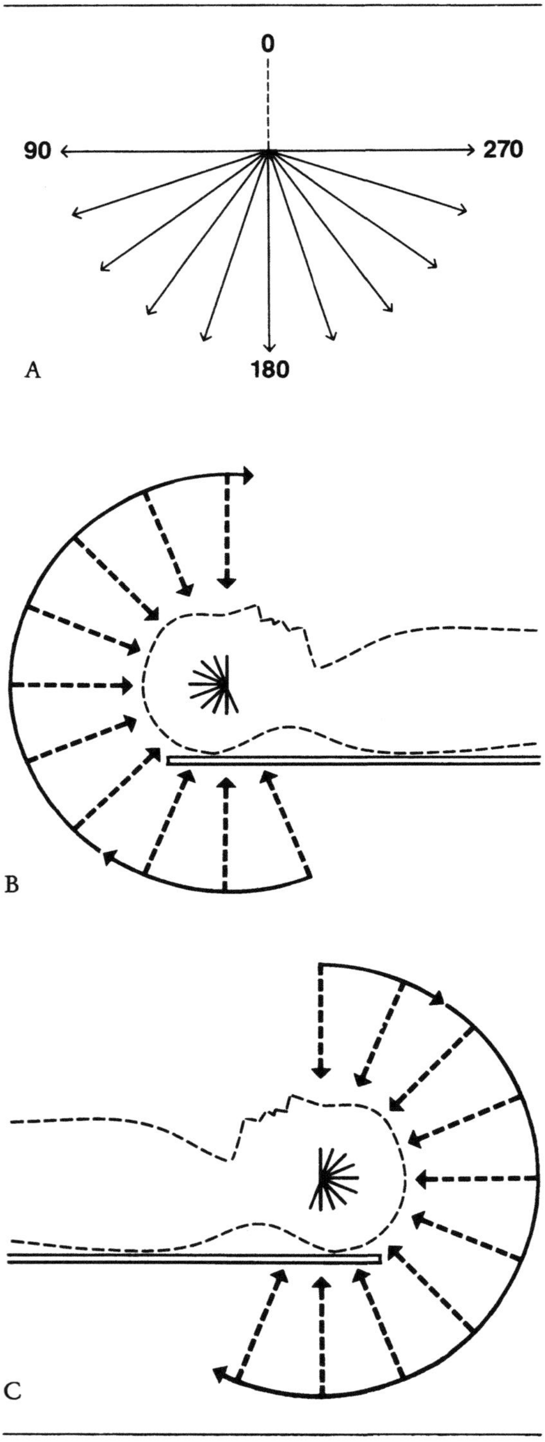

FIGURE 37–4. Various table positions are possible (A). Extent of the arc at the 90° table position (B). Extent of the arc at the 270° table position (C).

Other Stereotactic Adaptations to Linear Accelerators

Greitz, Steiner and associates (see Chapter 39) have adapted the Leksell stereotactic frame device to the linear accelerator. Instead of delivering radiation at one sitting, they have elected to use multiple radiation sessions. Initially, a mold of the patient's head is made. This allows identical head positioning at each session without the need to repeat the stereotactic procedure.

Colombo and colleagues have reported adapting a linear accelerator to the Riechert stereotactic system [1]. These investigators have used specialized computer programs to calculate the stereotactic coordinates from CT images. At the CT console, the CT coordinates of the selected target and of three radiopaque reference points (e.g., bony landmarks, calcified pineal gland, or artificially placed radioopaque markers) are identified. These points are also identified on stereoradiographs, and then the coordinates are calculated geometrically. The coordinates, the reference points, and the CT coordinates of the target are entered into a computer that calculates the coordinates of the target in stereotactic space. The computer also reconstructs the tumor volume. After centering the target within the stereotaxic sphere, an extracranial ruler is used to measure the depth of radiation and to determine the isodose curves. Then, using a phantom and the coordinates obtained, the tumor is set at the isocenter of the accelerator. Multiple arcs of radiation are delivered according to the previously described technique. Radiation is delivered in two sittings, eight to ten days apart. Twenty-two patients were treated in this manner, and no undesirable effects were seen. Six patients were followed up for at least six months; four of these patients showed significant decrease in tumor size.

A semi-stereotactic irradiation for AVM has been described by Zeilstra [14], who molded an individual head-fixation device for each patient. Exact localization of the target was obtained using angiography and CT scans. Conventional radiotherapy (total dose of 50 Gy) was delivered in 25 sessions. Excellent shrinkage of the lesion was observed in 10 out of the 20 cases followed for 15 months. In the remaining 10, no shrinkage was seen. In none of these 20 cases were undesirable effects produced.

TABLE 37–1. Stereotactic Irradiation Using a Linear Accelerator (1 cm Photon Beam)

Distance from Target	Average Radiation Received	Percentage of Total Radiation Receiver*
At target	1.06 μC	100
4 mm	0.883 μC	93.5
1.5 cm	68.6 ηC	6
2 cm	27.6 ηC	2.6
3 cm	14.3 ηC	1.35
4 cm	8.3 ηC	0.8

*Target received 100% of dose. ηC = nanocoulomb; μC = microcoulomb.

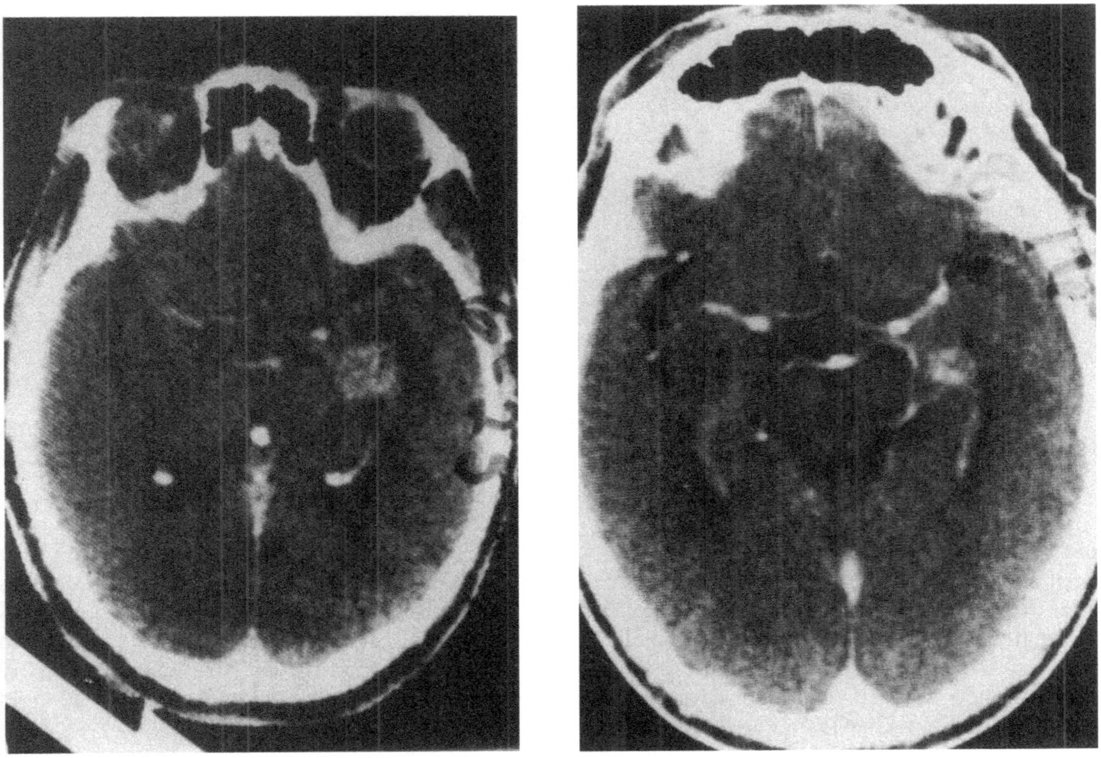

A B

FIGURE 37–5. Malignant astrocytoma in the temporal lobe before radiation (A). Eight weeks following the initial focal radiation. The tumor mass shows significant reduction (B).

Precautions

The following factors are mandatory during stereotactic linear accelerator treatment: (1) accurate coordinate determination; (2) transfer of the patient without movement of the head in relationship to the base platform of the linear accelerator table; (3) firm fixation of the head to the stereotactic system; (4) perfect parallel alignment of the base platform to the CT table during measurement of the coordinates and to

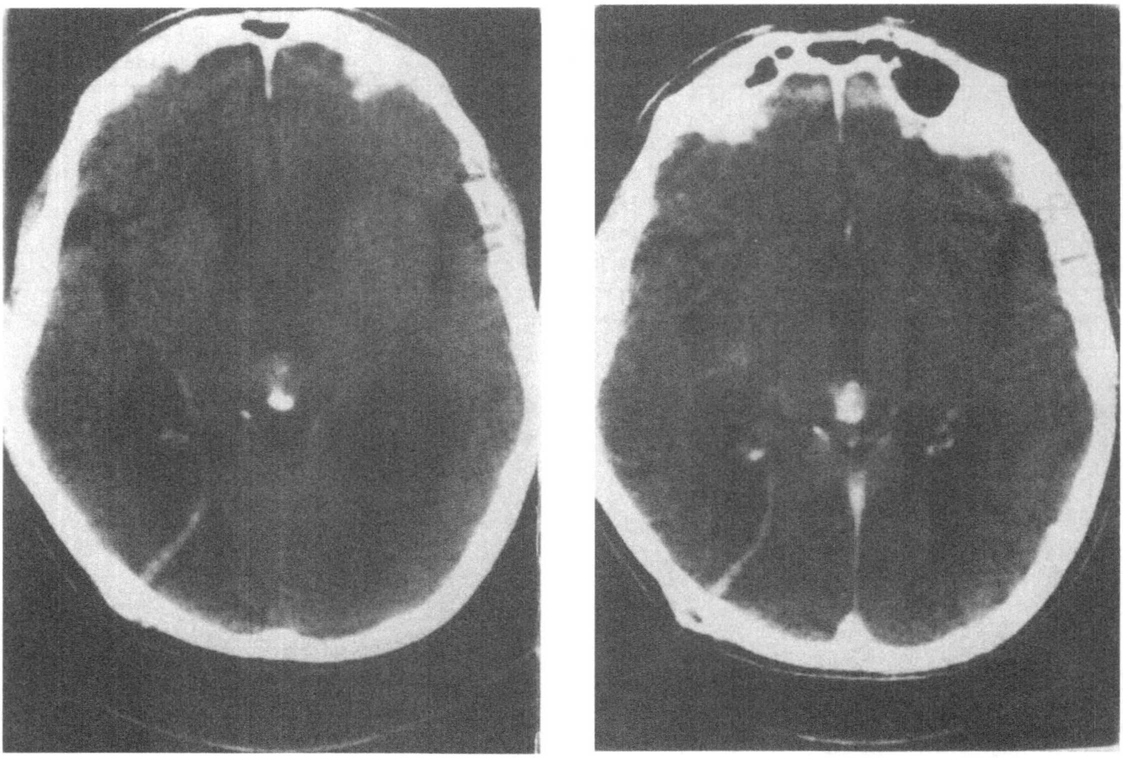

A B

FIGURE 37–6. Metastatic pineal tumor before radiation (A). Significant reduction in tumor mass is seen three weeks after radiation (B).

the accelerator table during alignment of the coordinates; (5) avoiding drift of the accelerator and/or CT table that could change the coordinates. (The tables should be watched, and if such drifts are seen, a leveling screw should be incorporated in the stereotactic system.); (6) frequent checks for accuracy of the positioning lights of both the scanner and accelerator; and (7) the accuracy of the accelerator beam around the isocenter should be confirmed. The current accuracy of most accelerators is believed to be ± 2 mm^2, which means that the radiation point at the isocenter could vary by 2 mm.

Advantages

1. Although radiosurgery using the gamma knife system has proven to be effective and safe, it requires special instrumentation that is expensive and totally dedicated to this procedure. In contrast, linear accelerators and CT scanners are becoming standard in most major hospitals, are used for many other procedures, and can be easily adapted with minimal cost.
2. This radiosurgical technique is noninvasive and can obviate the need for surgical intervention in carefully selected cases.
3. The total radiation dose can be delivered in a short time.
4. Radiation can be precisely focused; thus, irradiation of the entire brain can be avoided.

Indications for Use

Direct surgical excision is the best form of treatment in most intracranial lesions. When lesions are either surgically inaccessible or dangerous to approach, or when the patient declines surgical excision, radiosurgical treatment is a good alternative. In general, the procedure can be used for deep malignant primary tumors, single metastatic tumors, deep AVM, and deep benign tumors. Radiosurgery can also be used for pituitary tumors and acoustic neuromas if the patient rejects direct surgery. With the technique described in this chapter, the side of the head can be marked by a cross, using a skin marker to indicate the Z and Y coordinates; the forehead is marked by a line to indicate the X coordinate. These marks are then aligned with the three coordinates of the isocenter to focus the radiation beam during conventional radiation therapy.

Comments

The concept of radiosurgery in the treatment of intracranial lesions has been employed in the past with the use of multiple sources of gamma radiation [6, 7, 9, 13] or with heavy particle proton radiation [3–5, 8]. Both techniques have been found to be effective but have been used in only a few selected centers due to the complexity of the techniques and the high cost of the systems. Because it can rotate to deliver radiation at the isocenter, the linear accelerator can produce similar effects and is available in many more medical centers.

The critical part of the procedure is the precise placement of the isocenter. In the system that we have described, fixation of the head in the stereotactic system is maintained during measurements of the coordinates on the scanner table, and fixation remains during the transfer of the patient to the linear accelerator table and during radiation. The use of metal pins for skeletal fixation of the head guarantees absolute immobility of the head in the stereotactic system. Alignment of the target at the isocenter is easily accomplished with the use of the positioning light afforded by the linear accelerator. This alignment is further simplified because the Patil stereotactic system uses the circular attachment as the external marker, making the alignment of the Z and Y coordinates simple [10–13].

As demonstrated by Heifetz and co-workers [2] radiation is better localized if the beam is small. Therefore, we have preferred not to use a beam larger than 3 cm. In cases of oblong tumors, it is better to use two target points than to increase the size of the beam to minimize the radiation reaching surrounding normal brain structures. Using incomplete arcs, this system prevents critical areas surrounding the tumor from receiving radiation.

With this technique it is possible to obtain radiosurgical "debulking" of intracranial lesions. Malignant and deep-seated tumors receive, additionally, a small dose of conventional radiation, a treatment that may eliminate open surgical debulking. In large lesions, the necrotic part of the tumor may not get absorbed after irradiation and may cause mass lesions that require open surgical debulking. As our study dealt mainly with patients having malignant tumors, long-term follow-up is limited. Good short-term results have been reported by Colombo and colleagues [1] using the Riechert stereotactic frame.

Conventional radiotherapy uses fractionated radiation doses spread over a period of four to six weeks to avoid swelling and other side effects. Despite the high dose we delivered at a single sitting, the surrounding brain received only a fraction of radiation, and no swelling of the brain was seen. Those who have used the gamma knife technique [6, 7, 9, 13] have delivered radiation in doses up to 15,000 rad at one sitting. We have given an average of 5,500 rad for focal radiation, primarily because tumors were large and malignant and needed additional whole-brain radiation. In the case of smaller, benign lesions, higher doses of radiation can be used, providing the size of the beam is small and accuracy of the isocenter can be assured. Such lesions could include acoustic neuromas and deep-seated AVM. This form of treatment might not be suitable for tumors that have a large necrotic center, mainly because the maximum effect of this radiation is at the center. Although in the current report, the number of cases is small and follow-up relatively short, further evaluation of this technique for deep malignant tumors is worthwhile.

References

1. Colombo F, Bennetti A, Pozzo F, et al: External stereotactic irradiation by linear accelerator. *Neurosurgery* 16:154–160, 1985
2. Heifetz MD, Wexler M, Thompson R: Single-beam radiotherapy knife: A practical theoretical model. *J Neurosurg* 60:814–818, 1984

3. Kjellberg RN, Davis KR, Lyons S, et al: Bragg peak proton beam therapy for arteriovenous malformation of the brain. *Clin Neurosurg* 31:248–290, 1983
4. Kjellberg RN, Preston WM: The use of a Bragg peak of a proton beam for intracerebral lesions. In *Proceedings of the Second International Congress of Neurological Surgeons*, 1961, 36 E103
5. Larsson B, Leksell L, Rexed B, et al: The high-energy proton beam as a neurosurgical tool. *Nature* 182:1222–1223, 1958
6. Leksell L: Stereotactic radiosurgery. *J Neurol Neurosurg Psychiatry* 46:797–803, 1983
7. Leksell L: The stereotaxic method and radiosurgery of the brain. *Acta Chir Scand* 102: 316–319, 1951
8. Leksell L, Larsson B, Rexed B: The use of high-energy protons for cerebral surgery in man. *Acta Chir Scand* 125:1–7, 1963
9. Norén G, Arndt J, Hindmarsh T: Stereotactic radiosurgery in cases of acoustic neurinoma: Further experiences. *Neurosurgery* 13:12–22, 1983
10. Patil AA: Computed tomography (CT) oriented rotary stereotactic system: A technical note. *Acta Neurochir* (Wien) 68:19–26, 1983
11. Patil AA: Isocentric placement of target in the linear accelerator using CT stereotaxis: A technical note. Abstract presented at the annual meeting of the Scandinavian Neurosurgical Society, Stockholm, Sweden, September 16, 1984
12. Patil AA, Knudsen D: Single-beam radiosurgery using the linear accelerator and CT stereotaxis. Abstract presented at the 8th International Congress of Neurological Surgery, Toronto, Canada, July 7–11, 1985
13. Steiner L, Leksell L, Forster DMC, et al: Stereotaxic radiosurgery in intracranial arteriovenous malformations. *Acta Neurochir [Suppl]* (Wien) 21:195–209, 1974
14. Zeilstra DJ: Semi-stereotactic irradiation of inoperable intracranial AVM's by linear accelerator: Preliminary results in 45 patients. Abstract presented at the 8th International Congress of Neurological Surgery, Toronto, Canada, July 7–11, 1985

38. STEREOTACTIC RADIOSURGICAL TREATMENT OF ACOUSTIC NEURINOMAS

Georg Norén
Jürgen Arndt
Tomas Hindmarsh
Anita Hirsch

Stereotactic radiosurgery with the "gamma knife" was used for the first time in the treatment of acoustic neurinomas in 1969 [5, 7]. At that time, very little was known about the radiosensitivity of neurinomas to either fractionated or single high-dose irradiation. The radiosensitivity of adjacent structures such as cranial nerves, the brain stem, the cerebellum, and blood vessels also was unknown.

In the first 20 patients, pneumoencephalography, metrizamide cisternography, or computed tomography (CT) were used to outline the intracranial part of the tumor [11]. This information was then transferred onto plain stereotactic skull radiographs using the internal auditory canal and porus as aiming points. In 1976, the development of a stereotactic CT system enabled direct coordinate determination using the CT display and software [1, 8].

The whole procedure gradually has become more accurate with improvements in CT technology, dose planning, and stereotactic technique. More than 180 patients have been treated with radiosurgery. This experience has greatly expanded our knowledge about the response of both the tumor and the adjacent structures to single high-dose radiation.

Localizing Procedure

A standard CT-adapted Leksell stereotactic frame is attached to an aluminium ring that is fixed to the skull under local anesthesia with four pointed screws (figure 38–1). Alternatively, a stereotactic frame especially designed for radiosurgery is used. The patient is scanned with the frame attached to the scanner table. The tumor is visualized after intravenous or intrathecal contrast injection using metrizamide or iohexol. Air CT cisternography is less practical because the head has to be moved to positions not optimal for the stereotactic system. The tumor is mapped carefully with multiple thin-slice (105-mm) CT scans performed to visualize the entire volume, including the intracanalicular portion of the tumor. The relationship of important surrounding structures such as cranial nerves 5, 7, and 8 and the brain stem are defined, as is the site of the tumor within the skull.

Irradiation Parameters

When planning the irradiation procedure, one should aim for a single homogeneous and selective high dose to the tumor. With the collimator options available, a spherical intracranial tumor volume with a diameter equal to or less than 18 mm is treated with the head in one position within the radiosurgical unit. Larger tumors are treated by several irradiations between which the head is repositioned. The intracanalicular portion is irradiated separately. Tumors with a diameter exceeding 30 mm generally are not treated because increasingly inhomogeneous dose distribution eliminates the desirable selectivity that radiosurgery provides. The approximately spherical dose distribution can be modified in size and shape by changing the set of secondary (inner) collima-

L.D. Lunsford (ed.) *MODERN STEREOTACTIC NEUROSURGERY*.
Martinus Nijhoff Publishing. Boston/Dordrecht/Lancaster.

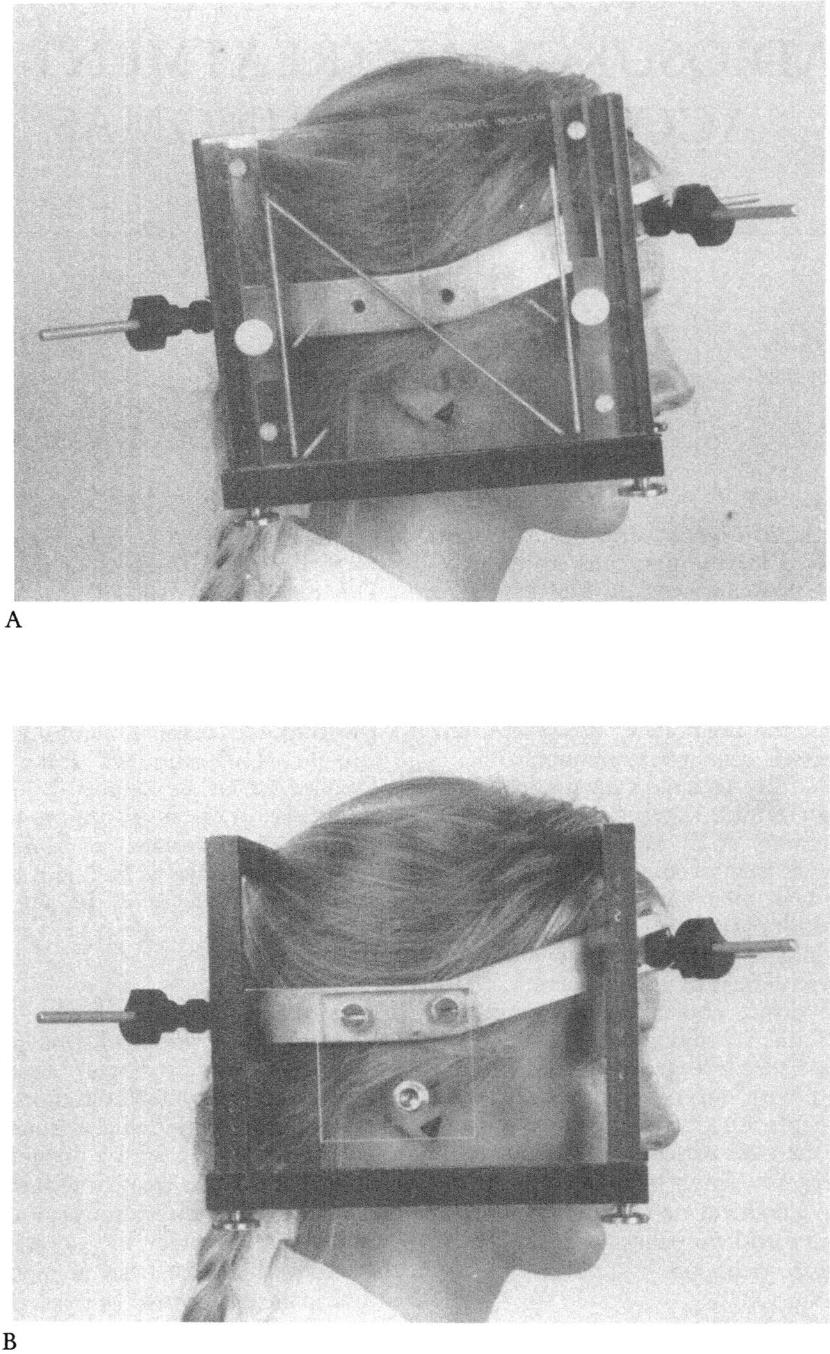

FIGURE 38–1. The stereotactic radiosurgical coordinate frame is adapted for radiographic localization and head fixation in an acoustic neurinoma patient. The two vertical and the 45° diagonal aluminum bars (A) are coordinate indicators, which are displayed as fiducials on the CT picture. According to the coordinate values a pair of holes are drilled in acrylic plates fixed on each side of the aluminum ring (B). Bearings put into these holes fit to trunions in the gamma knife collimator helmet.

tors and by plugging any combination of the collimators within the set.

The tumor periphery should coincide with 90% to 50% of the central dose in order to achieve the steepest possible dose gradient at the border of the tumor. The exact location of the gradient in relation to the tumor is dependent on the size and shape of the tumor.

The radiosensitivity of the critical structures closely surrounding the tumor will primarily determine the highest tolerable dose to the tumor periphery. Empirically, this dose was found to be 18–25 Gy. The 18-Gy dose is delivered to the periphery of the largest tumor. Some other factors such as the patient's age and coexistent vascular disease might implicate a lower tolerance of adjacent structures. The maximum dose within the tumor will usually range from 22–50 Gy.

The exact location of certain critical structures (facial and cochlear nerves, smaller arterial branches) cannot be determined from the radiographic studies. The risk of radiation-induced damage to these structures is consequently lowest when the dose distribution throughout the whole tumor is as homogeneous as possible.

Dose Planning

The distribution of the radiation dose absorbed within and around the tumor is calculated in three dimensions. The calculation is primarily based on the preliminary locations of the irradiation foci selected during the localizing procedure. Dose distributions are summarized from each individual irradiation and presented as isodose curves in planes of the stereotactic frame. If the same magnification is used, these isodose curves can be superimposed onto the tumor as defined on the hard-copy CT scan film. If the dose distribution is unsatisfactory, the locations of the radiation foci are modified until tumor volume is covered in an acceptable way.

Irradiation Procedure

After the radiographic localizing procedure is finished, the stereotactic frame is removed from the aluminum ring and the patient is positioned in the gamma knife unit according to the calculated X, Y, and Z coordinates. After the first irradiation is completed, a new irradiation begins with a new focus position within the head. This sequence is repeated until all irradiations prescribed by the dose plan are performed. The whole treatment including the localizing procedure usually takes four to six hours. The patient often is discharged a few hours after the irradiation.

Results

This chapter is based on our experiences with 110 patients (115 acoustic neurinomas) who were treated, with stereotactic radiosurgery at the Karolinska Hospital, Stockholm between 1969 and 1984. Adequate radiological, audiological, and clinical follow-up evaluations were available in these cases. An additional 16 patients were treated during this same period but were not included in this series because of insufficient data.

RADIOLOGY

Several examples of the response to radiosurgery are demonstrated by CT images in figure 38–2 through figure 38–4. In 60% of the cases, a loss of intravenous contrast enhancement developed in the center of the tumor and spread gradually to the periphery. This process occurred usually from six to 24 months after the irradiation and persisted for several months to years. Usually, however, the residual tumor regained at least some of its contrast-enhancing property over the next one to two years. This was accompanied by a more or less pronounced tumor shrinkage.

In six patients the tumors actually increased in size during the time of loss of enhancement, possibly indicating some radiation-induced swelling. These patients subsequently had permanent shrinkage of their neurinomas and did not require further treatment.

Changes in the tumor contrast enhancement pattern did not necessarily indicate decrease in tumor size. Some patients exhibited marked shrinkage of their neurinomas without enhancement changes (see figure 38–2).

Decrease of tumor size or no change was found in 86% of these cases. Decrease of tumor size was a slightly more frequent finding than no change (table 38–1). Eighty-four percent of patients treated between 1969 and 1981 showed arrest of growth or shrinkage in comparison to 88% of patients who were irradiated between 1982 and 1984 (table 38–2). The latter

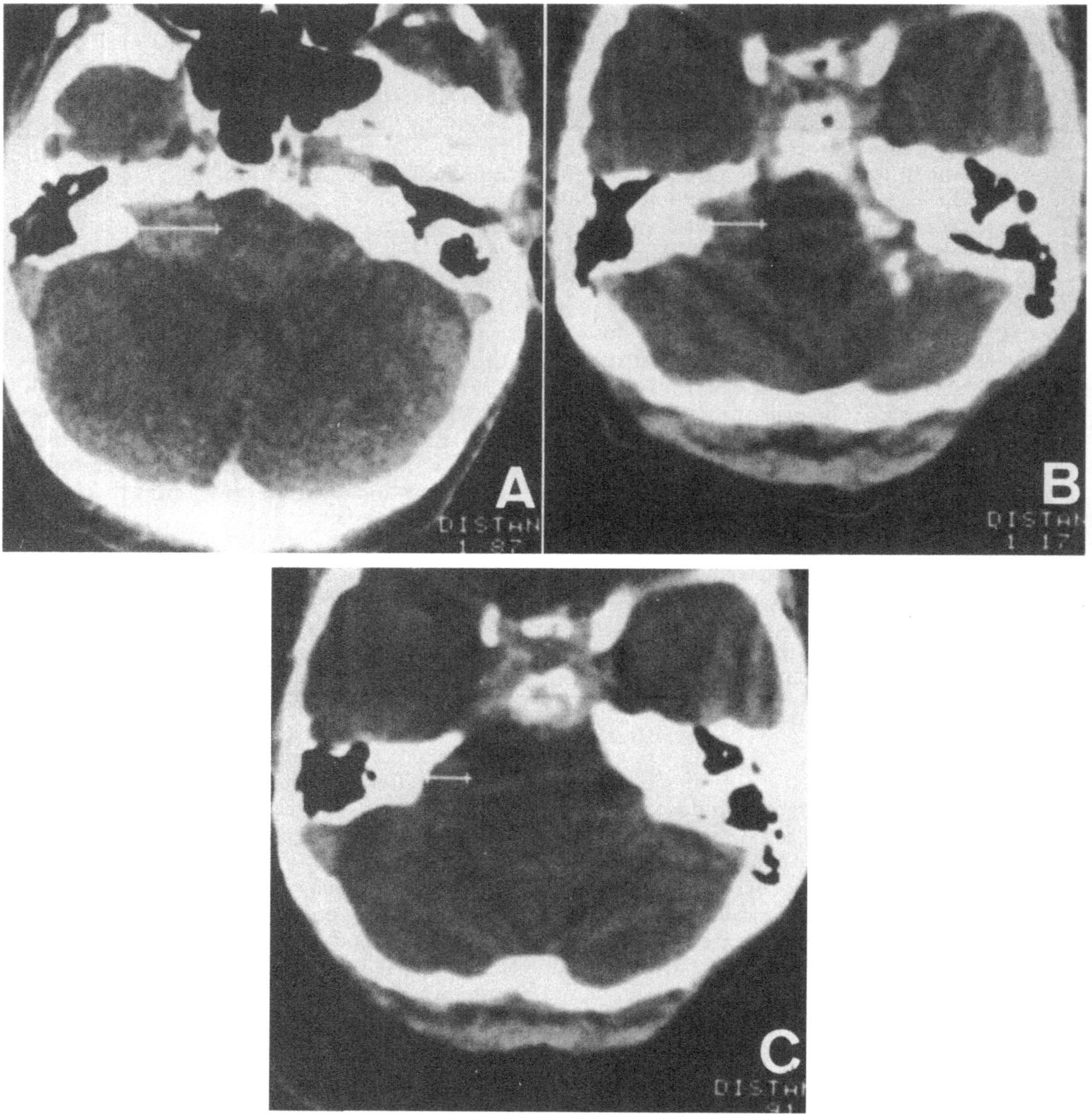

FIGURE 38–2. CT of acoustic neurinoma before (A), 14 (B), and 25 (C) months after stereotactic radiosurgery. A gradual decrease of the tumor size is seen. No obvious change in the CT attenuation pattern followed intravenous contrast administration.

group had the benefit of homogeneous dosimetry; the performance of the stereotactic procedure in this group also corresponded well to our current routine. Ninety-one percent of unilateral tumors responded to the radiosurgery; 67% of tumors associated with neurofibromatosis (all bilateral except for one) responded well (table 38–3).

FACIAL NERVE FUNCTION

Facial weakness, usually mild but in a few cases severe, developed in 15% of all patients (9% during the period of 1982 to 1983, 3% in the period of 1983 to 1984). We noted a marked correlation between the maximum dose of radiation to the tumor and the appearance of facial weakness: no patient who received less

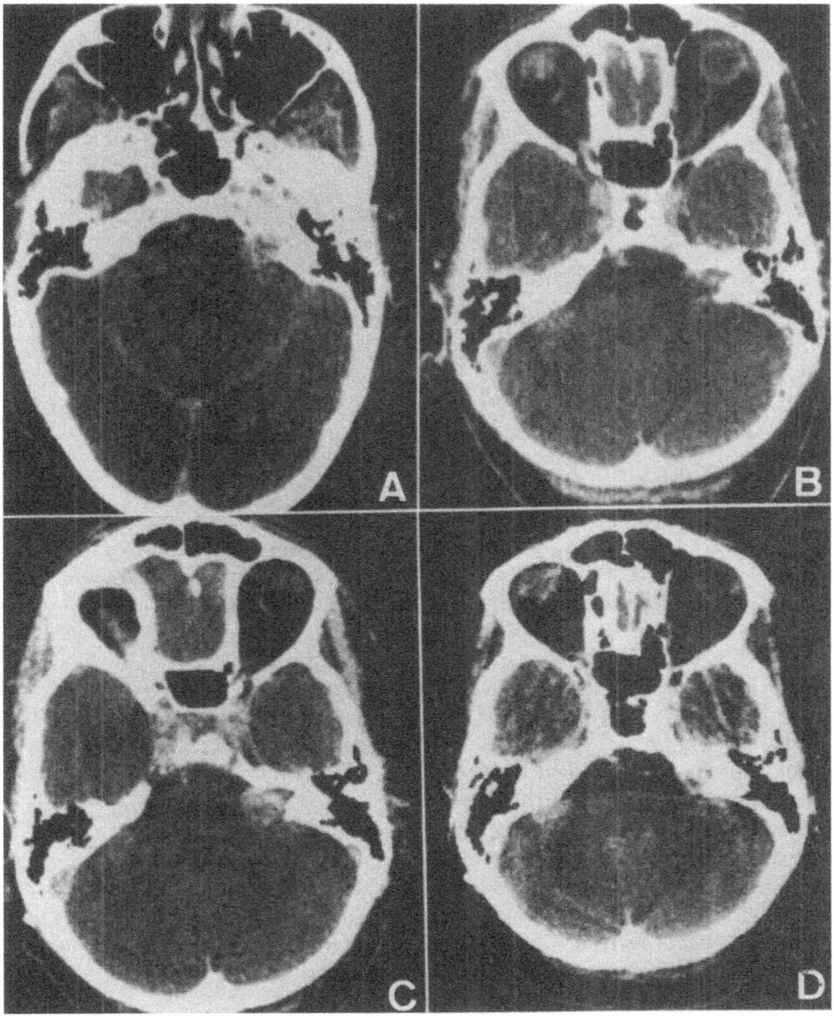

FIGURE 38-3. CT of acoustic neurinoma before (A), 5 (B), 18 (C), and 48 (D) months after stereotactic radiosurgery. At 5 months, reduction in intravenous contrast enhancement was noted. At 18 months, the CT scan showed an increase in tumor size and even more contrast staining. At 48 months definite shrinkage of the tumor is seen. The tumor no longer protruded into the cistern.

than 27 Gy developed weakness and only one who received 27–30 Gy did so. When facial weakness developed, the dose was usually 40 Gy or more.

The onset of facial palsy always appeared with a latency period of four to 15 (usually six to nine) months after radiosurgery. Facial nerve function improved within a few months in mild cases and within six months in more severely affected patients in whom electromyogram (EMG) studies showed signs of total or subtotal denervation.

The facial weakness was transitory in all patients. In the densely paretic cases, synkinesis appeared during the process of reinnervation as seen in equally severe cases of Bell's palsy.

HEARING

Sixty-four patients were evaluated fully prior to radiosurgery; in these patients adequate follow-up data were available, and all had hearing thresholds better than 90 dB pure tone averages (PTA, 0.5, 1.0, 2.0 kHz) before treatment. Fifty-four patients had unilateral tumors.

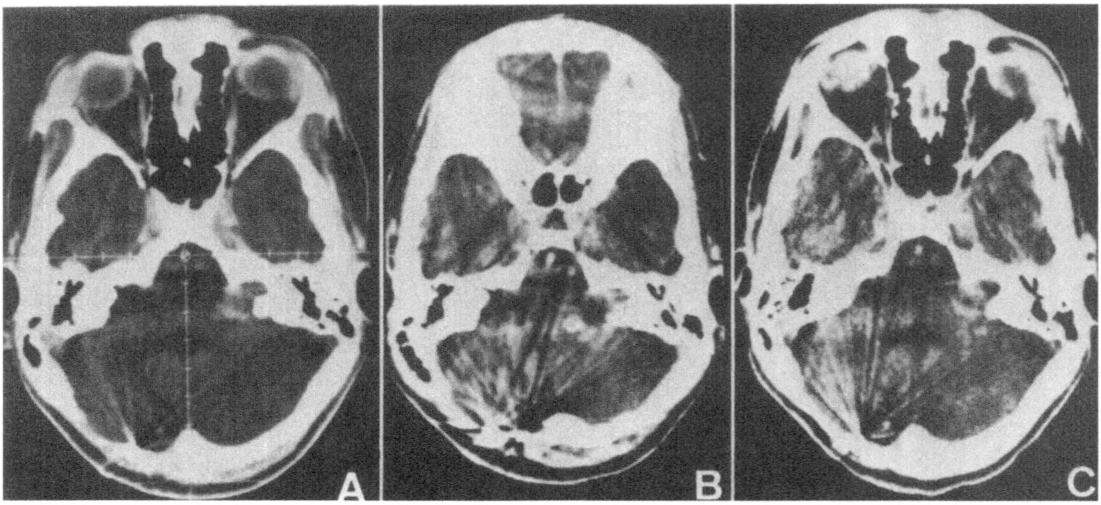

FIGURE 38-4. CT scan of a patient with bilateral acoustic neurinomas. The right-sided tumor was removed earlier via suboccipital surgery. The left-sided tumor was examined before (A), 5 (B), and 18 (C) months after stereotactic radiosurgery. Loss of contrast enhancement (B) and subsequent shrinkage (C) were seen.

Ten patients had bilateral tumors, and one patient was treated on both sides, a total of 65 "ears."

One year after radiosurgery, 26% of the patients had no change in hearing, defined as a change in PTA of less than 5 dB and a discrimination score equal to the value before treatment at a significance level of 5% (table 38-4) [3]. Two patients had significant improvement in hearing, which was verified by tone threshold and speech audiometry tests. Complete deafness (PTA $\geq$ 90 dB) was found in 20% of patients. All other patients showed a deterioration of hearing thresholds and/or loss in the discrimination scores.

One patient with bilateral neurinomas experienced sudden deafness within 24 hours of the irradiation. Corticosteroids were adminis-

TABLE 38-1. Change of Tumor Size after Radiosurgery in 110 Cases (115 Tumors), 1969-1984[a]

Change of Size	No. of Tumors (%)
Decrease	51 (44)
No change	48 (42)
Increase	16 (14)

[a] Follow-up period, 0.5-12.8 years (mean 4.0 years).

TABLE 38-2. Change of Tumor Size After Radiosurgery, 1969-1981 and 1982-1984

Period	Change of Size	No. of Tumors (%)
1969-1981 (57 tumors)	Decrease	29[a] (51)
	No change	19[b] (33)
	Increase	9 (16)
1982-1984 (58 tumors)	Decrease	22[c] (38)
	No change	29[d] (50)
	Increase	7 (12)

[a] Decrease after initial increase of 3 tumors, decrease after re-irradiation of 2 tumors.
[b] No change after initial increase of 1 tumor; no change after re-irradiation of 1 tumor.
[c] Decrease after initial increase of 2 tumors.
[d] No change after re-irradiation of 1 tumor.

tered but had no appreciable effect. With this exception, postoperative hearing in patients with bilateral tumors followed the same general course as noted in patients with unilateral tumors.

Over the subsequent years further deterioration of hearing was seen in most cases. We defined limited hearing loss of 20 dB PTA or less from the preoperative value as "preserved hearing": 56% at one year, 54% at two years, and 28% at six years had preserved hearing after radiosurgery. Speech discrimination scores usually decreased as pure tone thresholds declined, although rarely improvement of discrimination scores paralleled a more "cochlear" profile that was noted in the audiometric test battery. Our most successful patient in this series showed a discrimination score of 85% ten years after radiosurgery.

TRIGEMINAL NERVE FUNCTION

Overall 18% of the patients developed mild facial hypesthesia (9% during the period 1982 to 1984). As similarly noted in those patients who developed facial palsies, a latency period of six to nine months preceded the onset of trigeminal symptoms. The trigeminal motor division was involved very rarely, as checked clinically and by EMG. Several patients already had some facial numbness before the treatment, indicating pressure by the tumor on the trigeminal nerve root.

Complete or partial return of trigeminal function was noted in the mildly affected cases within several months or sometimes more than one year after treatment. Early in the series, five patients developed severe permanent facial anesthesia; in some of these patients, treatment was complicated further by the development of deafferentation pain. All tumors in these latter cases had received a high maximum dose of 50–100 Gy.

LONG-TERM CONSIDERATIONS

Twenty tumors had definite radiographic signs of subsequent growth; four responded favorably to re-irradiation and 11 were removed using standard microsurgical technique. Radiation-induced changes were verified histologically within the central part of most of these tumors. Five tumors so far have not required further treatment.

Cerebrospinal fluid (CSF) shunt operations were performed in 10% of the patients. In most of these cases the hydrocephalus was believed to be communicating in nature. It was sometimes evident at the time of the tumor diagnosis, whereas in other cases, it developed

TABLE 38–3. Change of Tumor Size After Radiosurgery: Unilateral and Neurofibromatosis tumors

Type	Change of Size	No. of Tumors (%)
Unilateral (91 tumors)	Decrease	45 (49)
	No change	38 (42)
	Increase	8 (9)
Neurofibromatosis (24 tumors)	Decrease	6 (25)
	No change	10 (42)
	Increase	8 (33)

TABLE 38–4. Audiologic Findings One Year After Radiosurgery

	Change of Hearing[a]						
	No Change		Deterioration		Deafness		
	No.	Percent	No.	Percent	No.	Percent	Total No.
Unilateral tumors	13	(24)	29	(54)	12	(22)	54
Bilateral (neurofibromatosis) tumors	4	(36)	6	(55)	1	(9)	11

[a] For definition, see text.

one to two years after irradiation. These patients uniformly had markedly elevated (up to fifteen-fold) CSF protein measurements. Peritumoral edema developed in 5% of patients, usually six to 12 months after irradiation. The degree of edema formation varied from a thin rim in the cerebellum adjacent to the tumor to involvement of most of the cerebellar hemisphere. These patients developed varying degrees of balance problems as well as trigeminal symptoms, possibly indicating a radiation-induced disturbance of the circulation of the anterior inferior cerebellar artery (AICA) branches. Corticosteroids provided little relief of this edema [4]. Usually gradual improvement occurred within six to 12 months. No mortality related to the radiosurgical treatment was noted in this series.

Discussion

Acoustic neurinomas generally are regarded as poorly responsive to radiation therapy. This assumption seems to be based more on the availability of satisfactory alternative surgical treatments; very little real experience or knowledge about the radiosensitivity of this kind of tumor exists. Newman and co-workers reported no tumor "recurrences" in 15 patients who underwent subtotal removal of acoustic neurinomas followed by 42–50 Gy of fractionated irradiation [10]. Doses below 32 Gy failed to control growth. This report suggests that acoustic neurinomas in fact are responsive to radiation doses similar to those used in the management of malignant intracranial tumors.

Based on our present knowledge, acoustic tumors are treated with a minimum single dose of radiation of approximately 20 Gy. To minimize the risk of radiation-induced cranial nerve disturbances, the maximum dose to the tumor should not exceed 30 Gy. A 20-Gy dose will inhibit further tumor growth in more than 90% of the unilateral cases and in 67% of the bilateral tumors.

In this study we treated several patients with bilateral tumors generally considered too large for radiosurgical treatment. These patients were accepted for irradiation as a last resort in an attempt to preserve hearing. We believe that if patients are selected with strict size criteria, arrest of growth will be achieved in a higher percentage of these bilateral tumors.

Linthicum noted a different relationship between the seventh and eighth nerves and the tumor tissue in unilateral as opposed to bilateral tumors [9]. In unilateral tumors, the nerves are located on the surface of the tumor; in bilateral tumors, the nerves frequently are divided and extend through the tumor tissue itself. Because the center of the tumor will always receive the highest radiation dose in radiosurgery, in bilateral tumors an excessive central dose should be avoided in order to preserve hearing. This feature was exemplified by the patient with bilateral tumors who experienced sudden deafness within 24 hours of irradiation.

In this series most patients had slow deterioration of hearing. This hearing loss may reflect a gradual impairment of the cochlear nerve and the cochlear system induced most likely by vascular insufficiency. During the 15-year period within which patients in this study were treated major improvements in radiological imaging techniques and in dosimetry occurred. These advances ultimately may improve the prospects of hearing preservation in future patients.

Our results regarding hearing compare well with the results obtained after microsurgical tumor removal. We believe that the slow deterioration of hearing after stereotactic radiosurgery is definitely preferable to immediate deafness, since the patient will have time to adapt to the deafness.

Successful radiosurgical treatment of an acoustic neurinoma cannot be defined in the same way as standard surgical results. The ideal microsurgical result (total tumor removal, normal facial nerve activity, and no complications [2]) does not apply to radiosurgery since the tumor itself is not removed. Gradual and eventually permanent tumor regression must be regarded as a successful or even ideal radiosurgical result, especially if hearing also is preserved. Without radiosurgery, the likelihood of spontaneous permanent shrinkage of acoustic tumors is very low. We regard preservation of facial nerve function as a major benefit of radiosurgery. The incidence of facial paresis after radiosurgery now is only 3% and it is always transient.

In certain patients, the growth rate of an acoustic tumor can be established before treatment [6]. Several patients in the present series had serial CT scans prior to stereotactic radiosurgery. Conceivably if the preirradiation tumor growth rate is unknown, lack of tumor regression after radiosurgery may reflect only the normal behavior of a specific tumor: a few small acoustic tumors show no signs of growth for years, even without treatment. However, recent evidence indicates that the vast majority of untreated tumors show growth when studied for one or more years [5]. We believe that tumors that remain "unchanged in size" [11] one or more years after radiosurgery should be regarded together with those of "decreased size" as having had "successful treatment."

As seen in figures 38–3 and 38–4, an increase in tumor size is occasionally noted approximately one year after treatment and probably represents either true radionecrosis or at least a reaction to the irradiation within the tumor. Tumor regression usually occurs later in the course. A minimal follow-up period of two years is required before the final result of stereotactic radiosurgery can be assessed.

References

1. Bergström M, Greitz T: Stereotaxic computed tomography. *AJR* 127:167–170, 1976
2. DiTullio MV, Malkasian D, Rand RW: A critical comparison of neurosurgical and otolaryngological approaches to acoustic neuromas. *J Neurosurg* 48:1–12, 1978
3. Hagerman B: Reliability in the determination of speech discrimination. *Scand Audiol* 5:219–228, 1976
4. Hatam A, Bergström M, Norén G: Effects of dexamethasone treatment on acoustic neuromas: evaluation by computed tomography. *J Comput Assist Tomogr* 9:857–860, 1985
5. Hirsch A, Norén G, Anderson H: Audiologic findings after stereotactic radiosurgery in nine cases of acoustic neurinomas. *Acta Otolaryngol* (Stockh) 88:155–160, 1979
6. Laasonen EM, Troupp H: Volume growth rate of acoustic neurinomas. *Neuroradiology* 28:203–207, 1986
7. Leksell L: A note on the treatment of acoustic tumours. *Acta Chir Scand* 137:763–765, 1971
8. Leksell L, Jernberg B: Stereotaxis and tomography. *Acta Neurochir* (Wien) 52:1–7, 1980
9. Linthicum FH: Unusual audiometric and histologic findings in bilateral acoustic neurinomas. *Ann Otol* 81:433–437, 1972
10. Newman H, Sheline GE, Boldrey EB: Radiation therapy of tumors of the eighth nerve sheath. *AJR* 120:562–567, 1974
11. Norén G, Arndt J, Hindmarsh T: Stereotactic radiosurgery in cases of acoustic neurinoma: Further experiences. *Neurosurgery* 13:12–22, 1983

39. STEREOTACTIC RADIOSURGICAL TREATMENT OF ARTERIOVENOUS MALFORMATIONS

Christer Lindquist
Ladislau Steiner

Stereotactic radiosurgery for arteriovenous malformations (AVM) of the brain was introduced by Steiner in 1970 at the Karolinska Institute. However, the concept of radiosurgery was coined by Leksell in 1951, when he first described his technique for the irradiation of a sharply delimited intracranial target with stereotactically directed narrow beams of ionizing radiation [7]. Today, radiosurgery can be defined as single-session irradiation of a predetermined target volume, causing destruction or a desired biological effect in this tissue volume without damage to surrounding tissue.

The early experimental radiosurgical operations were performed with protons accelerated in a synchrocyclotron, but this was abandoned for clinical purposes because it was an impractical and expensive tool. The linear accelerator then was considered as an instrument for stereotactic radiosurgery, but it could not meet the requirements for precision and ease of handling. Subsequently the cobalt-60 gamma unit was designed [8]. The radiation field of the gamma unit and the target remain fixed throughout the radiosurgical procedure. The design avoids moving parts, which ensures constant accuracy during the procedure and eliminates focusing errors. The multiple radiation sources guarantee a sharply circumscribed field of irradiation. Equipment failure does not occur, and service is therefore minimal. In contrast to more complicated equipment such as the linear accelerator, the gamma unit is operated easily by the neurosurgeon and one assistant and thus has become a true surgical tool. Localization of the target for radiosurgery demands basic knowledge of stereotactic techniques that is easily obtained. The ability to use this device enables the neurosurgeon to choose between microsurgical and radiosurgical techniques to provide the most favorable therapy for a patient with an AVM.

Treatment Strategies for AVM

The choice of therapeutic strategy in the treatment of a cerebral AVM primarily should take into account the medical history and the clinical condition of the patient and the information available from neuroradiological studies. The risks projected because of the natural history of the malformation should be weighed against the risks inherent in the available treatment modalities. From our own studies and those of others, it is known that AVM patients presenting with a subarachnoid or intracerebral hemorrhage run a 2%–6% risk of rebleeding every year, whereas the risk of hemorrhage from an AVM that has never ruptured is only 1% per year [3, 4]. The interval between initial and later hemorrhages is unpredictable for AVM, and not clustered during the early period as with aneurysms. Therefore, surgical removal of an AVM in the acute stage has not been advocated, except for patients with voluminous hematomas. In recent years, microsurgical techniques have greatly lowered the mortality and morbidity in surgical removal of AVM, even when operations are performed in eloquent areas of the brain. Selective catheterization of feeding arteries and embolization cur-

L.D. Lunsford (ed.) *MODERN STEREOTACTIC NEUROSURGERY*.

rently are being developed as an additional technique that certainly has a place in the therapeutic arsenal. However, at the present time, microsurgical removal and radiosurgery are the only methods available that are curative in the majority of patients.

It is a truism that therapies short of total removal are not satisfactory in eliminating the risk of new hemorrhages. The neurosurgeon confronted with the therapeutic decision-making should thus compare the expected results of microsurgical or intravascular intervention with the morbidity of radiosurgery and the natural history of AVM following radiosurgical treatment. With such considerations, we have formulated and applied a general treatment strategy for AVM in our institution. Microsurgical removal is advocated for small and large ruptured AVM in noneloquent areas of the brain. (A small AVM is here defined as one that can be treated optimally by radiosurgery. At the present time, this corresponds to a diameter of approximately 30 mm.) Small ruptured AVM in eloquent areas and nonruptured AVM in all locations are best treated by radiosurgery. Large malformations present a treatment problem regardless of the treatment modality. In 28 cases, we have tried stereotactic radiotherapy (i.e., fractionated radiation) using the linear accelerator, but the results are discouraging [5]. Recently, a number of patients with remnants of AVM following embolization were examined, and some were suitable for stereotactic radiosurgery. In other cases, although the density of abnormal vessels decreased, the volume of the AVM did not decrease following embolization, and the AVM still was too large for an optimal radiosurgical attack. However, the potential of primary embolization followed by radiosurgery for large AVM should be investigated in close cooperation with interested neuroradiologists.

Radiosurgical Treatment Strategies

In 1970, when Steiner first attempted radiosurgical treatment of AVM, radiotherapy had been used as a last therapeutic resort by several physicians but was considered ineffective and was largely abandoned [6]. The effects of radiation on the vascular walls had been studied by several investigators (for review, see [9]), but the effects and dosage requirements of single-dose gamma irradiation were not well known. Thus, the successful treatment of the first two patients greatly influenced which treatment strategies were adopted.

According to accepted neurosurgical principles, the cluster of pathological vessels was considered the prime target for the radiation. However, the first person considered for radiosurgery was chosen because conventional surgery was a great risk. The patient had a rather large AVM, and with the small collimators available in the first gamma unit, it was not possible to cover the cluster of pathological vessels. Instead, the two terminal branches of the artery feeding the AVM in the medial part of the left occipital lobe were included within a single radiation field, and 50 Gy were delivered over about half an hour. The malformation could no longer be visualized on the arteriogram made 19 months later. This remarkable result indicated that "gamma ligation" of feeding arteries, in contrast to surgical ligation, could be an effective treatment. Although it is difficult to surgically ligate all feeding arteries, including those deeply located, all feeders can, at least theoretically, be reached by the radiosurgical beams. Feeding artery irradiation is an attractive concept, because it implies that the field of radiation covers only the arterial feeders and the radiation field can be kept at a minimum by using the smallest collimators available (4 or 8 mm). Unfortunately, the procedure has not been easy to develop, because feeding arteries are often multiple and widely dispersed around the cluster of pathological vessels. Furthermore, for accurate determination of the stereotactic coordinates of a feeding artery, the same point on the artery must be identified in at least two projections, which is often very difficult on an ordinary arteriogram. Digital angiography and multiple projections may be the future solution to this localization problem.

The second radiosurgical case was a small AVM in the right basal ganglia. It was possible to include almost the entire cluster of pathological vessels within a field of 50 Gy. One year later, the malformation could no longer be visualized by arteriography. "Total coverage" since has proven to be the most reliable radiosurgical treatment strategy for AVM. However, in larger AVM, "total coverage" often is impossible to achieve with a single field of irradiation, even with our largest available collimator (14 mm), and the use of overlapping fields is necessary. By the summation, the maximum dose to the tissue then may exceed the individual target doses and can jeopardize the integrity of functioning brain. It is also likely that the risk of radionecrosis in the surrounding brain exceeds the increase of the volume irradiated. Therefore, rather than using several fields of radiation, we occasionally have used a strategy of "partial coverage." In these situations, the priority is to enclose the area where feeding arteries enter with an optimal dose.

Encouraged by the good results in the group of patients treated by total coverage, we recently have ventured to treat even large AVM with up to six overlapping fields of irradiation in a single-stage procedure for total coverage. To minimize the risk for radionecrosis, the dose has been kept considerably lower than what has hitherto been considered optimal. This "low-dose total coverage" strategy should yield some success, which, however, probably will not match our current results. The low incidence of radiologically proved obliteration in Kjellberg's series (20%) is due to the use of low doses.

Procedure

Radiosurgery requires that the field of irradiation is delivered with great precision. It is therefore crucial that the orientation of the patient's head in relation to the stereotactic frame is maintained precisely throughout the localization procedure and that the spatial relationship between the target and the fixation points of the head in the collimator helmet is not disrupted during the irradiation.

The entire procedure is carried out in one day and does not need repetition if successful. Local anesthesia is used while fastening the stereotactic frame on the head, except in children, who may require general anesthesia. Sedatives and analgesics occasionally are needed.

DOSE PLANNING AND TARGET LOCALIZATION

Dosimetry can be planned using the available diagnostic angiograms. The dose distribution in the target area is influenced by the size and shape of the patient's skull and by the target location. The measurements of the mediolateral, anterosuperior and anteroposterior radii of the approximately elliptical skull are entered into a minicomputer along with the distance of the target from the midpoint of the skull. Until a more sophisticated program became available, a computer used this information to produce isodose curves in the lateral, frontal, and axial planes through the intended focal point (figure 39–1) [1]. The isodose curves were printed on transparent paper, which was placed on lateral and frontal films of a stereotactic angiogram showing the full extent of the malformation. The focal point of the gamma beams was selected so that the periphery of the malformation coincided with the steepest isodose gradient, that is, the 50%–90% isodose curves. The gamma ray focus then was marked on the arteriogram, and the respective coordinates were read from the projections of the frame on the film. Next, the true stereotactic coordinates were calculated graphically or with a computer, as previously described [2]. With our new computer program, dosimetry is planned directly from a rapid serial angiography performed while a conventional Leksell stereotactic frame is on the patient's head. The stereotactic coordinates of the midpoint of the skull and the target are determined as before, and these values are processed by the minicomputer. Empirically, a minimum dose of 20–25 Gy to the malformation provides the best prospect for obliteration, and the target dose is determined accordingly. The new program allows the surgeon to select the desired peripheral dose to the AVM, and the computer will suggest focal points and collimators for multiple targets to achieve that peripheral dose. The transparent paper with the isodose curves then can be placed on lateral and frontal films showing the full extent of the malformation, so that accurate target placement can be confirmed. To avoid human error, it is preferable that two individuals each obtain separate coordinate determinations. A larger malformation needs a larger target dose if the minimal dose is to reach the periphery. A large target dose or a high dose in an overlapping area of two or more radiation fields can increase the risk of unwanted radionecrosis; therefore the dose delivered to the periphery of the AVM should be limited. The risk of radionecrosis with a given target dose presumably increases with the total volume irradiated. Nevertheless, in nine cases, the target dose to a single field with the largest collimator (14 mm) reached 100 Gy with no

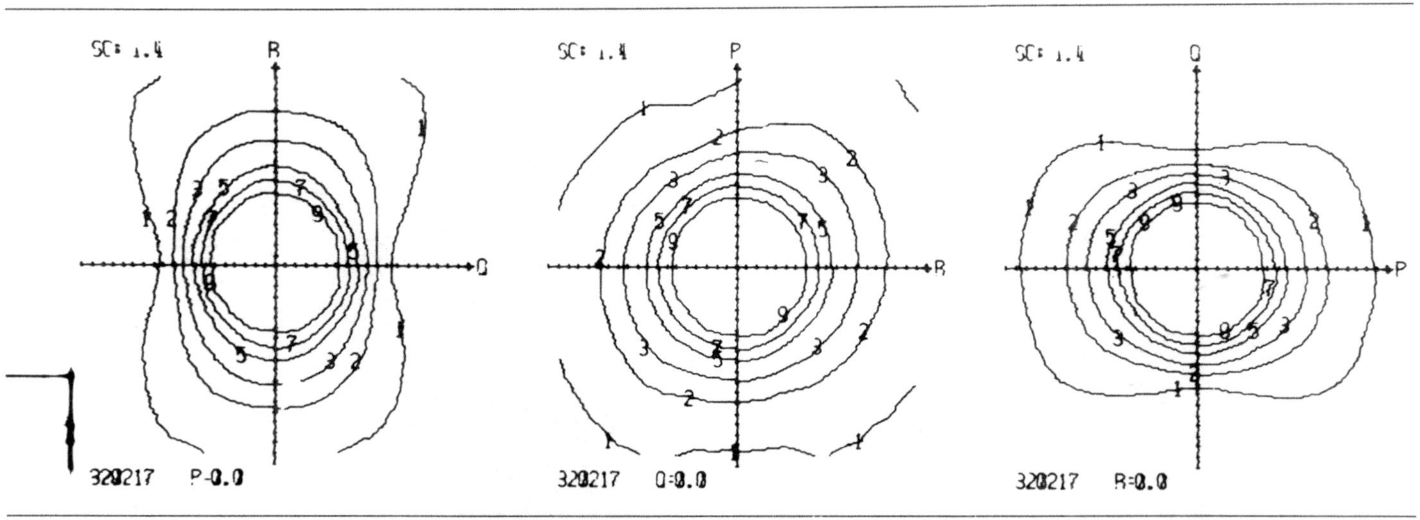

FIGURE 39–1. Isodose curves for 14-mm collimator in the lateral, frontal, and axial projections.

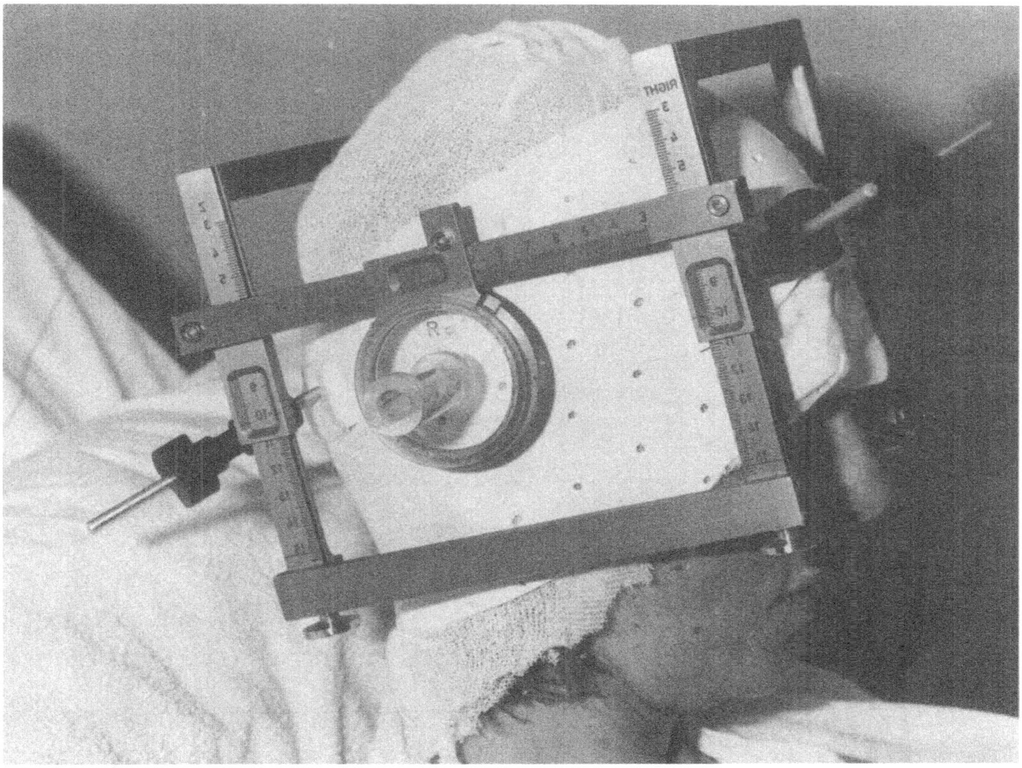

FIGURE 39–2. Leksell stereotactic frame in position for fixation of metal sockets on Orthoplast® helmet.

untoward effects. However, to emphasize the biological factors involved, radionecrosis occurred in a few cases in which the target dose in a single 14-mm field was only 50 Gy.

The standard Leksell frame does not fit into the collimator helmet of our gamma unit and, therefore, cannot be used to suspend the patient's head during treatment. This problem has been circumvented by using the standard frame for placement of bearings (sockets), at the correct Y and Z coordinates, on a metal ring or plastic helmet previously fixed to the skull (figure 39–3). The collimator helmet axis rods, which point to the focal spot of the gamma beams, are pushed into these sockets to suspend the head during treatment. The helmet is formed around the patient's head by using a commercially available plastic material* which is soft and pliable when warm, and hard and rigid at room temperature. To prevent rotation of the helmet, it usually is anchored to the skull by two metal plates previously screwed into the outer table of the skull while the patient is under local anesthesia. The axis rods are used to position the target point at the center of the collimator helmet, using the X coordinate determined from the angiogram. However, the X coordinate must be adjusted for the possible difference in distance between the midpoint of the frame and the midpoint between the bottoms of the bearings. This is easily done by measuring the distance from the outer edge of the frame to the bottom of the respective socket using the device shown in figure 39–3. Alternatively, a frontal projection with the sockets in place can be used to calculate the distance between the midpoint of the frame and midpoint between the bottoms of the bearings; this measurement then is used for adjusting the X coordinate.

The thermoplastic helmet has been used for the majority of AVM treatments and has proven reliable. However, a new fixation device for the Leksell stereotactic system has been developed and is used in the new generation gamma units. The new system incorpo-

Orthoplast® [Johnson & Johnson Products, Inc., New Brunswick, NJ]

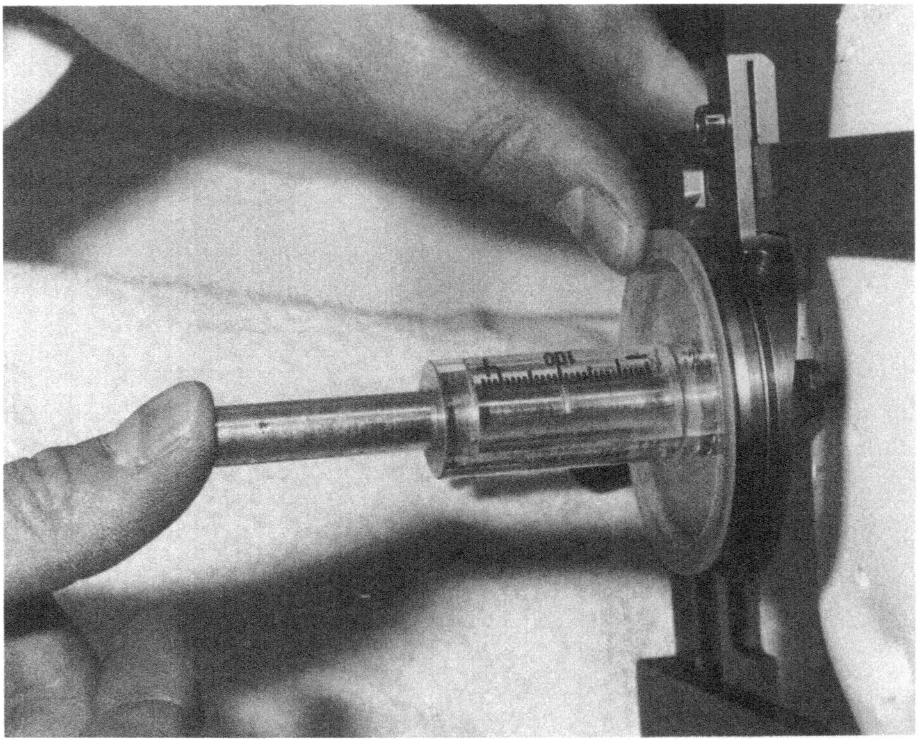

FIGURE 39–3. Close-up of device for application of metal sockets on plastic helmet. Note scale for measuring distance from frame edge to socket bottom. (Full description in text.)

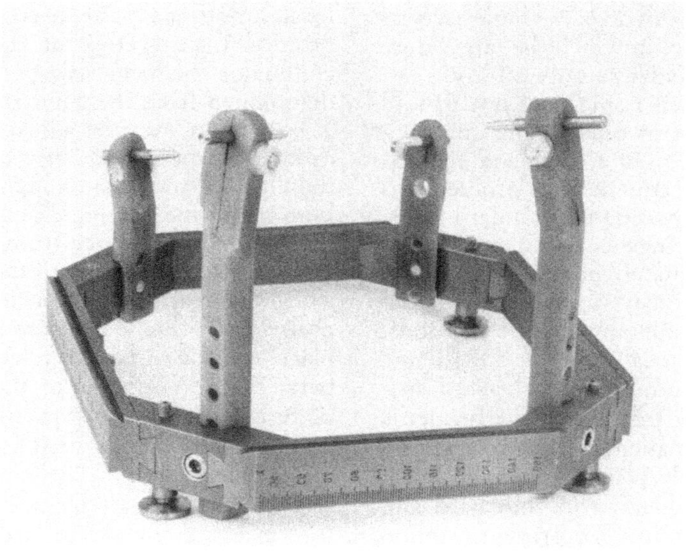

FIGURE 39–4. Base instrument for stereotactic target localization and fixation of patient in the gamma unit.

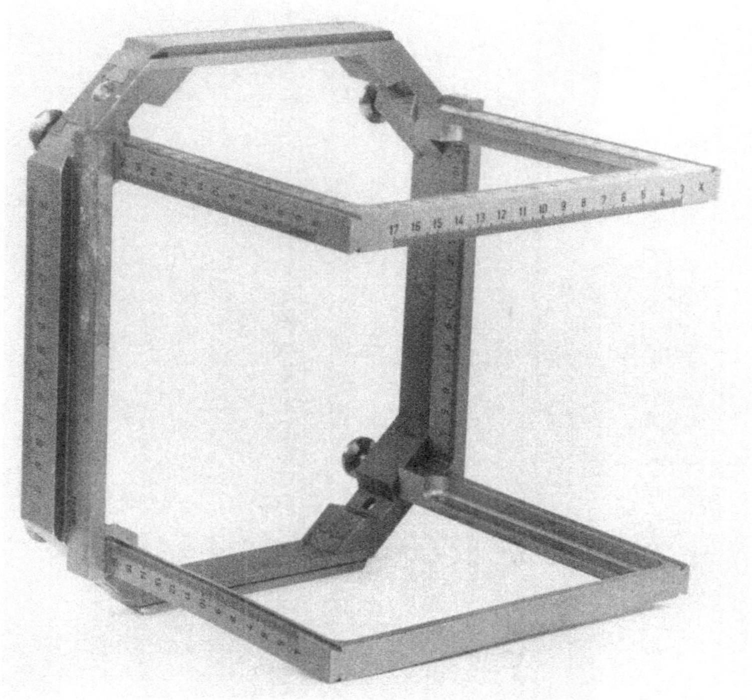

FIGURE 39–5. Leksell stereotactic frame attached to base instrument for stereotactic angiography.

rates the standard instrument and a base instrument. The base instrument (figure 39–4) is a rectangular, ring-like construction compatible with all modern imaging techniques. This structure is fixed to the skull, encircling the lower aspect of the face anteriorly and the upper cervical spine posteriorly. Fixation of the base instrument is provided by four fiberglass posts, each of which is anchored by a pin to a shallow drill hole in the skull. The standard Leksell stereotactic frame can be fastened to the upper surface of the base instrument via four metal or plastic screws (figure 39–5). On completion of target localization, the standard frame is removed, and adjustable side arms are set to the appropriate Y and Z coordinates, one on each side of the base ring. The base instrument is capable of providing spatial orientation by itself when the axis rods are connected to the sockets of the side arms. Because the midpoint between the side arms is also the midpoint of the frame coordinate system, the X coordinate determined can be used directly to position the patient correctly in the inner collimator helmet. After the irradiation shield of the gamma unit is opened, the operating table holding the patient slides into the unit. The inner helmet interconnects with the outer collimator helmet. The irradiation time is determined by the age of the cobalt sources and, to some extent, by the position of the malformation. In 1987, the dose rate was about 0.7 Gy/minute, or one-fourth of the original dose rate. Following irradiation, the helmet or other fixation device is removed, and the patient is returned to the ward. Discharge is deferred until the next day to monitor bleeding from the point of introduction of the angiography catheters in the femoral artery. There usually are no subjective complaints at the time of discharge, and the patient can resume normal activities immediately. A few patients have complained of nausea the day after treatment, and one patient with a brain-stem AVM had transient diplopia.

Follow-Up

Complete obliteration seems to be the only safeguard against hemorrhage from an AVM;

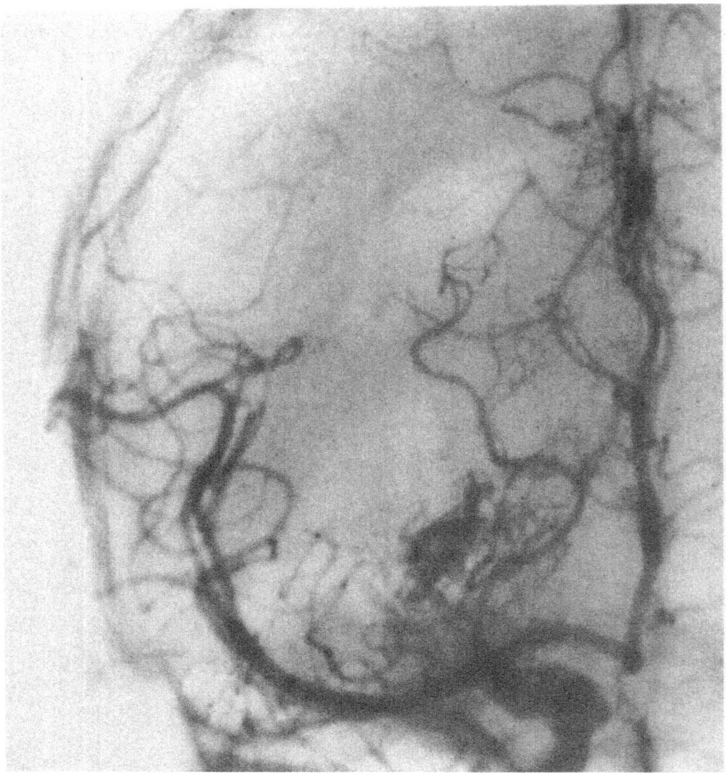

A

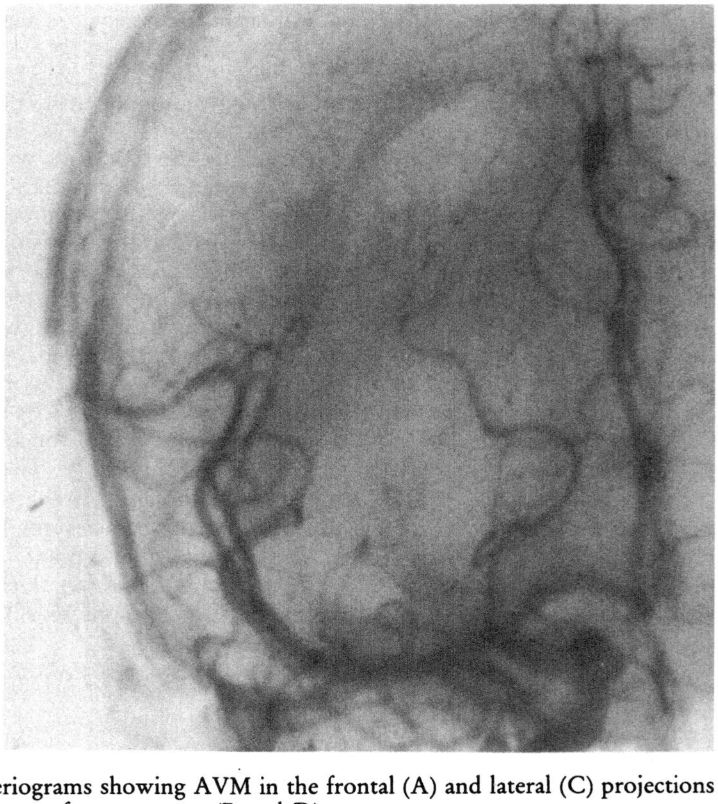

B

FIGURE 39–6. Arteriograms showing AVM in the frontal (A) and lateral (C) projections before radiosurgical treatment and one year after treatment (B and D).

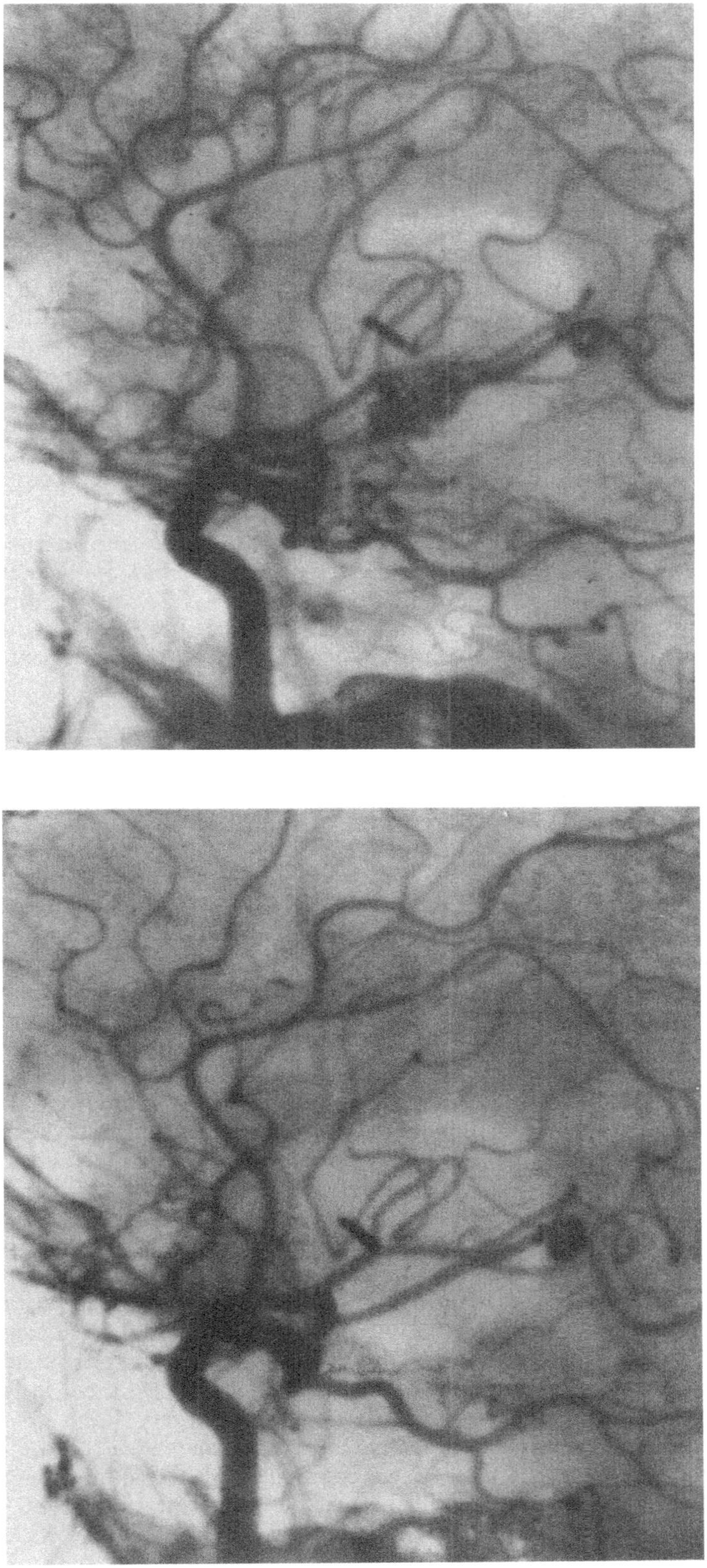

D

FIGURE 39–6. (cont.)

therefore, arterial angiography is necessary to confirm the effects of the radiosurgical treatment. In the beginning of the radiosurgical era, the first angiographic study often was done less than one year after treatment. However, in seven patients, arteriography performed within three months of treatment failed to reveal any obliteration, and in 18 patients studied within six months, only three obliterated AVM were seen. On the other hand, among 104 patients examined one year after radiosurgery, 39 were rid of their malformations. In consideration of the low benefit of early angiography and the relative risks involved, we now routinely recommend that the first follow-up angiography be performed one year after treatment. Digital subtraction angiography is an alternative for a follow-up study, but even if this indicates that the malformation was obliterated, we still recommend conventional serial arteriography for definite proof of a successful result. When the malformation is seen clearly on computed tomography (CT) or magnetic resonance imaging (MRI) scans, these imaging techniques, of course, offer an attractive primary imaging procedure for follow-up. In most cases, the arteriogram will show a definite effect of the radiosurgical treatment, but in only 40% of the optimally treated patients will complete obliteration be proved. In the other patients, a second postoperative arteriographic study is recommended two years after treatment. By then, the end result usually can be observed, but in a few patients, obliteration may be subtotal, and a third arteriogram then may be warranted after an additional year. Occasionally, the arteriograms performed at both one and two years will show minimal or no decrease of the AVM. In such cases, additional radiation or alternative treatment should be considered.

The angiographic criteria for an acceptable result are not yet fully elucidated. Until now, we have considered a result satisfactory only when the arteriogram has shown a normal circulation time, complete absence of pathological vessels in the former nidus of the malformation, and the disappearance or normalization of draining veins from the area. Although other, less satisfactory, results may be of some benefit to the patient, we contend that the criteria mentioned should be met before the malformation can be called obliterated and the patient declared cured.

Of course, the patient also should be monitored postoperatively for any undue effects of the radiosurgical treatment. Radiation-induced edema, delayed radiation necrosis, and obliteration of normal vessels (one case only) are the negative effects we have encountered so far. Any significant edema usually occurs within a few months. In some cases the edema resolves spontaneously, but in others, it heralds delayed radiation necrosis. Empirically, a CT scan performed six months after treatment will disclose any edema or early radionecrosis of importance while the process still can be influenced by steroid therapy. Therefore, we recommend that a CT scan be performed six months after radiosurgery as the first postoperative follow-up study. MRI shows postradiation-induced edema even better. Delayed radiation-induced necrosis is diagnosed using contrast-enhanced CT, on which this type of lesion appears as a central, low-attenuation area encircled by a contrast-enhanced high-density rim.

Patient Population and Results

Since the inception of radiosurgery, nearly 600 AVM have been treated by this method in Stockholm and 90 at Clinica del Sol in Buenos Aires. With the increased acceptance of the method, the number of patients treated every year in Stockholm has risen to approximately 100 per year, which is our present capacity for stereotactic angiography but is insufficient for the increasing demand. By 1982, 137 patients had been treated, and by 1985, the total had reached 332. Experiences with these cases form the backbone of our current body of radiosurgical knowledge. Patients of all ages have been treated, but the majority have been young. Men and women are represented in equal proportions. The patient population is biased, not only by our own treatment strategies, but also by biases of the referring physicians. Of course, the proportion of small AVM is large. Only a small portion of AVM were larger than 30 mm in their largest diameter. It should come as no surprise that many of the malformations were located in areas difficult to access by surgery (table 39–1). The reason why more than 90% of the patients were referred after suffering a subarachnoid hemorrhage is less readily apparent, as our general treatment strategy for AVM encourages microsurgical removal of ruptured AVM whenever feasible. In contrast, only 4% of our patients presented

TABLE 39-1. Anatomical Site of 250 Arteriovenous Malformations Treated by Radiosurgery

Site	No. of Cases
Thalamus and basal ganglia	56
Periventricular	51
Brain-stem cisterns	43
Occipital lobe	22
Sylvian fissure, insula	16
Corpus callosum	15
Parietal lobe	13
Cerebellum	9
Frontal lobe	8
Brain stem	7
Temporal lobe	7
Dura	3

with epilepsy, which has been the main presenting feature in some other series of patients. It may be that subarachnoid hemorrhage, being a more dramatic and serious symptom, more easily prompts a physician to refer a patient abroad.

At an early stage, we concluded that better results were achieved when the entire malformation could be irradiated with an optimal dose. Consequently, a large majority of patients received at least 20–25 Gy of radiation designed to treat the entire volume. Of the 248 patients treated before 1984, the treatment specifications placed 188 in this group. For complete coverage, it was necessary to use more than one field in 49 patients, even with the 14-mm collimator. In 43 patients, two fields were needed; in five patients, three fields; and in one patient, four fields.

The angiographic findings in a typical patient treated by complete coverage before, and one year after, treatment are illustrated in figure 39–6. The patient was a woman who was in good health until the age of 32, when she suffered a subarachnoid hemorrhage without consequent neurological deficits. The cerebral arteriogram (figure 39–6A, C) revealed an AVM in the quadrigeminal cistern fed by the left posterior cerebral and left anterior choroidal arteries. The size of the malformation was 10 × 15 × 10 mm. Two months after the hemorrhage, the patient was in excellent condition and the treatment was carried out. Due to the small size of the malformation it was possible to cover it completely within the 50% isodose line, using one field and the 8-mm collimator. The target dose selected was 50 Gy, and the whole malformation thus received at least 25 Gy. The follow-up arteriogram performed one year after treatment revealed complete obliteration of the malformation (figure 39–6B, D). It should be emphasized that obliteration was accomplished without occlusion or disturbance of flow in the normal brain vessels. An arteriogram also was performed in this patient 67 months after treatment. The findings were still normal, and there were no signs of recanalization of the malformation or negative effects on the normal vessels.

Another example is given in Figure 39–7. The patient was a 47-year-old man who, for 17 years, had been suffering from headache and seizures, but never had a subarachnoid hemorrhage and was neurologically intact. The preoperative left carotid arteriogram showed the full extent of the malformation (figure 39–7A, C), which was fed by the left pericallosal and callosomarginal arteries. This malformation could have been removed safely by microsurgical techniques, but in light of the fact that the patient never had a hemorrhage, radiosurgical treatment was preferred. Also, using the 8-mm collimator, this malformation could be covered completely with an effective dose. The target dose in this case was 100 Gy. An arteriogram performed five months after the treatment showed a decrease of the malformation; the AVM did not appear at all on the next study, performed 27 months after treatment (figure 39–7B, D). Thus, the occlusion of the malformation occurred sometime between five and 27 months after treatment. In this case, a decrease and normalization of the caliber of the main feeding artery was obvious in the lateral projection of the carotid arteriogram (figure 39–7D).

The angiographic results after treatment of an AVM with complete coverage has been consistent throughout the years, as shown in table 39–2. This table summarizes the results from two previous reports and the accumulated results in 159 more recent patients for whom adequate angiographic follow-up studies are available. Satisfactory results, that is, complete obliteration of the pathological vessels, were obtained in approximately 80% of patients, whereas lack of effect was found in only 1%–5%.

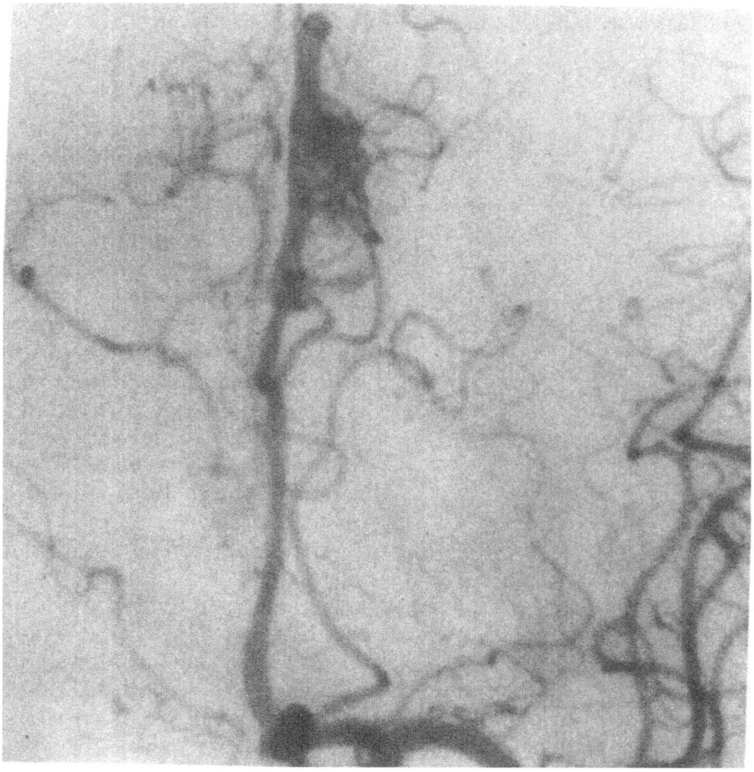

A

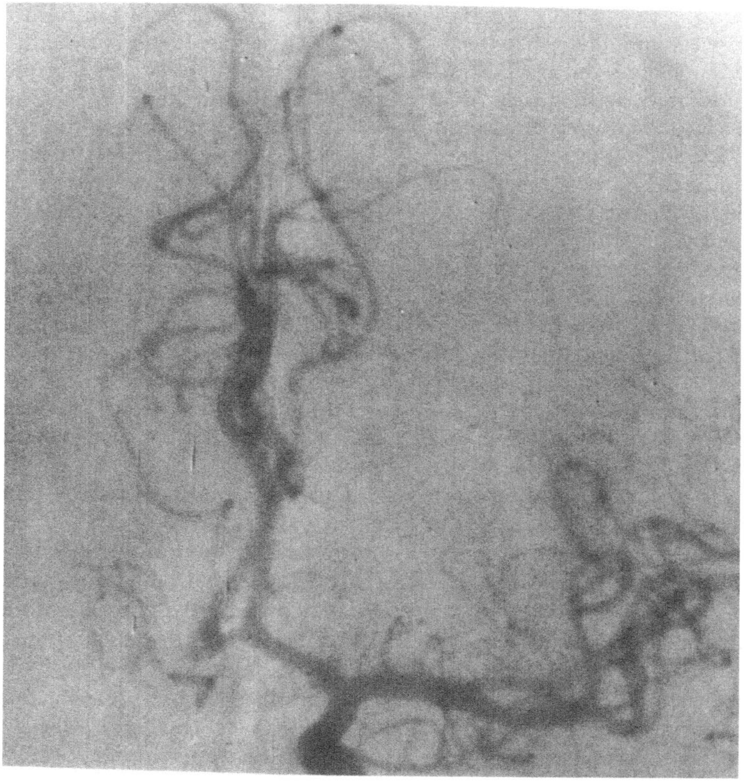

B

FIGURE 39–7. Left carotid arteriograms before (A and C) and after (B and D) radiosurgical treatment. Complete obliteration of AVM is demonstrated 27 months after treatment (B and D).

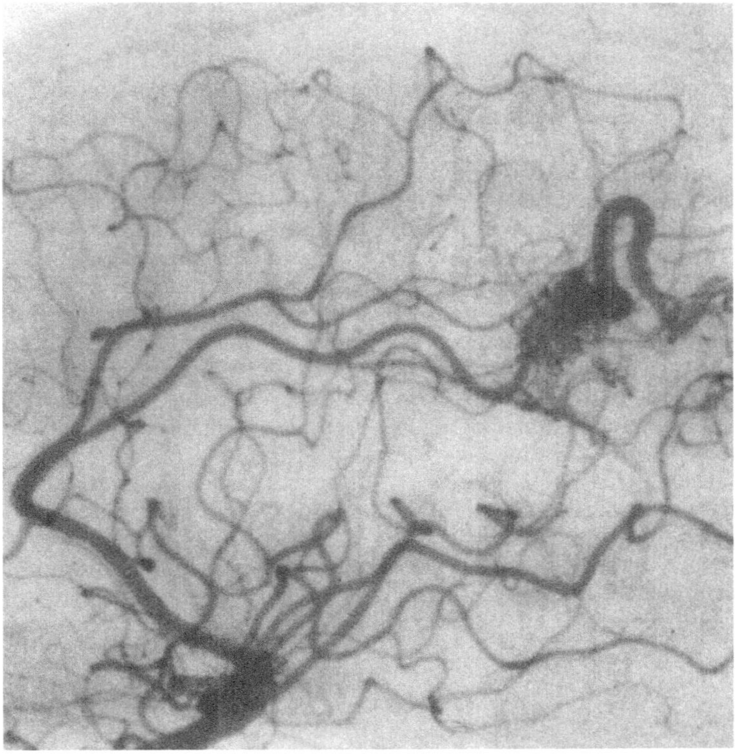

C

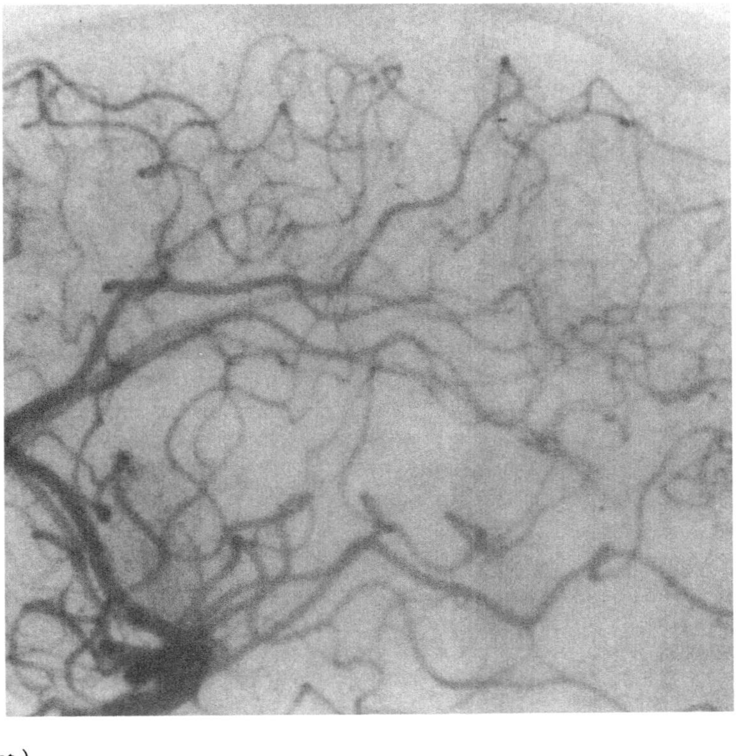

D

FIGURE 39–7. (cont.)

The percentage of malformations obliterated after incomplete coverage was much less satisfactory. However, in some cases, the malformation decreased to the extent that it could be completely covered in a second attempt. Therefore, some malformations recently were treated a second time, and the results are promising.

Irradiation of only the feeding arteries was tried in four of the patients treated before 1984. In one patient, the malformation was obliterated, in one it decreased, in one it was unaffected, and one patient has not been available for follow-up. With better imaging of cerebral vessels now possible, feeding artery irradiation deserves further trials.

The effect of radiosurgery on clinical symptoms is difficult to evaluate, as most of the patients were treated during a period after hemorrhage, when natural improvement was still to be expected. In recent follow-up questionnaires pertaining to the clinical outcome, information was obtained about 239 of 247 patients (97%), and this is now being analyzed. Preliminary findings indicate that the risk of rebleed following radiosurgery is not abolished until the malformation is completely obliterated and that recurrent hemorrhage or radionecrosis is the cause of new deficits following treatment. The first clinical sign of radionecrosis is headache occuring three to six months after treatment. The CT scan at this time reveals a low-density area with contrast enhancement at the location of the radiation field (figure 39–9). In five patients, the radionecrosis was accompanied by hemiparesis, but all five remain ambulatory. Improvement directly related to the radiosurgical treatment was more difficult to ascertain, but headache improved in many patients. In some patients, a seizure disorder was cured, but there were also a few cases in which seizures occurred only after treatment. The patients with radionecrosis and those with epilepsy soon will be scrutinized more carefully and findings will be presented in separate reports.

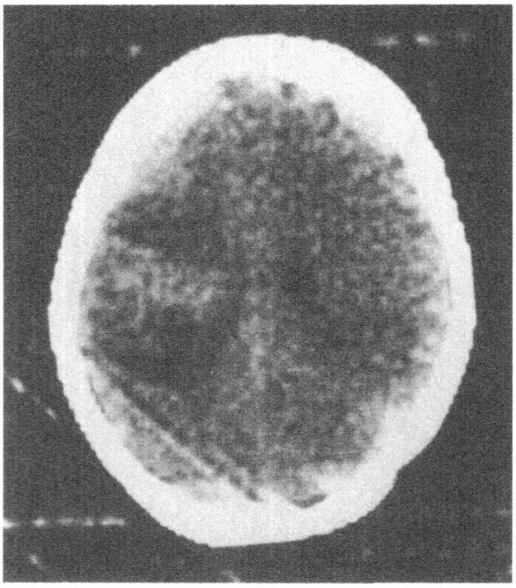

FIGURE 39–8. Contrast-enhanced CT image shows radionecrosis in right cerebral hemisphere.

Problems and Prospects

In selected patients with AVM, the overall results of stereotactic radiosurgery with the Leksell gamma unit are better, and complications are fewer, than with any other method of therapy so far described. However, only a fraction (maybe 30%) of AVM currently can be treated by radiosurgery. Most AVM are too large to be included completely within a radiation field without jeopardizing adjacent normal brain tissue. In addition, being dose-dependent, the risk is lessened by lowering the dose, but most likely, the chances of obliterating the malformation also will decrease. However, perhaps at a higher dose level the risk of radionecrosis parallels the likelihood of

TABLE 39–2. Results of Radiosurgical Treatment

Year of Report	No. of Cases	Percent Obliterated	Percent Unaffected
1984	63	84.1	4.7
1985	104	86.5	1.9
1987	159	79.2	1.3

obliteration. If this is so, malformations with larger volumes should respond to proportionately lower doses; unfortunately, there is little evidence to substantiate such a proposition at this time. However, Kjellberg claims that a small dose (10 Gy) to a large malformation may protect the patient from rebleeding by strengthening the vascular walls, even though the malformation is not obliterated. This claim has not been corroborated in our results.

Another approach to the large malformations has been tried in our institution: In 28 patients, stereotactic radiotherapy was attempted by using a linear accelerator to deliver 42 Gy in fractionated doses over a six-week period. The results have been dismal [5]. Further development is needed before we can treat effectively the larger malformations with radiosurgery. First, we need to find out more about the relationship between a high single dose, volume, and necrosis in the normal human brain; next, to define what is the minimum effective therapeutic dose. Then, attempts should be made to lower this minimum effective dose by using adjuvant agents to sensitize the vascular walls of the malformation. A better understanding of the reaction of normal vascular walls to single-dose ionizing radiation would be valuable in this context. Such studies are under way.

A special problem is presented by malformations in close proximity to eloquent areas, such as the brain stem, where even minute radionecrosis may be unforgiving. Up to now, some such malformations may have been given unnecessarily low and therefore nonoptimal doses simply because of ignorance about the radiosensitivity of the various brain structures. It also should be emphasized that the steep isodose gradients characteristic of the gamma unit must be exploited at these sites to spare structures seemingly more vulnerable than others, such as the cranial nerves.

The major threat to the patient after radiosurgical treatment is not the negative effects of the radiation itself, but the risk of rebleeding during the one- to three-year latency period of obliteration. Therefore, we have tried various ways of decreasing this latency period. In one series of patients, the radiosurgical treatment was supplemented by infusions of fresh frozen plasma was infused to promote thrombosis of the malformation, but no obvious latency decrease was noted. In another attempt, 50 patients were assigned randomly to a control group or to a group receiving a two-week course of postoperative treatment with tranexamic acid, again, in an effort to promote rapid AVM thrombosis. This adjuvant treatment also failed to achieve its purpose. It is our hope that in our search for vascular-wall sensitizers for the large AVM we also will find an agent to expedite the obliteration process.

References

1. Arndt J, Backlund EO, Dahlin H, et al: A computer-controlled dose planning system for irradiation of small volumes of the brain with a multicobalt unit. In *Proceedings of the Third Congress of the European Society of Radiology*, Edinburg, 1975
2. Bergstrom M, Greitz T, Steiner L: An approach to stereotaxic radiography. *Acta Neurochir* (Wien) 54:157, 1980
3. Crawford PM, West CR, Chadwick DW, et al: Arteriovenous malformations of the brain: Natural history in unoperated patients. *J Neurol Neurosurg Psychiatry* 49:1–10, 1986
4. Forster DMC, Steiner L, Hakansson S: Arteriovenous malformations of the brain: A long-term clinical study. *J Neurosurg* 37:562, 1972
5. Greitz T, Lax I, Bergstrom M, et al: Stereotactic radiation therapy of intracranial lesions: Methodologic aspects. *Acta Radiol* (Stockh) 25:81–89, 1986
6. Johnson RT: Radiotherapy of cerebral angiomas with a note on some problems in diagnosis. In Pia HW, Gleave JRW, Grote E, et al (eds): *Cerebral Angiomas: Advances in Diagnosis and Therapy*. Berlin: Springer-Verlag, 1975, pp 256–259
7. Leksell L: The stereotaxic method and radiosurgery of the brain. *Acta Chir Scand* 10:316, 1951
8. Leksell, L: *Stereotaxis and Radiosurgery: An Operative System*. Springfield, IL: Thomas, 1971
9. Steiner L: Treatment of arteriovenous malformations by radiosurgery. In Wilson CB, Stein BM (eds): *Intracranial Arteriovenous Malformations*. Baltimore/London: Williams & Wilkins, 1984, pp 295–313

INDEX

GPSR Compliance

The European Union's (EU) General Product Safety Regulation (GPSR) is a set of rules that requires consumer products to be safe and our obligations to ensure this.

If you have any concerns about our products, you can contact us on ProductSafety@springernature.com

In case Publisher is established outside the EU, the EU authorized representative is:

Springer Nature Customer Service Center GmbH
Europaplatz 3
69115 Heidelberg, Germany

Batch number: 10684222

Printed by Printforce, the Netherlands